P9-CAL-330

# Pediatric Therapy
## A Systems Approach

Philadelphia College of Pharmacy and Science
Occupational Therapy Department
600 S. 43rd Street, Box 24
Philadelphia, PA 19104-4495

# Pediatric Therapy
## A Systems Approach

**Susan Miller Porr, MEd, MS, OTR**
Occupational Therapist
Moore County Schools
Carthage, North Carolina

**Ellen Berger Rainville, MS, OTR, FAOTA**
Assistant Professor
Department of Occupational Therapy
Springfield College
Springfield, Massachusetts

*Pediatric Occupational Therapy Series Editor*
Shelly J. Lane, PhD, OTR, ATP, FAOTA

 **F. A. DAVIS COMPANY • Philadelphia**

F. A. Davis Company
1915 Arch Street
Philadelphia, PA 19103

Copyright © 1999 by F. A. Davis Company

All rights reserved. This book is protected by copyright. No part of it may be reproduced, stored in a retrieval system, or transmitted in any form or by any means, electronic, mechanical, photocopying, recording, or otherwise, without written permission from the publisher.

Printed in the United States of America

Last digit indicates print number: 10 9 8 7 6 5 4 3 2 1

*Publisher, Health Professions:* Jean-François Vilain
*Senior Editor:* Lynn Borders Caldwell
*Senior Developmental Editor:* Crystal Spraggins
*Production Editor:* Stephen D. Johnson
*Cover Designer:* Louis J. Forgione
*Watermark Artists:* Meghan Accorsi (Dedication Page), Gerald Summer (Part I), David Berger (Chapter 1), anonymous (Chapter 2), Kristen D'Angelo (Chapters 3, 11, and 13), Sara Rainville (Part II and Chapter 16), Carissa Rehbein (Chapter 4), David Rainville (Chapter 5), Lorisa Hasenbush (Chapter 6), Kelly Dupuis (Chapter 7), Robbie Johnson (Chapter 8), Nate Balser (Chapter 9), Anna Balser (Part III), Madeline C. (Chapters 10, 14, and 15), and Jessica Rainville (Chapter 12).

As new scientific information becomes available through basic and clinical research, recommended treatments and drug therapies undergo changes. The authors and publisher have done everything possible to make this book accurate, up to date, and in accord with accepted standards at the time of publication. The authors, editors, and publisher are not responsible for errors or omissions or for consequences from application of the book, and make no warranty, expressed or implied, in regard to the contents of the book. Any practice described in this book should be applied by the reader in accordance with professional standards of care used in regard to the unique circumstances that may apply in each situation. The reader is advised always to check product information (package inserts) for changes and new information regarding dose and contraindications before administering any drug. Caution is especially urged when using new or infrequently ordered drugs.

**Library of Congress Cataloging-in-Publication Data**

Porr, Susan Miller, 1952–
    Pediatric therapy : a systems approach / Susan Miller Porr, Ellen Berger Rainville.
        p.      cm. — (Pediatric occupational therapy series : 1)
    Includes bibliographical references and index.
    ISBN 0–8036–0259–6 (alk. paper)
    1. Occupational therapy for children.    2. Children—Diseases—Therapy.
    I. Rainville, Ellen Berger, 1955– .   II. Title.   III. Series.
    [DNLM: 1. Occupational Therapy—in infancy & childhood.    WS 368 P838p 1999]
RJ53.025P67    1999
615.8'515'083—dc21
DNLM/DLC
for Library of Congress                                                                      98–55693
                                                                                                            CIP

Authorization to photocopy items for internal or personal use, or the internal or personal use of specific clients, is granted by F. A. Davis Company for users registered with the Copyright Clearance Center (CCC) Transactional Reporting Service, provided that the fee of $.10 per copy is paid directly to CCC, 222 Rosewood Drive, Danvers, MA 01923. For those organizations that have been granted a photocopy license by CCC, a separate system of payment has been arranged. The fee code for users of the Transactional Reporting Service is: 8036-0259/99 0 + $.10.

to the children and families, especially our own, who have informed our practices and enriched our lives

SMP
EBR

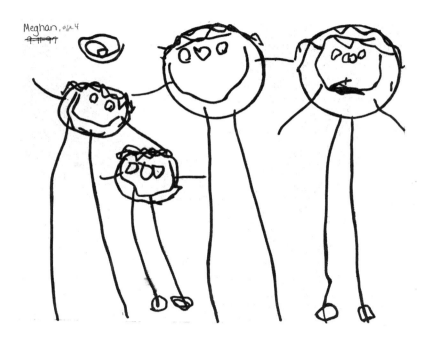

# Foreword

Since its inception, the field of occupational therapy has focused on the goal of assisting individuals to meet the demands of their roles in order to successfully enact meaningful occupations. Occupational therapists are schooled to recognize and address the physical, cognitive, emotional, and psychosocial demands that present themselves in the typical course of daily living and in the presence of disability, dysfunction, and disease. When occupational therapists work with children, they construct therapeutic interventions to facilitate success in childhood roles such as family member (sibling, daughter, son), student, friend, and playmate.

As early as the 1920s, occupational therapists began developing theories, models, and frames of reference as well as assessment and treatment techniques to address the occupational problems of their patients. Some of the perspectives and approaches that were developed were applicable to a select diagnosis and subscribed to narrow views of the problem and the potential for solutions. These included the biomechanical approach and the medical model perspective. Others were broader and more general, such as the developmental approach.

In the trade-off between specificity and generality the concept of occupation was often sacrificed for concepts and constructs that were more readily measurable in terms of establishing a level of dysfunction and plan for treatment. These concepts were also considered to be more straightforward and recognizable by others on the treatment team and in the treatment setting. In short, occupation was displaced by concepts that reflected ideas being developed in medicine, psychiatry, special education, and other larger fields that often named and framed the problems to be addressed by allied health professionals.

Occupational therapy scholars and researchers have often asked if it is necessary to relinquish a historical concept such as occupation to be compatible with other dominant concepts that are popular outside of the field. Must we give up occupation to be congruent with the times? Some have advocated a renaming of the field, whereas others have remained loyal to a concept that provides the depth and breadth of what occupational therapists do so well, namely, assist people to do the job of living. With this exciting new text, occupational therapy students and therapists alike will be able to remain true to the legacy of their field and embrace a contemporary perspective of occupational therapy for infants, children, adolescents, and their families.

Each chapter of this text deals with the multiple issues (medical, psychosocial, developmental, and familial to name a few) that threaten enactment of occupational roles. Additionally, the text offers a view of these issues in the situations and contexts where they are typically confronted by therapists who are assessing, treating, and/or consulting in pediatric-based practice. Along with a historical view of care for children, the text offers a contemporary analysis of occupation, family-centered care, and narrative to infuse an understanding of all that occupational therapy can be as we enter the 21st century.

The text contains innovative features within each chapter that telescope an array of information, including the availability of additional resources on selected topics ("From the Bookshelf "); the clinical manifestation of a pediatric need ("Case Story"); and the kinds of learning exercises and activities that allow students to develop skills and strategies for practice ("Real Life Labs") and allow therapists to develop strategies for treatment ("Therapeds Pointers").

With this collection of information the authors carefully demonstrate how far occupational therapy really has come as a profession and a science. Their commitment to occupation and the rapid development of occupation-oriented theory and science is present throughout the book. Numerous references are made to bodies of literature that address conceptual views of occupation including occupational behavior (Reilly, 1969; Matsutsuyu, 1971; Florey, 1969), the Model of Human Occupation (Kielhofner & Burke, 1980), and occupational science (Yerxa, 1989; Clark et al., 1991). The interweaving of occupation as theory within the realities of today's clinical demands give credibility and rigor to the unique value of occupational therapy in meeting the needs of children and their families. As a new generation of occupational therapists prepares for pediatric practice, this text provides a rich legacy of clinical examples that demonstrate how today's occupational therapist must think about and use occupationally grounded theory and research to enact practice.

**Janice P. Burke, PhD, OTR/L, FAOTA**
Chairman and Associate Professor
Department of Occupational Therapy
College of Health Professions
Thomas Jefferson University
Philadelphia, Pennsylvania

# Bibliography

Clark, F., Parham, D., Carlson, M. E., Frank, G., Jackson, J., Pierce, D., Wolfe, R. J., & Zemke, R. (1991). Occupational science: Academic innovation in the service of occupational therapy's future. *American Journal of Occupational Therapy, 45,* 300–310.

Florey, L. (1969). Intrinsic motivation: The dynamics of occupational therapy theory. *American Journal of Occupational Therapy, 23,* 319–322.

Kielhofner, G. & Burke, J. P. (1980). A model of human occupation, Part 1. Conceptual framework and content. *American Journal of Occupational Therapy, 34,* 572–581.

Matsutsuyu, J. S. (1970). Occupational behavior—A perspective on work and play. *American Journal of Occupational Therapy, 25,* 291–294.

Reilly, M. (1969). The educational process. *American Journal of Occupational Therapy, 23,* 299–307.

Yerxa, E. J. (1989). An introduction to occupational science: A foundation for occupational therapy in the 21st century. *Occupational Therapy in Health Care, 6,* 1–17.

# *Preface*

This text was conceived in response to a need for an uncomplicated, easy-to-use textbook for pediatric occupational therapists. Shelly Lane, the editor of this text, introduced us to each other and to the idea a few years ago. Sue (Porr), is a school-based occupational therapist, and Ellen (Rainville) is a college professor. At the time we began this book, Sue lived in Seattle and Ellen in Massachusetts. Since that time, we have each moved three times, Sue to another country and finally another coast, and Ellen to three different houses in the small western Massachusetts community she calls home. Sue was an elementary school teacher before she became an occupational therapist. Ellen practiced in early childhood intervention before she became a manager and then a graduate-level educator. We both believe in the innate capabilities of children and their families. We are also deeply committed to the provision of high-quality, innovative, and responsive services for children in their homes, schools, and communities.

We tell you these things to illustrate the similarities and differences in our experiences and in our perspectives and to let you know what an interesting journey the preparation of this book has been. We believe that our collaboration with each other, and with our remarkable contributors, reflects the broad range of knowledge in pediatric occupational therapy today. Our most sincere hope is that the final product demonstrates our appreciation for the complexities and gifts of this specialty.

In this book, we have attempted to present an informed source for understanding the illnesses and disabling conditions most commonly seen in the children we care for. We have attempted to offer a model for understanding the potential impact of these conditions on a child's ability to function and to suggest a framework for designing OT interventions that support the occupations of children in the many contexts they experience.

The book has three sections. The first section, "Childhood: The Complex, Fantastic Process of Birth and Becoming a Person," sets the stage for the sections that follow. The first two chapters describe the complex processes of prenatal and early development and introduce the reader to the essential interactions of professionals, team members, and families in pediatric care. The third chapter focuses on those current concepts of development and occupation that influence the practice of pediatric occupational therapy.

The second section, "Children's Bodies: Systems at Work and Play," relates the workings of various systems of a child's body and some of the more common diseases and disabilities associated with each system. The potential impact of these disabilities is framed from an occupational perspective in case story form. Process, content, and intervention are interwoven in each of these chapters. Examples of interventions are given, and the influences of environment, culture, and context on the child's occupation are recognized and respected. The possible roles of the occupational therapist on the "team" are highlighted, with the ever-present reminder that as the child changes, so do the occupational therapist's strategies and involvement.

The third section of the book, "Special Topics in Pediatric Occupational Therapy" grew out of the need to address some of the more specialized areas of pediatric occupational therapy that have emerged in the past decade. Increasing knowledge about development, increased recognition of the importance of collaborative service delivery as best practice, and continued medical technology for children at risk have all created new challenges and opportunities for pediatric occupational therapists. Children with multiple disabilities have chronic care needs that impact on their "kids will be kids" roles. Children with cancer live well into adulthood. Teenagers with head injuries continue to be vital community members after their accidents. Toddlers in powered wheelchairs enter preschool with their peers. Information in these special topic chapters allows a more in-depth look at these constantly changing areas.

What makes *Pediatric Therapy: A Systems Approach* different from other texts on the same topic? We have tried to include practical information ("Therapeds Pointers") that has been useful in providing services for children and families in our communities. "From the Bookshelf" is a guide for expanding one's knowledge on a particular topic beyond the scope of this text. These references add richness and often a new perspective or voice to the topic that each chapter addresses. The resources may be used for parent education, professional growth, or general reference.

The "Real Life Lab" and "Case Story" sections of each chapter are *growth* exercises to help readers process and integrate information provided in the text in a practical framework. These sections illustrate the real-world issues that pediatric therapists encounter. They are meant to emphasize the broad scope of knowledge and the complexity of the tasks involved in supporting children's everyday occupations.

We hope that you will find this a useful text for your education and/or your practice in pediatric occupational therapy. We look forward to hearing your responses, comments, and suggestions. Occupational therapy is fortunate to be a profession so intimately involved with the everyday activities of children. We hope that our work, and yours, will contribute positively to their lives.

**SMP**
**EBR**

# Acknowledgments

In a project of this magnitude one can never say "thank you" to too many people or enough times in the course of the endeavor. First and foremost I thank my family; to Darrel, my husband, for *not* editing and reviewing, as our styles are so different; and to Molly, my daughter, for tolerating "just a quick stop to check a reference" and "only 5 more minutes to finish a thought"—I love you both! To my parents, Frank and Barb Miller, my love and thanks, for always believing I could do anything I wanted to and for encouragement along the way. To my siblings, Tom Miller, Amy Bartlett, and Linda Cochran (my guardian angel) for listening to my gripes long distance for such a long time—I thank you (and so does Ma Bell).

A huge round of applause to the staff at F. A. Davis. To Lynn Borders Caldwell for supporting this project; to Crystal Spraggins, the most patient editor one could ever have, and to all the "pros" there who supported this fledgling author. To Shelly Lane, my friend, editor, and mentor—my deepest appreciation for presenting me with this "doable challenge" and reminding me constantly that it was doable! Kudos to the contributors, Jodi, Scott, Jayne, Judith, Shelly, Dianne, and Dianne, for enriching this text with their expertise. My appreciation to the reviewers for highlighting needs and offering valuable advice on numerous occasions. To Ellen, my co-author, my thanks for your humor, collaboration, and staying power!

To my personal friends, Linda Tyo and Molly Howard, my thanks for your consistent support in this lengthy process and intuition regarding *when* to ask "how's the book?" My appreciation to professionals in all arenas, from Germany to Washington State to North Carolina, who cheerfully answered questions, clarified points, and shared their knowledge in so many areas. And lastly, to the children (a.k.a. "my kids") and the families and staff with whom I have worked over the years—thanks "bunches" for sharing your practical knowledge, your contagious optimism, and above all your hopes and dreams.

**SMP**

As this project nears completion, I have been able to reflect upon the many people who have influenced, guided, and supported me. Although I will be unable to mention each of them, I am eternally grateful for their gifts. Among them, I especially acknowledge and thank:

- My mother, Ruth Berger, who taught me to believe in myself and who has provided incredible support, child care, apple pies, etc., etc., etc., so that I could have time to write, to study, to think. . . .

- My cousin, Janet Verner Platt Lambert, who introduced me to occupational therapy, and who has provided immeasurable encouragement.

- My children, Kellie, David, and Nicole, and my husband, Mike, just for being who they are, but also for understanding and for always caring.

- My sister Elizabeth and my Uncle Bill for being friends as well as relatives.

- My friend Diana Bailey, who introduced me to Jean-François Vilain and Lynn Borders Caldwell at F. A. Davis, and who first suggested that I consider writing a book.

- Crystal Spraggins, our developmental editor at F. A. Davis, for her incredible patience, persistence, and diplomacy.

- Sue Porr, my coauthor, for her indomitable spirit, her great work, and her dedication to this project.

- Our contributors *and* our reviewers for their very important contributions to this book.

- My colleagues in pediatric therapy, especially at Valley Infant Development Service and in the Massachusetts Early Intervention Consortium, who have taught me about collaboration and change for children and families.

- The faculty at Springfield College and at Boston University who have informed my understanding of human occupation, and who have helped me to continued to achieve professionally, as have my students, especially Sharon Koff and Marnie Sullivan.

- My colleague and friend Ellen Cohn, for listening and listening and listening.

- The teachers and children at the Springfield College Child Development Center, who have taught me much and who have helped my own children to learn and grow.

- My father, David Berger (1920–1966), who taught me to be respectful and creative. His artwork graces Chapter 1 of the book. My stepfather, Gerald Summer (1923–1996), who modeled a love of the written word. His artwork graces Part I of the book. My appreciation for them is eternal.

- Most of all, I thank the many exceptional children and families I have worked with and known over the years. Without them, this book would not be.

EBR

# Contributors

Judith Kytle Hanshaw, BS, OTR
Clinical Specialist
Virginia Commonwealth University-Medical College of Virginia
and
Clinical Instructor
Department of Occupational Therapy
School of Allied Health Professions
Virginia Commonwealth University
Richmond, Virginia

Shelly J. Lane, PhD, OTR, ATP, FAOTA
Professor and Chairperson
Department of Occupational Therapy
School of Allied Health Professions
Virginia Commonwealth University
Richmond, Virginia

Dianne Koontz Lowman, EdD
Assistant Professor
Department of Occupational Therapy
School of Allied Health Professions
Virginia Commonwealth University
Richmond, Virginia

JoAnn (Jodi) Petry, MEd, MS, OTR
Formerly, Occupational Therapist
C. S. Mott Children's Hospital
University of Michigan Health System
Ann Arbor, Michigan

Currently, Occupational Therapist
Duke Univerisity Health Systems
and
Lenox Baker Children's Hospital
Durham, North Carolina

Jayne T. Shepherd, MS, OTR
Assistant Professor
Department of Occupational Therapy
School of Allied Health Professions
Virginia Commonwealth University
Richmond, Virginia

Dianne Franklin Simons, MS, OTR/C
Assistant Professor
Department of Occupational Therapy
School of Allied Health Professions
Virginia Commonwealth University
Richmond, Virginia

Scott D. Tomchek, MS, OTR/L
Senior Occupational Therapist
Child Evaluation Center
Department of Pediatrics
School of Medicine
University of Louisville
Louisville, Kentucky

# Reviewers

Roselyn Armstrong, MA, OTR, Chair, Occupational Therapy Assistant Program, Pitt Community College, Greenville, North Carolina

Karin J. Barnes, MS, OTR, Associate Professor, University of Texas Health Science Center at San Antonio, San Antonio, Texas

Carmela M. Battaglia, MS, OTR, Assistant Professor, Department of Occupational Therapy, University of Pittsburgh, Pittsburgh, Pennsylvania

Christine Hencinski, MS, OTR, Program Director and Instructor, Occupational Therapy Assistant Program, Mt. Hood Community College, Memphis, Tennessee

Esther M. Huecker, MA, OTR, BCP, Assistant Professor, Department of Occupational Therapy, Loma Linda University, Loma Linda, California

Loretta Knutson, PhD, PT, PCS, Assistant Professor, University of Central Arkansas, Department of Physical Therapy, Conway, Arkansas

Sandra B. Levine, PhD, PT, OTR, Associate Professor, Department of Physical Therapy, University of Illinois at Chicago, Chicago, Illinois

Ruth D. Mulvany, MS, PT, Assistant Professor, Department of Physical Therapy, University of Tennessee, Memphis, Tennessee

Karen J. Opacich, MPHE, OTR, FAOTA, Education Coordinator and Assistant Professor, Department of Occupational Therapy, Rush University, Chicago, Illinois

Judith C. Vestal, PhD, MA, OTR, Associate Professor, School of Allied Health Professions, Department of Occupational Therapy, Louisiana State University, New Orleans, Louisiana

# Contents

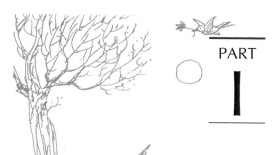

# CHILDHOOD
## THE COMPLEX, FANTASTIC
## PROCESS OF BEING BORN
## AND BECOMING A PERSON

by Gerald Simmer (1954)

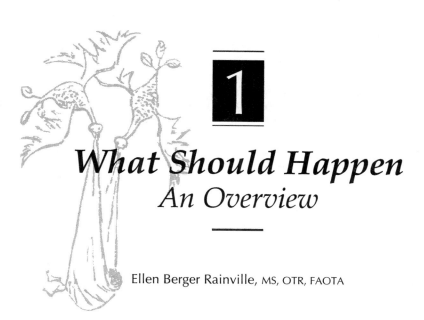

# 1

# *What Should Happen*
## *An Overview*

Ellen Berger Rainville, MS, OTR, FAOTA

*Aspirations may shape our vision of the future for new generations, but what realities will shape their lives? Prospects for the young vary widely in every corner of the world. Some will find privilege, while others will be born into environments with few opportunities. If we hope to prepare our children to meet the challenges of an ever-changing world, then we must show concern for their interaction with natural, manmade, and family environment; their physical and emotional well-being; their ability to survive a possible collapse of prevailing social or political systems; and their skills at meeting future needs and problems.*
—Adams, in Cohn & Leach, 1987

## KEY POINTS

- An understanding of prenatal growth and development is essential for the pediatric therapist. This understanding provides a solid foundation for the many complex mechanisms that underlie the developmental problems that come to our attention.

- The study of prenatal development is an emerging science with recent explosions in technology and hence knowledge. New methods for observing and recording even the most microscopic processes of conception and gestation have enabled scientists to understand what had only been imagined or hypothesized previously.

- The prenatal period is rich with opportunity—for potential parents as they anticipate their new family member(s), for health and social service providers as they work with families to assure the healthiest and smoothest prenatal course possible, and for the developing fetus as he or she prepares for a great adventure.

- Occupational therapists (OTs) may well be involved in providing support and education for families even before conception. Although they may provide limited direct care, OTs can be advocates for good, accessible prenatal care. They can advise and assist people to find and take advantage of such services. They can educate prospective parents about the advantages of prenatal care and preparation and can later help families adjust to problems they may be facing with their children by helping them to understand and make sense of their unique prenatal experience.

# BEGINNINGS

There is a long road from conception to birth and much can and does occur along that route. It is critical that professionals concerned with the development and the function of human beings, especially children, understand the prenatal course. Before we have even seen and touched the new baby, the majority of developmental and other disabling conditions begin. Our appreciation for the complexities of prenatal phenomena will help us understand not only what may have happened to cause a child to have a disability but also to be involved in efforts to prevent and ameliorate disability as early as possible.

This chapter provides an overview of the physiological processes that occur from conception to birth. Prenatal diagnostic testing procedures are reviewed in order for therapists to appreciate the sources of knowledge about young children that are available to families and professionals. Finally, the typical newborn is described and the important transitions experienced by families are explained. Because of the importance of these transitions, therapeutic service models that focus on the family are strongly recommended.

---

■ *THERAPEDS POINTER*

You may be wondering why a good understanding of prenatal development is important for the pediatric OT. In the same manner as anatomy and neuroscience help us to visualize certain impairments we see for treatment, a knowledge of prenatal development helps us to understand what may have occurred to cause the occupational problems we see in children. We can also hypothesize other potential problems that may be developmentally related. A good developmental and perinatal history will give us important clues. Here are some examples:

1. A child with myelodysplasia (spina bifida) experienced a failure in closure of the neural tube very early in gestation (30 days). An OT will want to watch for other midline and neurological defects that children with spina bifida may experience. Aside from systems that developed at that early time in gestation,

more generalized problems such as learning disabilities are also common in children with spina bifida.

2. A child who was born 5 weeks prematurely had good birth weight and Apgar scores. She did well medically and was discharged to home with her mother. Because of her prematurity, this infant completed her brain, lung, and other critical system development outside the safety and comfort of the womb. As a result, the child may have experienced stresses not known to her full-term peers. If you as an OT were involved with this family shortly after the birth, you would have the opportunity to make some preventive suggestions such as helping the family simulate the womb environment. Low lights, soft sounds, a water mattress, swaddling, rocking, holding, and gentle movement may help the baby's immature CNS cope with and learn from her environment.

## PRENATAL DEVELOPMENT

Human growth and development begin at conception or *fertilization*, when the female ovum, or egg, and male sperm unite. The fertilized egg, or conceptus, is referred to as a *zygote*. Through a process known as *mitosis*, the zygote changes from its single-cell form to multiple cells that join together in layers to form what is called a *blastocyst*, the foundation of a unique human being. More than 2000 years ago, Aristotle (Fig. 1–1) envisioned the process of gestation that will be explained here.

Approximately 2 weeks after conception, the blastocyst will have traveled through the fallopian tube to the uterus, where it attaches to the uterine wall. At this juncture, tremendous growth and development have already occurred, the newly implanted blastocyst being more than 1,000,000 times the size of the conceptus. At this stage the potential human being is known as an *embryo*. From the *villi*, which surround the blastocyst and form the attachment to the uterine wall, the *placenta* is formed. This membranous network connects the mother to the embryo. Although there is no direct blood or food supply via the placenta, the membranes of the mother and embryo, located contiguous to each other, do allow for the passage of certain substances. These include those necessary for the well-being of the embryo, such as nutrients and oxygen and carbon dioxide exchange, as well as those that may cause harm, such as toxins, drugs, and infection. These potentially harmful substances, known as *teratogens*, will be discussed in more detail in Chapter 2 (Batshaw & Perret, 1992; Eisenberg, Murkoff, & Hathaway, 1988; Enkin, Keirse, Renfrew & Neilson, 1995; Short-DeGraff, 1988; Visscher & Rinehart, 1990).

## ▟▌▐ FROM THE BOOKSHELF

Neilson, L. (1993). *A Child is Born: The Drama of Life Before Birth.* New York: Dell. This lovely book contains what are perhaps the most stuning photographs of intrauterine life. Nielson, a pioneer in this field, provides an accurate, compelling guide through gestation. The photographs are

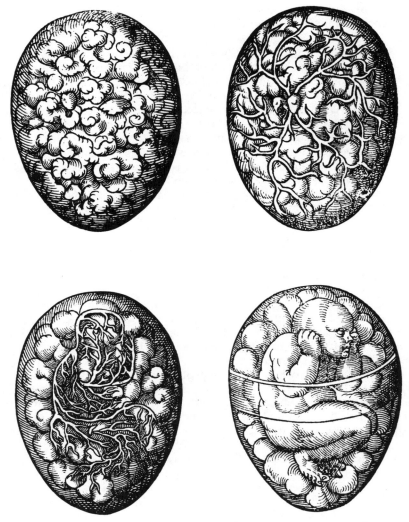

Figure 1–1 Prenatal development. (*Source:* The National Library of Medicine, Bethesda, MD.)

touching and realistic—this is a must read for people interested in this period of growth and development.

Video: NOVA: *The Miracle of Life.* This outstanding video, one of many excellent programs from the Public Broadcasting System's NOVA Series, also provides dramatic, beautiful photography and a fascinating narration of the process from conception to birth.

Growth and development occur in this stage at a continuing rapid rate. The embryonic layers further differentiate into the *amnion* and the *chorion,*

Table 1–1  **Layers of the Skin**

| | |
|---|---|
| Ectoderm | Skin, hair, nails, nervous system |
| Mesoderm | Skeleton and musculature |
| Endoderm | Internal organs |

which later form the amniotic sac, a fluid-filled structure in which the embryo is suspended. The amniotic sac provides protection against jarring and potential injury, as well as a regulated temperature that is just right for the embryo to grow into a fetus (Eisenberg et al., 1988; Kliegman, 1996).

Further differentiation of the embryo results in three layers that form the cellular basis for the various human systems (Table 1–1).

By the end of this first phase of prenatal development, the embryo is about 1 inch long and has the rudiments of human structure and function. The heart begins to beat as early as 4 to 5 weeks, and the facial features are present. Genitals have initially formed, as have tiny limbs with hands and feet. This tiny embryo will move in response to certain stimulation, indicating the existence of a neuromuscular system and sensory processing abilities (Lewerenz & Schaaf, 1996; Short-DeGraff, 1988). By 12 weeks of gestation, the basis for structural development is complete, and with the new development of bone cells, the embryo officially becomes a *fetus*. The fetal stage, which lasts from 12 weeks until birth, involves the growth, maturation, and functional development of the existing structures (Short-DeGraff, 1988).

Throughout gestation, the developing infant experiences incredibly rapid and substantive changes in size, form, and function as it expresses its predetermined individual genetic and species-specific codes and as it responds to its environment. During this period, the infant is especially vulnerable to external influences that may have significant effects on its ultimate outcome (Kliegman, 1996; Scheiner & Sexton, 1991, Short-DeGraff, 1988; Visscher & Rinehart, 1990). Some of these influences are positive and well within the control of the mother (parents). For example, many parents provide specific stimulation such as music or reading for their infant while it is still in utero. Other influences, specifically certain teratogens, may have a disastrous effect. Figure 1–2 illustrates the sequence of prenatal development and helps us to see when certain embryonic and fetal structures and systems are the most vulnerable to these teratogens.

## PRENATAL CARE

In today's world, prenatal care often begins *before* conception. A woman or couple will likely consult with their health-care provider prior to becoming pregnant so that they can be informed about the risks and benefits of certain health and lifestyle choices on the developing fetus (Blondel, Dutilh, Delour & Uzan, 1993; Gjerdingen & Fontaine, 1991; Williamson & Lefevre, 1992). Many women begin to take prenatal vitamins, become extra careful about nutrition, and limit their alcohol consumption prior to conception. These are not insignificant acts. It has been shown that ingesting just 1 mg of folic acid daily may entirely prevent certain defects of neural tube closure such as spina bi-

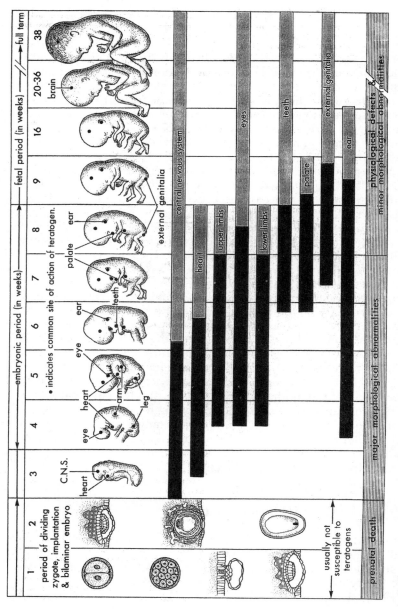

Figure 1–2 Embryonic and fetal development. (*Source:* Moore, K. L. [1983]. *Before we are born: Basic embryology and birth defects* [2d ed.]. Philadelphia: W. B. Saunders.)

fida (*Morbidity & Mortality Weekly*, 1992). The effects of alcohol and other substances on the fetus are also now well known to the public (Chiriboga, 1993; *Morbidity & Mortality Weekly*, 1995; Schorling, 1993).

In the United States, many pregnant women can access good prenatal care, either through private health insurance or Medicaid. Good prenatal care includes regular supervision throughout pregnancy, labor, delivery, and the neonatal period by a qualified physician and support personnel (nurses, social workers, and others) as needed. The American College of Obstetrics and Gynecology has developed guidelines for the frequency and content of such care (Visscher & Rinehart, 1990).

Programs do exist to provide additional supports for women, especially economically disadvantaged women, although the programs may not be adequately funded. These include the Women, Infants and Children (WIC) supplemental nutrition program, adolescent pregnancy and parenting programs, and Healthy Start pregnancy monitoring and support programs. In addition to qualified health-care personnel and specialty programs and services, a variety of technological resources are available to help women, families, and care providers understand and make decisions about each individual pregnancy. These procedures and tests are not routine; that is, they may not be performed on every pregnant woman. Each of these tests offers potentially valuable information, but each test also has risks. These valuable diagnostic tools are used by the physician based on the specific needs of the individual pregnancy. These tests are discussed below.

**Ultrasonography.** Ultrasonography is the use of sound waves that "bounce off" of internal structures and form a picture. In the case of a pregnant woman, they are used to form a picture of the uterine structures and the embryo or fetus (Fig. 1–3). This picture is quite specific, although special train-

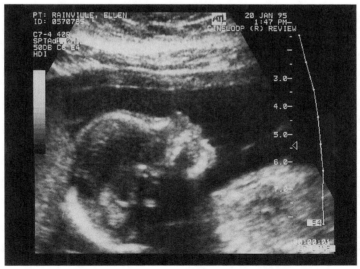

Figure 1–3 Ultrasonograph of a fetus at $18^{1}/_{2}$ weeks' gestation.

ing and expertise are needed to interpret results accurately, including the ability to visualize structures as small as the thalamus. Gestational age, gender, multiple pregnancy, intrauterine growth rate, fetal anatomy and position, and fetal heart rate are among the many things that can be determined with this painless, low-risk procedure. Multiple anomalies such as placenta previa, abruptio placentae, and insufficient amniotic fluid can be detected using this procedure. Early identification of structural anomalies in the fetus may be possible as well. Not only is this important for families to be able to prepare for the birth of a child with problems, but also, in some cases, to begin medical treatment before birth (Eisenberg, Murkoff & Hathaway, 1988; Enkin, Keirse, Renfrew & Neilson, 1995; Goncalves, Jeanty & Piper, 1994; Visscher & Rinehart, 1990). Ultrasound can be used safely from approximately the fifth week of pregnancy through delivery.

**Chorionic Villi Sampling (CVS).** At 8 to 12 weeks' gestation, a sample of the villi from the chorion can be obtained, usually through a catheter inserted through the vagina into the uterus. This sample is analyzed for genetic content and is used to predict genetic problems in the fetus. There is some risk of injury or infection involved in the invasive nature of the procedure itself. Also, the accuracy of this test has been questioned. CVS analysis takes only a few days after the sample is obtained. If CVS reveals potential anomalies, a more accurate procedure like amniocentesis may be recommended for confirmation of the diagnosis.(Eisenberg, Murkoff, & Hathaway, 1988; Enkin, Keirse, Renfrew, & Neilson, 1995; Visscher & Rinehart, 1990).

**Alphafetoprotein Screening.** Between 15 and 18 weeks, a sample of maternal blood may be drawn to test for the presence of a substance known as alphafetoprotein (AFP), which is produced by the fetus. The presence of high levels of AFP may indicate a defect of neural tube closure, such as spina bifida. Low levels of AFP have been associated with the presence of Down syndrome. For this procedure, lab analysis takes only a day or two. False-positive results are not uncommon with this test, so it is often repeated because it adds little or no risk to the mother. Should the risk of a birth defect in the fetus be high, an amniocentesis and/or a more detailed ultrasound examination may be pursued (Eisenberg et al., 1988; Enkin et al., 1995; Kellner et al., 1995; Visscher & Rinehart, 1990).

**Maternal Estriol Levels.** From the same blood drawn for AFP, the level of estriol can be evaluated. Since the concentration of this estrogenic hormone increases during gestation, serial measurements may help identify the condition of the uterus and placenta. If the estriol levels stabilize or decrease, this may indicate problems with the placenta, resulting in the mother requiring special care and perhaps induced delivery (Eisenberg, Murkoff, & Hathaway, 1988; Kellner et al., 1995).

**Amniocentesis.** Between 12 and 16 weeks' gestational age, a needle may be inserted through the mother's abdomen into her uterus and a sample of amniotic fluid obtained (Fig. 1–4). Ultrasound is used to monitor the needle placement so that it does not endanger the fetus. Over a 2-week period, the cells are

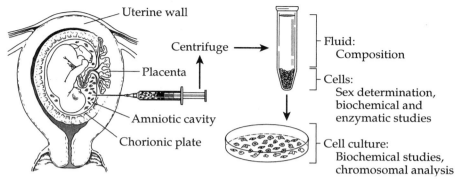

Figure 1–4  Amniocentesis. (*Source:* Friedman, T. [1971]. *Prenatal diagnosis of genetic disease. Scientific American* 225, 35.)

cultured to obtain a karyotype analysis of the fetus's individual genetics. This is a most accurate method of prenatally diagnosing biochemical and chromosomal disorders. Such disorders as Tay-Sachs disease, Down syndrome, and hemophilia may be identified. Also, from fluid drawn by amniocentesis, an analysis of the ratio of lecithin to sphingomyelin (L/S ratio) can yield an estimate of fetal lung maturity (Enkin et al., 1995; Visscher & Rinehart, 1990).

**Monitoring of Uterine Contractions, Fetal Movement, and Heart Rate.** Fetal movements can be felt by mothers starting at approximately 20 weeks' gestation and are often a source of great comfort and joy. Mothers should, however, notify their care providers if they feel a change in the patterns of fetal movement. In high-risk pregnancies, women are often trained to identify and monitor uterine contractions by learning to identify them by palpation. Mothers can count the number of felt fetal movements in a given time period and compare them to established norms. Also, tocolytic monitors (a 2- to 3-inch-diameter disk that monitors uterine contractions and is held over the uterus with a belt) are available for both clinical and home use. Uterine contractions can be indicative of impending labor. Monitoring enables early detection and intervention for pregnancies at high risk for preterm delivery. Fetal heart rate can be evaluated from about the seventh week using a fetal stethoscope or a special Doppler stethoscope (Eisenberg et al., 1988; Enkin et al., 1995; Visscher & Rinehart, 1990).

**Fetoscopy.** Sometime after the 16th week, it is possible to view the fetus through a miniature camera that is inserted through an abdominal incision. It is also possible to obtain tissue and fluid samples for analysis through this procedure. Much of the remarkable prenatal photography used throughout the information media has likely been obtained through fetoscopy (Eisenberg et al., 1988; Enkin et al., 1995; Visscher & Rinehart, 1990). Although it is not a common procedure, fetoscopy is also used for prenatal diagnosis and treatment.

**Nonstress Test.** Using a fetal monitor (which consists of an ultrasound transducer over the uterus), fetal heart rate (normally 120 to 160 beats per minute) can be measured during normal movement or in response to an external vibration or sound. A reactive response (normal) would show a slight acceleration of heart rate (10 to 20 beats per minute) in response to this stimulus. A nonreactive test, where there is no change, or a test during which a decrease is noted, would be cause for concern and further evaluation. This procedure is not routine, but it may be used in cases where the fetus's health status or position in utero is of concern (Eisenberg et al., 1988; Enkin et al., 1995; Visscher & Rinehart, 1990).

**Contraction Stress Test.** For this test, a baseline fetal heart rate is established using fetal monitoring. Mild contractions are then induced using an oxytocic drug. Within 10 minutes, three strong (40-second-duration) contractions should occur. If a decrease in fetal heart rate is noted at or after the peak of the contraction (called late deceleration), the condition of the placenta may be compromised. It may be necessary to determine the potential for the placenta to support fetal growth. If there are significant placental problems, delivery may be induced early to preserve fetal or infant health. This test is generally not used prior to 36 weeks' gestation because of the risk associated with preterm labor.

**Fetal Echocardiogram.** This sophisticated Doppler ultrasound evaluation examines blood flow through the placenta and fetal blood vessels in order to identify circulatory system deficits. This information may be essential for prenatal diagnosis and treatment as well as for planning for delivery and newborn care. Families who learn about heart or circulatory defects prenatally may be better able to cope with the realities of the diagnosis and the critical decisions that may need to be made.

**Biophysical Profile.** This test is often used as a follow-up to an atypical nonstress test. It consists of five independent measures:
1. Real-time ultrasound to monitor fetal respiration
2. Identification of a minimum of three fetal movements during a 30-minute period
3. Fetal heart rate acceleration with movement (as in the nonstress test)
4. Assessment of muscle tone through fetal movement
5. Amniotic fluid volume

Low scores in any or all of the subtests would indicate high risk for the safety of the pregnancy.

## WHY PRENATAL TESTING?

Prenatal diagnostics are useful for many reasons. They help to identify and facilitate the treatment of high-risk pregnancies (discussed in a later chapter), as well as identify fetal condition (Kuller & Laifer, 1995). This is helpful not only for families who wish to give consideration to termination of a pregnancy where the fetus may have a severe anomaly, but also for some innovative perinatal treatment. For example, recent technological advances have allowed for intrauterine treatments. One of the most successful has been the placement of a shunt to resolve bladder obstruction (Camosy, 1995; Flake & Harrison, 1995).

Also, prenatal diagnosis enables medical teams to be ready to conduct surgeries and other medical treatments as soon after birth as possible.

A word of caution, though. Although many conditions are identifiable through prenatal diagnosis, normal test results for any or all of these procedures do not ensure a healthy, typically developing child (Eisenberg et al., 1988; Visscher & Rinehart, 1990). Many developmental and other disabilities and diseases are not able to be diagnosed prenatally as yet. Medical researchers and clinicians continue to aim toward continuous improvement in ethical perinatal diagnosis and treatment.

## PREGNANCY AND DELIVERY

Human gestation is a rather miraculous process. For centuries, we were simply thankful when a healthy infant was born. Unfortunately, it was not unusual for families to experience the loss of a baby born too early, too late, or stillborn at the expected time. Our knowledge and technical resources have expanded so significantly during the past 20 years that we can now accurately track the most minute features of prenatal health and development, and we are sometimes able to intervene to prevent problems, in many cases prior to delivery (Gjerdingen & Fontaine, 1991). Table 1–2 illustrates some of the key features of prenatal development, month by month, and helps illustrate the remarkable capabilities of unborn humans.

## ▮▮▮ FROM THE BOOKSHELF

Eisenberg, H., Murkoff, H. E., & Hathaway, S. E. (1988). *What to Expect When You're Expecting.* New York: Workman. For many expectant parents, this very popular book has provided intelligent, clear, no nonsense information about pregnancy and delivery. The same authors also have written some other books as well: *What to Eat When You're Expecting, What to Expect During the First Year of Life,* and *What to Expect During the Toddler Years.* This collection is a valuable resource for parent(s) or professionals.

Pregnancy ends with the delivery of a baby. This process follows a fairly predictable sequence, although the particular characteristics of each stage vary a great deal from person to person and from delivery to delivery.

Childbirth, or labor, is divided into three stages (Eisenberg et al., 1988; Enkin et al., 1995; Visscher & Rinehart, 1990). The first stage is characterized by contractions that proceed from mild to strong. This stage may last as long as 24 hours, but it culminates in the opening of the cervix and the pelvic bones and the descent of the baby's head in preparation for its passage into the birth canal. Many women can actually remain at home during this stage. At home or in the hospital, most women continue to move around during much of this stage.

The second stage of labor lasts far less time than the first and is characterized by full dilation of the cervix, descent of the baby through the birth canal, and presentation of the baby's head at the vaginal opening.

The third stage of labor culminates in the complete delivery of the infant

Table 1–2  **Characteristics of the Developing Embryo/Fetus**

| By the end of the: | The Embryo/Fetus Will |
| --- | --- |
| First month | Be smaller than a pea and shaped like a tadpole. It will have been implanted in the uterus for only 2 weeks and will have developed a placenta, and will be safely inside the amniotic sac. The embryo will be $1/2$ in. long and weigh less than 1 oz. |
| Second month | Be approximately $1^1/4$ in. long and weigh $1/3$ oz. The neural tube, which forms the basis for the central nervous system, and the cardiac, gastrointestinal, and sensory systems will be developed. Arm and leg buds will have begun to form and the heart will be beating. |
| Third month | Be approximately 3–4 in. long and weigh about 1 oz. Reproductive systems, including genitals, will be formed. Vascular and urinary systems are functioning. The head is much smaller than the body. Early independent and reflexive movements are seen. |
| Fourth month | Be approximately 6–7 in. long and weigh 5 oz. Bones are visible and the body growth begins to exceed that of the head. Sucking, swallowing, and other reflexes are present. Movements may be self-initiated or initiated in response to stimulation. Flexion, extension, and rotation are noted and the head moves separately from the body. The fetus is very humanlike in appearance with fully formed limbs, fingers, toes, and facial features. The fetus may be able to hear now. |
| Fifth month | Be approximately 8–12 in. long and weight 8–16 oz. Its movements are strong enough to be felt by its mother. A soft, moist vernix and hairlike lanugo cover and protect the body. Hair, nails, eyelashes, and eyebrows are developing. The fetus now hiccups, swallows, sucks its thumb, and actively moves its arms and legs. |
| Sixth month | Be approximately 11–14 in. long and weigh about $1$–$1^3/4$ lb. Eyes begin to open and close, finger and toe prints emerge. Hearing is believed to be intact. The fetus at this age very much resembles a newborn infant but is able to survive outside the womb only with significant support (intensive care), since all of its systems are still quite immature. |
| Seventh month | Be approximately 15 in. long and weigh 3 lb. At this time, it is believed that the fetus cries, differentiates tastes, and responds to pain, light, and tactile stimulation. The placenta and amniotic fluid are diminishing in volume in preparation for delivery. |
| Eighth month | Be approximately 18 in. long and weigh 5 lb. Nutrition is especially important now since brain growth and maturation is foremost in this period. A typically developing fetus born now would likely survive, although she or he may need extra assistance because of lung immaturity. |
| Ninth month | Be approximately 20 in. long and weigh 6–9 lb. It is ready for birth. Lungs are fully mature. The relatively large size of the fetus in the uterine space may limit fetal movements. |

*Source:* Adapted from Kliegman, 1996; Short-DeGraff, 1988; Visscher & Rinehart, 1990.

and the expulsion of the placenta. Current obstetrical practices generally allow for the parents to see and perhaps hold the new infant quite soon after delivery (Enkin et al., 1995). Initial suctioning of nose and mouth are commonly done, special eye drops are applied, and Apgar scores are noted (see Table 1–3). Vital signs (temperature, pulse, and respiration) and statistics (measurements of height, weight, and head circumference) are taken, and quick physical and neurological exams are conducted within minutes of delivery (Eisenberg et al., 1988; Enkin et al., 1995).

If problems arise during labor, delivery, or after, most medical centers have highly trained technical teams who can respond quickly and appropriately to these situations. In some situations, labor may not be progressing, so an oxytocic drug known as *pitocin* is used to induce a more efficient labor (Enkin et al., 1995). If the infant is in distress, as evidenced by abnormal tracings on the fetal monitor and/or by examination, delivery may have to be assisted with instruments such as forceps or a vacuum extractor. More extremely, delivery may be performed surgically by a procedure known as a cesarean section. The Apgar score (Table 1–3) is the standard "quick" measure for evaluating the health status of a newborn. It is used for every infant born in the United States. If the newborn has a very low Apgar score or is otherwise in distress, he or she may be transferred to a neonatal intensive care unit (NICU). Most areas have a regionalized emergency transport system using ambulances, helicopters, and so on to ensure the most immediate transfer of the baby and attention to his or her medical needs. In certain situations, it is possible to transport the mother to a high-risk obstetrical facility with NICU resources prior to delivery (Enkin et al., 1995; Visscher & Rinehart, 1990).

---

■ *THERAPEDS POINTER*

In the prenatal history of a child receiving occupational therapy services, you may discover information pertaining to risk factors. For example, the use of drugs during labor and delivery has been linked to hearing impairment. In some states, infants with this exposure may be eligible for a free audiological screening. The early identification of problems in hearing may make an immeasurable difference in the child's ability to learn to speak.

---

Table 1–3 **Apgar Score**

| | Score | | |
|---|---|---|---|
| **Criteria** | **0** | **1** | **2** |
| Color | Blue, pale | Body pink, extremities blue | All pink |
| Heart rate | Absent | <100 | >100 |
| Respiration | Absent | Irregular, slow | Good, crying |
| Reflex response to nose catheter | None | Grimace | Sneeze, cough |
| Muscle tone | Limp | Some flexion of extremities | Active |

*Source:* Adapted from Apgar, V., & Beck, J. (1972). *Is my baby all right?* New York: Simon & Schuster.

# THE NEWBORN

The normal newborn does not much resemble the baby seen in most television shows, magazine ads, and movies. (Such babies are often months old.) The newborn's head may be unusually shaped because of the molding that occurred as he or she descended through the birth canal (Enkin et al., 1995). Sometimes the pressure from the birth may cause scalp bleeding, which looks like a slight bruise or bump on the head. The baby may also have swollen eyelids and/or broken blood vessels in the whites of the eyes or on the skin. Some of the instruments used in delivery, such as internal fetal scalp monitors or forceps, may also leave superficial marks.

The newborn baby's head is large in contrast to the baby's body, and the face is small in contrast to the head size. This disproportion is interpreted by adults as quite appealing and is believed to help the infant obtain adult attention and care. The baby's eyes may be open or shut.

Healthy full-term newborns are able to breathe independently and to feed as soon as moments after delivery. Physiological reflexes (rooting and sucking) enable babies to seek the source of food (breast or bottle), latch on, and suck from it to obtain nourishment. Infants need and benefit from sensory stimulation such as holding, cuddling, rocking, talking, touching, and music (Eisenberg et al., 1988; Krajicek & Tompkins, 1993; Short-DeGraff, 1988; Vergera, 1993). They communicate quite effectively with adults using nonverbal language, eye contact, cries, and coos. Infants are charming, delightful, and challenging. They change the life of a family forever.

Newborns' bodies will be covered with a cheesy substance called vernix and some lanugo. Their breasts and genitals may initially be swollen because of a surge in maternal hormones. The umbilical cord will jut out and will be a dark purple from the disinfectant dye used to coat it until it falls off. Babies have sensitive skin and may discolor easily or have birthmarks and other skin features such as cradle cap or milia (harmless small, white, pimplelike skin eruptions). Their initial pigmentation may change over the first year of life. Despite all this, adults generally find newborn infants irresistible. Newborns have fully intact hearing and good vision, with normal visual actuity within 8 to 12 inches (just the right distance to be cradled in adults' arms). Babies' inherent sensory capacities as well as their interactional abilities are believed to contribute to adults' desire to hold and care for them, thus meeting their essential needs.

Some newborns may have trouble processing the large volume of red blood cells, previously needed in utero, through their still-immature livers. An excess of bilirubin, which is the by-product of this blood, may therefore remain in the bloodstream. This condition is referred to as *hyperbilirubinemia* and may manifest as *jaundice,* a yellow appearance of the skin and eyes. Untreated, jaundice may be dangerous, causing a condition known as *kernicterus,* which may result in damage to the central nervous system. Once diagnosed, treatment is readily available for hyperbilirubinemia and consists of exposure to ultraviolet light for a sustained period of time, generally no longer than a few days (Kliegman, 1996). Once the liver matures and red blood cell supplies are stabilized, jaundice should no longer be a problem.

Premature infants and others at risk may have special needs. These unique situations, often requiring the expertise of an occupational therapist and other professionals, are discussed in further detail in Chapter 3.

---

■ *THERAPEDS POINTER*

Whether you are working alone or on a team, a developmental history can be very helpful to your understanding of child and family needs. The information is best obtained by one person (often the social worker if there is one on the team) so that the family does not have to keep repeating its story. This information can, however, be obtained by the occupational therapist. A personal interview format is best. The interviewer should make certain that the parents are comfortable and aware of the purpose of the interview. Practice and training in interviewing can help the professional to ask questions in the least threatening and invasive manner.

Some professionals or teams have the family read and fill out part of the history form themselves, perhaps before an interview. If you choose this option, be sensitive to the diversity of families. Make sure to present written and verbal information in the family's native language and always offer to read written information and write down answers for them. For a variety of reasons, many adults do not read well and may be uncomfortable disclosing this. Anticipating the needs of families will increase their comfort and confidence and you will, in return, receive richer information to help you plan and provide good care for their children.

---

# THE FAMILY

From almost the moment of conception, baby, mother, father, and siblings' lives change as they become a family. A new family is in fact created with each new infant. Parental independence, freedom, and time management are immeasurably altered by the addition of children. For all families, a new baby changes the family members' relationships with each other. In fact, without a "family," a group of loving, caring adults and others, babies generally will not thrive. From conception into adulthood, the family is the most appropriate context for intervention. For infants this is especially important. Important considerations in working with families include:

1. *The Members of the Family.* These may include the traditional members—mother, father, siblings, and grandparents, or may include others, such as close friends, aunts or uncles, or foster parents. What is important to know is who is responsible for the care of the child and who cares about him or her. Characteristics of each family member, age, vocation, marital status, level of education, and so on, influence the family as a whole. It is helpful to know the roles of different family members as well as to

understand their styles of interaction. Each family has its own unique interests, values, and traditions. Understanding cultural context goes a long way toward being able to offer useful support and assistance.

2. *Family History.* It is helpful to know how long the family has been together, as well as what problems and successes this group of people has experienced, and how have they coped. It is helpful to know where people have "come from" in order to help them to get where they would like to go. The history of a family provides a rich context for understanding their unique resources as well as their needs. This, coupled with an appreciation of ethnic origins, religion or spiritual systems, and family rituals and beliefs, gives great insight into family functioning.

3. *Resources.* These include financial resources as well as social supports such as friends and relatives, agencies, and service providers. It is helpful to know about each family's health-care and educational resources as well. Use of some of the available public assistance programs can greatly ease family burdens. Too often families may be eligible for assistance, but they are unaware or uninformed that such assistance exists. Community support systems such as church or synagogue, clubs, and neighborhoods can also provide significant help (Krajicek & Tompkins, 1993).

4. *Family-Centered Care.* Occupational therapists and others have historically provided a somewhat hierarchical model of caregiving. In this model, professionals make the essential decisions and their patients or clients simply comply. In recent years, the caregiving system has shifted to allow much more involvement of individuals in their own care, even promoting collaborative decision making and goal setting. For children, a commitment to collaboration with families is reflective of this shift in professional practice. Family-centered care places *all* the individuals who care about and who have information and expertise in a partnership relationship. This type of care is believed to produce superior services as well as a greater satisfaction for all involved. The principles of family-centered care are listed in Table 1–4.

# WRAPPING IT UP

This chapter has provided an overview of the typical events that occur during pregnancy and delivery. Common prenatal diagnostics have also been reviewed. Since collaboration among professionals and families is essential to the provision of quality care, a discussion of the unique features of human newborns and the philosophy of *family-centered care* has been introduced. A good understanding of the prenatal experience is invaluable to practicing therapists. This chapter provides some strategies for attending to this essential stage of human development.

Table 1–4 **Principles of Family-Centered Care**

- Family is the constant in the child's life and has the greatest influence on the child.
- The family is the client.
- All service needs of the family are addressed.
- All information about services is shared with the family. The family decides what will remain confidential.
- The strengths, individuality, and methods of coping of the family are recognized and are the basis on which services are developed.
- Services to the family are flexible and responsive to the family's needs. The program fits the family, not the other way around.
- Family peer support is encouraged and facilitated.
- The team is composed of the family and all those service providers who serve the family.
- The family and the service providers collaborate on issues of direct care, program development, and policy.
- All services received by the family are delivered and coordinated by primarily one person on the team.

*Source:* National Center for Family-Centered Care. (1990). *What is family-centered care?* (brochure). Washington, DC: Association for the Care of Children's Health.

## CASE STORY

Wilhemina, an airline industry executive, was 34 years old when she finally became pregnant. After 5 years of infertility treatments, she and her husband, Ed, a professional musician, were more than delighted. She began prenatal care early in the pregnancy—actually before it began because her infertility treatment was provided by obstetrical specialists. She read everything she could get her hands on about prenatal nutrition and exercise, and she followed as much of the advice as she could.

At 15 weeks of pregnancy, a blood test revealed increased AFP levels. Her doctor recommended an amniocentesis, which was done at 17 weeks. The test revealed a fetus with Down syndrome. Although they were heartbroken to learn this, Wilhemina and Ed chose to continue the pregnancy and learn all they could about what they could do to help their new baby. A fetal echocardiogram done subsequently was normal.

At 22 weeks, Wilhemina began to experience elevating blood pressure and some leaking of amniotic fluid. Ultrasound evaluation revealed that the fetus was healthy and thriving. However, Wilhemina's doctor put her on medical bed rest just to make sure.

As part of this family's exploration of resources for their child, they have contacted you, a community OT.

1. What assistance might an OT be able to offer for Wilhemina during her period of bed rest?

2. How could you help Wilhemina and Ed prepare for their new roles as parents of a child with Down syndrome?

> ## Real-Life Lab
>
> 1. Interview your own parents about their pregnancy and childbirth experience. It will be interesting for you to see how much of what happened long ago they still remember. You may also be able to see how much prenatal care has changed over recent years.
>
> 2. Visit friends or relatives who have a new baby. Interview them about their prenatal experience. Make sure to note any similarities and differences between their expectations and the realities. Ask them to show you the results of any prenatal tests that they have. (Many parents now make the prenatal ultrasound pictures a central part of the photo album.)
>
> 3. Visit a maternity center. Many maternity centers provide tours for the general public. Hopefully you will have the opportunity to see some prenatal testing areas, as well as the labor, delivery, and recovery rooms, and the newborn nurseries.
>
> You might wish to ask if there is an OT involved in perinatal services, perhaps in the NICU or through home-care services for high-risk mothers or infants.

# References

Batshaw, M. L., & Perret, Y. M. (1992). *Children with disabilities: A medical primer.* Baltimore: Paul Brooks.

Blondel, B., Dutilh, P., Delour, M., & Uzan, S. (1993). Poor prenatal care and pregnancy outcomes. *European Journal of Obstetrics, Gynecology, & Reproductive Biology, 50*(3), 191–196.

Camosy, P. (1995). Fetal Medicine: treating the unborn patient. *American Family Physician, 52*(5), 1385–1392.

Chiriboga, C. (1993). Fetal effects. *Neurological Clinics, 11*(3), 707–728.

Cohn, A., & Leach, L. (1987). *Generations: A universal family album.* New York: Pantheon Books.

Eisenberg, A., Murkoff, H. E., & Hathaway, S. E. (1988). *What to expect when you're expecting.* New York: Workman.

Enkin, M., Keirse, M., Renfrew, M., & Neilson, J. (1995). *A guide to effective care in pregnancy and childbirth* (2d ed.). New York: Oxford University Press.

Flake, A. W., & Harrison, M. R. (1995). Fetal surgery. *Annual Review of Medicine, 46,* 67–78.

Gjerdingen, D. K., & Fontaine, P. (1991). Preconception health care: A critical task for family physicians. *Journal of the American Board of Family Practice, 4*(4), 237–50.

Goncalves, L. F., Jeanty, P., & Piper, J. M. (1994). The accuracy of prenatal ultrasonography in detecting congenital anomalies. *American Journal of Obstetrics & Gynecology, 171*(6), 1606–1612.

Kellner, L. H., Weiss, R. R., Weiner, Z., Neuer, M., Martin, G. M., Schulman, H., & Lipper, S. (1995). The advantages of using triple-marker screening for chromosomal abnormalities. *American Journal of Obstetrics & Gynecology, 172*(3) 831–836.

Kliegman, R. (Ed). (1996). *Nelson textbook of pediatrics.* Philadelphia: W. B. Saunders.

Krajicek, M., & Thomlinson, A. (1983). *Detection of developmental problems in children* (2d ed.). Baltimore: University Park Press.

Krajicek, M., & Thompkins, R. (Eds.). (1993). *The medically fragile infant.* Austin, TX: Pro-ed.

Kuller, J., & Laifer, S. (1995). Contemporary approaches to prenatal diagnosis. *American Family Physician, 52*(8), 2277–2283.

Lewerenz, T. L., & Schaaf, R. C. (1996). Sensory processing in at-risk infants. Sensory integration special interest section newsletter. *American Occupational Therapy Association, 19,* 1–4.

Plouffe, L., Jr., & Donahue, J. (1994). Techniques for early diagnosis of the abnormal fetus. *Clinics in Perinatology, 21*(4), 723–741.

"Recommendations for the use of folic acid to reduce the number of cases of spina bifida and other neural tube defects." (1992). *Morbidity & Mortality Weekly Review, 41* (RR-14), 1–7.

Schorling, J. B. (1993). The prevention of prenatal alcohol use: A critical analysis of intervention studies. *Journal of Studies on Alcohol, 54*(3), 261–267.

Short-DeGraff, M. (1988). *Human development in occupational therapy and physical therapy.* Baltimore: Williams & Wilkins.

"Trends in fetal alcohol syndrome—United States, 1979–1993." (1995). *Morbidity & Mortality Weekly Report, 44*(13), 249–251.

Vergera, E. (1993). *Foundations for practice in the neonatal intensive care unit in early intervention.* Rockville, MD: American Occupational Therapy Association.

Visscher, H. C., & Rinehart, R. D. The American College of Obstetrics & Gynecology. (1990). *Planning for pregnancy, birth and beyond.* New York: Penguin Books.

Williamson, H., Jr., & LeFevre, M. (1992). Tangible assistance: A simple measure of social support predicts pregnancy outcome. *Family Practice Research Journal, 12*(3), 289–295.

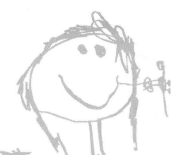

# 2

# *Prenatal and Perinatal Risk Factors*

Ellen Berger Rainville, MS, OTR, FAOTA

**Risk** *(risk), n. 1 exposure to the chance of injury or loss . . .*
**Prenatal** *(pre nat' l) adj., previous to birth or giving birth . . .*
**Perinatal** *(per'e nat'l) adj., occurring during or pertaining to the phase*
*surrounding the time of birth, from the twentieth week of gestation to the*
*twenty eighth day of newborn life*
—*Random House Dictionary,* 1987

## KEY POINTS

- It is amazing that babies are conceived, grow, and develop in their mother's wombs and are born—most without complications. For some, however, the *prenatal* and *perinatal* periods are laden with problems and risks, some of which may result in serious consequences for the baby.

- It is important to understand the risks encountered in pregnancy before becoming pregnant, in order to anticipate care needs and options; during pregnancy, in order to actively minimize risk; and after pregnancy, in order to make sense of problems experienced by the offspring as well as to mediate the emotional impact of risk on the family.

- Understanding prenatal and perinatal risk factors is critical to occupational therapists and other caregiving professionals because:

  1) An understanding of the precursors to developmental delay and deviation is essential for medical/health-care providers to best assess current and future problems.

  2) Risk factors give us a good idea of which children might benefit from close monitoring in order to enhance their development and function.

3) Early identification of actual delays and deviations in development allow us to provide the earliest possible interventions.

- For families, it is also important to understand what has and what might yet happen to their children. Making sense of the experience of becoming a family is an essential occupational task for family members.

- It is also important for care providers to understand family, gestational, and other histories in order to best empathize with each family's unique experience. Using techniques of narrative in therapy, where therapists help families to construct and tell their own "stories," families can make sense of their past and present and imagine the future that is most realistic and desirable for them (Mattingly & Fleming, 1994).

- Occupational therapists (OTs), especially, need to be aware of risk factors, because the emphasis of our intervention will be on reducing the impact of certain risk factors; on supporting families in identifying their own values, interests, and needs; in assisting family members to feel competent in their chosen roles, especially in light of caretaker demands; and in improving performance in daily life activities.

## ▰▰▰ FROM THE BOOKSHELF

For further information on the use of narrative in therapy, the following resources are suggested:

Clark, F., Ennevor, B. L., & Richardson, P. L. (1996). A grounded theory of techniques for occupational storytelling and occupational story making. In Zemke, R., & Clark, F. (1996). *Occupation science: The evolving discipline.* (pp. 373–392). Philadelphia: F. A. Davis.

Fazio, L. (1992). Tell me a story: The therapeutic metaphor in the practice of pediatric occupational therapy. *American Journal of Occupational Therapy, 46(2), 112–119.*

Higgs, J., & Jones, M. (Eds.). (1995). *Clinical reasoning in the health professions.* Oxford: Butterworth-Heinemann.

Mattingly, C. (1991). What is clinical reasoning? *American Journal of Occupational Therapy, 45(11), 972–978.*

Mattingly, C., & Fleming, M. (Eds.) (1994). *Clinical reasoning: Forms of inquiry in a therapeutic practice.* Philadelphia: F. A. Davis.

# BEGINNINGS

This chapter provides a brief overview of the most common prenatal and perinatal risk factors facing families today. The reader is directed to "From the Bookshelf" or toward the very broad prenatal and perinatal literature available for more indepth coverage.

For ease of understanding, the concept of risk is addressed. The specific risks discussed will be categorized as genetic, environmental and lifestyle, maternal, and pregnancy-specific. The relevance of risk assessment for therapists is explained, and specific procedures for history taking are provided. It is certainly possible to have what is known as *multifactorial risk*, where factors from any or all of these categories interact to present a unique type of risk. As history has demonstrated, there are also undoubtedly many risk factors that are as yet unknown or unidentified.

To best appreciate the potential impact of various risk factors, a good knowledge of typical prenatal and perinatal development is essential (see Chapter 1) to appreciate the critical importance of such factors as timing, frequency, duration, and amount of exposure to risk factors on potential outcomes. For example, exposure to certain environmental hazards or toxic substances during the first trimester of pregnancy (when the embryological systems are forming) has very different consequences for the infant than exposure later in pregnancy.

# RISK

Why is risk important for occupational therapists? Risk implies danger. Sometimes that danger presents a climate of thrill, excitement, or challenge, such as skiing, race car driving, or making one's first public presentation. In pediatric therapy, risk also involves danger, but the spirit is far more sedate. Many potential risks exist before, during, and after pregnancy, each of which can affect the developing fetus, the newborn, the child, and the family. In these cases, risk implies danger or potentially poor outcome—problems for infants and families that might be preventable.

There are three levels of prevention:

*Primary prevention* aims to intervene *prior to the occurrence of a disability or problem in order to prevent it from happening or decrease its impact.* An example is the provision of affordable, accessible prenatal health and nutrition services that are known to improve pregnancy outcomes. Another example is educational programs about the effects of drugs and other toxins on developing fetuses. These might prevent women from using substances such as tobacco, alcohol, or drugs, especially if they think they might be pregnant.

*Secondary prevention* aims to intervene *as soon as possible after the identification of a problem in order to eliminate the problem or reduce its undesirable effects.* This serves to lessen the impact of a disability and may improve future function. An example of secondary prevention might be screening programs to identify sometimes "hidden" but treatable conditions that could cause functional problems. A hearing screening program, for example, could identify children with otitis media (middle ear infections), which may delay language development and create associated vestibular problems. Otitis media is a common childhood problem that can be treated medically. Another example is a vision screening program, which could identify children who need glasses, a highly successful means of reducing the impact of many visual acuity problems.

*Tertiary prevention* aims intervention *after the problem has occurred.* The types of problems that require tertiary prevention cannot be entirely prevented or eliminated, but efforts are made to reduce the impact and to prevent secondary complications. An example of tertiary prevention might be found in the same program mentioned earlier. Here, children with sensorineural hearing loss could be identified and specialty services, including hearing aids, could be initiated. Another example applies to children with cerebral palsy. For many of these children, therapists work to reduce the impact of atypical movement patterns on a child's function. This is believed to not only improve the child's performance but also to reduce the incidence or severity of the secondary orthopedic problems common to children with this diagnosis.

Inherent in a preventive perspective is an emphasis on *promotion*, where the interventions are focused on enhancement of the capabilities of children and families rather than on the elimination or reduction of disability (Brown & Brown, 1993).

---

■ *THERAPEDS POINTER*

A preventive approach promotes child and family function.

Within the context of an individual's culture, biological factors interact with environmental factors in different ways. Disease and disability have very different meanings for different people, families, and communities. This means that in designing and implementing their interventions, therapists must:

- Understand the risks that potentially jeopardize child and family function
- Identify functional and developmental problems
- Focus on the unique values, beliefs, strengths, and resources of each child and family

Therapists must also be diligent at their attempts to understand a range of perspectives and experiences. This means that a nonjudgmental approach to families is essential. For example, it is best to temper any feelings of anger or disgust that you may have with a mother who abused drugs during her pregnancy, even if the baby you are treating has disabilities that resulted from the drug abuse. It is essential that you step back from your own biases and take a more holistic approach. The mother may not have understood the potential effects of her prenatal drug use on her infant, or maybe she was so ill she could not change her behavior. Perhaps she was not even aware of her pregnancy until it was too late. If your relationship with her is strong and trusting, it may be appropriate to discuss this. However, early on, as you plan your interventions, perhaps you could consider how a *preventive* approach, including child-focused activities as well as support and education for the mother, might help to:

- Reduce the effects of the child's disability
- Improve the child's ability to function in the environment
- Help the mother feel better about herself, which in turn might help her to facilitate her child's optimal development and function or help her to avoid drug abuse in subsequent pregnancies

Your knowledge of risk helps you to appreciate the context of the child's disability and allows you to aim accurately at family function and prevention. Your focus can be on promoting the bond between mother and child. A collaborative effort between therapists and parents is far more likely to promote developmental gains in children.

# RISK ASSESSMENT

The importance of recording or documenting risk cannot be overemphasized. A careful and detailed history addressing prenatal and perinatal risk factors; child and family health; and developmental, sociocultural, and economic factors is critical to obtaining a clear picture of each child's unique situation. This forms the basis for risk assessment—often an essential aspect of determining eligibility for services. It is also an essential component of the overall assessment and evaluation process.

---

■ *THERAPEDS POINTER*

A team approach to risk assessment has many benefits.

Generally, care providers, working either individually or as members of teams, develop a standardized format for collecting and recording relevant historical information. Usually there is a standard data collection or intake form kept with the records of each child and family served. Sample history-taking, data collection, and intake forms are provided in the Appendix for your review.

As a team member, what is the therapist's role in history taking? What is the therapist's responsibility? What can an OT learn from this process?

Therapists most often function as essential members of caregiving teams—multidisciplinary, interdisciplinary, or transdisciplinary. These teams can be found in almost every health-care, educational, and social service environment. On these teams there is *complementarity*, as each team member brings the unique perspective of his or her discipline and individual experience to the team effort. There are also many areas of *overlap* on teams. For example, all team members are concerned about comfort levels and behavior, since these so influence their intervention efforts. Teams often collaborate on strategies to manage these factors. Team members also provide specialized information to each other to help with the individual and collective understanding of the child and family.

For example, when the physical therapist explains to team members about the impact of a child's atypical muscle tone on balance, endurance, and efficiency, other team members are able to use special seating and positioning strategies to minimize the effects of that tone on performance. For the same child, the educator and speech pathologist may address the child's difficulty in processing auditory sensations. Team members then could work with the child in nondistracting environments using careful verbal and physical cueing.

In regard to history taking, team members also have both unique and overlapping needs. For example, the physical therapist may be concerned with the sequence and timelines for a child's acquisition of motor milestones, whereas the occupational therapist may want to know about the child's unique responses to sensory experiences. An individual child's history may reveal a tendency to avoid touch. This is described as discomfort with movements, such as rolling over, that require contact with surfaces, as well as aversion to cuddling and holding. As you can see, this information has relevance to each team member individually as well as to the team collectively.

As team members, it is appropriate for therapists to be involved in the development of the team's history-taking protocols. Working with their colleagues, therapists can assure that the appropriate data are collected in the most considerate and efficient manner possible. Therapists should work to assure that:

- Necessary information is collected.
- Data collection methods (written questionnaire, interview, record review, etc.) are the most considerate and effective for the data to be obtained.
- The timing and presentation of data collection are respectful to the privacy rights and needs of families.
- The data collected are used to help understand the child and family and to provide appropriate interventions, including both direct services and referrals to other resources that may be helpful.

Once a team has determined the essential information to be collected, they can allocate the responsibility of data gathering to the appropriate team member(s). Often the nurse or social worker takes the lead in this aspect of caregiving. Therapists may be directly or indirectly involved.

Although therapists may not be the primary team members responsible for history taking, they will be involved in interpretation of the information gathered. They will also need to talk with the families as they work with them; therefore, understanding the principles of history taking may be helpful.

Data collection forms such as history-taking (intake) forms (or portions of them) may be mailed or brought to families for them to review or fill out at their leisure. This practice may save time. However, a personal interview should be a significant part of data collection for the history. This interview could serve to summarize the information collected in writing, give opportunities to learn new information, or allow for verbal communication with individuals who do not or cannot read or write well. Personal contact with a warm, genuinely interested professional is more likely to help the family feel comfortable while revealing detailed personal information than filling out an impersonal form.

Personal interviews work best when they present questions in the native language of and at the level of most ready understanding for the family. The reading and comprehension levels of adults vary widely, so questioning should enhance the family's ability to tell its own story rather than inhibit or intimidate family members with complex terminology or judgmental attitudes. It is important also to recognize that families may be telling their story to many people, so minimizing the number of professionals asking the same questions is both considerate and cost-effective. Historical information, coupled with other evaluation data, such as observation and testing, guides us in making responsible judgments about intervention programming and support services.

# PERINATAL RISK FACTORS

Team members need to be familiar with the common risk factors encountered by the consumers of their care. This not only establishes a common language and understanding for team members but also helps to identify potential prevention, intervention, and case-finding efforts. For example, an early childhood intervention program might collaborate with a drug treatment program to provide prenatal support and education about drug use during pregnancy. This would be a primary prevention service. Team members might also provide postnatal monitoring of infants exposed to drugs during pregnancy. This is also a preventive service, at the secondary prevention level, as well as a case-finding one. Through developmental monitoring of high-risk infants, it is possible to identify children and families in need of intervention services at the earliest possible time.

The remainder of this chapter focuses on the more common risk factors encountered in pediatric practice. It primarily addresses biological and established risks that interact with environmental factors. Environmental risks are discussed in more detail in Chapter 3.

---

■ *THERAPEDS POINTER*

Classification of Risk Factors

**Established risk** includes those conditions that have a known range of problems with development and/or function (e.g., Down syndrome or cerebral palsy).

**Biological risk** includes those organic risk factors that are highly likely to result in developmental or functional problems (e.g., prematurity, prenatal toxin exposure).

**Environmental risk** includes psychological and/or environmental factors, such as insufficient caregiving, that are likely to contribute to adverse developmental and functional outcomes.

---

The following discussion of prenatal and perinatal risk factors is divided into four categories for ease of understanding: genetic, environmental and lifestyle, maternal, and pregnancy-related. In this categorization, the term environmental refers only to the inanimate environment and includes toxins, infections, and so on.

# GENETIC RISK FACTORS

It is estimated that 2 to 3 percent of infants have a major genetic defect and another 4 to 5 percent have less obvious or less serious defects (Visscher & Rinehart, 1990). Humans have 23 pairs of chromosomes: 22 autosomes, which are identical pairs, and 1 pair of sex chromosomes, which are identical (2 Xs) if the human is female, and disparate (one X and one Y) if the human is male. Deviations from this normal genetic map are responsible for genetic defects. Figure 2–1 illustrates the inheritance patterns that may result in certain genetic anomalies.

There are three types of genetic risks: multifactorial, chromosomal, and single-gene.

## MULTIFACTORIAL

These risks involve an interplay between the environment and the genetic code. Essentially, there are certain measurable traits (e.g., height, blood pressure, facial features) or disease states that are the result of the additive or interactive effects of one or more genes. These traits have a continuous, bell-shaped distribution and interact with environmental factors to produce the individual variability in individuals, families, and populations of people. Some disease states that are attributed to multifactorial inheritance include myelodysplasia, cleft lip, cardiac malformation, neural tube defects, clubfoot, and hip dislocations (Blackman, 1990; Kliegman & Arvin, 1996; Visscher & Rinehart, 1990).

## CHROMOSOMAL ABNORMALITIES

These are inherited defects that are caused by too few or too many chromosomes, extra or missing pieces of chromosomal material, and/or errors in the development of the egg or sperm. An infant's risk for chromosomal abnormalities increases with the age of the mother. For a 22-year-old mother, the likelihood of any chromosomal abnormality is 1 in 500 births. This risk remains stable until after age 29, and for a 35-year-old mother, the risk is 1 in 200. For a 40-year-old mother, the risk is 1 in 60 that her offspring will have some chromosomal abnormality (Blackman, 1990; Enkin et al., 1995; Visscher & Rinehart, 1990).

Specific types of chromosomal abnormalities include:

*Nondisjunction.* The chromosomes fail to divide properly, resulting in an error in number. An example of this would be where there are more than two chromosomes in a single cell, such as in the trisomies (e.g., Down syndrome is a trisomy of the 23rd chromosome).

*Deletions.* A part of a chromosome has broken or has been lost, such as in cri-du-chat syndrome, a deletion of the short arm of the fifth chromosome.

*Translocations.* A lost or broken part attaches to another chromosome. This is another mechanism that may create a trisomy, such as in Down syndrome (Batshaw & Perret, 1992).

| Inheritance Pattern | Characteristics | Examples |
|---|---|---|
| **X-linked recessive**<br><br>Carrier mother<br>Parents: X X (Carrier mother) — X Y (Father)<br>Gametes: X  X  X  Y<br>Children: X X (Carrier daughter) — X Y (Affected son) — X X (Normal daughter) — X Y (Normal son)<br><br>Affected father<br>Parents: X X (Mother) — X Y (Affected father)<br>Gametes: X  X  X  Y<br>Children: X X (Carrier daughter) — X Y (Normal son) — X X (Carrier daughter) — X Y (Normal son) | Either parent may have the gene present on the X chromosome.<br>Since females have two X chromosomes; in order to be affected they must have a pair of altered genes.<br>If a woman has an altered gene on only one X chromosome, she is a carrier (usually not affected) and has a 25% risk of having an affected son.<br>Since males have only one X chromosome, they need only a single, altered gene to be affected. (There are no male carriers.)<br>If a man is affected, all of his daughters will be carriers and not affected, and all of his sons will be normal. | Duchenne and Becker muscular dystrophies; hemophilia; Hunter's syndrome; color-blindness; Lesch-Nyhan syndrome |
| **Autosomal recessive**<br><br>Parents: A a (Carrier) — A a (Carrier)<br>Gametes: A  a  A  a<br>Children: A A (Normal, 25%) — A a (Carrier, 50%) — a A — a a (Affected, 25%) | Disorders are caused by a pair of altered genes on the autosomes.<br>Both parents are carriers of the altered gene (though they are clinically normal).<br>When both parents are carriers, there is a 25% risk of having an affected child (male or female) with each pregnancy. | Cystic fibrosis; galactosemia; limb-girdle muscular dystrophy; maple syrup urine disease; PKU; sickle-cell anemia; Tay-Sachs disease |
| **X-linked dominant (rare)**<br><br>Affected mother<br>Parents: X X (Affected mother) — X Y (Father)<br>Gametes: X  X  X  Y<br>Children: X X (Affected daughter) — X Y (Affected son) — X X (Normal daughter) — X Y (Normal son)<br><br>Affected father<br>Parents: X X (Mother) — X Y (Affected father)<br>Gametes: X  X  X  Y<br>Children: X X (Affected daughter) — X Y (Normal son) — X X (Affected daughter) — X Y (Normal son) | Either parent may be affected because of an altered gene on their X chromosome.<br>If a mother is affected, she has a 50% risk of having an affected son or daughter with each pregnancy.<br>If a father is affected, all of his daughters will be affected, and all of his sons will be normal. | Hypophosphatemia (vitamin D–resistant rickets) |
| **Autosomal dominant**<br><br>Parents: A a (Affected) — a a (Normal)<br>Gametes: A  a  a  a<br>Children: A a (Affected, 50%) — A a — a a (Normal, 50%) — a a | Disorders are caused by a single altered gene on one of the autosomes.<br>Either parent may have the gene, or the disorder may be caused by a new gene alteration (mutation).<br>If one parent is affected, there is a 50 % risk of having an affected child (male or female) with each pregnancy. | Achondroplasia; Huntington's disease; tuberous sclerosis; neurofibromatosis; Stickler's syndrome; myotonic dystrophy |

Figure 2–1 Mechanisms of inheritance. (*Source:* Blackman, J. A. [1997]. *Medical aspects of developmental disabilities in children birth to three* [3d ed.]. Gaithersburg, MD: Aspen.)

## SINGLE-GENE DEFECTS

Unlike chromosomal abnormalities, where there is an inadequate amount of genetic material, in single-gene defects, there is adequate material, but there is an alteration in the gene or gene pair itself. This results in inaccurate decoding of the specific DNA. Single-gene defects are also known as inborn errors of metabolism (Blackman, 1990).

Table 2–1 provides a listing of common genetic syndromes and the resultant disorders.

It is possible to determine the incidence of a particular genetic disorder occurring in the general population by analysis of data that are required to be reported on all newborns in the United States. This type of information, which includes birth weights, neonatal and infant mortality, and birth defects, is called *vital statistics* and is usually maintained by the public health department in each state and by the federal government's Bureau of Vital Statistics. Table 2–1 includes a summary of the incidence (the rate or range of new occurrences) of particular genetic disorders in the general population. For individuals and families at risk for, or concerned about, potential genetic disorders, genetic counseling is available and recommended. This service analyzes individual risk and enables families to make important decisions as they plan and prepare for their individual family needs.

# MATERNAL HEALTH
# AND NUTRITION

Maternal age, general health, and maternal stress are potential risk factors. For example, adolescent mothers face a very special set of risks and problems. Because they are still growing themselves, they are placed in the position of competing with the fetus for nutrition and therefore they may need extra attention to diet. Because of the developmental issues associated with adolescents, it is not uncommon for women and men at this stage to have unrealistic expectations for themselves and their children, to have financial and emotional stresses, and to have lifestyle demands (such as high school) that are not compatible with the demands of child-rearing. Adolescent parents also face a higher rate of infant morbidity and mortality for reasons that are still unclear. However, with support and education in child-rearing, day care, alternative high school programs, sufficient prenatal and postnatal health care, and family and community support, adolescents can be competent, caring parents (Short-DeGraff, 1988).

Women over the age of 35, while perhaps more emotionally and financially prepared for parenthood, face significantly increased risk for genetic anomalies and for problems in conception, pregnancy, and delivery. However, more women than ever are having children later in life with very good outcomes (Prysak, Lorenz, & Kisly, 1995). With the proper prenatal and postnatal supports, women and men of all ages can be effective parents.

Maternal health is critical. If a mother is exerting a great deal of effort to recover from illness or to cope with stress, vital nutrient and energy stores

Table 2–1 Some Chromosomal Syndromes and Their Sequelae

| Syndrome | Incidence | Mechanism | Description | Developmental/Functional Sequelae |
| --- | --- | --- | --- | --- |
| Cornelia de Lange syndrome | 1/10,000 | Possible chromosome 3q mutation | Short stature, microcephaly, characteristic facial appearance, hypertrichosis | Autistic-like behaviors, language delays, feeding abnormalities, mental retardation (MR) |
| Cri-du-chat syndrome | 1/20,000 | Partial deletion of short arm of chromosome 5 | Catlike cry at infancy, prenatal and postnatal growth retardation, MR, congenital heart defects, microcephaly, simian creases | Severe respiratory and feeding abnormalities in infancy, hypotonia, inguinal hernias |
| Down syndrome | Variable | Trisomy 21 or, rarely, mosaicism or translocation | Hypotonia, flat facial profile, upwardly slanted eyes, small nose and ears, short stature, MR, simian creases, congenital heart disease | Atlantoxial instability, ligamentous laxity, visual and auditory deficits, thyroid disease, premature senility |
| Duchenne muscular dystrophy (DMD) | 1/3,300 | Mutation in dystrophin gene located on the short arm of X chromosome | Progressive pelvic muscle weakness and atrophy, with enlargement of thigh muscles, tight heel cords | Contractures, scoliosis, wheelchair dependence (usually by age 10–12 years), progressive weakness, pneumonia, ECG abnormalities |
| Fragile X syndrome | 1/1250 male births, 1/200 female births | Defect in X chromosome | Prominent jaw, large ears, large testes, mild connective tissue abnormalities | Behavior problems, hyperactivity, and autistic features common to both sexes; learning disabilities in females only; MR in males only |
| Marfan syndrome | 1/10,000 | Abnormality in the fibrillin gene, located on chromosome 15q | Tall, thin stature, spiderlike limbs, hypermobile joints, dislocation of lens, aortic aneurysm, usually normal intelligence | Joint instability, thoracic deformities, loss of vision |

| | | | | |
|---|---|---|---|---|
| Neurofibromatosis (type I, von Recklinghausen disease) | 1/3000 | Defect in chromosome 17q11 | Multiple *café-au-lait* spots on body; nerve tumors in body and on skin | Optic gliomas, glaucoma, macrocephaly, hypertension, learning disabilities (attention-deficit–hyperactivity disorder) |
| Hurler's syndrome (Mucopolysaccharidosis I-H) | 1/100,000 | Deficiency of enzyme alpha-iduronidase, located on chromosome 4 | Short stature, progressive MR, coarse facial appearance, full lips | Visual and hearing deficits, progressive joint limitation, kyphosis, hernias, progressive cardiac failure |
| Lesch-Nyhan syndrome | 1/100,000 | Deficiency of enzyme HGPRT necessary for purine metabolism | Progressive neurological disorder, self-injurious behavior, MR, progressive choreoathetoid cerebral palsy, excessive uric acid in blood | Urinary uric acid stones, kidney disease, mild anemia, arthritis, dysphasia, vomiting |
| Spinal-muscular atrophy (Werdnig-Hoffman syndrome) | 4/100,000 | Deletion in chromosome 5q | Progressive respiratory failure and severe muscle weakness in infancy; normal intelligence; survival unusual past 2 years of age | Contractures, cardiomyopathy, respiratory infections, scoliosis |
| Tay-Sachs disease | 1/3800 in Ashkenazic Jews | Deficiency of enzyme hexosaminidase; located on chromosome 15 | Progressive nervous system disorder, deafness, blindness, seizures; rapidly fatal, usually by 4 years | Feeding abnormalities, aspiration |
| Treacher Collins syndrome (mandibulofacial dysostosis) | Unknown | Defect in chromosome 5q3 | Characteristic facial appearance, malformation of external ear, flattened area near cheekbones | Choanal atresia, respiratory and feeding problems in infancy, obstructive apnea |
| Trisomy 13 | 1/8000 births | Nondisjunction resulting in extra chromosome 13, rarely translocation | Microphthalmia, cleft lip and palate, and polydactyly, dysmorphic appearance | Multiorgan system involvement; profound MR, visual impairment, cerebral palsy |

Table 2–1  **Some Chromosomal Syndromes and Their Sequelae**—*Continued*

| Syndrome | Incidence | Mechanism | Description | Developmental/Functional Sequelae |
|---|---|---|---|---|
| Trisomy 18 | 1/6000 | Nondisjunction resulting in trisomy for chromosome 18 | Small for gestational age, low-set ears, clenched hands with overriding fingers, congenital heart defects | Feeding problems, aspiration, diaphragmatic hernia; most do not survive first year of life |
| Tuberous sclerosis | 1/10,000–1/50,000 | Defect on chromosome 9 or 16 | Hypopigmented areas, acnelike facial lesions, infantile spasms, calcium deposits in brain | Malignancies, hydrocephalus, tumors of the heart |
| Turner's syndrome (XO syndrome) | 1/5000 | Chromosomal non-disjunction resulting in a single X chromosome | Short stature; female; broad chest with widely spaced nipples; congenital heart disease; ovarian dysgenesis; usually normal intelligence | Thyroid abnormalities, diabetes mellitus, kidney abnormalities, learning disabilities |
| Williams syndrome (hypercalcemia-elfin facies syndrome) | 1/10,000 | Deletion on chromosome 7q11 (elastin locus) | Short stature, full lips and cheeks, periorbital fullness, hoarse voice, MR | Cardiac abnormality, renal abnormalities, contractures |
| XYY syndrome | 1/1000 | Chromosomal nondisjunction | Tall stature, poor fine motor coordination, aggressive behavior | Slow nerve conduction velocities, learning disabilities |

*Source:* Kurtz, L., et al. (1996). *Handbook of developmental disabilities.* Gaithersburg, MD: Aspen.

needed by the infant may be unavailable. Preconceptive and pregnant women are encouraged to maintain a healthy, active lifestyle, including good nutrition, careful health practices, rest, and exercise.

Women have special nutritional needs during pregnancy. Additional calories are needed to help the mother do the work of digestion and breathing for the fetus as well as to supply the necessary nutrients. Pregnant women are typically advised to add approximately 300 calories to their diet each day for each fetus. They are advised to expect a 25- to 35-pound weight gain for a typical pregnancy, more if they have twins. Given the physical demands of pregnancy, it is understandable that many women report unusually large appetites during pregnancy.

Specific nutrients are also needed, often at specific times during pregnancy, to support embryonic and fetal growth and development. Extra iron and protein are needed throughout pregnancy for fetal growth and increased blood volume. Folic acid is needed in the first 5 weeks to prevent neural tube defects. Calcium and phosphorus are needed in the final trimester for bone growth (Eisenberg et al., 1988; Visscher & Rinehart, 1990).

# MATERNAL DISEASE

As an OT you and your colleagues will encounter many adults who have disabling conditions. Like others, they may be parents or may wish to become parents. Depending on the nature of their conditions, the latter may be possible, especially with the myriad of medical technologies available today. If biological childbearing is not feasible, adoption and foster parenting are also options. If you can, make yourself available to those who serve adults with disabilities. You can provide training, consultation, and resources to help these individuals understand the possibilities for becoming parents as well as the services and supports available to parents with disease or disability.

Once an adult with a disability has become a parent, or a parent has become disabled, he or she may need varying degrees of assistance in order to feel competent and satisfied in the occupational role of parent. OTs can assist with the physical, cognitive, and psychosocial aspects of parenting. Here are some examples:

- For adults with physical disabilities, OTs can recommend home modifications for safe, easy access; adaptive techniques and equipment for child-care activities; energy conservation techniques; and strategies for managing assistants (family members, personal care attendants, etc.).
- For adults with psychosocial disabilities, OTs can assist with strategies for stress management, use of support systems (friend, family, and professional), and health maintenance (medication and treatment compliance).
- For adults with cognitive disabilities, OTs can assist with structuring daily schedules and routines for child care and home management, helping with realistic expectations for child development, and assisting with child care provided by others (family, day care, school, etc).

There is no reason why having a disease or disability should prevent a person from having a successful parenting experience, although there will certainly be challenges. The OT can play an important role in reducing the risks associated with adult disease and disability, thus improving the quality of the child's experience within his or her own family.

The following poem eloquently shows that the relationship between parent and child transcends disability. In fact, it shows how our memories are enhanced by the unique attributes of our parents.

## A Special Place

*Susan Russo*

A special place on my mother's lap—
She was soft and embracing.
We were both enclosed by the steel of her chair.
Even this took on her warmth, and I used to play beneath
her wheels.
I would wheel myself around the house for hours,
negotiating the turns and doorways.

Everything was done on her lap—
I placed my head there for what seemed like an eternity,
while she painstakingly set my hair in pin curls.
My cheeks pressed against her thighs, her skirt pattern
imprinted on my face.
I rested and slept.
I was there in all new situations.
It was like my secret cave.
I could look out, but no one could see me.
She would read books, sing songs, tell me stories.
Preparing dinner was done there. I handed her the food and
utensils that took up my space.
Outside I had my personal limousine:
Soft seating, great views, constant companionship, wheeled
to the front of long lines at Radio City Music Hall . . .
even for the holiday shows.
We could sit in the aisle, looking at the high kicks, our
vision unblocked by any strange heads.

Now I am too big, I seek out enclosing spaces.
I like to be quietly next to someone, feeling their
breathing.
I watch my children investigate my mother.

They hold onto her chair for balance and first steps.

She is a jungle gym as they explore ways to climb up.

Now they discover the lap.

From: AOTA Physical Disabilities Special Interest Section Newsletter, 12(2),
June 1989.

## ▰▰▰ FROM THE BOOKSHELF

Here are some reading ideas for adults and children on the topic of disabilities.

For adults:

AOTA Physical Disabilities Special Interest Section Newsletter Vol. 12 No. 2 Special Issue on Childbearing and Parenting by Persons with Disabilities. Katherine Post, Editor

*This publication includes the following articles:*
### Childbearing issues for women with physical disabilities
*by M. Freda, H. M. Cioschi, C. Nilson*

From conception through delivery and postpartum care, the authors present a comprehensive review of the special needs of women with such disabilities as spinal cord injury, multiple sclerosis, and rheumatoid arthritis. The potential role of the occupational therapist in promoting a positive pregnancy and childbirth experience for these women is clear.

### Raising children from a wheelchair
*by C. Stewart*

The author is an occupational therapist who uses a wheelchair. She shares her experiences in parenting her three young children. She discusses useful furnishings and equipment, mobility, play, and interaction.

### HELP: When the parent is handicapped
VORT Corporation
Palo Alto, CA

This companion to the popular HELP (Hawaii Early Learning Profile) pediatric assessment provides specific program and support ideas for working with parents with disabilities.

### Retraining housekeeping and child care skills
*by Cara Stewart*

In Occupational Therapy for Physical Dysfunction, fourth edition C. Trombly, Ed.
Williams & Wilkins, 1995

This chapter provides clear guidance and practical strategies for therapists who are working with homemakers and parents with disabilities from an author who has special expertise (see above).

### Parenthood with limitations
In Living with Chronic Illness: Days of Patience and Passion
*by Cheri Register*

This sensitive autobiography highlights the logistical and emotional realities of parenting with a disability.

*For children:*

The following three titles are examples of well-written and well-illustrated children's books that provide straightforward information about adults with disabilities. There are many books on disabilities that are written for children. Many bookstores and libraries have a special section; a visit to this section is highly recommended.

### My mommy's special
*by Jennifer English*
Children's Press, 1985

### The snailman
*by Brenda Silvers*
Little Brown & Co., 1978

### Grandma drives a motor bed
*by Dianne Hamm Johnson*
Whitman, 1987

---

Disease processes in the mother pose potential dangers to the fetus from the illnesses themselves as well as from the medical effects of the treatments. In these cases, careful planning with the prenatal care provider is indicated. Regarding treatment approaches, the risks and benefits for both mother and fetus must be carefully evaluated from both a medical and ethical perspective. Specific diseases are discussed here.

## DIABETES

For mothers with uncontrolled pre-existing insulin-dependent diabetes mellitus, there is a 10 percent risk, three times that of the general population, of fetal anomalies, including those of the spine, the skeleton, and the cardiovascular system. There is also a slightly greater risk of fetal death and a higher incidence of macrosomia (where the infant is quite large for gestational age and thus at risk for cephalopelvic disproportion during delivery). The incidence of juvenile diabetes in the offspring of diabetic mothers is less than 2 percent.

Also of concern are associated diabetic conditions in the mother during pregnancy, specifically retinopathy, nephropathy, and hypertension. For example, for mothers with diabetic retinopathy, pregnancy may worsen the condition. The best prevention of these negative effects is careful control of the maternal diabetes through medication and diet. This in itself reduces the risks to the offspring to near those of the general public (Batshaw & Perret, 1992; Enkin et al., 1995; Visscher & Rinehart, 1990).

## GESTATIONAL DIABETES

Some women develop pregnancy-related diabetes. This seems to be more likely in women who are 30 years of age or older, who are obese, who have a family history of diabetes, or who have a history of stillbirth. Gestational diabetes is most often diagnosed by a glucose-tolerance test administered at the end of the second trimester. If the diabetes remains uncontrolled, there is a higher risk of macrosomia, hydramnios (an excess of amniotic fluid), and a higher incidence of miscarriage and pre-eclampsia. Because of the macrosomia, these babies tend to have more problems during delivery and have a higher incidence of shoulder problems such as shoulder dystocia and brachial plexus injuries. Shoulder dystocia is an atypical situation where, during delivery, the infant's shoulder presses on the symphysis pubis. This can compress the chest and impede breathing. Excessive stretching during delivery, such as in shoulder dystocia or breech delivery, may cause bleeding, tearing, or avulsion of the nerves of the brachial plexus and result in upper-extremity paralysis. Gestational diabetes can usually be controlled with diet, and although symptoms usually disappear after pregnancy, these women may be at greater risk for nongestational diabetes (Enkin et al., 1995; *Merck Manual*, 1997; Visscher & Rinehart, 1990).

## HYPERTENSION

Hypertension, or high blood pressure, can be pre-existing or chronic or can arise during pregnancy. Symptoms include headache, edema, dizziness, visual disturbances, and sudden weight gain. Chronic hypertension needs to be controlled with diet and/or medication in order to reduce the mother's risk of heart attack and stroke, in addition to her risk for placental separations and for delivering babies who are small for gestational age.

A dangerous condition caused by increased maternal blood pressure, known as *pre-eclampsia* or *toxemia*, may first occur in the second trimester, with symptoms of protein in the urine and fluid retention. Because of the mother's risk for liver, kidney, cardiac, and central nervous system (CNS) problems, including seizures, these infants may need to be delivered early. Pre-eclampsia can, however, usually be controlled with bed rest or medication. Should it progress to the even more serious *eclampsia*, this situation is considered an emergency and the baby is generally delivered by cesarean section or induction (Batshaw & Perret, 1992; Visscher & Rinehart, 1990)

## MATERNAL HEART DISEASE

Pregnancy is characterized by increased cardiovascular work and stress, as well as blood volume increases of up to 40 percent. For women with cardiac disease, pregnancy and delivery can place both mother and infant at high risk. As an example, the infants of women with heart disease may be premature or small for their gestational age, a situation that is attributable to the mother's difficulty in maintaining cardiac function sufficient to support fetal circulatory needs.

Women with cardiac disease should seek specialized medical care for a high-risk pregnancy, if possible prior to conception, and certainly during pregnancy and delivery. Only 4 or 5 percent of mothers with congenital heart disease actually pass on the disease to their infants. However, congenital heart disease is not an insignificant concern in obstetrics or pediatrics (Visscher & Rinehart, 1990).

## MATERNAL LUNG DISEASE

Typically, respiration becomes more difficult in pregnancy because of the position of the uterus, which causes changes in the shape of the chest cavity. Individual assessment and careful management of mothers with lung disease is essential to reduce the potentially negative effects of diminished maternal respiratory function (Visscher & Rinehart, 1990).

## EPILEPSY

Children of mothers with epilepsy face two to three times greater risk for birth defects, especially for heart defects or cleft lip and palate. The specific reason for this risk is yet unclear; however, it has been suggested that an important factor may be the medications used to treat the mother's seizures. A specific fetal hydantoin (Dilantin) syndrome has been described in 10 to 33 percent of exposed infants. This syndrome includes growth deficiencies, microcephaly, mental retardation, dysmorphic features, and congenital heart disease. The obstetrical care providers must work with the family to reach a delicate balance between the dangers to both mother and fetus of repeated seizures and the risks and benefits of the necessary medications (Batshaw & Perret, 1992; Visscher & Rinehart, 1990).

## MULTIPLE SCLEROSIS (MS)

This demyelinating disorder of the CNS can involve an array of clinical features. The disease is characterized by difficulty in diagnosis and prognosis, in part because of remissions and exacerbations that yield unpredictable, changing symptoms. Disorders of voluntary movement, muscle tone, balance, sensation, bowel and bladder function, vision, and cognition are associated with MS (Blaslin, 1989). MS often begins to appear clinically, and to impede function, in women between 20 and 40 years old.

Interestingly, MS seems to have little or no effect on conception, gestation, or delivery. It does not seem to affect or be affected by delivery method or by breastfeeding. In fact, disease symptoms have been noted to decrease significantly during pregnancy. Unfortunately, MS symptoms do appear to reoccur, often with exacerbation, during the 3-month period following delivery (Cook, Troiano, Bansil, & Dowling, 1994; Weinreb, 1994). Mothers and fathers with significant functional impairments from MS will need extra support in their parent and caregiver roles.

## SYSTEMIC LUPUS ERYTHEMATOSUS (SLE)

This autoimmune disorder can affect any and all body systems. It is characterized by joint pain and dysfunction ranging from arthralgia to arthritis. There is a characteristic skin rash. Cardiac, respiratory, spleen, and kidney involvement are not uncommon. CNS involvement ranges from none to headache to epilepsy and psychosis. In women with cardiac or kidney disease, pregnancy significantly increases the risk of maternal morbidity and mortality (*Merck Manual*, 1992).

SLE is treated with corticosteroids, which do not appear to harm the fetus. In cases where the disease is in remission and there is no kidney involvements, a healthy pregnancy is possible. However, in 30 percent of women with SLE, pregnancy causes an exacerbation of symptoms. Although the disease does not impair fertility, there is a higher risk of first- and second-trimester miscarriage, intrauterine growth retardation, and prematurity (*Merck Manual*, 1992; Visscher & Rinehart, 1990)

## RHEUMATOID ARTHRITIS

This disease is characterized by episodes of joint inflammation, pain, tenderness, and swelling, as well as generalized fatigue. Pathology involves either a cycle of acute exacerbations and remissions or a continuing deterioration, including involvement of other body systems. Arthritis can be safely treated during pregnancy with certain anti-inflammatory drugs. Some women report improvement in their arthritis with pregnancy, perhaps because of gestational increases in cortisols (hydrocortisones) (*Merck Manual*, 1992; Visscher & Rinehart, 1990).

---

■ *THERAPEDS POINTER*

The occupations of families are an appropriate and essential target for therapeutic interventions.

To be helpful to children, therapists must focus their efforts not only on the occupations of children but also on the occupations of the family. Within the context of the family children develop their sense of self, their sense of safety and security, and their ability to explore and learn from their world.

Parenting is a vital human occupation. As such, it is essential that OTs direct their attention toward promoting the most optimal and healthy parenting experiences. To accomplish this, OTs focus on supporting parental roles and functions that may be at risk owing to:

1. Child disease or disability (the primary focus of this book) and/or
2. Parental disease or disability

---

# PREGNANCY-SPECIFIC FACTORS

The experience of pregnancy has been outlined in Chapter 1, and the reader must appreciate the complexities of gestation. There are some well-known gestational risks that have to do with atypical structure and function of the female reproductive system during pregnancy. The more common of these pregnancy-specific risk factors are discussed here.

## PLACENTA PREVIA

In placenta previa, the placenta lies in the uterus in such a way that it partially or completely obstructs the cervix. This condition is believed to be related to maternal age, hypertension, and multiple pregnancies (Batshaw & Perret, 1992).

Placenta previa makes vaginal delivery impossible and may result in bleeding and impairment of fetal circulation. This can create an emergency situation, and early delivery by cesarean section may be necessary (Visscher & Rinehart, 1990).

The incidence of placenta previa is estimated at 1 in 200 pregnancies, and the fetal mortality rate is an alarming 15 percent (Batshaw & Perret, 1992).

## ABRUPTIO PLACENTAE

In this situation a normally placed placenta precipitously detaches from the uterine wall prior to delivery, thus causing decreased oxygen supply to the baby. This is an emergency situation for which early delivery by cesarean section is often required (Visscher & Rinehart, 1990).

This condition is believed to be related to hypertension, a short umbilical cord, or trauma. The incidence of abruptio placentae is estimated at 1 per 100 pregnancies. The fetal mortality rate is 30 percent. The mother's health is also at significant risk. Surviving infants face the risks of preterm delivery, which include higher incidence of respiratory distress, low Apgar scores, patent ductus arteriosus, and anemia (Batshaw & Perret, 1992; Enkin et al., 1995).

## UTEROPLACENTAL INSUFFICIENCY

In this condition, there is inadequate exchange of nutrition and respiration across the placenta. This could be the result of a number of factors such as maternal illness, substance abuse, or hypertension. As a result of uteroplacental insufficiency, the infant may experience intrauterine growth retardation (IUGR), which has serious health and developmental consequences (Batshaw & Perret, 1992). Good prenatal care enables early identification of this condition. Since the causes are many, treatment options are related to each individual cause.

# DYSTOCIA

This condition refers to structural abnormalities of the reproductive organs or pelvis that may cause problems for the fetus. One example is *cephalopelvic disproportion,* a condition in which the maternal pelvis is too small or too misshapen or the infant's head too large to allow safe delivery. This places the infant at high risk for intracranial hemorrhage and sepsis. This condition is not related to the physical size of the mother and in fact cannot be predicted until labor begins.

Another example of dystocia is *incompetent cervix.* Here the cervix tends to open too early in pregnancy and, depending on when this occurs, may cause a premature delivery or miscarriage. This can be treated with surgical suturing of the cervix, known as cerclage (Batshaw & Perret, 1992; Enkin et al., 1995).

## UTERINE DYSFUNCTION

For a variety of reasons, the uterus may not function normally, especially during labor. In the case where contractions are too rapid, the infant is at risk for hypoxia from poor fetal circulation, intracranial hemorrhage from a precipitous delivery, or abruptio placentae. If labor begins too early, tocolytic agents (contraction-inhibiting drugs) such as ritodrine may be used along with bed rest or activity restriction.

If, on the other hand, contractions are too weak, labor may not progress. In this case, oxytocic (labor-enhancing) drugs, such as pitocin, may be used to increase the strength and frequency of contractions or delivery may occur by cesarean section. These drugs are generally believed to be safe for the fetus (Batshaw & Perret, 1992).

## BLOOD GROUP INCOMPATIBILITY

Each blood type, A, B, AB, and O, has what are known as antigens that mark the blood type and bring on immune responses. An important type of antigen is the Rh factor. If the mother's blood does not have the Rh antigen but the father's does, and the infant inherits the father's blood type, the blood of mother and infant will be incompatible. This is a problem because during pregnancy, the mother's and infant's blood will likely mix. In this case, the mother's blood undergoes a process known as *sensitization,* during which it develops antibodies to the fetal blood. Biochemically, the mother's blood perceives the infant's blood as the enemy. Antibody cells from the mother's blood supply will actually attack the infant's blood supply. This is called erythroblastosis fetalis Rh or hemolytic disease. Without intervention, the infant can become severely anemic and may die. In order to prevent sensitization, blood type testing is routinely conducted prior to or during pregnancy, and when necessary, Rh immunoglobulin is administered. If sensitization has occurred, the infant may need transfusions, which can even be performed in utero (Visscher & Rinehart, 1990).

## PREMATURE RUPTURE OF MEMBRANES (PROM)

One in ten women will experience the rupturing of the membrane that holds in the amniotic fluid prior to 37 weeks' gestation. Although amniotic fluid will be released, it is still being manufactured until delivery, so if the rupture is minor, there may still be an adequate fluid supply.

The cause of membrane rupture is usually not known for full-term pregnancies or for premature rupture. However, in approximately 50 percent of cases of PROM, labor begins within 24 hours; it begins within 1 week in 85 percent of all such cases. PROM presents two risks—one of infection and the other of umbilical cord compression (in the absence of shock-absorbing amniotic fluid). In most cases of PROM, the mother is hospitalized and preventive antibiotic therapy is initiated. Care providers must balance the risks of infection with the risks of prematurity. If the fetus is significantly premature, cautious management to continue the pregnancy may be the course elected (Visscher & Rinehart, 1990).

### PREMATURE LABOR AND DELIVERY

There are many reasons why a woman may begin labor in advance of her due date. If labor begins prior to 36 weeks' gestation, it is considered premature labor. The risks of prematurity for infants are significant. Medical interventions such as early identification of preterm labor, activity restriction, hospitalization for bed rest, and tocolytic drugs are used to prevent premature deliveries whenever possible (Visscher & Rinehart, 1990).

### POSTTERM LABOR AND DELIVERY

Approximately 10 percent of pregnancies extend longer than 42 weeks. These are considered postterm pregnancies. Infants of postterm pregnancies are at risk mostly because of an aging, insufficient placenta. Specific risks include meconium aspiration, macrosomia, and cardiac rhythm abnormalities. Careful monitoring of the pregnancy is helpful in identifying postterm pregnancies (Visscher & Rinehart, 1990).

## ENVIRONMENTAL AND LIFESTYLE RISK FACTORS

This category of risk includes prenatal exposure to external substances that may interfere with fetal development, often in quite specific, predictable ways. Here, environmental risk refers to a one-time exposure to an infection, a toxin, or other environmental substance during a specific pregnancy that is unlikely to be repeated in subsequent pregnancies. Lifestyle risks include repeated exposure to similar external substances that are part of an individual's lifestyle. Such lifestyle risks may include misuse of tobacco, drugs, or alcohol. In addition, inadequate nutrition presents a lifestyle risk. These risks are likely to be repeated in subsequent pregnancies unless behavioral changes are made (Eisenberg et al., 1988).

Specific environmental and lifestyle agents that place fetuses at risk are known as *teratogens*. Approximately 8 percent of birth defects are clearly linked to this cause of structural and functional abnormalities in the developing embryo and fetus; however, the actual percentage may be higher (Blackman, 1990). Teratogen is a broad term that encompasses infections, drugs and medications, and radiation. Maternal chronic illnesses may also be considered teratogens. However, these will be dealt with in a separate section of this chapter.

For teratogen exposure, the timing and amount (dosage) of exposure as well as the genetic condition of the mother and embryo or fetus are critical in determining outcome. In some cases, a substance is not harmful at certain levels or at certain times, or is harmful to animals and not to humans, or to humans and not to animals, or is harmful to one person and not another. In general, for humans, the higher the dosage of a teratogen and the closer the exposure is to the first trimester, the more serious the damage (Batshaw & Perret, 1992; Blackman, 1990; Kliegman, 1996). As stated in Chapter 1, during the first weeks of gestation vital body parts and organ systems are forming, so exposure to teratogens at this time could have significant impact on the embryo. After the structures are formed, however, the impact of the teratogen exposure would be less likely to affect the structure itself and may affect function only. In regard to certain teratogens, such as medications that may be critical to a mother's health, difficult decisions must be made about dosages and timing. Consideration must be given to risks and benefits for both mother and fetus. It is also notable that in many cases, teratogen exposure is often unknown—another reason why careful history taking is so important (Batshaw & Perret, 1992; Blackman, 1990; Kliegman, 1996).

## INFECTION

Although the placenta acts as a protective barrier for some substances, infections still pass from mother to fetus. The fetus is most vulnerable to infection and other teratogens during embryogenesis, the first 5 weeks of pregnancy. Although both viral and bacterial infections are possible, viral infections are more commonly contracted during pregnancy. Bacterial infections are more common in the newborn period (Batshaw & Perret, 1992; Blackman, 1990).

There are three methods of transmission of infection from mother to fetus or infant. The first is *transplacental,* where the infection is carried through the maternal circulatory system and crosses the placenta to the fetal blood supply. Approximately 2 percent of infants are infected in this manner. The second is referred to as *ascending* or *vertical* transmission of infection, where the infant is exposed to the infection as it passes through the mother's cervix, often after rupture of membranes, or the infant contracts the infection as he or she passes through an infected vaginal canal. The third is called *neonatal,* where infection is transmitted after birth, through contact with people or materials (Eshner & Clark, 1994; Gotoff, 1996). Figure 2–2 illustrates the possible routes of infectious transmission.

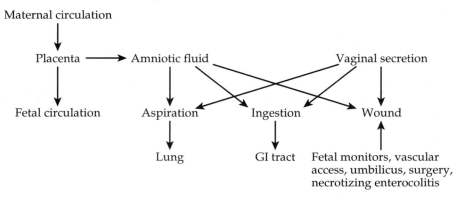

Figure 2–2 Mechanisms of perinatal infection transmission. (*Source:* Kliegman, R. M. [1996]. The fetus and the neonatal infant. In Nelson, W. E., Behrman, R. E., Kliegman, R. M., Arvin, A. M. [Eds.]. *Nelson textbook of pediatrics.* Philadelphia: W. B. Saunders, p. 514.)

There are many infectious diseases that place infants at great risk. Some of the more common ones are briefly reviewed in Table 2–2. There are many other infectious processes that place mother and infant at risk. Parvovirus, enterovirus, influenza, malaria, mononucleosis, and others are believed to place the fetus at risk for miscarriage but not for developmental or other abnormalities (Batshaw & Perret, 1992). Human immunodeficiency virus (HIV), acquired immunodeficiency syndrome (AIDS), and group B *Streptococcus* are discussed separately here.

**HIV AND AIDS.** HIV, the causative agent of AIDS, an ultimately fatal disease, is believed to be transmitted by direct contact with a person's blood or other body fluids, including sperm and breast milk. AIDS causes deficiencies in the immune system that increase an individual's susceptibility to repeated serious bacterial and viral infections. It was first identified in adults in 1981, and in children in 1982. In adults, it is most often transmitted during sexual contact or during shared use of intravenous needles. Once transmitted, HIV may lay dormant for many years, later emerging as AIDS-related complex (ARC) or as "full-blown AIDS" (Enkin et al., 1995).

For children, transmission is possible by infection of blood products used in a transfusion, but most commonly it is transmitted from an infected mother during pregnancy. For an untreated mother with HIV, there is as high as a 30 percent risk of transmission to the fetus, by the virus crossing the placenta, by the child being exposed during a vaginal delivery to the mother's blood and body fluids, or more rarely through breast milk (Grose, 1996). Recent developments in HIV treatment indicate that it is possible to reduce the risk of prenatal transmission significantly with medical treatment (Frenkel et al., 1997; Simpson et al., 1997). This has resulted in an increased impetus for HIV testing of pregnant women.

Maternal-to-fetal transmission rates in the past have varied from 25 to 70 percent, depending on the severity of the disease and when, whether during pregnancy or prior, it was contracted. Certainly prevention of disease is the

Table 2–2  Infectious Diseases during Pregnancy

| Disease | Description | Incidence | Method of Fetal Transmission | Perinatal Exposure Outcome |
|---|---|---|---|---|
| Syphilis (parabacterial spirochete) | In the adult, symptoms include genital chancres, flulike illness, low-grade fever, headache, weight loss, malaise, enlarged lymph nodes. May see kidney, liver, eye, and CNS symptoms as disease progresses.<br><br>This disease is sexually transmitted and can be treated if detected in the early stages | The maternal-fetal transmission rate is 100%.<br><br>Fetal or perinatal death occurs in 40% of infants | Transplacental or ascending (vaginal) during delivery | In utero, 25% of babies will die by the second trimester, 25% will die at birth, and 50% will survive after birth. Of the survivors, 25% may have anemia, pneumonia, skin rash, bone inflammation (osteochondritis), and other skeletal abnormalities. The remaining 75% will have no problems at birth but later will have dental or skeletal abnormalities, blindness, mental retardation, and/or seizure disorders |
| Gonorrhea (bacterium) | In adults, uncomplicated gonorrhea has urogenital symptoms only. In disseminated (complicated) gonorrhea, there is fever, arthritis, and dermatitis. Gonococcal ophthalmitis occurs frequently. If untreated, it may result in corneal rupture and blindness. | 1 million cases/yr reported.<br><br>Prevalence is estimated at <1% in perinatal populations | Vaginally, during delivery | Symptoms appear 2–5 days after birth and without treatment can result in corneal damage. |

Table 2–2 **Infectious Diseases during Pregnancy**—*Continued*

| Disease | Description | Incidence | Method of Fetal Transmission | Perinatal Exposure Outcome |
|---|---|---|---|---|
| Chlamydia (intracellular parasites) | The form of chlamydia that is sexually transmitted causes genitourinary symptoms, and may cause pelvic inflammatory disease. | 3 million new cases of chlamydia are reported annually. The incidence of cervical chlamydial infection in pregnant women is estimated at 20–30% The risk of transmission from mother to infant is 50% | Vaginally, during delivery | Of infants born to mothers with chlamydia, 30–50% will have neonatal inclusion conjunctivitis, 50% will have nasopharyngeal infection, and 20% will develop chlamydial pneumonia |
| Herpes (virus) | There are two types of the herpes simplex virus, type I, in which sores appear around the mouth, and type II, in which sores are found in the genital area. Approximately 60% of affected people will experience recurrent episodes of active lesions. Some of these recurrences are | In the general population, estimates vary widely; from 16 to 25% are believed to have the herpes virus. Risk of transmission from mother to infant varies from 3% (in recurrent infection) to 44% (in primary infection) | During vaginal delivery, however, it can be transmitted through the placenta. | When herpes is transmitted during delivery, symptoms, including skin and mucous membrane lesions, appear within 5–9 days. In the more severe cases, all organs and systems are involved. In this case, sequelae include growth delay, brain atrophy, scarring, and retinal lesions. |

This disease is sexually transmitted and can be treated in the early stages.

|  | Description | Incidence | Transmission | Effects |
|---|---|---|---|---|
|  | believed to be in response to the stress of pregnancy | In general, the incidence in newborns is estimated at 0.1 to 0.5/1000 |  | If herpes is transmitted via the placenta, it can result in prematurity; CNS, skin, eye lesions; and even death. |
| Toxoplasmosis (parasite) | A parasitic infection caused by a protozoam. Toxoplasmosis is acquired by contact with infected sources such as raw meat, cat feces (>24 h old), and/or the eggs of infected animals.<br><br>Symptoms range from mild or subclinical to enlarged lymph nodes, muscle pain, and fever, to pneumonia, hepatitis or encephalitis. | True incidence is unknown, yet it is estimated at 2/1000 live births. | Transplacental, especially during a primary infection.<br><br>The overall maternal-fetal transmission rate is 39%. | It is believed that 40% of children of affected mothers will develop symptoms. Sequelae may include spontaneous abortion, prematurity, hydrocephalus, microcephalus, other CNS disorders, fever, jaundice, and/or eye problems.<br><br>Of infants exposed during first trimester, 17% will become ill compared to 65% of infants exposed during the third trimester. However, the disease is far more severe in those cases where exposure was during the first trimester. |
| Cytomegalovirus (CMV) (virus) | Caused by a member of the herpes family, CMV, this flulike, often asymptomatic virus, is believed to be transmitted through contact with body fluids. It is estimated that 75% of the general population | In adults, the prevalence of CMV is estimated at 40-70%.<br><br>In infants, the incidence has been estimated at 2-20/1000 live births<br><br>There is a 1-2% risk of | The virus is passed through the placenta, the vagina, and in breast milk. | Infants born with CMV will carry the virus for up to 2 years, placing caregivers at some risk if they are not immune.<br><br>Only 5–10% of infected infants will be symptomatic at birth. For these children, the |

Table 2–2 Infectious Diseases during Pregnancy—*Continued*

| Disease | Description | Incidence | Method of Fetal Transmission | Perinatal Exposure Outcome |
|---|---|---|---|---|
| | have had CMV infection, yet only 10% have ever been ill. Symptoms may include fever, swollen glands, enlarged liver, and spleen. In immuno-suppressed patients, CMV can be extremely dangerous. | infection for pregnant women. If the CMV is a primary infection, there is a 40% chance of maternal-fetal transmission. If it is a recurrent infection, there is a 0.5–1.45 risk. | | mortality rate is 12% and survivors will have permanent disability. Symptoms include eye problems, low birth weight, jaundice, rash, anemia, liver and spleen enlargement, and encephalitis, which can result in motor and/or visual problems. Of the 90–95% of exposed infants with no symptoms at birth, 15–20% will experience progressive sensorineural hearing loss and learning disabilities |
| Rubella (virus) | In adults, rubella, or German measles, presents a mild, salmon colored rash and upper respiratory infection. The mother may only report a mild flulike disease during her pregnancy. | If the mother is infected within the first 28 days prior to conception, the infant has a 43% chance of being infected. During the first trimester, there is a 51–75% chance of infection; | Transplacental | In infants, congenital infection symptoms include low birth weight, intrauterine growth retardation, blindness, deafness, microcephalus, CNS disorders, heart defects, thyroid disease, and hepatosplenomegaly. Infants born with rubella will |

|  | Description | Mode of transmission | Risk of transmission | Effects |
|---|---|---|---|---|
| Varicella zoster (Chickenpox) (virus) | One of the herpesviruses, a primary infection causes chickenpox. The disease then remains dormant in the CNS. If reactivated, it will result in shingles (herpes zoster). The majority of children contract this common childhood disease. Although, if they do not, they are vulnerable into adulthood. There is presently a preventive immunization for this disease. | Transplacental until the ninth month. Exposure during the ninth month or after birth will, after the 10–14 day incubation in the infant, result in postpartum varicella, which can be a very serious disease. | during the second trimester, 23%; and during the third, almost none. There is an estimated 25% risk of maternal-fetal transmission. This risk is greatest in the first half of the pregnancy. Of infected fetuses, less than 5% will have the symptoms of congenital varicella. | carry the virus for up to 2 years, placing caregivers at some risk if they are not immune. There is a typical presentation of congenital varicella syndrome involving the brain, eyes, skin, and extremities. Specific symptoms in newborns include skin lesions; eye problems; shortened or malformed extremities; motor, sensory, and CNS deficits. |
| Hepatitis B (HBV) (virus) | Hepatitis is an infection of the liver. It is transmitted through the blood and body tissues. There are a number of strains of the virus; however, HBV is believed to be the most serious during pregnancy. Its onset is often slow and symptoms include | Transplacental, vaginal, breast milk | As many as 80% of infants born to women with chronic HBV will become infected during delivery; of these, most will become chronic carriers who are at risk for the long-term effects of this disease. | Symptoms in newborns include jaundice, decreased appetite, nausea, and fatigue. Chronic hepatitis and other liver disease are long-term effects. |

Table 2-2 **Infectious Diseases during Pregnancy**—*Continued*

| Disease | Description | Incidence | Method of Fetal Transmission | Perinatal Exposure Outcome |
|---|---|---|---|---|
| | malaise, fever, weight loss, nausea, joint pain, fatigue, and headache. If untreated at this stage, the disease will progress to liver enlargement and jaundice. | | | |

*Source:* Adapted from Behrman, R. E., Kliegman, R. M., & Arvin, A. M. (1996). *Mechanisms of perinatal infection transmission.* Philadelphia: W. B. Saunders.

primary goal. However, in those instances where the child has contracted HIV, there are some typical outcomes. If untreated, approximately 80 percent of children infected with HIV perinatally will develop full-blown pediatric AIDS within the first 2 years of life, with symptoms perhaps beginning to emerge late in the first year. Survival is generally less than 5 years. Because infants will carry maternal antibodies to HIV for some time, the presence of the virus in their blood will be difficult to detect, and diagnosis may not be reliable through blood testing only (Gordon, Schanzenbacher, Case-Smith, & Carrasco, 1996; Grose, 1996). Again, there have been tremendous advances in the treatment of pediatric HIV infection and AIDS, with both longevity and quality of life increasing daily.

Clinical symptoms of HIV infection or AIDS in children include *Pneumocystis carinii* pneumonia, recurrent bacterial infections and sepsis (invasive bacterial infection), persistent or recurrent thrush, failure to thrive, neurological abnormalities, and developmental delays. As the disease progresses, occupational performance, or function, decreases, and the child is weakened by respiratory, skin, gastrointestinal, and nervous system impairments. This disease is particularly complex, since it involves not only the health and development of affected children but also that of their mothers and perhaps other family members, if they too have HIV or AIDS (Enkin et al., 1995; Gordon et al., 1996; Grose, 1996).

The use of specific medications during gestation and immediately after delivery has significantly reduced the risk of fetal infection (Frenkel et al., 1997; Simpson et al., 1997). There appears to be no risk of transmission of the virus through normal caregiving activities, only through direct contact with blood and body fluids. Universal precautions are appropriate not only to protect care providers from the virus but also to minimize the risk of secondary infection to the person with HIV or AIDS whose immune system is likely suppressed (Gordon et al., 1996; Grose, 1996).

Each day, prevention and treatment of HIV improves. Although AIDS has been considered a fatal disease, some professionals are beginning to refer to it as a "chronic disease," because the progression of symptoms has been successfully delayed and the duration and quality of life increased by some of these treatments (Batshaw & Perret, 1992; Enkin et al., 1995). It is important that therapists remain up to date on breakthroughs in the diagnosis and treatment of this devastating disease, as well as the community and health supports available.

**Group B Streptococcus.** Group B *Streptococcus* (GBS) is the most frequent cause of sepsis in newborns. Its most severe form is characterized by the rapid onset of respiratory distress, sepsis, and shock. GBS is a common inhabitant of the human gastrointestinal and genitourinary tracts. During pregnancy, GBS is often asymptomatic, although urinary tract or other infections may be seen.

The rate of maternal-fetal transmission is estimated at 50 percent. The incidence is believed to be approximately 0.7 to 3.7 per 1000 live births, or 0.5 to 2 percent of all newborns. The risk is highest in infants with a birth weight of less than 2500 g, and in women who present with PROM and/or fever.

Sequelae vary from intrauterine death to bacteremia (systemic infection, which may or may not be present, with symptoms typical of infection), to respiratory disease, meningitis, and sepsis. Prevention includes routine screening of pregnant women at 28 weeks' gestation or a quick antigen screening at the onset of labor, especially for high-risk mothers. Treatment with intrauterine and postpartum antibiotics is believed to reduce the transmission to the infant and the severity of the disease (Enkin et al., 1995; Gotoff, 1996).

## DRUGS AND MEDICATIONS

Many medications have been well tested and determined to be safe during pregnancy. Women should work with their prenatal care provider to determine which of these may be useful to them, if for some reason medication is necessary just prior to or during pregnancy.

Drugs and medications, natural or manufactured, are powerful chemicals. It is therefore advisable to consider all such substances as teratogenous and to use them only with the guidance and supervision of skilled and knowledgeable prenatal care providers. Table 2–3 provides a brief outline of the effects on the fetus from these types of teratogens. Most of the effects of medications on infants have been determined since the thalidomide tragedy in the 1960s, and much is still unknown.

Transmission of drugs has been assumed to be from mother to infant through the placenta; however, direct effects on the genetic makeup of the egg should also be considered. Evidence suggests that paternal exposure to a given drug may result in the drug being transported directly into the egg via an exposed sperm (Visscher & Rinehart, 1990).

For legal drugs, rigorous testing, including determination of safety for pregnant women, is required for Food and Drug Administration (FDA) approval. However, it is important to recognize that the long-term effects of these substances may not be able to be known for some time.

There are many new drugs, licit and illicit, available each day. It is estimated that each year as many as 100,000 newborns are exposed prenatally to cocaine or other street drugs (Batshaw & Perret, 1992), yet the actual outcomes of prenatal exposure to these substances is still unclear (Lane, in press; Visscher & Rinehart, 1990).

## RADIATION

Research on the devastating effects of the Hiroshima and Nagasaki atomic bombs, as well as nuclear power plant accidents like the Chernobyl incident, have indicated that radiation is indeed harmful to fetuses, infants, and children. In these studies, aftereffects included miscarriage, microcephaly, and childhood cancers (Batshaw & Perret, 1992; Blackman, 1990; Short-DeGraff, 1988).

In fetuses and embryos of women exposed to large amounts of medical radiation, multiple malformations, mental retardation, and growth problems were also noted. Chromosomal abnormalities, structural defects in the embryo and fetus, and CNS insult also characterize the outcomes of radiation exposure. For this teratogen, dosage and timing are exceptionally important. During the first trimester, fetuses are most vulnerable, particularly to the lethal effects of radiation exposure. As pregnancy progresses, the outcomes

Table 2–3  **Effects of Teratogens on the Fetus**

| Substance | Effect on Fetus |
|---|---|
| Accutane (isotretinoin) | Facial and ear anomalies, heart disease |
| Alcohol | Developmental abnormalities in childhood |
| Amphetamines | Congenital heart disease, IUGR |
| Anesthetic agents (volatile) | CNS depression |
| Anticoagulants, e.g., warfarin (Coumadin, Panwarfin) and dicumarol | Abnormalities in bones, cartilage, and eyes; CNS defects |
| Aspirin | Neonatal bleeding, prolonged gestation |
| Bromides | Rash, CNS depression |
| Chemotherapeutic drugs, e.g., methotrexate (Mexate) and aminopterin | Increased rate of miscarriage, various abnormalities |
| Cocaine | Abnormal brain development, microcephaly, low birth weight, IUGR, behavioral disturbances |
| Dilantin | Fetal hydantoin syndrome (growth and mental deficiency, abnormalities of the face, anomalies of the hands) |
| Lead | Reduced intellectual function, increased rate of miscarriages and stillbirths |
| Lithium | Ebstein anomaly, congenital heart disease |
| Lysergic acid diethylamide (LSD) | Spontaneous abortions, chromosomal changes, suspected anomalies |
| Methyl mercury | Minamata disease, microcephaly, deaf, blind, mental retardation |
| Morphine and its derivatives (addiction) | Withdrawal symptoms (poor feeding, vomiting, diarrhea, restlessness, yawning and stretching, dyspnea and cyanosis, fever and sweating, pallor, tremors, convulsions) |
| Oxytocin | Hyperbilirubinemia, hyponatremia |
| Phenobarbital | Bleeding diathesis (vitamin K deficiency) |
| Polychlorinated biphenyls | Poor neurological development |
| Radiation therapy | Congenital anomalies, growth retardation, chromosomal damages, mental deficiency, stillbirth |
| Radioactive iodine | Destruction of fetal thyroid |
| Reserpine | Drowsiness, nasal congestion, poor temperature stability |
| Stilbestrol (diethylstilbestrol [DES]) | Vaginal adenocarcinoma in adolescence, reproductive abnormalities |
| Thalidomide | Phocomelia, hearing loss, cardiac anomalies |
| Toluene (solvent abuse) | Preterm labor, fetal alcohol-like syndrome, dysmorphology |
| Valproate | Spina bifida |

*Source:* Adapted from Behrman, R. E., Kliegman, R. M., and Arvin, A. M. (1996). *Mechanisms of perinatal infection transmission.* Philadelphia: W. B. Saunders.

are less likely death of the fetus and more likely to be the abnormalities noted (Batshaw & Perret, 1992; Blackman, 1990; Short-DeGraff, 1988).

## CHEMICAL TOXINS

Prenatal exposure to heavy metals (e.g., lead, mercury) has been associated with cerebral palsy as well as fatal neurological syndromes. In utero exposure to polychlorinated biphenyls (PCBs) in food sources has been associated with infants who are small for gestational age and who have disorders of the skin, teeth, and hair. A 125 percent increase in the rate of congenital malformation was reported for children exposed prenatally to the toxic waste dumped into the Love Canal in the early 1980s. Skin disorders have been associated with dioxin exposure. Cigarette smoke is associated with low-birth-weight infants and has been tenatively linked to sudden infant death syndrome (SIDS). Prenatal exposure to diethylstilbestrol (DES), which resulted in an increased rate of vaginal adenocarcinoma in daughters, suggests that some chemicals may be cross-placental carcinogens. Chemotherapy treatment for maternal cancers can also have significant negative effects of the fetus (Miller, 1996).

Exposure to chemicals should be kept to a minimum for all pregnant women. Although exposure is not always intentional or direct, second-hand cigarette smoke can be avoided, as can exposure to work clothing permeated with chemicals or asbestos fibers. Air and water pollutants are also potentially harmful to the fetus (Miller, 1996).

## WRAPPING IT UP

As you review this material, remember that for many people, much of the first trimester of pregnancy passes without signs, symptoms, or even awareness of the pregnancy. For low-risk mothers, there may only be one prenatal visit during this critical period. For those who are able to plan ahead and prepare for pregnancy, preconceptive care is now available, including counseling on diet, lifestyle, and other health behaviors that can significantly reduce risks to fetuses, especially during the first trimester. For many people, though, there is guilt and anger at what they might have done differently to prevent problems with their infants. Bear in mind as you work with families that risk factors are just that, risks. They are not direct causal connections. Families will need support as they explore the possible causes of their children's developmental problems. They may be examining and re-examining their own behaviors as well as the behaviors of their caregivers. At the very least, knowledge of prenatal risk factors can help families of children with special needs plan for subsequent pregnancies.

The potential risks to a fetus are extensive and certainly seem overwhelming. Babies are so fragile, so vulnerable, and so innocent. Adults have so much responsibility—and so little control. According to the authors of the popular pregnancy guide *What to Expect When You're Expecting*, worry is one of the most common complaints of pregnancy, even more common than morning sickness. They cite research that found that

94 percent of women worry that their children will not be normal and 93 percent worry that their children will not survive through delivery. The authors assure their readers that although a little worry is normal, pregnancy should be a pleasant time, and too much worry is unhealthy. They point out that "despite all that we hear, read and worry about, never before in the history of reproduction has it been safer to have a baby" (Eisenberg et al., 1988, p. 16).

Furthermore, even if the infant does experience problems, never before in the history of childhood has there been as much knowledge, technology, and caring within families, communities, and service systems to help children to achieve their personal best. For many of us, parenthood is a chance we simply have to take.

## CASE STORY

Mary Margaret was 24 years old when she married 26-year-old Jonathan. Within a year, they were delighted to be expecting their first child. Because of their young ages, good health, and reportedly uneventful family history, Mary Margaret received routine prenatal care, took great care of her health and diet, and eagerly anticipated the first grandchild for both sides of the family. Katherine was born at full term, with Apgar scores of 8 at 1 minute and 9 at 5 minutes. Labor and delivery proceeded uneventfully. Katherine was indeed a lovely infant and she provided great joy to her family.

When Katherine was approximately 6 months of age, Mary Margaret had a nagging feeling that something wasn't right. Her pediatrician and her family assured her that all new parents worry but that Katherine was doing fine—there was nothing to be concerned about.

At her 9-month checkup, Mary Margaret and Jonathan told the pediatrician that it seemed as though Katherine was getting weak. She was able to sit but she did not seem to be able to move in and out of sitting and she was not interested in moving around by herself. Even when they held up toys or books she had enjoyed, she no longer seemed interested unless they were held within her reach.

This report concerned the doctor. She did a very thorough physical examination and referred the family to a neurologist who confirmed her suspicions that Katherine had Tay-Sachs disease. This came as a tremendous shock to all, because although Jonathan was of Eastern European Jewish origin, Mary Margaret's family were Catholics from Italy. The genetic counselor explained that although Tay-Sachs disease was most prevalent among people of Ashkenazic origin, others from nearby European areas occasionally expressed the disease as well.

Katherine was immediately referred to an early childhood intervention program for family support and developmental assistance. The occupational therapist (OT) on that team, working closely with the nurse and social worker, was able to help the family anticipate Katherine's developmental regression, vision loss, and ultimate death. The OT used carefully selected sensorimotor toys and developmental activities, therapeutic handling and positioning techniques, adaptive techniques, and therapeutic equipment to help the family make Katherine's life as full as possible. For example, the OT initially provided toys with simple cause-and-effect features that were easy for Katherine to activate, such as busy boxes and simple switch toys. As Katherine's health declined, the OT and family collaborated to select toys with easier activation and more pronounced auditory and tactile feedback. At first, the OT and family worked on understanding infant feeding, including the impact of different food textures on oral motor functioning. As Katherine's abilities declined, the OT helped with adaptive positioning and feeding techniques to support Katherine's nutrition and keep the mealtime experience an enjoyable one for all.

The OT needed to work closely with her team members not only to understand the realities of Katherine's disease but also to receive support for herself as she experienced sadness and grief for Katherine and her family. As a result, the family felt competent as parents in a highly complex situation. They reported that they would not have been able to cope without the early intervention team. Not only had the team helped them care for Katherine, but they felt so satisfied with their parenting experience that they went on to have two more children.

1. If you were working with the family described in the case story about Katherine, what prenatal services would you expect them to receive prior to having their second and third child?

## Real-Life Lab

1. List some activities you might use to help the following hypothetical parents.

a.   A mother who is wheelchair-bound because of spastic diplegic cerebral palsy needs help with managing her newborn's daily care routine. Describe some strategies you might suggest for feeding, bathing, diapering, and dressing the baby.

b.   A father of newborn twins had had a traumatic head injury a few years before these infants were born. He is able to walk, talk, and care for himself, but he was not able to keep his previous job as an electrician. He does work full time days in a supervised employment setting where he does repetitive factory work. His wife is also employed part time nights as a pediatric nurse. They both enjoy their jobs and are excited but a bit anxious about managing work and child care—especially with twins. They especially need your assistance with helping the father to participate in the rearing of their children. What suggestions might you make for feeding, dressing, and playing with these babies?

**2.** Using an existing developmental history form or a form that you develop, interview a friend or relative who has a young child. What prenatal risk factors were present for this family?

**3.** Be very honest with yourself now. How do you feel about working with families who:

    **a.** Have children with terminal diseases?

    **b.** Have abused drugs during their pregnancy?

    **c.** Have HIV, AIDS, or other sexually transmitted disease?

**4.** What other risk factors or perinatal situations make you uncomfortable?

**5.** In situations like those in question 3, or in other situations where you have felt similar discomfort, what have you done to change your feelings?

**6.** What could you do in the specific situations described in question 3?

**7.** Working with friends, fellow students, or colleagues, role play some initial interviews (history taking) as well as some intervention sessions with hypothetical families who have any of the above risk factors. You will need people to play the parents, the OT, and as many other team members as you have players for. It is also helpful to have one or two people play the role of observer and recorder, or you could videotape your role playing so that you can get feedback on your verbal and nonverbal actions.

# References

Batshaw, M. L., & Meyer, G. (1996). The syndromes. In Kurtz, L. A., Dowrick, P. W., Levy, S. E., & Batshaw, M. L. (Eds.). *Handbook of developmental disabilities* (pp. 12–24). Gaithersburg, MD: Aspen.

Batshaw, M. L., & Perret, Y. M. (1992). *Children with disabilities: A medical primer.* Baltimore: Paul Brookes.

Bhasin, C. A. (1989). Occupational therapy in the management of multiple sclerosis. *American Occupational Therapy Association Physical Disabilities Special Interest Section Newsletter, 12*(4), 1–3.

Blackman, J. A. (1990). *Medical aspects of developmental disabilities in children birth to three* (2d ed.). Gaithersburg, MD: Aspen.

Brown, W., & Brown, C. (1993). Defining eligibility for early intervention. In Brown, W., Thurman, S. K., & Pearl, L. F. (Eds.). *Family-centered early intervention with infants and toddlers: Innovative cross disciplinary approaches.* Baltimore: Paul Brookes.

Cook, S. D., Troiano, R., Bansil, S., & Dowling, P. C. (1994). Multiple sclerosis and pregnancy. *Advances in Neurology, 64,* 83–95.

Eisenberg, A., Murkoff, H. E., & Hathaway, S. E. (1988). *What to expect when you're expecting.* New York: Workman.

Enkin, M., Keirse, M., Renfrew, M., & Neilson, J. (1995). *A guide to effective care in pregnancy and childbirth* (2d ed). New York: Oxford University Press.

Ensher, G. L., & Clark, D. A. (1994). *Newborns at risk: Medical care and psychoeducational intervention.* (2d ed.). Gaithersburg, MD: Aspen

Gordon, C. Y., Schanzenbacher, K. E., Case-Smith, J., & Carrasco, R. C. (1996). Diagnostic problems in pediatrics. In Case-Smith, J., Allen, A. S., & Pratt, P. N. (Eds.). *Occupational therapy for children* (pp. 113–164). St. Louis: Mosby.

Gotoff, S. P. (1996a). Unique aspects of infection. In Nelson, W. E., Behrman,

R. E., Kliegman, R. M., & Arvin, A. M. (Eds.). *Nelson textbook of pediatrics* (pp. 514–520). Philadelphia: W. B. Saunders.

Gotoff, S. P. (1996b). Neonatal sepsis and meningitis. In Nelson, W. E., Behrman, R. E., Kliegman, R. M., & Arvin, A. M. (Eds.). *Nelson textbook of pediatrics* (pp. 528–535). Philadelphia: W. B. Saunders.

Grose, C. (1996). Viral infections of the fetus and newborn. In Nelson, W. E., Behrman, R. E., Kliegman, R. M., & Arvin, A. M. (Eds.). *Nelson textbook of pediatrics* (pp. 523–527). Philadelphia: W. B. Saunders.

Kliegman, R. (1996). The fetus and the neonatal infant. In Nelson, W. E., Behrman, R. E., Kliegman, R. M., & Arvin, A. M. (Eds.). *Nelson textbook of pediatrics* (pp. 431–472). Philadelphia: W. B. Saunders.

Krajicek, M., & Tompkins, R. (Eds). (1993). *The medically fragile infant.* Austin, TX: Pro-ed.

Lane, S. J. (1996). Cocaine: An overview of use, actions, and effects. In Chandler, L. S., & Lane, S. J. (Eds.). *Children with prenatal drug exposure.* New York: Haworth.

Mattingly, C., & Fleming, M. (Eds.) (1994). *Clinical reasoning: Forms of inquiry in a therapeutic practice.* Philadelphia: F. A. Davis.

Melvin, A. J., & Frenkel, L. M. (1997). Pediatric HIV-1 infection. *Obstetrics and Gynecology Clinics of North America, 24,* 911–924.

*The Merck manual of diagnosis and therapy.* (17th ed). (1997). Rahway, NJ: Merck & Co.

Miller, R. W., (1996). Chemical pollutants. In Nelson, W. E., Behrman, R. E., Kliegman, R. M., & Arvin, A. M. (Eds.). *Nelson textbook of pediatrics*

(pp. 2004–2006). Philadelphia: W. B. Saunders.

Miller, R. W., & Merke, D. P. (1996). Radiation injury. In Nelson, W. E., Behrman, R. E., Kliegman, R. M., & Arvin, A. M. (Eds.). *Nelson textbook of pediatrics* (pp. 2002–2004). Philadelphia: W. B. Saunders.

Part XII: Infections of the neonatal infant. (1996). In Nelson, W. E., Behrman, R. E., Kliegman, R. M., & Arvin, A. M. (Eds.). *Nelson textbook of pediatrics* (pp. 514–540). Philadelphia: W. B. Saunders.

Prysak, M., Lorenz, R. P., & Kisly, A. (1995). Pregnancy outcomes in nulliparous women 35 years and older. *Obstetrics and Gynecology, 85,* 65–70.

*Random House dictionary of the English language.* (1987). New York: Random House.

Short-DeGraff, M. A. (1988). *Human development in occupational therapy and physical therapy.* Baltimore: Williams & Wilkins.

Thomas, C. L. (1997). *Taber's cyclopedic medical dictionary.* Philadelphia: F. A. Davis.

Vergera, E. (1993). *Foundations for practice in the neonatal intensive care unit and early intervention.* Rockville, MD: American Occupational Therapy Association.

Visscher, H. C., & Rinehart, R. D. (Eds.). (1990). *The American College of Obstetrics and Gynecology: Planning for pregnancy, birth and beyond.* New York: Penguin Books.

Weinreb, H. J. (1994). Demyelinating and neoplastic diseases in pregnancy. *Neurologic Clinics, 12*(3), 509–526.

Williamson, W. D., & Demmler, G. S. (1992). Congenital infections: Clinical outcome and educational implications. *Infants and Young Children, 4,* 1–10.

# 3

# *The Special Vulnerabilities of Children and Families*

Ellen Berger Rainville, MS, OTR, FAOTA

"I believe the children are our future,
teach them well and let them lead the way,
show them all the beauty they possess inside,
give them a sense of pride,
to make it easier,
let the children's laughter,
remind us of how we used to be . . ."

—George Benson

## KEY POINTS

- Children and their caregivers are engaged in essential co-occupations. To enhance the functioning of children, it is important that pediatric therapists appreciate concepts of child development and family functioning as well as the factors that may help them to withstand stress and adversity.

- Children are occupational beings. The occupations of children are different from those of adults. Families have distinct occupations, as do teachers and other caregivers. Therapy can therefore be focused at many aspects of occupational performance, such as those of the children, their caregivers, and/or their environments.

- Some families and children seem to be better able to function than others. This is evident in each family's ability to overcome obstacles, to set and achieve reasonable goals, and to use its own strengths and resources. There are certain factors that may account, at least in part, for these differences.

- There are some situations that place children and families at great risk. These include economic stress, social isolation, abuse and neglect, domestic violence, parental illness, and parental substance abuse. Although these situations may not be the primary reason for a child's referral to occupational therapy, they may be causative factors (e.g., a child's head injury may be the result of a beating) or may be influential (a parent's inability to carry through on therapy activities may be a result of illness or disability). It is important for pediatric therapists to be familiar with these family issues, because they will likely be operating in the lives of many of the children we serve.

# BEGINNINGS

This chapter is intended to frame this book's perspective on children and on the appropriate domain of pediatric occupational therapy practice. As a foundation for the material in the chapters that follow, the reader is provided with a review of the history of our understanding of childhood, a discussion of the occupations of children and families, and a review of child development. This information, coupled with knowledge of specific diagnoses, will enable you to understand the unique impact of disabling conditions on individual children and families. The concepts of risk, resilience, and vulnerability are also introduced, because it may be these factors, more than diagnosis, prognosis, or other determinants, that account for individual success in managing the stressors of disability. Finally, some significant family stressors are presented to help the reader to understand those experiences or situations that may make it difficult for families to function effectively. Therapists' expectations may be more realistic and their interventions more helpful if a broad view of family functioning is provided.

# THE HISTORY AND CULTURE OF CHILDHOOD

Childhood has only recently been recognized and appreciated as a distinct and valued phase of the life cycle. In earliest recorded history, it seems that there was no real conception of childhood. First-born male children were sacrificed to the gods, unhealthy children were destroyed at birth, parents had no responsibility for their offspring, and infanticide or abandonment was socially acceptable. As time went on, there was a shift toward greater parental responsibility for children. However, abandonment (to orphanages, convents, etc.) continued to be common (Zeanah, 1993).

By the Middle Ages, things had not improved much. Health care was such that deaths of mothers or children were not uncommon, with each newborn having less than a 50 percent chance of surviving to age 5. Abandonment of infants was also common. In fact, if a child survived, he or she was likely to be working and married early in adolescence. Although there were probably exceptions, the prevailing attitude toward children was negative and unemotional (Black, Puckett, & Belle, 1992; LeFrancois, 1993; Zeanah, 1993).

It was during the Renaissance that the concept of childhood began to emerge. The relationship between parents and children began to involve love and caring, and there was an interest in the unique qualities of young people. Ambivalence about children did still prevail, because some perceived children as inherently evil, needing to have the "devil" purged out of them (Black, Puckett, & Belle, 1992; LeFrancois, 1993; Zeanah, 1993).

During the late 1600s, philosopher John Locke encouraged a more compassionate attitude toward children. He recommended removing the tight swaddling cloths that had been thought to prevent children from tearing off their ears and to keep them from walking like animals. He suggested that the infant is a *tabula rasa* (a blank slate), who is highly responsive to information, kindness, and punishment (Black, Puckett, & Belle, 1992; LaFrancois, 1993; Zeanah, 1993).

During the 18th century, following Locke's initiative, there was a growing recognition of the importance of childhood, especially the early years. Nonetheless, the punishment of children was taken to what we would now consider to be abusive extremes. Children were still believed to be evil and were severely punished for delays in toilet training, masturbation, or other transgressions.

It was at this time that philosopher Jean-Jacques Rousseau advocated the view that children are not inherently good or evil; rather that they respond to their environment. He suggested that play, experiential learning, freedom to explore, supportive adults, and compassionate treatment are essential to promoting goodness in children (Black, Puckett, & Belle, 1992; LeFrancois, 1993; Zeanah, 1993).

The 19th century brought some more improvements for children, who were not only loved and cared for more often than they were abandoned, but who were recognized for their economic value. Children often were put to work at young ages, often in mines or on farms where they sustained the injuries and illnesses associated with hard labor in unsafe conditions (Black, Puckett, & Belle, 1992; LeFrancois, 1993; Zeanah, 1993).

The Industrial Revolution caused families to shift from rural, agricultural environments to urban, industrial ones. This created a new set of issues. Because parents no longer worked at home (on the farm), there needed to be schools, nurseries, and so on to provide care and guidance for children. In fact, it was at this time that abuse of children began to be perceived as inappropriate. The first laws protecting children from abuse were passed early in the 20th century.

Over the past 50 years, we have seen a dramatic shift to at least having espoused beliefs that children are valued members of our society with needs that are distinctly different from those of adults. Parents are recognized as having essential responsibilities to nurture, protect, and facilitate the development of their children. It has also been recognized that parenting requires a great deal of knowledge, time, energy, and emotional maturity.

Despite advances in our understanding, we still have too many children who are hurt, abandoned, or even killed by their caregivers. We also still have too many public policies that do not respect the unique needs of children and families. OTs and other child-development professionals can and do contribute daily to improving the status of children in our country. They do this through service, education, and community action. These activities help to increase people's understanding of the distinctive capabilities and needs of children and families.

---

■*THERAPEDS POINTER: THE ROLE OF THE PROFESSIONAL IN HELPING PARENTS*

A major role of the child-development professional, including the OT, is helping parents and other caregivers to understand child development. If caregivers understand what is developmentally appropriate behavior, they can respond to it in ways that are helpful to children.

For example, a 2-year-old child's temper tantrum will only be made worse by punishment. Instead, if the caregiver (parent, daycare teacher, clinician) understands that a temper tantrum is an expression of frustration, perhaps because the child does not yet have sufficient language to express her feelings, then the adult can provide an environment that is safe and quiet for the child to calm down and regain control. The adult can use words to express an understanding of the child's frustration—"Yes, Judy, I know that you want to have that toy. Tamarra is playing with it now. When she is all done, perhaps we can ask her if you may have a turn with it."

For all children, but especially for children with disabilities, the expectations of child development must be adapted to each child. The role of OTs and other child-development professionals in interpreting child development and behavior is an essential one. In doing so, not only are we fostering healthy parent-child interaction and promoting good child development, but we are also preventing some types of child abuse and neglect.

Children with disabilities may not walk or speak or be able to care for themselves until much later than their peers, if they are able to do these things at all. When adults, or even peers, inaccurately perceive behaviors that result from the disability as intentional "bad" behavior, these children may suffer such inappropriate consequences as punishment, humiliation, and isolation.

For example, imagine a 6-year-old child with mild sensory impairment and learning disabilities who "acts out" in the classroom. A teacher who does not understand the impact of this child's disability on behavior might reprimand the child, assign him to a timeout, or report the behavior to the parents and principal. This teacher's approach may cause the child to feel that he is bad and may even increase the acting out. On the other hand, the OT can avert these consequences by helping the teacher to understand that because of the child's disabilities, he cannot make sense of the teacher's spoken or written instructions. They can work together to modify the environment to meet the child's needs. Perhaps a seat closer to the black-board and written instructions from the teacher would be enough for the child to understand the teacher's expectations. These interventions would foster the teacher's sense of occupational fulfillment as well as help the child partake in the learning environment.

By reframing the caregiver's view of the child to be more accurate, more empathic, and more individualized, it empowers both caregiver and child in their respective occupations and results in a win-win situation.

## OCCUPATION IN CHILDHOOD

Occupation is meaningful, purposeful activity and is the focus of the therapeutic process for our profession. Our knowledge of human occupation informs our understanding of the impact of illness or disability on a particular person and those people involved in the person's life. Occupations are also the means by which we facilitate adaptation to disease or disability and through which we hope to restore health and wellness. Children are distinctly different from adults, and so is their occupation.

There is evidence that occupation is a developmental phenomenon (Keilhofner, 1995) because different occupations are engaged in by persons at different ages and stages of life. For example, play is a major occupation for young children, yet older children, adolescents, and adults also are expected to work.

In childhood, children's volitions involve choices of activity, and children learn about their capacity to affect their environment (personal causation). As interpersonal, motor, and language abilities develop, children's experiences may lead them to feel competent or inadequate. Feedback from adults and peers, competition, and challenge provide the environmental stimuli necessary for this developing sense of self. Cultural messages are quite powerful in childhood. Parental or community values are transmitted to children directly or indirectly and will influence the child's occupational choices. For example, in families that value contribution, a child may choose to have a paper route or sell Girl Scout cookies to practice and be reinforced for work behaviors.

Children find tremendous pleasure and gratification in the mastery of new learning and activity. They are drawn to activities that provide rich sensory experience, that provide continuity or repetition during mastery, and that involve exploration and/or social interaction (Keilhofner, 1995). Adolescents focus on preparation for independence in adult life. The interests of children and adolescents reflect those activities that provide a sense of challenge that is evenly matched to their level of developing capability (Csikszentmihalyi, 1990), or, those activities that provide a "just right challenge" (Ayres, 1979).

Habituation involves roles and routines. The roles of player and family member are key in childhood. As children move beyond infancy and toddlerhood, the roles of student and friend become important. The role of player involves not only exploration and mastery of activity, but also experimentation in social roles. The pretend play so characteristic of preschoolers, the dramatic play of school-aged children, and the rule-governed play of games and sport are examples of the developmental and social roles for children. As family members, children integrate the values and routines of their family's culture as they play out the roles of child, sibling, and so on. As children develop, they acquire habits and routines that help them adapt to biological and environmental demands. The routines and skills of self-care, sleeping and waking, eating, and leisure are formed in childhood, within the family context. The foundations of other roles and routines are laid down in childhood as well, through school and other frequented activities (Kielhofner, 1995). In adolescents, school, work, and social and volunteer activities provide opportunities for mastery of independent skills and expression of individuality. The peer group can take on an importance equal to that of the family. Table 3–1 provides an overview of occupation at various stages of development.

Obviously, play and self-care and learning activities are appropriate occupations for the therapist to address and employ. Of interest is also the idea of using narrative in therapy (see Chapter 2) with children as well as with adults. Storytelling is a central aspect of childhood in most cultures. Children listen and observe as adults read and tell stories about real and imagined worlds. As children grow, they integrate aspects of the stories into their lives and they learn to tell their own stories, real or imagined. This natural development of narrative lends itself to our understanding of occupations and can be an effective therapeutic activity (Kielhofner, 1995; Mattingly & Fleming, 1994).

The integration of imaginative play into therapy is a central component of pediatric therapy. A glance inside any sensory integration clinic will reveal children riding imaginary whales, jumping across imaginary chasms, and conquering the wildest of imaginary "bucking broncos."

For a variety of reasons, occupation in childhood can be problematic. Disease or disability can directly impact the child's inherent ability to engage in activity. Dysfunctional or impoverished environments, including troubled families, can make the healthy expression of human occupation difficult at best. Pediatric OTs concern themselves with the child, the child's environment, and the transactions between child and environment, to promote healthy occupational functioning.

A focus on the occupations of children provides meaning and purpose in the therapy experience. Burke (1993) says that

> an occupational therapist, using the occupation-based perspective . . . observes, assesses, interprets, and intervenes in the child's role performance as a player as well as the other roles of the child (e.g., family member, brother, or sister). Thus, intervention includes analysis of the environments that the child interacts in and the human nonhuman objects the child relates to in everyday functioning. (p. 203)

## THE CONTEXTS OF CARE: OCCUPATIONS OF FAMILIES AND CAREGIVERS

We are all occupational beings who function in specific environments. As pediatric therapists we need to be knowledgeable about the various contexts in which children function so as to best promote their occupational perfor-

Table 3–1 **Occupational Performance in Childhood and Adolescence**

| | Infancy and Toddlerhood (Birth to 2 yr) | Early Childhood (3 to 5 yr) | Childhood (6 to 12 yr) | Adolescence (13 to 19 yr) |
|---|---|---|---|---|
| Occupational Roles | Son, daughter, brother, sister grandchild, niece, nephew | Same as prior stage, also peer, friend | Same as prior stage, also best friend, student | Same as prior stage, also employed worker, volunteer |
| Adaptive Behaviors | Responding to nurturing, taking nourishment Learning to move, communicate, and control body functions Developing emotional attachment to caregiver(s) | Refining and mastering abilities learned in the first 2 years of life | Refining perception and organization Learning social skills Acquiring skills for daily living Developing attitudes toward self and others Mastery of reading and writing Learning calculation and conceptual thinking | Building relationships Defining occupational and social roles Learning socially responsible behavior Achieving emotional independence Preparing for financial independence Acquiring personal values and ethics Making career and work choices |
| Self-Care and Self-Maintenance | Receiving nurturance Self-sufficiency and competence, especially in feeding | Developing self-sufficiency in eating, dressing, washing, toileting | Continuing mastery of ADL skills Developing individual preferences expressed in clothing, food, etc. Value of money begins to be appreciated, with jobs like baby-sitting, newspaper route | Mastery or independence in ADLs and IADLs continues as does individual expression Having some of one's own money from job or allowance is important |

*Continued on following page*

**Table 3–1  Occupational Performance in Childhood and Adolescence—*Continued***

| | Infancy and Toddlerhood (Birth to 2 yr) | Early Childhood (3 to 5 yr) | Childhood (6 to 12 yr) | Adolescence (13 to 19 yr) |
|---|---|---|---|---|
| Play and Leisure | Skill development through engagement with objects and caregivers | Continual exploration and investigation of the environment Repetitive activity and imitative play Parallel to cooperative play | Focused on group and team activities Rules are important Peer influence gains importance | Enjoyment, attention, and recognition are the focus of activities Team and group activities are common Various interests, i.e., arts, music, academics, sports, etc. Solitary time is important |
| Work and Education | Play groups, day care possible | Preschool, kindergarten | Mastery of academics, including decision making and problem solving Socialization and extracurricular activities are an important focus of school | School, some paid and/or volunteer work, extracurricular activities |
| Rest and Relaxation | 11–16 hours of sleep per day | Sleeping through the night; restlessness is associated with stress | Influenced by the environment Home and school routines foster balance in occupational performance areas | More controlled by the adolescent than the environment Balance is important |

*Source:* Adapted from Llorens, L. A. (1991). Performance tasks and roles throughout the life span. In C. Christiansen and C. Baum (Eds.). *Occupational therapy: Overcoming human performance deficits.* Thorofare, NJ: Slack.

mance. As therapists, our interventions can be oriented toward promoting change in the child, promoting change in the environment, or some combination of the two. We need to be knowledgeable about each. This section will address the animate environment for children, families, and others.

The most obvious context for children's function is of course within families. In their landmark work on occupational science, Zemke and Clark (1996) discuss the relevance of the family perspective:

> Occupational scientists must learn to listen more carefully to the story of mothering and respect more highly the validity of the individual experience. As occupational therapists, we can learn, in the same way, to listen with respect to the experience of the parents of children in our care. Although we may have a resource of treatment knowledge, parents have a depth of knowledge of their lives as it is entwined with that of their child. They must make realistic decisions about the . . . programs developed and given to them by occupational therapists and the techniques recommended that they apply. As Bernheimer, Gallimore, and Weisner suggest, strategies must be meaningful and sustainable when they fit the family activity pattern. They can only do that when they become part of the family's valued routine occupations. (p. 215)

The family is clearly the most important context for child development and function and hence for pediatric therapy. It is recommended that pediatric therapists become familiar with current literature and clinical practice relating to family development and functioning. This knowledge is essential to a relevant pediatric practice.

It is also important to recognize that children function in a myriad of social and cultural contexts, to some extent independent of their families. As therapists we need to be cognizant and involved with these contexts because they are also important settings for pediatric therapy. These include child care, school, churches, teams, and social clubs. We also need to recognize that many characteristics of family interaction also apply to children interacting with nonfamily caregivers. For example, a classroom teacher's values, beliefs, and behaviors powerfully influence a child's performance, self-esteem, and self-confidence. Therefore, the teacher, like the parent, is an appropriate target for our interventions with the child.

Zemke and Clark (1996) describe occupation as an "activity of one individual and its meaning to him or her" (p. 213). They go on to describe co-occupation as an occupation that could be carried out by one person, but instead is carried out by those involved in social interactions in which occupations are shared. Barn-raising is given as an example of shared occupations that are community-building. Community awareness campaigns, neighborhood watches, and cooperative food drives are more modern examples of such co-occupations. Parents and children are described by Zemke and Clark as engaging in the co-occupations of caregiving. In other words, the child is not a passive recipient of the parents' caregiving; he or she in fact participates, perhaps by engaging parents in interaction and/or responding to their efforts. This author interprets the work of Zemke and Clark as suggesting that the co-occupations of children and parents are in fact what builds a family. The co-occupations of children and teachers, therefore, are those that build communities of learning. Pediatric therapists must focus on these essential co-occupations as well as the individual occupations of children.

## ABOUT CHILDREN

Children grow and develop along a fairly predictable course. Without duplicating the many excellent resources available on this topic, Figure 3–1 provides a graphic illustration of growth expectations, whereas Table 3–2 provides a summary of major developmental milestones.

Childhood can be divided into the following stages, which reflect fairly significant phases in the development process: infancy, and toddlerhood, early childhood, childhood, and preadolescence. Pediatric occupational therapy practice appreciates the unique characteristics and issues at each stage, and provides services in settings that are most appropriate for each child and family.

| Stage | Age | Practice Setting |
|---|---|---|
| Infancy and toddlerhood | Birth to 3 years | Early-intervention hospital, home health |
| Early childhood | 3 to 6 | Preschool, day care Head Start, public school, home, hospital, clinic |
| Childhood (school age) | 7–11 | Elementary school, home, hospital, clinic |
| Preadolescence | 12–14 | Junior high or middle school, home, hospital, clinic, community recreation: YMCA, YWCA, scouting, band, sports, church |
| Adolescence | 15–20+ | High school, college, home, hospital, clinic, community recreation, workplace, church |

It is recommended that pediatric therapists keep up their knowledge of typical child growth and development through reading, continuing education, formal course work, clinical observation, and supervision. This knowledge of "normal" growth and development is essential to therapy practice. Coupled with a knowledge of disease and disability, this enables the therapist to understand the impact of disability on an individual child and his or her occupational capability and dysfunction. Obviously, this underlies any successful intervention.

The nature of occupational therapy assessment and intervention is complex. With children, it goes beyond training children to perform developmental milestones. Havighurst's (1972) description of the developmental task as "a task which arises at or about a certain period in the life of the individ-

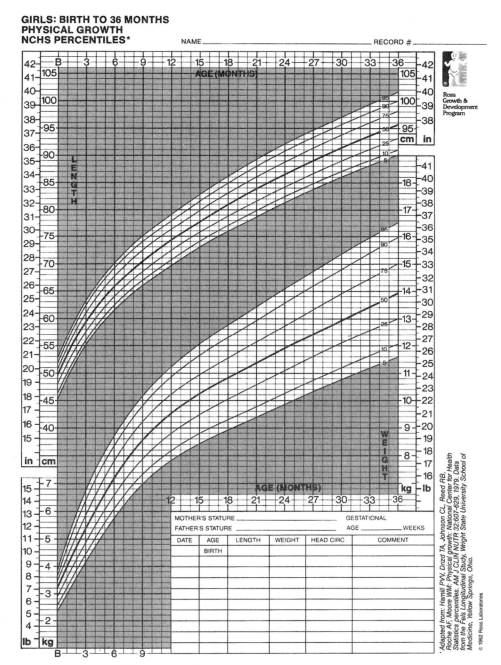

Figure 3–1 Physical growth NCHS percentiles.

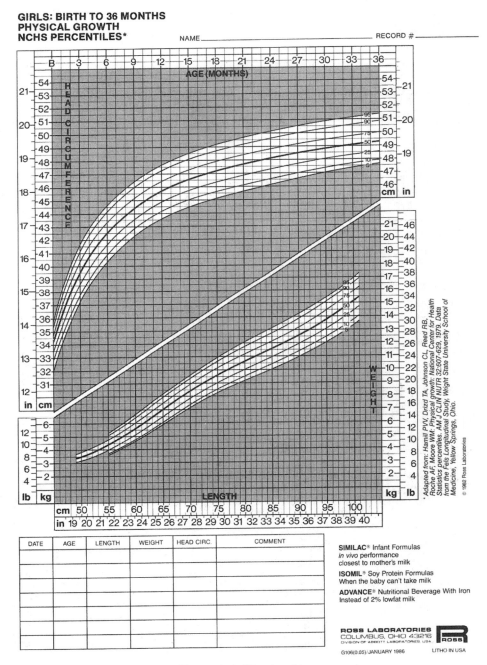

Figure 3–1 (*Continued.*)

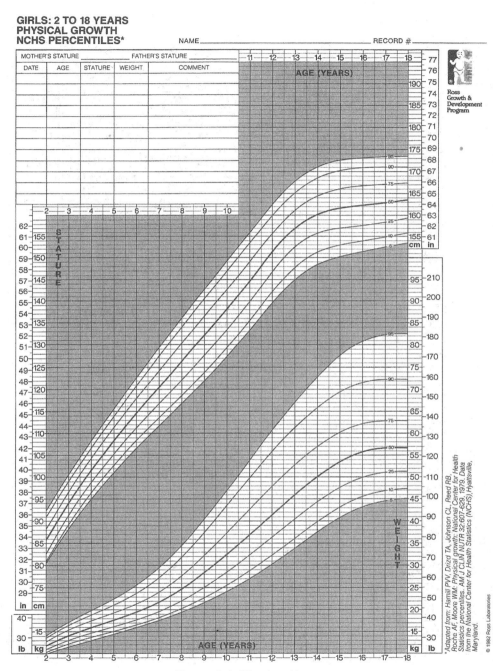

Figure 3–1 (*Continued.*)

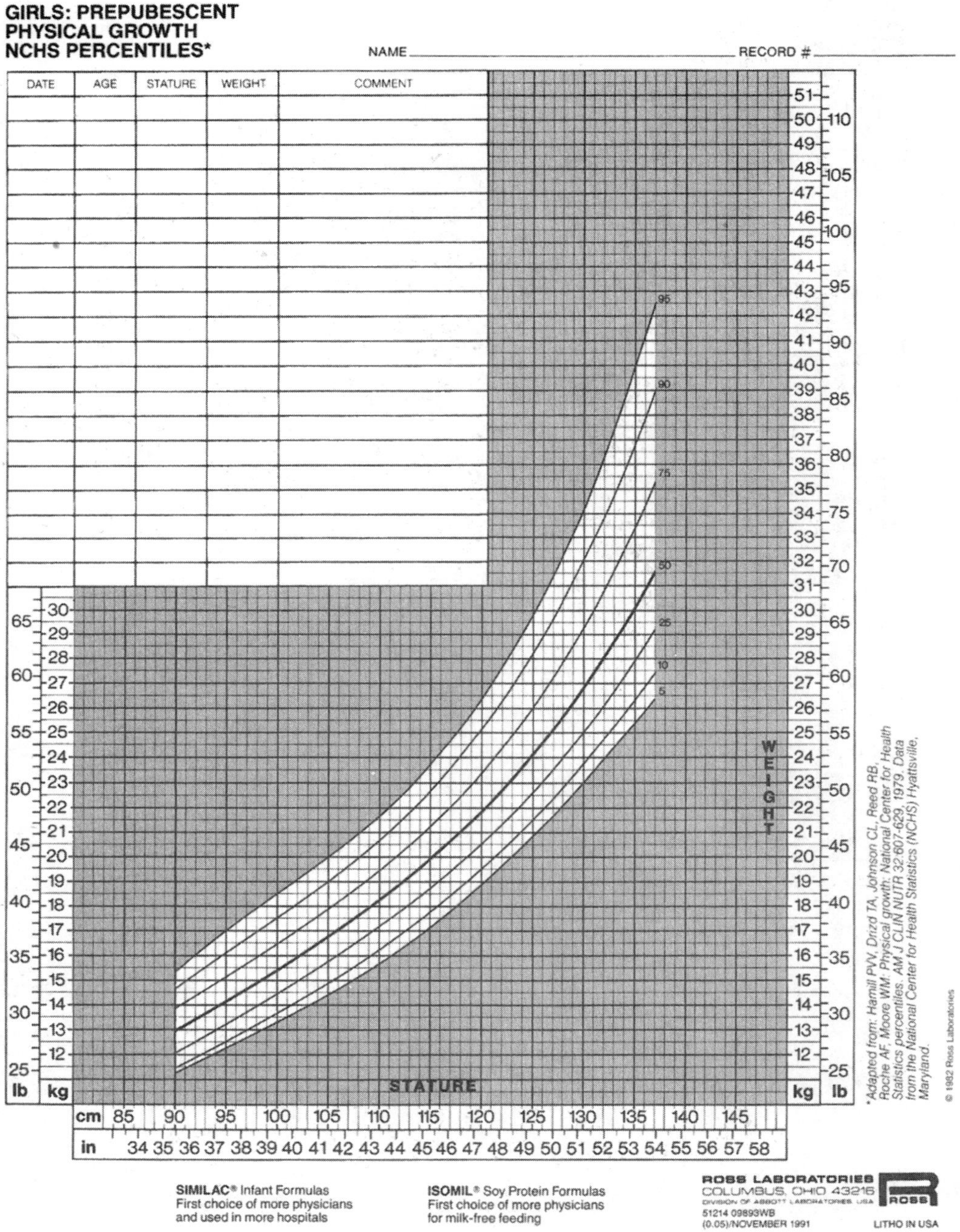

**GIRLS: PREPUBESCENT
PHYSICAL GROWTH
NCHS PERCENTILES***

NAME_____ RECORD #_____

Figure 3–1 (*Continued.*)

**BOYS: BIRTH TO 36 MONTHS**
**PHYSICAL GROWTH**
**NCHS PERCENTILES***

NAME _____ RECORD # _____

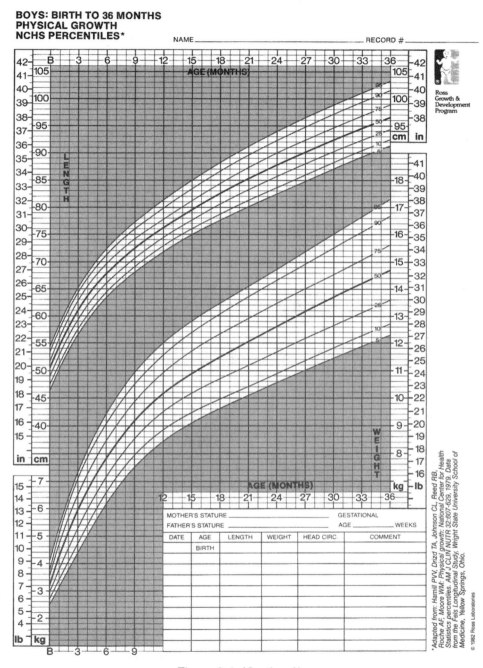

Figure 3–1 (*Continued.*)

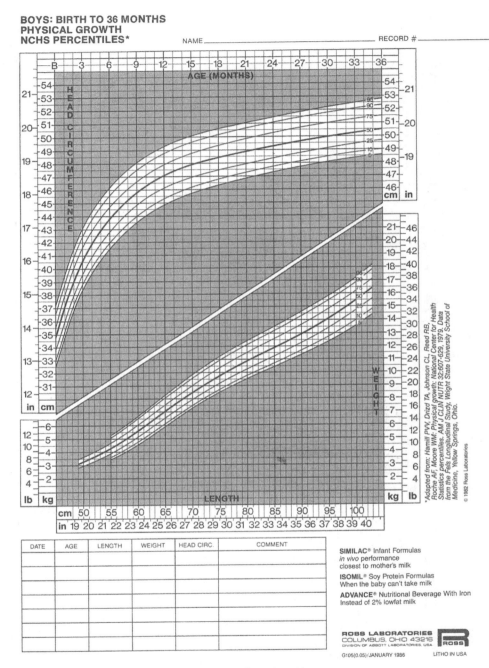

Figure 3–1 (*Continued.*)

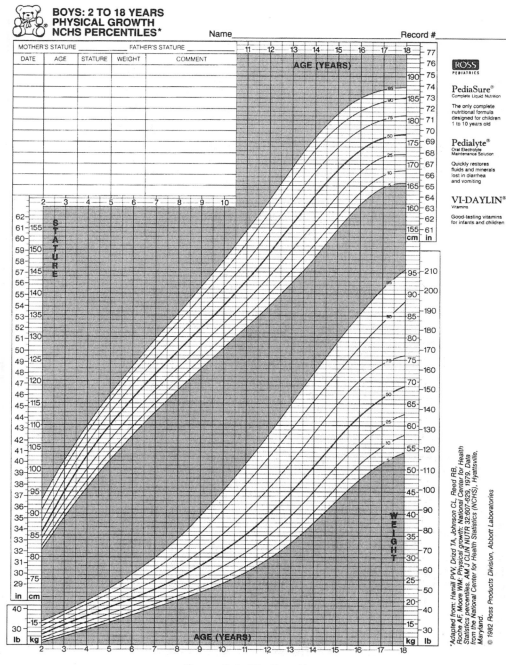

Figure 3–1 (*Continued.*)

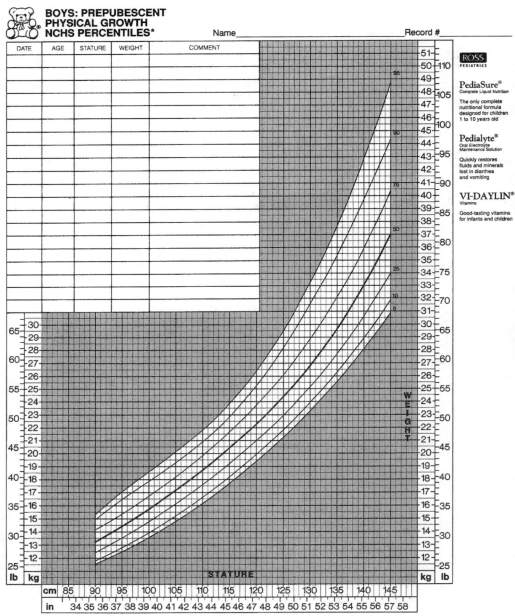

Figure 3–1 (*Continued.*)

**Table 3–2  Milestones in Child Development**

| Age | Physical | Cognitive | Language | Social-Emotional |
|-----|----------|-----------|----------|------------------|
| 0–6 mo | Holds head up when on stomach<br>Rolls over from front to back<br>Reaches for objects<br>Exhibits many reflexes | Demonstrates primary circular reaction stage of sensorimotor intelligence<br>Scans within a face<br>Shows preference for contrast in visual displays<br>Prefers looking at normal face | Cries and coos<br>Recognizes human voice, prefers "baby talk"<br>Can discriminate /d/ from /t/ | Signals needs with crying and gazing<br>Becomes attached to caregiver<br>Smiles in sleep<br>Smiles at people but indiscriminately |
| 6–12 mo | Demonstrates fewer reflexes<br>Gets first tooth<br>Sits up<br>Develops pincer grasp<br>Creeps, crawls<br>Stands holding on | Demonstrates secondary circular reaction<br>Demonstrates coordination of secondary circular reactions<br>Imitates new behavior if scheme is familiar<br>Searches for completely hidden object<br>Looks longer at scrambled face | Repeats consonant-vowel syllables<br>Varies intonation<br>Says first word<br>Says mama, dada<br>Uses single words to express complex thoughts, i.e., "juice?" for "I want some juice." | Smiles selectively<br>Begins to use social referencing<br>Shows stranger anxiety<br>Responds to distress of other by showing distress, crying |
| 12–18 mo | Walks<br>Climbs stairs | Demonstrates tertiary circular reactions<br>Includes others as recipients of play behaviors | Uses expressive jargon | Experiences peak of separation distress |
| 18–24 mo | Begins to run | Demonstrates invention of new means through mental combinations<br>Finds hidden objects through invisible displacement<br>Shows deferred imitation<br>Activates toy or doll in pretend play | Understands multiword utterances<br>Uses multiword utterances to express complex thoughts, i.e., "Daddy go," "Baby up" | Demonstrates less separation distress<br>Begins to show empathic responses to another's distress |

*Continued on following page*

Table 3-2  Milestones in Child Development—*Continued*

| Age | Physical | Cognitive | Language | Social-Emotional |
|---|---|---|---|---|
| 24–36 mo | Jumps<br>Begins to ride a tricycle | Shows ability to substitute objects in pretend play<br>Shows greater ability to substitute objects in pretend play<br>Shows ability to integrate themes in play | Uses verbal strategies to start a conversation<br>Uses two-part sentences (i.e., "me go home") | Begins to respond verbally to another's distress<br>Includes others in pretend play |
| 3 yr | Demonstrates true run, with both feet leaving ground<br>Walks upstairs alternating feet<br>Walks downstairs using marked-time climbing<br>Can take most clothes off | Begins to demonstrate pre-operational thinking<br>Knows conventional count-ing words up to 5<br>Can solve nesting cup prob-lem by reversing two cups or by insertion | Understands *in*, *on*, and *under*<br>Speaks in more complete sentences<br>Distinguishes graphics that are writing versus graph-ics that are pictures<br>Begins to overgeneralize rules for creating verb tenses and plurals | May begin preschool<br>Uses physical aggression more than verbal aggression |
| 3 yr, 6 mo | Can hop a few steps on pre-ferred foot<br>Can button large buttons<br>Can put easier clothes on | Can't easily distinguish real-ity from fantasy<br>Can count five objects before making a partition-ing error | Might use syllable hypothe-sis to create written words<br>Rereads favorite storybooks using picture-governed strategies<br>Often uses scribble-writing | Has difficulty generating alternatives in a conflict situation<br>Will learn aggressive behav-ior rapidly if these means succeed |
| 4 yr | Appears thinner due to longer trunk<br>Can walk a curved line<br>Walks downstairs alternat-ing feet<br>Can gallop<br>Can cut straight line with scissors | Can make a row of objects equal to another row by matching one to one<br>Puts shorter and longer sticks together in piles but can't create a series | Creates questions and nega-tive sentences using cor-rect word arrangement<br>Might create "mock" letters | Watches, on average, 2 to 4 hour of TV per day |

| | | | | |
|---|---|---|---|---|
| 4 yr, 6 mo | May begin to hold writing tool in finger grip<br>Leans forward more when jumping from a height<br>Can button smaller buttons | Knows conventional counting words up to 15<br>Is better able to distinguish reality from fantasy | Often reverses letters when writing<br>Understands *beside, between, front,* and *back*<br>Doesn't notice or grasp print conventions | |
| 5 yr | Can stop and change direction quickly when running<br>Can hop 8 to 10 steps on one foot | Selects own view in three-mountain task<br>Can create a series through trial and error<br>Creates classes of objects based on a single defining attribute | Understands passive sentences<br>May begin to use invented spellings | Is still poor at self-control; success depends on removal of temptation or diversion by others |
| 5 yr, 6 mo | Can connect a zipper on a coat<br>May be able to tie shoes | Can count 20 objects without making a partitioning error | May begin to make print-governed reading attempts with favorite books | Uses more verbal aggression |
| 6 yr | Has 90% of adult-size brain<br>Reaches about two-thirds of adult height<br>Begins to lose baby teeth<br>Moves a writing or drawing tool with the fingers while the side of the hand rests on the table top<br>Can skip<br>Can tie a bow | Begins to demonstrate concrete operational thinking<br>Demonstrates conservation of number on Piaget's conservation tasks<br>Can create series operationally rather than by trial and error | Might use a letter-name spelling strategy, thus creating many invented spellings<br>Appreciates jokes and riddles based on phonological ambiguity | Feels one way only about a situation<br>Has some difficulty detecting intentions accurately in situations where damage occurs<br>Demonstrates Kohlberg's preconventional moral thinking |

*Continued on following page*

Table 3–2  Milestones in Child Development—*Continued*

| Age | Physical | Cognitive | Language | Social-Emotional |
|---|---|---|---|---|
| 7 yr | Is able to make small, controlled marks with pencils or pens due to more refined finger dexterity<br>Has longer face<br>Continues to lose baby teeth | Begins to use some rehearsal strategies as an aid to memory<br>Becomes much better able to play strategy games<br>May demonstrate conservation of mass and length | Appreciates jokes and riddles based on lexical ambiguity<br>Might have begun to read using a print-governed approach, but coordination of cueing systems might be imbalanced | May express two emotions about one situation, but these will be same valence<br>Demonstrates Kohlberg's conventional thinking<br>Understands gender constancy |
| 8 yr | Plays jacks and other games requiring considerable fine-motor skill and good reaction time<br>Jumps rope skillfully<br>Throws and bats a ball more skillfully | Still has great difficulty judging if a passage is relevant to a specific theme<br>May demonstrate conservation of area | Begins to sort out some of the more difficult syntactic difficulties, such as "ask" and "tell"<br>Might be able to integrate all cueing systems for smooth reading<br>Becomes more conventional speller | May express two same-valence emotions about different targets at the same time<br>Understands that people may interpret situation differently but thinks this is due to different information |
| 9 yr | Enjoys hobbies requiring high levels of fine-motor skill (sewing, weaving, model building) | May demonstrate conservation of weight | Interprets "ask" and "tell" correctly | Can think about own thinking or another person's thinking but not both at the same time. |
| 10 yr | May begin to menstruate | Begins to make better judgments about relevance of a text<br>Begins to delete unimportant information when summarizing | Becomes more sophisticated conventional speller | Can take own view and view of another as if a disinterested third party |
| 11 yr | May begin preadolescent growth spurt if female | May demonstrate conservation of volume | Begins to appreciate jokes and riddles based on syntactic ambiguity | Still has trouble detecting deception<br>Spends more time with friends |

| Age | | | | |
|---|---|---|---|---|
| 12 yr | Has reached about 80% cent of adult height if male, 90% if female<br>Has all permanent teeth except for two sets of molars<br>Plays ball more skillfully due to improved reaction time<br>Probably has begun to menstruate | Shows much greater skill in summarizing and outlining<br>May begin to demonstrate formal operational thinking | | May begin to demonstrate Kohlberg's postconventional moral thinking |
| 13 yr | Has reached and passed peak of growth spurt if female<br>Has probably reached puberty (begun menstruation) if female | May demonstrate formal operational thinking | Speaks in longer sentences, uses principles of subordination<br>Understands metaphors, multiple levels of meaning<br>Increases vocabulary | Still has weak sense of individual identity, is easily influenced by peer group<br>Spends more time with friends, usually of same sex<br>May begin sexual relationships, especially if male |
| 14 yr | Is reaching peak of growth spurt if male<br>Is gaining muscle cells if male, fat cells if female<br>May develop anorexia or bulimia, especially if female<br>Is getting deeper voice if male<br>Has probably reached maximum height if female | Continues to gain metacognitive abilities and improve study skills | Improves reading comprehension abilities and study skills<br>Writes longer, more complex sentences | Seeks increasing emotional autonomy from parents |

*Continued on following page*

**Table 3–2  Milestones in Child Development—*Continued***

| Age | Physical | Cognitive | Language | Social-Emotional |
|---|---|---|---|---|
| 15 yr | Has probably reached puberty (begun sperm production) if male<br>May reach fastest reaction time | Can think in terms of abstract principles<br>May demonstrate dogmatism-skepticism | | Seeks intimate friendships and relationships<br>May have had sexual intercourse but may not use contraception |
| 16 yr | Has probably reached maximum height if male<br>May reach peak performance level in some sports | Can argue either side in a debate<br>Shows growing interest in social and philosophical problems | May fail to develop writing ability if not instructed | Is actively involved in search for personal identity<br>Is likely to be sexually active<br>May use alcohol and cigarettes<br>May have dropped out of school |
| 17 yr | Is still gaining muscle strength if male | May demonstrate post-skeptical rationalism<br>May take SAT or ACT test as part of college admissions process | With instruction and practice, metacognitive abilities and study skills continue to improve | Likely to be involved in continuing process of identity formation<br>May have part-time job<br>May make decisions that bear on later occupational choices<br>May be preparing to leave home, separate from parents |

*Source:* Schickendanz, J. A., Schickendanz, D. I., Hansen, K., and Forsyth, P. D. (1993). *Understanding children.* Mountain View, CA: Mayfield.

ual, successful achievement of which leads to happiness and to success with later tasks, while failure leads to unhappiness in the individual, disapproval by the society, and difficulty with later tasks" (p. 2) nicely illustrates the focus of pediatric therapy.

According to Havighurst, developmental tasks arise from physical maturation, culture and society, personal values and aspirations, or from combinations of these factors. Disease or disability can interfere with a developmental task, and it is here that the focus of therapy lies. Table 3–3 provides a summary of the developmental tasks of childhood and adolescence, according to Havighurst.

### Table 3–3 Havighurst's Developmental Tasks

| Period | Developmental Tasks |
|---|---|
| Infancy and early childhood (birth through preschool period) | 1. Achieving physiological stability<br>2. Relating emotionally to parents, siblings, and others<br>3. Learning to take solid foods<br>4. Learning to talk<br>5. Learning to walk<br>6. Learning to control elimination of body wastes<br>7. Learning sex differences and sexual modesty<br>8. Learning to distinguish right from wrong |
| Middle childhood (the elementary school period) | 1. Learning skills necessary for games<br>2. Building a positive sense of one's self<br>3. Deveoping culturally appropriate masculine or feminine roles<br>4. Learning to get along with peers<br>5. Developing values, morality, and a conscience<br>6. Learning basic reading, writing, and arithmetic skills<br>7. Developing an understanding of the social world |
| Adolescence | 1. Learning conceptual and problem-solving skills<br>2. Achieving mature relationships with male and female peers<br>3. Developing a system of values and ethics to guide one's behavior<br>4. Aiming toward socially responsible behavior<br>5. Accepting one's changing physique and using one's body effectively<br>6. Preparing for a career<br>7. Achieving emotional independence from parents and other adults<br>8. Preparing for marriage and family life |

*Source:* Adapted from Havighurst, R. J. (1972). *Developmental tasks and education* (3rd ed.). New York: Longman.

## ABOUT DEVELOPMENT

There are many theorists who offer important perspectives on child growth and development. The pediatric OT needs to be familiar with developmental theory. The reader is referred to the vast array of information in this area. Tables 3–3 through 3–5 and Figure 3–2 provide a sampling of some useful developmental theories. The theories of Jean Piaget, Erik Erikson, L. S. Vygotsky, and Urie Bronfenbrenner were selected because of their emphasis on the interaction between person and environment, a concept central to OTs. There are many other developmental theories that pediatric OTs might want to be familiar with as well. In fact, many occupational therapy educational programs require course work in human development or developmental psychology.

Piaget (Table 3–4) describes in elegant detail the processes by which children learn. His theory is therefore considered to be a cognitive one. However, it can be applied to learning of new movements or social skills as well. Because Piaget's theory is based on observation of his three grandchildren (albeit rigorous and intense observation), his research methodology has been questioned over and over. However, this description of cognitive development remains central to today's understanding of child development.

Erikson (Table 3–5) describes a series of psychological conflicts that must be dealt with at each stage of life. According to his theory, resolution of each

Table 3–4 **Piaget's Stages of Cognitive Development**

| Stage | Approximate Age | Some Major Characteristics* |
|---|---|---|
| Sensorimotor | 0–2 yr | Ability to use reflexes to satisfy own needs<br>No distinction between sensation and action<br>Awareness of cause and effect<br>Action for pleasure only<br>Beginning of tool use |
| Preoperational | 2–7 yr | Thinking remains egocentric<br>Children learn to organize their environment through classification, sensation, and conservation<br>Vocabulary and language expand<br>Early use of inductive reasoning |
| Concrete operations | 7 to 11–12 yr | Understands number concepts, reversibility (related to conservation), and rules<br>Understands whole/part relationships<br>Thinking remains concrete—bound by stimulus and experience |
| Formal operations | 11–12 to 14–15 yr | Able to think abstractly<br>Development of idealism<br>Able to hypothesize |

conflict permits advancement to the next stage, where resolution of the next conflict is the challenge. Table 3–5 provides a list of the Erikson stages as well as a comparison to Freudian stages. Further, the developmental tasks and important influences of each stage are given.

**Table 3–5 Erikson's Psychosocial Stages**

| Erikson's Psychosocial Stage | Corresponding Freudian Psychosexual Stage | Principal Developmental Task | Some Important Influences for Positive Developmental Outcome |
| --- | --- | --- | --- |
| Trust vs. mistrust | Oral (0–18 mo) | Developing sufficient trust in the world to explore it | Mother: warm, loving interaction |
| Autonomy vs. shame and doubt | Anal (18 mo to 2–3 yr) | Developing feeling of control over behavior; realizing that intentions can be acted out | Supportive parents; imitation |
| Initiative vs. guilt | Phallic (2–3 to 6 yr) | Developing a sense of self through identification with parents and a sense of responsibility for own actions | Supportive parents: identification |
| Industry vs. inferiority | Latency (6–11 yr) | Developing a sense of self-worth through interaction with peers | Schools, teachers: learning and education: encouragement |
| Identity vs. identity diffusion | Genital (11 yr and older) | Developing a strong sense of identity—of ego (self); selecting among various potential selves | Peers and role models; social pressure |
| Intimacy vs. isolation | Genital (young adulthood) | Developing close relationships with others; achieving the intimacy required for marriage | Spouse, colleagues, partners, society |
| Generativity vs. self-absorption | Genital (adulthood) | Assuming responsible adult roles in the community; contributing; being worthwhile | Spouse, children, friends, colleagues, community |
| Integrity vs. despair | Genital (older adulthood) | Facing death; overcoming potential despair; coming to terms with the meaningfulness of life | Friends, relatives, children, spouse, community and religious support |

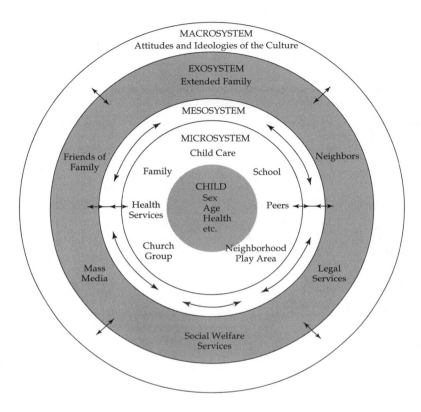

| Level | Type of Interaction |
|-------|---------------------|
| Microsystem | Child in immediate, face-to-face interaction |
| Mesosystem | Relationships between two or more microsystems |
| Exosystem | Linkages and relationships between two or more settings, one of which does not include the child |
| Macrosystem | The totality of all other systems, evident in the beliefs, the options, the life-styles, the values, the more of a culture or subculture |

Figure 3–2 Levels of context in Bronfenbrenner's Ecological (Open) Systems Theory.

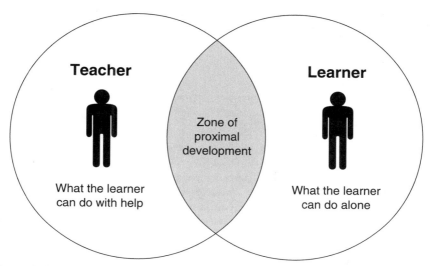

Figure 3–3   Vygotsky's Theory: The Zone of Proximal Development. Vygotsky hypothesized that between a child's actual development level and ability to problem-solve and perform with assistance, there is a "zone of proximal development." This area of learning is most responsive to adult intervention.

Vygotsky (Fig. 3–3) describes the essential human abilities to use tools and symbols to create culture. His theories emphasize the important influence of culture on human development, the important functions of language, and the vital interaction between the developing child and his or her environment. In essence, Vygotsky hypothesized that development is the outcome of the interaction between an individual child's inherent biological and maturational capabilities and an environment or culture that provides opportunities and demands that are appropriate for that child. This is similar to the concepts of flow (Begun, 1996; Csikszentmihayli, 1990) and the just-right challenge (Ayres, 1979) described earlier.

Bronfenbrenner (see Fig. 3–2) has taken an ecological view of human development. He has hypothesized that the interactions between the person, the context, and the process account for development change. He described an ecological system as the context of human performance that takes into account those influences nearest to the individual (microsystem) to those furthest away (macrosystem).

Pediatric therapists are encouraged to keep up to date in regard to human development because research and theoretical developments in this area can and should have tremendous influence on our practice.

## MORE ABOUT CHILDREN

Each individual child comes with a unique personality and temperament. And for each child, a secure attachment to an adult caregiver forms the basis for adult interactions. Temperament contributes to attachment. The interactions between adults and children build the foundation for self-esteem and coping. Understanding of these aspects of children's individuality complements one's knowledge of child development.

## Temperament

Temperament is a style of interacting with the environment that may in fact be a component of personality. Temperament is believed to have a biological basis that changes over the life span as the individual interacts with his or her environment. Table 3–6 provides an outline of the most common descriptors of temperament as well as an illustration of three personality and temperament patterns. An understanding of temperament can help us to appreciate the potential fit between the individual and his or her environment. For example, for a parent who is orderly, predictable, and reliant on routine, the fit with a "difficult" child will be challenging at best.

Therapists can use their understanding of temperament to help caregivers reframe their view of children. Imagine for a moment the way a very persistent child might handle a classroom activity. He or she might be so focused on that activity that everything else goes unnoticed. The parents may say things like "When J.J. is working on something interesting, the house could burn down and he'd never notice!" If J.J.'s teacher understands J.J.'s unique temperament, his lack of response to the teacher's instructions will be attributed to concentration and *not* disrespect or disobedience. This understanding can go a long way in shaping the child's view of himself or herself.

## Attachment

Attachment, simply defined, is the emotional connection between two people, in this case between child and caregiver. An essential occupational task of infancy and early childhood is the development of attachment. This involves complex transactions between children and adults, most often parents.

Attachment is believed to develop in stages. The first stage, *preattachment* involves social responsiveness, synchrony in movement, crying, smiling, grimacing, and so on. The second stage, *attachment in the making*, involves more directed efforts of the child toward the selected primary attachment objects and persons. The third stage, *clear-cut attachment*, involves intentional use of social communications with the attachment object or person. The fourth and last stage, *goal-directed attachment*, involves the use of cause and effect in the relationship—manipulation of the other through communication and social cues as well as taking the perspective of the other. The attachment relationship is believed to be the medium through which language and cultural understanding is developed.

There are three types of attachment (Table 3–7). If a child does not develop a secure attachment with at least one adult, the consequences can be significant. Failure to thrive and some social communication disorders have been linked to early problems with attachment (LeFrancois, 1993). Table 3–8 provides some behavioral indicators of problems associated with attachment.

Table 3–6 **Parameters and Patterns of Temperament**

### Parameters of Temperament

- *Activity level* (general arousal level as expressed by motor reactions). Some children squirm and move a good deal, whereas others are much more relaxed and calm.
- *Rhythmicity* (regularity in biological functions such as sleeping, eating, or defecating).
- *Approach/withdrawal* (the readiness of the child to approach new situations and new people). Some children appear to enjoy new situations, whereas others seem to recoil from every new experience.
- *Adaptability* (the extent to which the child adjusts to changes in routine). Some children adjust quickly to changes in their routine, but others appear unhappy at any minor disruption of their activities.
- *Threshold of responsiveness* (initial sensitivity to light, noise, or other sensory stimuli).
- *Mood* (unhappiness, cheerfulness, and so on).
- *Intensity of reactions* (strength of child's responses). For example, some children cry loudly, and others have a more subdued cry.
- *Distractibility*. For example, when hungry, some children can be diverted and calmed with a pacifier, whereas other children remain distressed until they are given food.
- *Persistence* (duration of interests). For example, some children are quite content to play with an object for a relatively long period of time compared with others, who move quickly from one toy to another.

### Patterns of Temperament

| | |
|---|---|
| Easy | Regularity in eating and sleeping (high rhythmicity); high approach tendencies in novel situations; high adaptability to change; preponderance of positive moods; low or moderate intensity of responses |
| Difficult | Irregularity in eating and sleeping (low rhythmicity); withdrawal in novel situations; slow adaptation to change; preponderance of negative moods; high intensity of reactions to stimulation |
| Slow to warm up | Low activity level; high initial withdrawal from unfamiliar; slow adaptation to change; somewhat negative mood; moderate or low intensity of reaction to stimulation |
| Varying mixtures | Combinations and variations of the described patterns |

*Sources: **Parameters** adapted from Schiamberg, L. B. (1988). Child and adolescent development. New York: Macmillan. **Patterns** adapted from Lefrancois, G. R. The lifespan (4th ed.). Belmont, CA: Wadsworth.*

## Temperament and Attachment

Temperament and attachment are interrelated in a way that is important to pediatric therapists. The unique temperament and personality characteristics of each adult (caregiver) and each child interact to produce powerful relationships that form the basis of attachment. For example, a withdrawn, quiet parent may have very different dynamics with a very active, distractible child

Table 3–7 **Types of Attachment**

| Attachment Classification | Common Behavior When Mother Leaves or Returns | Approximate Percentage of Population |
|---|---|---|
| Secure | Uses mother as base from which to explore; upset when she leaves; greets her return positively and reestablishes physical contact | 68 |
| Anxious avoidant (insecure) | Rarely cries when mother leaves; ignores mother when she returns or actively avoids her, sometimes pushing her away or pointedly not looking at her | 20 |
| Anxious ambivalent (insecure) | Very upset when mother leaves; often angry when she returns; may push her away while seeking proximity (hence, ambivalence) | 12 |

*Source:* Adapted from Lefrancois, G. R. (1993). *The lifespan* (4th ed.). Belmont, CA: Wadsworth.

Table 3–8 **Attachment Disorders—Behaviors**

| Behaviors | Signs of Attachment Disorders in Young Children |
|---|---|
| Showing affection | Lack of warm and affectionate interchanges across a range of interactions; promiscuous affection with relatively unfamiliar adults |
| Comfort seeking | Lack of comfort seeking when hurt, frightened, or ill, or comfort seeking in odd or ambivalent manner |
| Reliance for help | Excessive dependence, or inability to seek and use supportive presence of attachment figure when needed |
| Cooperation | Lack of compliance with caregiver requests and demands by the child as a striking feature of caregiver— child interactions, or compulsive compliance |
| Exploratory behavior | Failure to check back with caregiver in unfamiliar settings, or exploration limited by child's unwillingness to leave caregiver |
| Controlling behavior | Oversolicitous and inappropriate caregiving behavior, or excessively bossy and punitive controlling of caregiver by the child |
| Reunion responses | Failure to re-establish interaction after separations, including ignoring/avoiding behaviors, intense anger, or lack of affection |

*Source:* Zeanah, C. H. (Ed.). (1993). *Handbook of infant mental health.* New York: Guilford.

than with one who is easygoing, adaptable, and persistent. Sometimes just describing the different characteristics and styles of caregiver and child, and affirming their biological nature and interactional possibilities, can be a very effective intervention.

The more people know and understand about each other, the more they can interact effectively. If an anxious parent can learn to wait for the response of a shy child, or if a zealous caregiver can learn to modulate his or her instructions so that the child can focus and attend, their interactions and relationships will be greatly enhanced. The foundation of a secure attachment between caregiver and child underlies the acquisition of developmental milestones and learning. A healthy interaction between caregiver and child enhances and extends the utility of therapy programs and recommendations. It is an important focus for the pediatric therapist.

The interaction of the child with the world that he or she lives in and experiences results in the child's having a certain feeling about his or her worth or self-esteem. It also results in the child's having a unique set of strategies for coping with that world (Garbarino, 1990). It is our hope that children will have high self-esteem and effective coping. Our efforts can contribute to that reality.

## ▟▙▌ FROM THE BOOKSHELF

> For interesting, relevant reading on the coping skills of children and families, refer to the work of J. Gordon Williamson, an OT who has done extensive research and clinical work in this domain. With this colleague Shirley Zeitlin, a psychologist, Williamson developed a set of very useful standardized assessments (*The Coping Inventory* and the *Early Coping Inventory*) of coping as well. Both coping inventories are published by the Scholastic Testing Services.

## LEARNING ABOUT CHILDREN THROUGH OBSERVATION AND INTERVIEW

Although formal and informal assessment strategies are available for therapists working with children, pediatric OTs are reminded that perhaps the most important aspects of a child's occupation occur in naturalistic contexts. Formal testing coupled with informal observation and interview (talking with the child and caregiver[s]) will likely yield the most accurate picture of an individual child's occupations.

Table 3–9 provides a summary of the various methods for structured observation of children. As you can see, each affords different types of information. It is a good idea to become familiar with a variety of methods because no two children or observation sites are the same.

Interviewing is another method of obtaining important information from children. It can capture a child's thoughts, feelings, and attitudes in a way that testing and observation cannot. Table 3–10 is an example of an interview that seeks to understand the meaning of reading in a particular

Table 3–9 **Methods for Observing and Recording Data about Child Development**

| Method | Purpose | Advantages | Disadvantages |
|---|---|---|---|
| **Anecdotal Record:** A narrative of descriptive paragraphs, recorded *after behavior occurs* | To detail specific behavior for child's record; for case conferences; to plan for individuals | Open-ended; rich in details; no special observer training | Depends on observer's memory; behavior taken out of context; difficult to code or analyze for research |
| **Running Record:** A narrative written in sequence over a specified time, recorded *while behavior is occurring* | To discover cause and effects of behavior; for case conferences; to plan for individuals | Open-ended; comprehensive; no special observer training | Time-consuming; difficult to use for more than one child at a time; time-consuming to code and analyze for research |
| **Specimen Record:** A detailed narrative written in sequence over a specified time, recorded *while behavior is occurring* | To discover cause and effects of behavior; for child development research | Open-ended; comprehensive and complete; rich in details | Time-consuming to record; time-consuming to code or analyze for research; difficult to observe more than one child at a time |
| **Time Sampling:** Tallies or symbols showing the presence or absence of specified-behavior during short time periods, recorded *while behavior is occurring* | For behavior modification baseline data; for child development research | Objective and controlled; not time-consuming; efficient for observing more than one child at a time; provides quantitative data for research | Closed; limited to observable behaviors that occur frequently; no description of behavior; takes behavior out of context |
| **Event Sampling:** A brief narrative of conditions preceding and following specified behavior, recorded *while behavior is occurring* | For behavior modification input; for child development research | Objective; helpful for in-depth diagnosis of infrequent behavior | Closed; takes event out of context; limited to specified behavior |

| | | | |
|---|---|---|---|
| **Rating Scale:** A scale of traits or behaviors with check marks, recorded *before, during, and after behavior occurs* | To judge degree to which child behaves or possesses certain traits; to diagnose behavior or traits; to plan for individuals | Not time-consuming; easy to design; efficient for observing more than one child at a time for many traits; useful for several observers watching same child | Closed; subjective; limited to specified traits or behaviors |
| **Checklist:** A list of behaviors with check marks, recorded *before, during, and after behavior occurs* | To determine presence or absence of specified behaviors; to plan for individuals; to give observer an overview of child's development or progress | Efficient for observing more than one child at a time for many behaviors; useful for an individual over a period of time; a good survey or inventory tool; useful for several observers at once; no special training needed | Closed; limited to specified behaviors; no information on quality of behavior |

*Source:* Beaty, J. (1990). *Observing the development of the young child.* New York: Merrill.

Table 3–10 **A Sample Interview with a Child**

NAME: _____

AGE: _____ GRADE: _____

1. Do you like to read?

2. What kinds of things do you like to read?

3. What are your favorite books or stories?

4. Do your parents read? Do they read to/with you?

5. Do you think that you are a good reader?

6. Who do you know who is a good reader (your parent(s), teacher(s))?

7. What makes him or her a good reader?

8. When you are reading and you come to something you don't know, what do you do? What else could you do?

9. If you know someone was having trouble reading, what would you do to help them?

10. What might someone else (your parent(s) or teacher(s)) do to help them?

11. How did you learn to read?

12. What would you like to do better as a reader?

13. If you wrote a book or story, what would it be about?

14. What would you like to read about next?

_____

*Source:* Adapted from Burke, C. (1992). In Black, J. K., Puckett, M., & Bell, M. J. (Eds.), *The young child: Development from prebirth through age eight.* New York: Merrill.

child's life. As you can see, information gained through interview and observation complements the highly specialized data available through standardized testing. In fact, interviewing can help to bring the child's occupation into context.

## ▮▮▮ FROM THE BOOKSHELF

Garbarino, J., Stott, F. M., and the faculty of the Erikson Institute. (1990). *What children can tell us: Eliciting, interpreting and evaluating information from children.* San Francisco: Jossey-Bass.

This thoughtful and comprehensive book provides a framework for interaction with children. It reviews children's communication, contexts for communication with children, and strategies for eliciting accurate information. It is highly recommended for the bookshelf of anyone who wishes to truly include children in their service delivery.

# THE CONCEPTS OF VULNERABILITY, RISK, AND RESILIENCE

Why is it that two families, with many apparent similarities, have different responses to a child with special needs in their family? Why do two children, of the same age, same gender, same diagnosis, from the same neighborhood even, have such different occupational abilities?

Let's take a look at two scenarios.

The first scenario involves a family with two professional, well-educated, apparently loving parents. They have a good home, adequate financial resources, and a supportive extended family and community.

The second scenario involves another family, this one headed by a single teenage mother and an absent father. Conditions of poverty, poor health care, and possible substance abuse place the mother and child at great risk.

Many people would guess that the family described in the first scenario will cope effectively and the other family will not. Although much of the literature attributes what is called socioeconomic status (SES), or the parents' financial, educational, and marital status, to the outcomes for children, the relationships between child and family characteristics and child and family outcomes are not that clear. In fact, it is quite complex and is not well understood at all. While the family in the first scenario may in fact "do well," it may just as likely not. And although the family in the second scenario does not seem to have much in its favor, it is quite conceivable that it will adjust and thrive.

As therapists, we need to understand what factors might influence these outcomes. We need to have the most current knowledge about which strategies are most likely to help families achieve the successful outcomes they each desire and deserve. We need to know how to best help families muster their resources, minimize their risks, and achieve their own goals. What factors should we attend to accomplish this?

An individual family's economic and social status, its values and beliefs, its social and cultural systems, and its behaviors all contribute to its uniqueness. It is helpful for therapists to be familiar with these factors for each child they serve. It is also within these factors that an individual family's risk, vulnerability, resilience, and protective factors can be found.

*Risk* refers to internal and external factors that increase the likelihood of certain, usually undesirable, outcomes. Chapter 2 explores certain risks in greater detail.

*Vulnerability* refers to the characteristics that a particular family brings to a situation. It specifically refers to how protected from or accessible to the potentially negative effects of risk factors each family is. For example, if a family is flexible (i.e., is able to easily accommodate change), it is less vulnerable to stress than a family who is rigid in its responses. A family that is too disorganized to mobilize its own resources is more vulnerable than one that is in more control. For example, a young woman who has a history of mental illness, who lives with her infant in substandard housing, and who has little family or community interaction is more vulnerable to many dangers than another young mother who has adequate finances and lives in safe housing with one or more supportive adults (Scarr & McCartney, 1983).

Begun (1996) provides a framework for determining the probability of problems based on these factors (Table 3–11).

*Resilience* is the ability of the child or family to resist the effects of the risks. Resilience is a concept that emanates from the field of public health. In the case where an entire population of people may be equally exposed to a potentially harmful substance yet only a small percentage are actually affected, those who are not affected are considered to be resilient. This is an important concept for therapists because it offers a new perspective on the impact of disability and disease. It may not be the disease or disability itself that determines the outcome, but each child and family's resilience (Scarr & McCartney, 1983, Werner, 1990).

In children, resilience involves a sense of self-efficacy, self-esteem, and self-confidence, a range of social problem-solving abilities, and a belief in one's own ability to affect change and to adapt. It is likely that these same characteristics would contribute to resilience in family units. It is important to remember, however, that risk, vulnerability, and resilience change as time passes and as life circumstances change (Werner, 1990).

Resilience is *greatest* for families whose vulnerability and risk are lowest and is *least* for those whose risk and vulnerability is high. Moderate resilience is found in families where one dimension is high and the other is

**Table 3–11  Likelihood of Family Problems**

| Risk | + | Vulnerability | = | Likelihood |
|------|---|---------------|---|------------|
| Low  |   | Low           |   | Low        |
| Low  |   | High          |   | Moderate   |
| High |   | Low           |   | Moderate   |
| High |   | High          |   | High       |

*Source:* Adapted from Begun, A. L. (1996). Family systems and family centered cared. In Rosin, P., Whitehead, A. D., Tuchman, L. I., Jesien, G. S., Begun, A. L., & Irwin, L. (Eds.), *Partnerships in family centered care: A guide to collaborative early intervention* (pp. 33–65). Baltimore: Brooks.

low. Interventions for highly resilient families can focus on supporting and maintaining the things that keep their risk and vulnerability low. On the other hand, as resilience decreases and the likelihood of problems increases, interventions would focus on reducing the risk and vulnerability by reduction of environmental risk and by the enhancement or addition of protective factors.

*Protective factors* are the characteristics that a child or family bring to a situation that actually shield their response to risk or stress. Scarr and McCartney (1983) identified certain genetic characteristics (temperament, intelligence, activity level, and sociability) in resilient children. Werner's (1990) extensive review of the literature on risk and resilience indicates that protective factors consist of:

1. Characteristics of the child that elicit positive interactions between the child and the environment. These include physical capability, easygoing temperament, and intelligence.
2. A family system characterized by warmth and nurturance where trust, initiative, and independence are facilitated.
3. Environmental support systems that offer positive values and reinforcement of competence and capability.

A word of caution though. A very thorough assessment of a child's and family's strengths, resources, and needs (usually conducted by an interdisciplinary or transdisciplinary team) is essential to determining their risk, vulnerability, and resilience. All is never as it appears. For some families, poverty is not an obstacle, but for others it is. What one person considers to be substandard housing may be more than adequate for another person. A family whose interaction is characterized by loud verbalization may simply be passionate in their expressive style or they may be argumentative and dysfunctional. Very careful attention to each child and family's own stories, their values, their beliefs, and their behaviors will give you the best picture of their ability to withstand stress.

It is our responsibility to remain aware of how families and children are when we come to know them, how they had been, and how they are changing. Armed with this knowledge, we can address our interventions toward their present and future strengths and needs.

Werner (1990) says that "the life stories of resilient individuals have taught us that competence, confidence, and caring can flourish even under adverse circumstances, if young children encounter persons who provide them with a secure basis for the development of trust, autonomy, and initiative" (p. 113).

## ▟▊▊ FROM THE BOOKSHELF

Here's some recommended reading on the topics of attachment, temperament, risk, vulnerability, and resilience. These concepts provide a helpful framework for assessment and intervention with many populations, but especially with children and families.

Challener, D. D. (1997). *Stories of resilience in childhood: The narratives of Maya Angelou, Maxine Hong Kingston, Richard Rodriguez, John Edgar Wideman & Tobias Wolff.* New York: Garland Publishing.

Haggerty, R., Rutter, M., Garmezy, N., & Sherrod, L. R. (Eds.). (1994).

*Stress, risk, and resilience in children and adolescents: Processes, mechanisms, & interventions.* Englewood Cliffs, NJ: Cambridge Books.

Haggerty, R., Rutter, M., Garmezy, N., & Sherrod, L. (Eds.). (1996). *Stress, risk, and resilience in children and adolescents.* Englewood Cliffs, NJ: Cambridge Books.

Simeonsson, R. J., (Ed.). (1995). *Risk, resilience, & prevention: Promoting the well-being of all children.* Baltimore: Paul Brookes.

Carey, W. B., & McDevitt, S. C. (1995). *Coping with children's temperament: A guide for professionals.* New York: Basic Books.

Carey, W. B., & Jablow, M. (1997). *Understanding your child's temperament.* New York: Macmillan.

## FAMILIES AT RISK

This section provides an overview of particular risks and vulnerabilities for children and families. Table 3–12 provides a synthesis of some rather startling statistics that reflect the status of children and families today. It is well known that the two-parent nuclear family is no longer in the majority. We have come a great distance in appreciating the diversity of family structures as well as their functioning. Today, children are living in two- as well as one-parent homes. They may also live in two or more homes as a result of single parenthood by choice or because of divorce, remarriage, or death. They are parented by biological parents, adoptive parents, grandparents, foster parents, and close relatives and friends. Children are parented by heterosexual parents and by parents who are gay, lesbian, or bisexual. Families may be inherent members of cultural communities, they may draw their members from a single common ethnic background, or their backgrounds may reflect multiple ethnicities and cultures. Children seem to function quite well in any of these family contexts. What seems to matter the most is that the children are at the center of the adult family members' concern, caring, and loving. What is distressing about the statistics in Table 3–12 is that they illustrate the reality that many factors make it difficult for families today to provide adequate food, shelter, and clothing, not to mention love and care.

Table 3–13 provides a brief overview of those family situations that present the greatest risks to children. Parental illness or disability can interfere with the ability to perform the occupations of families successfully. This can range from the difficulties a parent might experience in managing the physical aspects of caregiving (see Chapter 2 for a discussion of physical disability and parenting) to the emotional unavailability of parents who abuse substances such as alcohol or drugs.

Pediatric therapists will encounter these situations, regardless of the community or setting in which they practice. At times, these risks will cause a child be referred to occupational therapy to diminish or monitor the risk itself or to address its consequences. For example, many early-childhood intervention programs provide routine developmental monitoring and family and child support services to reduce the potential impact of these risks. As an OT, you may provide developmental screening, special consultation, or training to staff and participants in special programs for families at risk. For children who have developmental difficulties, occupational therapy evaluation

Table 3–12  **Portrait of the American Child, 1995**

**THERE ARE ABOUT** 57 million children under 15, about 22 percent of the population. About 79 percent are white, 16 percent black and 5 percent Asian or Pacific Islander, American Indian, Eskimo or Aleutian. About 12 percent of the population is of Hispanic origin.

**IN 1994, THERE** were an estimated 3,949,000 births. This was the first time since 1989 that the total has fallen under four million. The decline indicates an echo effect, as the outsize number of baby-boom mothers start to pass out of their childbearing years.

**THE NUMBER OF** children per woman has decreased from 3.6 in 1960 to 2.0 today. Nearly 1 potential mother in 10 now says she never expects to bear a child.

**THE AVERAGE AGE** of a first-time mother is 23.7, only slightly higher than the average age of first-time mothers in 1940 but nearly two years higher than in 1960. First-time fathers then and now are typically three or four years older.

**THE INFANT MORTALITY** rate decreased from 10.6 per 1,000 births in 1985 to 8.5 in 1992. This has been attributed to expanded Medicaid coverage, better nutrition and better medical technology. Even so, a recent report found that the rate is still lower in 22 other developed countries.

**AMERICAN RANKS 31ST** in the percentage of low-birth-weight babies, behind Turkey, Iran and even Romania. Washington, D.C., had the highest U.S. concentration of low-birth-weight births, 14.3 percent as of 1991, compared with 10 percent for New York City and 7.1 percent for the country.

**THE PROPORTION OF** multiple births to all births in America is still very small, 2.4 percent in 1992. Nonetheless, since the early 70's the multiple-birth rate has increased by a third. The increase is attributable to an increase in births to older women, an increase in infertility service seekers and new drugs and treatments.

**RECENT DATA SHOW** that 42 percent of families with children under 18 have only one child in the household. In 1960, the figure was only 32 percent. Now, 6 percent have four or more children. Then, the figure was 17 percent.

**SINCE 1950, THE** number of American children living in mother-only families has quadrupled, from about 5 million to nearly 20 million, and since 1970 the number of single parents has tripled, from about 4 million to about 12 million. About 26 percent of households with children under 18 now have only a mother at home, and another 4 percent have only a father. The highest concentrations of such single-parent households are in Louisiana, Mississippi, Tennessee and Washington, D.C.

**ONE OF EVERY** six children is a stepchild. One of every eleven adults is divorced, three times the proportion in 1970.

**IN 1991, OF** the total amount of child support supposed to be paid, only 67 percent was actually paid.

**AS OF 1992,** the median income of families with children was $35,100. The official poverty level for a family of four was $14,763. There are more than 14 million children living in poverty in the U.S. In a recent study, the U.S. ranked worst among 18 Western industrialized nations for the percentage of children living in poverty.

**AN ESTIMATED 464,000** children were in foster homes, group homes or residential treatment centers on any single day in 1993. That's only 0.5 percent of all children, but it represents an increase in 77 percent since 1982.

*Continued on following page*

Table 3–12 **Portrait of The American Child, 1995—*Continued***

**ABOUT 200,000 WOMEN** a year are trying to adopt a child.

**IN RECENT YEARS,** about 200,000 children 14 and under immigrate to the United States annually. Nearly a quarter of the children come from Mexico, with high concentrations from the former Soviet Union, Vietnam, India and China. New York City's public-school student body represents children from 188 countries.

**IN CONSTANT DOLLARS,** in 1959–60 public schools spent $1,765 per student in average daily attendance. By 1980, that amount had more than doubled. By 1990, it had more than tripled.

**STUDENT-TEACHER RATIOS** in public schools have been decreasing steadily nationwide. In 1940, there were 29 students per teacher; in 1950, 27; in 1960, 25.8; in 1970, 22.3; in 1980, 18.7; and in 1990, 17.2. New York City's ratio of 18 is only slightly higher than the national average, but with current budget cuts, the number of students per classroom in the city is on the rise.

**OVER 25 YEARS,** national averages for reading and math at the grade-school level have not changed significantly. The most recent report indicates that 42 percent of fourth graders scored below the basic reading level, and 41 percent scored below the basic math level.

**AVERAGE COMBINED SCORES** on the Scholastic Aptitude Test have dropped 78 points since 1963. The latest national average S.A.T. scores are 424 in verbal and 478 in math.

**THE NO. 1** foreign language studied in public schools is Spanish, with 443,000 students in 1948 and more than 2.5 million by the early 90's. Only French has come close.

**SINCE 1978, THE** number of children receiving home schooling has jumped from 12,500 to 1 million.

**FROM 1985 TO 1994,** the number of reported cases of child abuse nationwide increased 64 percent. More than three million cases were reported in 1993. It's estimated that a third of all cases reported are substantiated. It is also estimated that three children died each day in the U.S. in 1994 as a result of maltreatment.

**IN A RECENT** study, the U.S. ranked in the lower half of Western industrialized countries in providing services for family support.

**PUBLIC CONCERN ABOUT** teen-age pregnancy appears to be having an effect. The Government reported last month that the birthrate among teen-agers dropped 2 percent in 1993. That followed a drop of 2 percent in 1992. Even so, teen pregnancy rates are significantly higher in the U.S. than in many developed countries—twice as high as in England, France and Canada, and nine times as high as in the Netherlands and Japan. Every day in America, 1,340 teen-agers give birth.

**THE PERCENTAGE OF** first births to American teen-agers that occur out of wedlock has increased over 30 years from 33 percent to 81 percent. The percentage of teen-age first-time mothers in America nearly equals the percentages in Jordan, the Philippines and Thailand.

**IN 1991, MORE** teen-agers and young adults died from suicide than from cancer, heart disease, H.I.V. infection or AIDS, birth defects, pneumonia, influenza, stroke and chronic lung disease combined.

**IN 1994, ABOUT** one in five high-school seniors smoked. In 1975, it was about one

*Continued on following page*

Table 3–12 **Portrait of The American Child, 1995—*Continued***

in four. More than half the three million adolescent smokers are male. Another one million use smokeless tobacco.

**EVERY DAY, 135,000** children take guns to school.

**EVERY DAY, 1,200,000** latchkey children go home to a house in which there is a gun.

**THE PERCENTAGE OF** mothers using organized day care for children under 5 rose from 13 percent in 1977 to 30 percent in 1993.

**ALTHOUGH REPORTED CRIMES** of violence have decreased nationwide in the past 10 years, arrest rates for violent crimes committed by juveniles ages 10 to 17 doubled between 1983 and 1992. The majority of juvenile violent crimes are committed between 3 P.M. and 6 P.M.

**IN 1994, 99 PERCENT** of the 850,000 children reported missing were found.

*Source:* Sweeney, C. (1995). Portrait of the American child. *The New York Times Magazine,* October 8.

and intervention within the context of understanding the child's unique circumstances can be central to a child's recovery process. These are important opportunities to help children and families. Reviewing typical child development may help a child-abuse investigator substantiate a report of abuse. Teaching young parents about appropriate toys and activities may foster a child's learning and growth as well as attachment to caregivers. It is essential in dealing with these risk factors that therapists become very aware of their own experiences, feelings, values, and beliefs. As with any unknown, knowledge is the key. It is incumbent upon you as pediatric therapist to learn about these risks and vulnerabilities. it is important to be aware of resources in your community and professional network that can help to reduce these risks for families and children. The few moments it takes to refer a family to Parent's Anonymous will pay itself back a hundredfold in stress reduction for that family. By taking this action, you are supporting the parents in their essential family occupations, and in so doing you may be saving the life of a child.

Appendix 3–1 provides some information on indicators of child abuse and neglect. More information and specific training are available through the governmental agency in your area with responsibility for child protection.

## FROM THE BOOKSHELF

Here are some books written for children. They provide calm, realistic illustrations and narrative about situations many children face. The selections provided here focus on particular family risks.

PARENTAL ILLNESS
Sherkin-Langer, F. (1995). *When mommy is sick.* Morton Grove, IL: Albert Whitman.

FAMILY ALCOHOL AND SUBSTANCE ABUSE
Vigna, J. (1988). *I wish Daddy didn't drink so much.* Morton Grove, IL: Albert Whitman.

**Table 3–13  Family Risk Factors**

| Population/Risk | Possible Outcomes | Support/Intervention Strategies |
|---|---|---|
| Adolescent parents | Greater risk for toxemia and anemia in pregnancy, Greater risk for prolonged labor, birth complications<br>Greater school dropout rates<br>Greater risk of prematurity<br>Increased risk of genetic disorders<br>Increased likelihood of poverty, divorce, suicide | Support completion of education<br>Prevent/plan future pregnancies<br>Encourage mature, stable marriage<br>Encourage support from adolescent(s) own parents/family |
| Parent(s) with mental illness | Children are at increased risk of mental illness themselves<br><br>Maternal depression and schizophrenia are associated with other risks, e.g., poverty, psychosocial stress, relationship disturbances<br>Decreased parent-child interaction is common<br>Insecure attachment, parent-child conflict are more common<br>Children tend to be more impulsive, more "difficult," have more problems with peer interactions<br>Ill parents tend to perceive their children as more difficult than well mothers do | Single risk factors are not associated with specific outcomes<br>Multiple risks must be considered simultaneously, e.g., interactional problems, family beliefs and values, and economic status |
| Parent(s) with substance abuse | Children are at great risk for developmental and behavioral problems<br>Children exposed to substances prenatally have a twofold predicament:<br>1. A biological vulnerability because of the prenatal biochemical exposure<br>2. Dysfunctional interactions may decrease the child's ability to recover from the biological vulnerability<br>Addictions by nature imply a loss of control and a possible preoccupation with the substance, thus making the parent unavailable to the child and unable to care for himself or herself | Comprehensive treatment of family, including appropriate alcohol or drug treatment as well as attention to the child's health, development, and behavior |

| | | |
|---|---|---|
| | Parent(s) who are not sensitive or responsive to the needs of their child(ren) may participate in a cycle of neglect that can lead to failure to thrive. This neglect, coupled with stress, increases the risk of violence and depression, both of which can have tragic outcomes for children and families | |
| Children exposed to violence | Outcome(s) dependent on: the *intensity* of the violent act(s), *proximity* to violent event(s), *familiarity* with the victim(s) or perpetrator(s), *the developmental status of the child*, and the *chronicity* of exposure to violent acts<br><br>Children who have been traumatized may have posttraumatic stress syndrome (PTSS), which is characterized by re-experiencing trauma, avoidance or hyperarousal at reminders of trauma, development of new fears, development of aggressive behaviors, nightmares, dissociative reactions, and decreased emotional responsiveness | Positive interactions with caregiver(s)<br>Learning to relate to others in positive ways<br>Positive role models<br><br>Adequate housing, area lighting, safety services<br>Prompt professional evaluation, treatment, and counseling of children can decrease developmental harm |
| Poverty | Increased likelihood of inadequate health care, inadequate nutrition, chronic illness<br>Increased infant mortality and morbidity<br>Increased maternal depression<br>Parents who must focus on the physical aspects of caregiving, as well as the issues of survival and safety, may have limited resources left to attend to the other essential needs of their children (e.g., emotional, social, etc.);<br>this is of particular concern in the presence of other familiar risk factors<br>Homeless children (25% of homeless people) are at greatest risk for being depressed, excessively shy and withdrawn, anxious | "Breaking the cycle" of poverty, through increasing socialization, motivation, parent involvement, preparation for school success, provision of health care, food, shelter, and job training and placement |

*Continued on following page*

Table 3-13 **Family Risk Factors**—*Continued*

| Population/Risk | Possible Outcomes | Support/Intervention Strategies |
|---|---|---|
| Children who are maltreated | Child maltreatment may include physical abuse, sexual abuse, emotional abuse, neglect, and inadequate parenting Families with parental mental illness, parental cognitive disability, parental illness, family poverty, and/or parental substance abuse are at greatest risk for child maltreatment | Decrease family stress Increase knowledge of typical child development and appropriate discipline Psychotherapy, professional counseling, self-help organizations such as Parents Anonymous Separation of the perpetrator from the child may be necessary, thus placing the child in the care of relatives or in foster care |

*Source:* Adapted from Barnard et al., 1993; Crockenberg et al., 1993; Halpern, 1993; Mrazek, 1993; Osofsky & Fenichel, 1996; Schickendanz et al., 1993; Seifer & Dickstein, 1993; Zeanah et al., 1993; Zigler et al., 1993; and Zuckerman & Brown, 1993.

Vigna, J. (1990). *My big sister takes drugs.* Morton Grove, IL: Albert Whitman.

DOMESTIC VIOLENCE
Trottier, M. (1997). *A safe place.* Morton Grove, IL: Albert Whitman.
Girard, L. W. (1984). *My body is private.* Morton Grove, IL: Albert Whitman.
Hochban, T. and Krykorka, V. (1994). *Hear my roar: A story of family violence.* Buffalo, NY: Annick Press.

---

■ *THERAPEDS POINTER: DEALING WITH CHILDREN AT RISK*

Many therapists are uncomfortable with the notion of children and families at risk, especially for maltreatment. It is possible to avoid attending to these issues, saying that they are not the appropriate domain for OTs. This is unfortunate. If a therapist focuses only a child's movement, or on the acquisition of specific skills or milestones, while ignoring the context in which a child functions, the therapy lacks meaning and value. A therapist's own comfort is not the objective of therapy; rather it is the enhancement of the child's ability to be a successful occupational being. A brave and realistic look at some of the difficult situations children and families face will enhance your practice. It will also deeply affect your understanding of the world. The ability of children and families to rise above significant risks and vulnerabilities is oftentimes remarkable. It is a privilege to be a professional whose work has helped people to achieve their own goals. It is also tragic to see children hurt by their own families or by strangers. The pain and discomfort associated with the reality that this happens too often, even in our own backyards, can be overwhelming. OTs can contribute to improving the status of children through their direct and indirect service to families and children, by their sharing of their knowledge with others, and by their efforts at advocating for children's rights and family supports.

---

# WRAPPING IT UP

If one takes the "long view," the reason for providing therapy services for children is to improve their occupation. By reducing risk and vulnerability; by facilitating resilience and protective factors; by recognizing the importance of development in context; and by supporting the family members, teachers, and others in their essential caregiving occupations, we can help children to realize a life that has hope, challenge, and choice. Although attention to specific problems in performance and provision of specific types of therapy treatments is certainly helpful to children, it is best to include these within the overall context of the child's occupation. When our actions have real meaning and purpose (relevance) in the lives of the children we serve, their impact is greatest. I am reminded of the song by the children's folk singer, Raffi, that goes like this:

"Will I ever grow up mama,

will I ever grow up papa,

will I be just like you,

so big and so strong

will I wear grown up clothes,

will I have a grown up voice,

going off to work someday,

all by myself.

Having babies of my own,

in my family home,

will I ever grow up

will I be just like you

will I ever grow up,

say that I can."

Our responsibility as role models, coaches, teachers, helpers, advocates, and caregivers is enormous. Through our work with children, we have the opportunity to shape the future. It is an opportunity we must embrace, for through these transformations, we grow and change as well.

## CASE STORY

Pam is the youngest of five brothers and three sisters. Her mother and father began having children when they were only teenagers. Both worked outside the home, and there is some question of alcoholism and possible neglect or abuse in Pam's family. As a young teenager, Pam managed to maintain good grades in school, and she had many friends. Sometimes Pam baby-sat to make extra money.

When Pam was 15, she met and fell in love with 18-year-old Jeff. His family was well-to-do. Jeff did well in school and was to graduate soon. He was planning to go away to college. Jeff worked at the golf course part time and was active in afterschool sports.

By Christmas vacation, Pam and Jeff knew that she was pregnant. They decided to tell their families, who were angry at first, but then encouraged them to get good health care and to sign up for a program that would help them to stay in school and still have the baby. The next spring Sarita was born. She was a healthy, beautiful 7 lb, 6 oz newborn. Jeff stayed in town and commuted to a local college. Pam lived with her older sister and finished high school. When Sarita was 5 years old, Pam and Jeff moved in together and married.

A year after they were married, Pam and Jeff had a son, Paul. Jeff was now employed at the local electric company and Pam worked part-time in a law office. Sarita was starting kindergarten. Their extended families have been involved and supportive.

Paul is now 6 years old. He has been referred to occupational therapy for problems with learning, behavior, and attention. He has been very disruptive in kindergarten class. His parents report that he is constantly crying or screaming at home. He seems fearful when you meet him.

Your testing reveals tactile, visual, and auditory processing deficits and delays in all areas of development. Your observations at school and home confirm the parent and teacher reports. You have noticed that Paul does not often maintain eye contact and that he resists both deep and light touch, even from his parents. While you were working on a dressing task, you notice bruises on his arms, as though someone had held him too tightly, and scratches on his neck and back. Pam reports that Jeff is often away from home, that they are fighting frequently, and that he is impatient with the children. Pam seems to shift from being very alert to being inattentive or even sleepy. She seems to have lost a great deal of weight in the few weeks you've known her, and her complexion is sallow. She wears only long-sleeved, high-necked clothing, even though it is summertime. She often wears dark glasses, even when she is indoors. When you called the doctor's office to discuss your findings, you learned that Paul and Sarita have not been to the doctor for their annual physical examination that was scheduled for 3 months ago.

1. What do you think might be causing Paul's problems? List three possible causes.
2. From the above information, list three risks or vulnerabilities.
3. From the above information, list three protective factors.
4. What additional information would you like to have?
5. What occupational therapy interventions would you recommend at this point?
6. What feelings do you have about this family?
7. Who might you discuss these feelings with?

## Real-Life Lab

1. Visit a local preschool program or child development center and, with the permission of teachers and parents, practice using the various observation strategies provided. Start with children whose development and behavior are typical for their age range.

2. Make up some notes for yourself about which observation strategies provide which types of information. Try to write a brief narrative description on these observation tools.

3. Try the same observation strategies and activities for:

   a. A child in his or her home environment

   b. A child in a hospital environment

   c. A child whose development and behavior are atypical

4. Try using the interview about reading with a child you know.

5. Ask a child to tell you a story.

6. Tell a story to a child.
7. Listen to a professional storyteller.
8. Go to the children's section in the library or bookstore. Sit on the floor. *Read.*
9. Go to a great children's toy store. Get on the floor. *Play.*

# References

Answorth, M. (1979). Infant mother attachment. *American Psychologist, 34,* 932–937.

Ayres, J. (1979). *Sensory integration and the child.* Los Angeles: WPS.

Barnard, K. E., Morisett, C. E., & Spieker, S. (1993). Preventive intervention: Enhancing parent-infant relationships. In Zenach, C. H. (Ed.), *Handbook of infant mental health* (pp. 386–401). New York: Guilford Press.

Bauchner, H. (1996). Failure to thrive. In Behrman, R. E., Klugman, R. M., & Arvin, A. M. (Eds.), *Nelson textbook of pediatrics* (p. 122). Philadelphia: W. B. Saunders.

Beaty, J. (1990). *Observing the development of the young child.* New York: Merrill.

Begun, A. (1996). Family systems and family centered care. In Rosin, P., Whitehead, A. D., Tuchman, L. I., Jesien, G. S., Begun, A. L., & Irwin, L. (Eds.), *Partnerships in family centered care: A guide to collaborative early intervention* (pp. 33–65). Baltimore: Brooks.

Black, J. K., Puckett, M. B., & Belle, M. J. (1992). *The young child: Development from prebirth to age eight.* New York: Macmillan.

Bolding, D., & Forman, M. A. Impact of violence. In Behrman, R. E., Klugman, R. M., & Arvin, A. M. (Eds.), *Nelson textbook of pediatrics* (p. 112). Philadelphia: W. B. Saunders.

Burke, J. (1993). Play: The life role of the infant and young child. In Case-Smith, J. (Ed.), *Pediatric occupational therapy and early intervention* (pp. 198–224). Boston: Andover.

Christiansen, C., & Baum, C. (1991). *Occupational therapy.* Thorofare, NJ: Slack.

Crockenberg, S., Lyons-Ruth, K., & Dickstein, S. (1993). The family context of infant mental health: II. Infant development in multiple family relationships. In Zenach, C. H. (Ed.), *Handbook of infant mental health* (pp. 38–55). New York: Guilford Press.

Csikszentimhalyi, M. (1990). *Flow: The psychology of the optimal experience.* New York: Harper Collins.

DeMause, L. (Ed.) (1974). *The history of childhood.* New York: Harper & Row.

Egeland, B., & Farber, E. (1984). Infant mother attachment: Factors related to its development and changes over time. *Child Development, 55,* 753–771.

Freier, M. C., Griffin, D. R., & Chasnoff, I. J. (1991). In utero drug exposure: developmental flu and maternal infant interaction. *Seminars in Perinatology, 15,* 310–316.

Garbanno, J., Stoff, F. M., and the Faculty of the Erikson Institute. (1996). *What children can tell us.* San Francisco: Jossey-Bass.

Garbarino, J. (1990). The human ecology of early risk. In Meisels, S. J. & Shonkoff, J. P. (Eds.), *Handbook of early intervention.* Cambridge: Cambridge University Press.

Halpern, R. (1993). Poverty and infant development. In Zenach, C. H. (Ed.), *Handbook of infant mental health* (pp. 73–86). New York: Guilford Press.

Havighurst, R. J. (1972). *Developmental tasks and education* (3rd ed.) New York: Longman.

Hunter, J. G., & Powell, G. F. (1990). Failure to thrive. In Semmler, C. J., & Hunter, J. G. (Eds.), *Early occupational therapy intervention* (pp. 185–196). Gaithersburg, MD: Aspen.

Johnson, C. F. (1997). Abuse and neglect of children. In Behrman, R. E., Klugman, R. M., & Arvin, A. M. (Eds.), *Nelson textbook of pediatrics* (pp. 112–119). Philadelphia: W. B. Saunders.

Kielhofner, G. (1995). *A model of human occupation theory and application,* (2nd ed.). Baltimore: Williams & Wilkins.

Lefrancois, G. R. (1993). *The lifespan,* (4th ed.). Belmont, CA: Wadsworth.

Mattingly, C., & Fleming, M. H. (1994). *Clinical reasoning: Forms of inquiry in a therapeutic practice.* Philadelphia: F.A. Davis.

Miller, H. (1997). Prenatal cocaine exposure and other-infant interaction: implications for occupational therapy intervention. *American Journal of Occupational Therapy, 51* (2), 119–131.

Mrazek, P. J. Maltreatment and infant development. In Zenach, C. H. (Ed.) (1993). *Handbook of infant mental health* (pp. 159–170). New York: The Guilford Press.

Osofsky, J. D., & Fenichel, E. (Eds.) (1996). Islands of safety: Assessing and treating young victims of violence [special issue]. *Zero to Three, 16* (5).

Raffi (Performer). (1993). Will I ever grow up. In *Raffi on Broadway: A family concert* (CD, MCAD 10709; Cassette, MCAC 10709). Universal City, CA: MCA Records.

Rosin, P., Whitehead, A. D., Tuchman, L. I., Jesien, G. S., Begun, A. L., & Irwin, L. (1996). *Partnerships in family centered care: a guide to collaborative early intervention.* Baltimore: Brooks.

Scarr, S., & McCartney, L. (1983). How people make their own environment. *Child Development, 54,* 424–435.

Schiamberg, L. B. (1988). *Child and adolescent development.* New York: Macmillan.

Schickendanz, J. A., Schickendanz, D. I., Hansen, K., & Forsyth, P. D. (1993). *Understanding children.* Mountain View, CA: Mayfield.

Seifer, R., & Dickstein, S. (1993). Parental mental illness and infant development. In Zenach, C. H. (Ed.), *Handbook of infant mental health* (pp. 120–142). New York: Guilford Press.

Semmler, C. J. (1990). Child abuse and neglect. In Semmler, C. J., & Hunter, J. G. (Eds.), *Early occupational therapy intervention* (pp. 197–217). Gaithersburg, MD: Aspen.

Sweeney, C. (1995). Portrait of the American child. *The New York Times Magazine,* October 8.

Werner, E. E. (1990). Protective factors and individual resilience. In Meisels, S. J. & Shonkoff, J. P. (Eds.), *Handbook of early intervention.* Cambridge: Cambridge University Press.

Wood, W. (1996). Legitimizing occupational therapists' knowledge. *American Journal of Occupational Therapy, 50,* 626–634.

Zeanah, C. H. (Ed.) (1993). *Handbook of infant mental health.* New York: Guilford Press.

Zeanah, C. H., Mammen, O. K., & Lieberman, A. F. (1993). Disorders of attachment. In Zeanah, C. H. (Ed.), *Handbook of infant mental health* (pp. 332–349). New York: Guilford Press.

Zemke, R., & Clark, F. (Eds.) (1996). *Occupational science the evolving discipline.* Philadelphia: F. A. Davis.

Zigler, E., Hopper, P., & Hall, N. W. (1993). Infant mental health and social policy. In Zenach, C. H. (Ed.), *Handbook of infant mental health* (pp. 480–492). New York: Guilford Press.

Zuckerman, B., & Brown, E. B. (1993). Maternal substance abuse and infant development. In Zenach, C. H. (Ed.), *Handbook of infant mental health* (pp. 143–158). New York: Guilford Press.

# *Appendix 3–1*

Table 1  **Risk Factors for Child Maltreatment**

| Characteristics of the Caregiver | Characteristics of the Immediate Environment | Characteristics of the Community | Characteristics of the Culture or Society |
|---|---|---|---|
| *Compensatory Factors* | | | |
| High IQ Awareness of past abuse History of a positive relationship with one parent Special talents Physical attractiveness Good interpersonal skills | Healthy children Supportive spouse Economic security/ savings in the bank | Good social supports Few stressful events Strong, supportive religious affiliation Positive school experiences and peer relations as a child Therapeutic interventions | Culture that promotes a sense of shared responsibility in caring for the community's children Culture opposed to violence Economic prosperity |
| *Risk Factors* | | | |
| History of abuse Low self-esteem Low IQ Poor interpersonal skills | Marital discord Children with behavior problems Premature or unhealthy children Single parent Poverty | Unemployment Isolation; poor social supports Poor peer relations as a child | Cultural acceptance of corporal punishment View of children as possessions Economic depression |

*Source:* Schickendanz et al., 1993.

Table 2  **Physical Indicators of Child Abuse for Medical Professionals**

The following injuries and conditions are often seen in cases of abuse or neglect. These warning signals or indicators should be considered in light of explanations provided, medical history (especially if inconsistent), and the developmental abilities of the child to engage in activities that might have caused the injury.

**Bruises and welts that may be indicators of physical abuse:**

Bruises on any infant, especially facial bruises.

Bruises on the posterior side of a child's body.

Bruises in unusual patterns that might reflect the pattern of the instrument used, or human bite marks.

Clustered bruises indicating repeated contact with a hand or instrument.

Bruises in various stages of healing.

**Burns:**

Immersion burns indicating dunking in a hot liquid ("sock" or "glove" burns on the arms or legs or "doughnut" shaped burns of the buttocks and genitalia).

Cigarette burns.

Rope burns that indicate confinement.

Dry burns indicating that a child has been forced to sit upon a hot surface or has had a hot implement applied to the skin.

**Lacerations and abrasions:**

Lacerations of the lip, eye, or any portion of an infant's face.

Any laceration or abrasion to external genitalia.

**Skeletal injuries:**

Rib fractures.

Fracture of the mandible, sternum or scapulae.

Skull trauma.

Spinal shaft fracture or spinal trauma.

Recurrent injury to same site.

Injuries caused by twisting or pulling:

Metaphyseal or corner fractures of long bones;

Epiphyseal separation;

Periosteal elevation;

Spiral fractures.

**Head injuries:**

Absence of hair and/or hemorrhaging beneath the scalp due to vigorous hair pulling.

Subdural hematomas—hemorrhaging beneath the outer covering of the brain (due to shaking or hitting).

Retinal hemorrhages or detachments (due to shaking).

Jaw and nasal fractures.

Loosened or missing teeth.

**Internal injuries caused by blows to midline of abdomen:**

Duodenal or jejunal hematomas.

Rupture of the inferior vena cava.

Peritonitis—inflammation of the lining of the abdominal cavity.

Laceration of liver, spleen, or pancreas.

Renal injury.

Rigid abdomen; tenderness in abdomen.

*Source:* From the National Center for Child Abuse and Neglect Specialized Training.

---

## Table 3  Behavior Indicators of Child Abuse

Children who are abused physically or emotionally display certain types of behavior. Many of these are common to all children at one time or another, but when they are present in sufficient number and strength to characterize a child's overall manner, they may indicate abuse. More than simple reactions to abuse itself, these behaviors reflect the child's response to the dynamics of the family. Children learn to deny, suppress, or exaggerate parts of themselves as they struggle to get their needs met the best way they can in a disturbed, stressful household. These learned survival mechanisms become a child's "mode of operation" used to cope with the world at large. The behaviors which characterize abused children fall into four categories:

Overly compliant, passive, undemanding behaviors aimed at maintaining a low profile, avoiding any possible confrontation with a parent which could lead to abuse. The child has adapted to the abusive situation by trying to avoid any behavior which the abusive parent notices at all.

Extremely aggressive, demanding and rageful behaviors, sometimes hyperactive, caused by the child's repeated frustrations at not getting basic needs met. The child has adapted by seeking to provoke the needed attention with whatever behavior it takes to get that attention.

Role-reversed "parental" behavior, or extremely dependent behavior. Abusive parents have been unable to satisfy certain of their own needs appropriately and so turn to their children for fulfillment, which can produce two opposite sets of behavior in the children. If a parent needs parental attention, the child may be expected to assume this task, and become inappropriately adult and responsible. Other parents, with a need to keep their child dependent, will produce clinging, babyish behavior in the child long after a child in a healthy family would have become more self-reliant.

Lags in development. Children who are forced to siphon off energy, normally channeled towards growth, into protecting themselves from abusive parents may fall behind the norm for their age in toilet training, motor skills, socialization and language development. Developmental lags may also be the result of central nervous system damage caused by physical abuse, medical or nutritional neglect or inadequate stimulation. There may, of course, be organic or congenital causes for such lags in development.

Some abused children live in an uncertain environment where requirements for behavior are inconsistent and unclear. In some families, abuse is frequent and severe enough to be emotionally and physically harmful but insufficient to threaten physical survival. Frequently, discipline is meted out arbitrarily in response to the parent's needs and feelings at the moment, rather than to punish a child for transgressing clear limits. Children may receive some love, affection and security from their parents but are also often frustrated in attempts to fulfill their needs. This inconsistency creates anger and frustration in the child which is frequently expressed indirectly with the parents, or by explosions with others outside the home.

Other abused children have learned to do what the abusive parent wants or expects. At the other end of the spectrum from overly aggressive children, some adapt quickly to others' expectations. Unlike children who act out their frustration and

*Continued on following page*

## Table 3  **Behavior Indicators of Child Abuse—*Continued***

rage, these children may have learned not to expect anything in the way of love or support. Their best efforts are directed at avoiding conflict which, in the context of the abusive family, can be triggered by expressing almost any kind of personal need, curiosity, anger or playfulness.

Ultimately, a list of specific behaviors to identify child abuse is useful only if the family dynamics which produce those behaviors are clearly understood. The behaviors, verbal and physical, indicate both the survival techniques the child has learned in order to exist in the family, and attempts—frequently inappropriate in kind or intensity—to get from others what the parents do not provide. The greater the abuse, the less the child will trust other people and the greater the child's difficulty in responding to love and care.

*Source:* From the National Center for Child Abuse and Neglect Specialized Training.

## Table 4  **Indicators of Sexual Abuse**

**Physical indicators**
>    Difficulty in walking or sitting
>    Torn, stained, or bloody underclothing
>    Pain or itching in genital area
>    Bruises or bleeding in external genitalia, vaginal, or anal areas
>    Venereal disease
>    Pregnancy

**Behavioral indicators**
>    Unwilling to change for gym or participate in physical education class
>    Withdrawn, regressive, or infantile
>    Sophisticated or unusual sexual behavior or knowledge
>    Poor peer relationships
>    Delinquent; truant; runaway
>    Reports sexual assault by caretaker

*Source:* From the National Center for Child Abuse and Neglect Specialized Training.

Table 5 **Indicators of Child Neglect**

**Lack of supervision**
  Very young children left unattended
  Children left in the care of other children too young to protect them
  Children inadequately supervised for long periods of time or when engaged in
    dangerous activities
**Lack of adequate clothing and good hygiene**
  Children dressed inadequately for the weather
  Persistent skin disorders resulting from improper hygiene
  Children chronically dirty and unbathed
**Lack of medical or dental care**
  Children whose needs for medical or dental care or medication
    and health aids are unmet
**Lack of adequate education**
  Children who are chronically absent from school
**Lack of adequate nutrition**
  Children lacking sufficient quantity or quality of food
  Children consistently complaining of hunger or rummaging
    for food
  Children suffering severe developmental lags
**Lack of adequate shelter**
  Structurally unsafe housing or exposed wiring
  Inadequate heating
  Unsanitary housing conditions
**In identifying neglect, be sensitive to:**
  Differing cultural expectations and values.
  Differing child-rearing practices.
  Issues of poverty vs. neglect. Neglect is not necessarily related
    to poverty; it reflects a breakdown in household management,
    a breakdown of concern for and caretaking of the child.

*Source:* From the National Center for Child Abuse and Neglect Specialized Training.

---

Table 6 **Characteristics of Abuse Families**

---

We all have the capacity to strike out in anger, fear, pain or frustration and this capability defines all of us as potential child abusers. Yet most of use are able to control these violent impulses. This profile concerns the broad categories of experience and dynamics that contribute to the abusive parent's inability to control these impulses. An increasingly comprehensive and authoritative body of literature defines seven general problem areas: 1) unfulfilled needs for nurturance and dependence, 2) fear of relationships, 3) lack of support systems, 4) marital problems, 5) life crises, 6) inability to care for or protect a child, and 7) lack of nurturing child-rearing practices. The following is not intended as a definitive profile of factors contributing to physical abuse. Rather, it is designed as an overview and reference guide to the special problems which can contribute to abusive behavior.

THE INFLUENCE OF PERSONAL FACTORS

| | |
|---|---|
| Unfulfilled Needs for Nurturance and Dependence | Many abusive parents were significantly and consistently deprived of emotional support as children. They were unable to depend consistently on the adults in their lives for support, physical or emotional care, or love. The abusive parent's own needs to be parented were essentially unsatisfied. These unmet needs may carry over into adulthood and shape relations with family, friends and especially children. Fear, frustration and anger are associated with these unmet needs and abusive parents are more likely to act on impulses. The degree of fear, frustration and anger generally corresponds to the level of deprivation experienced in childhood. |

Abusive parents often lack the skills and abilities necessary to provide emotionally for themselves. They have not learned to identify and obtain the emotional support they need from others nor have they learned how to cope with the anger, fear and frustration they feel in relation to these unmet needs. As a result they experience a severe lack of self-esteem or sense of self-worth. Abusive parents feel unloved, unappreciated and unwanted. This negative self-image often leads to perceptions of themselves as insignificant, unattractive or stupid.

Low self-esteem can lead to low expectations. Abusive parents are likely to expect, even to invite rejection. A vicious cycle of negative self-image may lead to behavior which denies satisfying or fulfilling relationships with others. Some of this behavior is focused on avoiding most social interactions as a method of avoiding rejection and failure. Other, more aggressive or offensive behaviors may actually provoke rejection—abusive parents may actually make themselves difficult to like.

While they still desperately need the support and reinforcement denied during childhood, they are at a loss as to how to achieve it, and may, in fact, act in ways which serve to deny them the sense of belonging and worth they so strongly need.

In addition, many abusive parents were themselves physically

*Continued on following page*

Table 6 **Characteristics of Abuse Families—*Continued***

|  |  |
|---|---|
|  | or sexually abused as children. They tend to accept extreme forms of physical punishment as normal aspects of parent-child interactions. |
| Isolation | Abusive parents expect very little from others in the way of friendship or support. They avoid rejection and anger by breaking off close personal relationships. They avoid committing themselves to caring relationships with neighbors, friends, and even family. They are afraid to reach out to make contact. If both parents have a sense of personal isolation, the problem is compounded. The family will be cut off from all outside sources of support. This internal dependency exerts added pressures on the family unit which may further increase the likelihood of abuse. |
| Lack of Ability to Care for and Protect a Child | The abused child may fill one of many roles in the family and in a parent's life. She/he may represent an attempt on the parent's part to fulfill needs for love, acceptance and dependence. This situation constitutes a type of role-reversal in which the child becomes the nurturer of the parent, the life-giver. When the child is unable to fulfill the parent's emotional needs, the resulting frustration and disappointment can lead to abuse. |
|  | The child may also be perceived by the parents as an extension of self. The parent's lack of self-esteem and negative self-image may be projected onto the child as well. The child becomes a scapegoat and is made to pay for the parent's sense of inadequacy and failure. |
|  | The special child—one who is mentally, physically or developmentally handicapped and may have special needs or require extra parental attention—may provoke feelings of resentment in the parent. In these cases, parent-child bonds may be too weak to protect the child from parental frustration and anger. In addition, the children may react to abusive dynamics in the family by developing personality or behavior traits that are unattractive. These traits may actually heighten the likelihood of abuse and place these children in constant danger. |
| Lack of Nurturing Child-Rearing Practices | Abuse may also be contingent on the child-rearing practices used by the family. Child-rearing skills are acquired by observing family, social and cultural role models. Abuse may result from child-rearing practices which, while considered unacceptable by community standards, are seen as normal within the family unit. |
|  | Various cultures and sub-cultures have a variety of child-rearing patterns and methods of punishment which are considered appropriate for unacceptable behavior. These methods may be passed from generation to generation even after they become unacceptable by community standards. In some cases, these punishment practices can result in injuries or conditions that are considered abusive by the community even though the family may consider them to be normal child-rearing. |

*Continued on following page*

## Table 6  **Characteristics of Abuse Families—*Continued***

| | |
|---|---|
| Unrealistic Expectations | In addition, parents may have unrealistic expectations of a child's developmental abilities. They may be unfamiliar with what a child can be expected to do at a certain age. Punishment is inevitable when a child fails to meet inappropriate expectations. In other cases, performance or developmental standards may reflect parental attempts to control the child. The parent may be acting out a need for dominance by demanding high levels of performance from a child. When the child fails to perform at these inflated levels, the parent's frustration results in abuse. |

It is important, in looking at this kind of overview and reference guide for the special problems which can contribute to abusive behavior, to recognize that no one abuser suffers from all of the problems noted, nor does any one abuser have all of the characteristics cited. Some characteristics are even contradictory. Abusers do, however, tend to have a number of problems and characteristics in common and represented here.

### THE INFLUENCE OF ENVIRONMENTAL FACTORS

| | |
|---|---|
| Lack of Support Systems | Frequently, abusive parents are emotionally unable to establish or utilize outside support systems even when the opportunity is available. They have not learned how to ask for and receive the kind of help they need to provide for themselves and their children. This inability intensifies the danger in times of crisis. With outside lifelines cut off, the abusive parent has nowhere to turn during periods of heightened stress. Often, it is during these periods that the potential abuser becomes the actual abuser. |
| Marital Problems | The lack of support systems often extends to marital relationships. Abusive parents frequently find themselves locked into a non-nurturing, noncommunicative marriage in which neither spouse is able to support or adequately meet the other's needs. Children are involved in the process of the parents' acting-out of anger and frustration. The child may be ignored or abandoned because he constitutes a painful reminder of marital dissatisfaction. A child who reminds one parent of the other may become the target of displaced anger. The parents may use the child as a seesaw, tugging and pulling at both ends for attention. Mutual abuse of a child may represent the only common ground established between parents. Regardless of the dynamics, the child becomes a conduit for indirect, often angry communications between two frustrated adults. If physical violence is part of parental interaction, this violence is likely to extend to the child as well. A pattern is established in which frustrations are dealt with physically and restraint of impulses to physically violent behavior is diminished by all family interactions. |
| Life Crises | External stress is frequently a contributing factor in abuse. Loss of employment or housing, lack of food or clothing, indebtedness, or any domestic crisis which precipitates fear |

*Continued on following page*

## Table 6 **Characteristics of Abuse Families—*Continued***

or anxiety, can push the parents into abuse. Significant personal loss such as the death of a close relative or the relocation of a friend or neighbor can strip the parent of precious support mechanisms, heighten the sense of futility and create a feeling of inability to control one's own life. This loss of control can in turn lead to abuse and neglect.

On the other hand, external stress can be a way of life for some abusive families. Some families are crisis-ridden; it is a life-style posture. Everything is a crisis; and the parents are unable to deal with daily pressures or control their environment.

*Source:* From the National Center for Child Abuse and Neglect Specialized Training.

## Table 7 **OT Role in Child Maltreatment**

- Educating oneself and one's colleagues about child maltreatment
- Reporting cases of suspected abuse of neglect, as required by law
- Evaluating and treating abused or neglected children
- Educating and training the biological, foster, or adoptive parents about their child's special needs
- Preadoption assessments of special needs infants
- Providing records or consulting reports for court testimony
- Testifying in court
- Researching the implications of abuse for children's future functioning and interventions with neglected or abused children
- Collaboration with state-mandated child protective service agency
- Participating in community activities to prevent child maltreatment

*Source:* Adapted from Semmler, C. J. (1990). Child abuse and neglect. In Semmler, C. J., & Hunter, J. G. *Early occupational therapy intervention* (pp. 185–196). Gaithersburg, MD: Aspen.

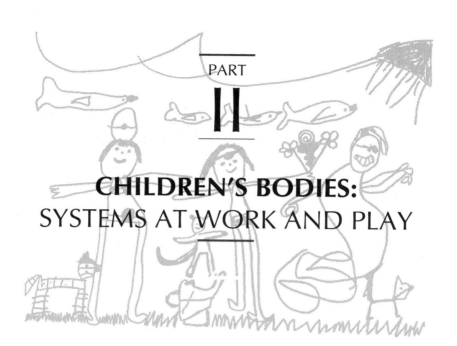

PART

II

# CHILDREN'S BODIES:
## SYSTEMS AT WORK AND PLAY

# 4

# *The Cardiovascular and the Pulmonary Systems*

Joann (Jodi) Petry, MEd, MS, OTR
Ellen Berger Rainville, MS, OTR, FAOTA

*It's hard to explain how it feels to have cystic fibrosis. Because I've had it all my life I don't know how it feels not to have it . . . If anything good has come out of having this disease, it's that it has brought our family closer together. It's made our relationship better and strengthened our ties because we have to depend on one another . . .*
—Jimmy O'Neill, age 15 (Krementz, 1991, p. 100)

*Having open-heart surgery has definitely changed my thinking. One thing I can say for sure is that now I know how to fight for my life and never give up hope . . .*
—Joseph Buck, age 14 (Krementz, 1991, p. 5)

## KEY POINTS

- Children born with heart and lung disease have a better prognosis than at any other time in history. This is in part a result of improved surgical techniques, intensive care nursing, medications, and respiratory support. Pediatric heart and/or lung disease requires that caregivers respect and understand the unique characteristics of these life-threatening illnesses. Children with heart and/or lung disease may be classified as "medically fragile."

- Most children with heart and lung disease receive hospital treatment at various times in their lives. They may also require specialized home care such as respiratory, therapeutic, and nutritional support. Therapists are quite likely to encounter these medically fragile children in their practice, in hospitals, in schools, or at home.

- As a result of their cardiac and/or pulmonary disease, or as a result of

123

repeated hospitalization, medically fragile children may experience delays or deviations in their growth and development. These areas are appropriate targets for pediatric therapy.

- Because of the complexity in managing cardiac and pulmonary disease and disability, the family may be *teaching the therapist* about the specialized care of their child. This exchange of expertise can enhance the collaborative relationship between parent(s) and professional(s).

- The severity and hence the outcome of cardiac and pulmonary disease varies considerably, so over time, children who are medically fragile may: (1) Resolve many of their problems, (2) have persistent complex medical issues, or (3) despite technological advances, have a shortened life.

- Unfortunately, children with heart and lung disease are somewhat more likely than other children to die during infancy or childhood. Therapists who work with these children may therefore experience their own grieving, as well as that of each child's family.

# BEGINNINGS

Pediatric therapists will have many opportunities to work with children with cardiac or pulmonary disease. Quite often, children with neurological, developmental, or orthopedic disability have secondary heart or lung disease. For example, approximately 40 percent of children with Down syndrome have congenital cardiac anomalies (Batshaw, 1992). Some children have central nervous system (CNS) dysfunction caused by anoxia or other complications of heart or lung disease. Also, children whose primary diagnosis is heart or lung disease may be referred directly to occupational therapy.

Referral to occupational therapy may occur early in the newborn period or at any time throughout childhood. It is important to ascertain each child's specific cardiac, pulmonary, and neurodevelopmental status. Depending on the child's age, diagnosis, family and community support, and specific occupational performance dysfunction(s), therapy is tailored to meet the unique needs of each child.

Providing therapy services for children with cardiac and/or pulmonary dysfunction does require specialized clinical skill and knowledge. To serve these children effectively, it is necessary to understand the structure and function of the heart and lungs, clinical pathology and treatment, postoperative care, and the developmental issues. Knowledge of the signs and symptoms of distress are extremely important as a precaution for successful therapeutic intervention with the child. This chapter serves as an entry point for improving the therapist's knowledge base in this domain.

# CARDIAC DISEASE

## THE CARDIAC SYSTEM

A normal pediatric heart is a hollow, muscular pump approximately the size of a child's hand fisted into the other hand. It is divided by a muscular septum into right and left sides, and valves separate each side into upper and lower chambers. The right side of the heart relates to pulmonary circulation and the left side of the heart supports systemic circulation. Deoxygenated venous blood returns to the heart into the low-pressure right atrium. The blood is then pumped through the tricuspid valve into the low-pressure right ventricle to be pumped to the lungs for oxygenation. The blood returns from the lungs into the left atrium and passes through the mitral valve into the high-pressure left ventricle. The blood is then pumped up through the aorta to the rest of the body (Fig. 4–1).

The heart has a posterior surface known as the base and an apex oriented to the left side. The inferior border runs along the bottom or diaphragm. On the left it borders the left lung and on the right it borders the right lung. The back is known as the diaphragmatic side and the front as the sternalcostal side. The heart is protected by the sternum and rib cage. In a normally functioning heart, the two sides do not directly communicate with one another. The heart's structures include the endocardium (lining of the chambers), myocardium (heart muscle), and pericardium (the area around the heart) (Moller, Neal, & Hoffmann, 1988).

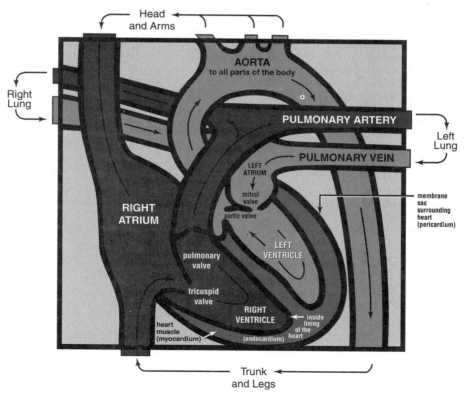

Figure 4–1 The cardiovascular system. (American Heart Association. [1995]. *Your heart and how it works.* Author, with permission.)

Table 4–1 lists some common cardiac terminology.

Typical cardiac (pulse) and respiration rates are given in Table 4–2. There will be variations in these rates following exercise or other exertion; however, sustained deviations should be reported to the physician or primary health-care provider. Many persons today are able to monitor their own pulse and respiration rates and know their limitations. This self-awareness and self-care ability is even more important for people with cardiac or respiratory disease. As a result, patient education is an important function of the health-care team.

The heart is a pump made up of specialized cardiac muscle tissue. It has four electrophysiological impulse functions that are essential to health:

1. Automatic response to stimulation with spontaneous impulses
2. Regular rhythm of impulses
3. Conductive ability (to transmit impulses)
4. Quick response to excitability, with fast response to impulses

---

Table 4–1 **Common Cardiac Terminology**

**Arrhythmia**—abnormal heart rate
  **Blood vessels:**
  **Arteries**—transport blood from the heart to the body
  **Veins**—return blood from the body to the heart
  **Capillaries**—responsible for exchange of nutrients, gases and wastes
**Blood pressure**—the force of the heart pumping blood through the arteries
**Cardiac arrest**—when the heart stops beating
**Congestive heart failure**—an accumulation of fluid in and near the heart and
  throughout the body, caused by a problem in the heart's pumping ability.
**Electrocardiogram (EKG, ECG)**—a recording of the heart's electrical impulses
**Echocardiography**—ultrasound of the heart
**Myocardial infarction**—damage to an area of the heart muscle caused by reduced
  blood flow to that area. Often referred to as a heart attack.
**Pulse**—each contraction of the heart (heart beat) is felt as a "pulse." The heart rate
  varies based on activity (increases with exercise and decreases with rest).

---

Table 4–2 **Typical Pulse and Respiration Rates**

| HEART RATE | |
| --- | --- |
| **Age** | **Beats/minute** |
| Newborn | 70–170 |
| 2-year-old | 80–130 |
| 10-year-old | 70–110 |
| Adult | 60–80 |

| RESPIRATORY RATE | |
| --- | --- |
| **Age** | **Breaths/minute** |
| Newborn | 30–80 |
| 2-year-old | 20–30 |
| 10-year-old | 17–22 |
| Adult | 15–20 |

Functional classifications of heart disease (Criteria Committee, New York Heart Association) (Mullins & Mayer, 1988) include:

I No symptoms with normal physical activity
II Symptoms with normal physical activity
III Symptoms with restricted physical activity
IV Symptoms appear at rest

Specific symptoms of heart problems include:

*Bradycardia*—A heart rate of less than 60 beats per minute
*Tachycardia*—A rapid rise in heart rate in response to sympathetic stimulation
*Tachypnea*—Rapid breathing, often because of pulmonary congestion.
*Cardiomegaly*—Enlarged heart
*Cyanosis*—A bluish discoloration of the skin, generally throughout the body, which indicates lack of oxygen

Heart disease can be congenital or acquired. Each will be discussed separately.

## CONGENITAL HEART DISEASE

Congenital heart disease (CHD) occurs in approximately 10 of every 1000 live births. It includes a number of structural abnormalities of the heart that are present at birth and that disrupt the normal circulation of blood.

Causes of CHD are generally unknown; however, cardiovascular disease has been shown to have a familial link. Prenatal environmental factors such as rubella virus or other teratogens present at the critical period of cardiac development (<55 days in utero) may also be involved. Certain genetic syndromes such as trisomy 18, trisomy 21, and Turner's syndrome include CHD.

Of children born with CHD, more than half have symptoms that are severe enough to cause death unless treated. CHD can be classified into three types of problems (Callow & Wild, 1990).

---

Types of Congenital Heart Disease

1. Disorder of a *valve* of the heart that causes circulatory difficulties and hence fatigue.
2. A *shunt* (where blood flow is diverted) from the left to the right side of the heart. This causes oxygenated blood to mix with oxygen-depleted blood. Because the left side of the heart has greater pressure, this causes an increase in the work required of the right ventricle. As a result, pulmonary congestion, increased work of breathing, and diminished blood flow to the aorta may occur.
3. A *shunt* from the right to the left side of the heart. This will reduce the pulmonary flow and result in significant cyanosis.

Table 4–3 provides a description of some common CHDs and their associated symptoms.

In infancy, many of the congenital heart defects can be treated with "palliative" surgery until sufficient growth occurs to allow total surgical repair. Medications are used to assist with heart congestion and circulation, and with respiratory support when the work of the heart is great. It is important to note that postsurgical complications may include anoxia, cerebrovascular accident (CVA), seizures, fever, and infection. Each of these may result in secondary CNS damage. The subsequent neurological, developmental, and functional problems may necessitate the services of occupational therapy and other specialties.

## ACQUIRED HEART DISEASE

Although a child may be born with a healthy heart, he or she may experience disease, often bacterial or viral, which affects cardiac function and requires specialized care. Some of the more common pediatric acquired heart diseases include:

### Cardiomyopathy

Cardiomyopathy comprises a wide range of conditions that affect the heart muscle. Arrhythmias are common symptoms. Cardiomyopathies typically fall into three categories:

1. *Obstructive.* Thickening of the heart wall that reduces outflow and increases ventricular pressure. Symptoms include chest pains and fainting.
2. *Restrictive.* Heart walls are also thickened and inflow of blood is reduced; symptoms are similar to obstructive cardiomyopathy.
3. *Congestive.* The heart becomes quite large and the child develops congestive heart failure (CHF) symptoms.

### Rheumatic Fever

Rheumatic fever is a relatively rare acute illness that follows streptococcal infection. It may affect the heart. Most commonly the valves become inflamed and may leak. Later, scarring of the valves may interfere with function. Other areas of the heart may also be affected.

### Endocarditis

Endocarditis is an inflammation, usually bacterial, that is a complication of the other types of heart disease. This disease may cause damage to the heart itself or may result in emboli passed to other organs.

## Table 4–3 **Types of Congenital Heart Defects**

| Diagnosis | Description | Symptoms |
|---|---|---|
| **VALVULAR (OBSTRUCTIVE) DISORDERS** | | |
| • Aortic stenosis | • A constriction of the aortic valve | • Abdominal pain |
| • Pulmonary stenosis | • Obstruction of blood flow into the lungs | • Distal duskiness and coolness |
| | | • Lethargy and irritability |
| **ACYANOTIC DEFECTS (L TO R) SYNDROMES** | | |
| • Aortic stenosis | • A constriction of the aortic valve | • Labored breathing, possible pulmonary edema |
| • Atrial septal defect | • A hole in the wall between the atrium | • Fatigue |
| • Coarctation of the aorta | • Constriction of the aorta | • Greater likelihood of respiratory infections |
| • Endocardial cushion defect | • Defects in the atrial or ventricular septum, or the mitral or tricuspid valves | • Poor tolerance of prone position |
| • Patent ductus arteriosis | • The ductus arteriosis (the prenatal) passage between the aorta and the pulmonary artery fails to close within 48 hours of birth | • Decreased activity tolerance |
| | | • Slow weight gain the and failure to thrive |
| • Ventricular septal defect | • A hole in the wall between the ventricle | |
| **CYANOTIC DEFECTS (R TO L) SYNDROMES** | | |
| • Transposition of the great vessels | • A congenital malformation in which the aorta comes out of the right ventricle and the pulmonary artery out of the left (the exact opposite of typical heart structure) | • Crying worsens |
| | | • Cyanosis |
| | | • Tachypnea |
| | | • Fatigue |
| • Hypoplastic left heart syndrome | • A failure of the mitral or aortic valves in which the left ventricle is too small to sustain life | • Decreased tolerance for activity and prone positioning |
| • Pulmonary stenosis | • A constriction of the pulmonary artery as it emerges from the right ventricle | • Increased work of breathing (dyspnea) with increased respiratory rate |
| • Pulmonary atresia | • Closure of the pulmonary valve (between the right ventricle and the pulmonary artery) | • Poor weight gain |
| | | • Feeding difficulties |
| • Tetralogy of Fallot | • A ventricular defect and a pulmonary stenosis | |
| • Total anomalous pulmonary venous return | • Pulmonary veins connect to the left rather than the right atrium | |
| • Tricuspid atresia | • Absence of the tricuspid valve | |

## *Pericarditis*

Pericarditis is an inflammation, usually viral, of the pericardium, which sometimes follows open heart surgery. The major symptom is chest pain. A pericardial effusion (leakage of fluid) may also occur.

## ▋▌▊ FROM THE BOOKSHELF

> Here are some well-written, clear and comprehensive books about pediatric heart disease. They are useful references for both parents and professionals.
> Moller, J. H., Neal, W. A., and Hoffman, W. R. (1988). *A parent's guide to heart disorders.* Minneapolis: University of Minnesota Press.
> Neill, C. A., Clark, E. B., & Clark, C. (1992). *The heart of a child—What families need to know about heart disorders in children.* Baltimore: John Hopkins University Press.

## THE IMPACT OF CARDIAC DISEASE ON CHILD HEALTH AND DEVELOPMENT

Children with CHD are somewhat more susceptible to respiratory and bacterial illness, in part because of frequent visits to hospitals and clinics where there are other ill children. A flu shot as well as the routine childhood immunizations, minimal exposure to crowds during cold and flu season, and good handwashing are usually recommended to decrease the risk of illness. Children with heart disease should not be exposed to passive smoke or other pollutants (Yahav, Avigad, Frand, et al., 1985).

Children with congenital heart disease are at greater risk for CVAs, hypoxic and anoxic episodes, seizures, metabolic acidosis, and fever related to infection. Their health status is generally monitored closely by health-care providers. Although many children with CHD do experience normal growth and development, their development and learning should be also carefully monitored.

Perhaps in an effort to prevent cardiac stress, children with CHD have a tendency to remain sedentary even after successful repair or resolution of the cardiac disease process. Families also have a tendency to support restricted gross motor activity long after acute illness (D'Antonio, 1979). This is not necessary. A child's response to motor activity will vary. Activity should be gradually introduced and reactions carefully monitored. Callow (1995) reports that a child with CHD will typically realize the limits of his or her own body and stop to rest. Usual childhood activities such as riding a bike, swimming, and playing on a playground can be enjoyed without worry (Barton et al., 1994). Some gross-motor activities such as prolonged walking can remain fatiguing long after other activities are possible. Amusement park rides usually require some restrictions, as do contact competitive sports. Travel is also possible. With some cardiac diseases, however, flying may require in-flight oxygen.

The role of the pediatric OT varies depending on the strengths and needs of each individual child. However, occupational therapy can assist with stress management, energy conservation, strength and endurance training for functional activities, activity pacing, and developmental support. A child's ability to know his or her own disease and its impact enables the child to make choices about occupations. Knowledge also helps reduce the fears of others in the child's environment. For example, a simple inservice for classmates and teachers cannot only increase their understanding of and comfort with the child but can also provide constructive strategies to promote the child's best function within the classroom and playground.

Children with heart and lung disease will hopefully participate in school and community activities with their peers. Therapy, therefore, has a role in multiple settings.

---

■ *THERAPEDS POINTER*

Here's another helpful resource.
CHASER: Congenital Heart Anomalies Support Education &
    Resources

This is a national resource for the parent of a child with CHD. Families can be linked by a database and national registry to obtain information regarding local, state, and national resources. CHASER can be reached at 2112 North Wilkins Road, Swauton, OH 43558, (419) 825–5575

---

## INTERVENTIONS

### *The Child*

For the child with heart disease, keeping up with other children may be a challenge. Also, trying to manage multiple medical interventions, medications, and surgeries makes it more difficult to be a part of the "gang." Children with heart disease need strategies that will help them feel capable of those activities that interest and motivate them, even though they may need some special supports or have some restriction. Here's an example.

---

■ *THE STUDENT AND THE SITUATION*

A 10-year-old boy with multiple cardiac problems who also has age-level developmental and learning abilities, is seen by his teachers and classmates as whiny, lazy, and too easily tired. His participation in recess and after-school recreational activities has been minimal, and recently he seems to be withdrawing from others in the classroom.

### Possible Strategies and Solutions

1. Arrange an inservice (to be planned and presented with the child) for peers and teachers about the typical heart and about heart disease.
   a. Review typical cardiac symptoms and the physical demands that may cause fatigue, discomfort, or other problems.
   b. Teach the children about energy conservation techniques and other relevant prevention and health promotion strategies.
   c. Brainstorm about and discuss some ways that teachers and children can help the child with heart disease to conserve energy, pace activity, and develop strength and endurance.
2. Develop some fun group activities (perhaps in consultation with the physical education teacher) that children can do to increase their strength and endurance and to monitor their safe energy expenditure.
3. Develop "charts" that children can fill out to track their "training" activities.
4. Work with the child's parents to develop an understanding of their child's realistic capabilities and responses to his or her heart disease.
5. Develop strategies for grading and pacing activities so that the child can be as independent as possible without exacerbating symptoms. For example,
   a. Help the child select his or her clothing the night before. Select simple clothes that are easy to put on and take off (e.g., sneakers with Velcro closures, sweat pants).
   b. Wake the child a little earlier to allow sufficient time to incorporate rest into the morning routine. First, wash up and rest, then dress and rest, then eat and rest.
6. Develop a "buddy" system for helping the child with heart disease (and other students) to implement the ideas for energy conservation and symptom management generated by teacher and students.

## The Parent or Caregiver

A major concern of caregivers is to provide the most normal experiences of childhood without causing disease-related problems. Reaching a balance between overprotection and risk is a real challenge. The daily living tasks of parents and caregivers are appropriate targets of occupational therapy interventions. This is an example where occupational therapy interventions are focused on the occupations of parenting.

| Child Characteristic | Adult or Parent Issue | Possible Strategy or Solution |
|---|---|---|
| 10-year-old becomes too exhausted to dress himself each morning. Before school he usually cries because he is too tired to eat and often has chest pain and discomfort. | Concerns that parents' expectations for child may be creating disease symptoms. | 1. Teach parents about energy conservation techniques. 2. Provide multiple sources of information on heart disease, including diagnosis, prognosis, symptoms. 3. Refer parents for peer support through meeting other "cardiac" parents one to one or in support groups. |

■ *THERAPEDS POINTER: THE PSYCHOSOCIAL ASPECTS OF REPEATED HOSPITALIZATION*

Hospitalization early in life, sometimes at a distant hospital, has significant effects. Families will experience a multitude of emotions. Repeated adjustment and readjustment to disease, treatment, and disability can be challenging and stressful for families. Fear of death may be legitimate. Support and education are essential.

Consideration of each child's developmental level can help you to understand the family's perspective. The preschool child has a limited understanding of body function, which complicates treatment (Rybski & Gisel, 1984). For example, magical thinking, prevalent at this age, may produce pain and fears of death. At this age stress may result in developmental regressions, such as thumb sucking and loss of toileting skill (Shaker, 1990). The center of a preschool child's world is his or her family. Their support and guidance are essential.

The school-age child is concerned with peers and social contact. Because of their disease, children with CHD may face rejection and isolation. With each rehospitalization, children this age may withdraw, sleep more frequently, want to postpone rehospitalization, or intellectualize or physically resist it. The adolescent may fear loss of adult activities, and may experience regression, depression, and antisocial behaviors. An unnatural preoccupation with the procedure or illness may result (Wolf & Glass, 1992). Bowen (1985) offers a protocol for working with adolescents. The uncertainty of prognosis presents a dilemma for some families. The enormity of information they must deal with can be overwhelming. Not only must they contend with the ill child, but they must also attend to other family members, finances, and survival. Multifaceted support and education for children and their care-givers is essential.

Prolonged hospitalization can result in

- Delayed developmental progression
- Sensory and motor deprivation
- Poor strength and endurance for physical activity
- Physical deconditioning

Interventions need to be oriented toward preventing these undesir-able outcomes.

# PULMONARY DISEASE

## THE RESPIRATORY SYSTEM

The human respiratory system is divided into the upper and lower respira-tory tracts. The upper respiratory tract consists of the nose, mouth, throat, esophagus, and trachea. Its primary function is to "filter, warm and humid-ify inspired air" (Swanson & Brown, 1992, p. 69). The lower respiratory tract begins at the larynx and extends through the lungs (Fig. 4–2).

The function of the respiratory system is to exchange gases between blood and the air that we breathe. The heart then pumps the blood throughout the body. In typical pulmonary function, ventilation is the movement of air in and out of the lungs through the specific interactions of the lungs, rib cage, and res-piratory muscles. These muscles include the intercostals and accessory mus-cles and the diagphragm and abdominal muscles. A good example of this in-terdependence can be found in Wasserman et al. (1987, p. 2). Ribs serve as moving levers with fulcrums at the costotransverse articulation by increasing the anteroposterior size of the thorax with inspiration. Distortion of this move-ment by conditions such as scoliosis, spasticity, congenital diaphragmatic her-nia, and bronochopulmonary dysplasia change respiratory function.

Perfusion is blood flow through the lungs. Both ventilation and perfu-sion are essential to normal pulmonary function. A mismatch between venti-lation and perfusion leads to decreased oxygenation and, hence, pulmonary dysfunction.

Some genetic syndromes are associated with abnormal respiratory struc-tures. These include De Lange's syndrome, cleft lip and/or palate, Pierre Robin syndrome, Treacher Collins syndrome, and the trisomies. Disorders of the CNS may affect the control of breathing, as will congenital disorders of the chest wall and musculature. Other respiratory disorders are usually ac-quired. Other disease processes may cause respiratory dysfunction as well. Chest cysts, tumors, or malformations (such as scoliosis) may result in per-manent damage with residual respiratory problems. Table 4–4 provides some common respiratory terminology.

Pulmonary dysfunction falls into two main categories: obstructive and restrictive.

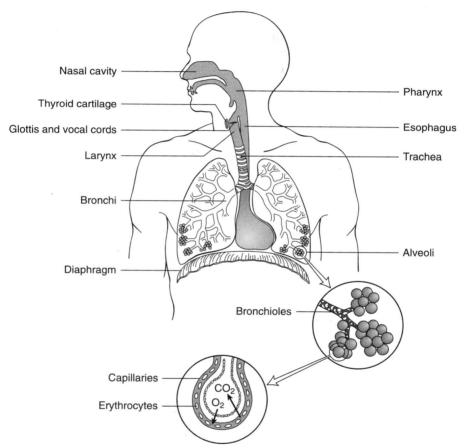

Figure 4–2 The pulmonary system. (Adapted from Chabner, D-E. [1996]. *The language of medicine*. Philadelphia: W.B. Saunders.)

Table 4–4 **Common Respiratory Terminology**

---

**Anoxia**—absence of oxygen in the blood
**Apnea**—absence of spontaneous breathing
**Breath Sounds**—during breathing, unusual sounds may be heard. These
  include:
  **Stridor**—a high-pitched, harsh sound
  **Wheezing**—a whistling sound
  **Grunting**—an expulsive sound
**Dyspnea**—decreased respiratory rate
**Hypoxemia**—decreased oxygen in the blood
**Lung compliance**—distensibility
**Nasal flaring**—exaggerated, effortful, opening of the nostrils in order to make the
  airway larger
**Negative inspiratory force**—the amount of muscle force necessary to take a deep
  breath
**Oxyhemoglobin saturation**—the amount of hemoglobin molecules bound to
  oxygen - an indirect measure of oxygenation
**Respiratory arrest**—breathing stops
**Respiratory rate**—the speed and rhythm of breathing
**Retractions**—sucking inward of the skin in the dorsal upper chest area indicating
  the use of accessory muscles
**Shortness of breath**—gasping for air, unable to fill lungs with air automatically,
  getting "winded"
**Tachypnea**—increased respiratory rate
**Tidal volume**—amount of air breathed in or out while at rest
**Vital capacity**—An indicator of pulmonary reserve, the amount of air that can be
  inhaled or exhaled with maximum effort
**Work of breathing (WOB)**—related to lung compliance as well as resistance to
  airflow, the work of breathing changes when the airway structure or function
  changes

---

# OBSTRUCTIVE LUNG DISEASE

*Obstructive impairments* indicate an increase in resistance to airflow through the lungs in two ways: (1) excessive pressure during expiratory airflow and (2) resistance encountered in narrowed airways. With obstructive disease, residual lung volume (air remaining after exhaling) is increased because air is trapped, thus resulting in less of the lung being available for breathing. Symptoms of obstructive processes include tachypnea, accessory muscle use, retraction, and nasal flaring. Narrowing of the airways can occur from an increase in mucus, bronchospasms, thickening of the walls of the airway, or inflammation. Children may experience one of the three types of chronic obstructive lung conditions:

- Asthma
- Bronchiectasis
- Cystic fibrosis

## Asthma

*Asthma* results from increased responsiveness to the stimulation of the tracheobronchial tree by a variety of stimuli. It is manifested as wheezing, coughing, dyspnea (labored breathing), and a failure to expel air completely. Asthma occurs in acute episodes between relatively symptom-free periods. Airway reactivity is increased to both internal and external stimuli with hyperinflation of the lungs and narrowing of the airway. Asthma may be triggered by airborn allergens, exercise, cold, and stress, either emotional, environmental, occupational, or pharmacological. Young children can have respiratory syncytial virus (RSV) and rhinoviruses that can precipitate attacks (Balfour et al., 1991). Prolonged asthma symptoms can leave a person exhausted from the work of breathing and sleep deprivation.

## Bronchiectasis

*Bronchiectasis* is chronic dilation (greater than four times normal size) of the bronchi with distortion of one or more bronchi. This is characterized by a persistent cough with mucopurulent sputum, recurrent pulmonary infections, and hemoptysis. In bronchiectasis, as the mucous glands dilate, necrotizing infection spreads. This damages the epithelial lining, elastic tissue, smooth muscle, and cartilage, and results in fibrosis or scarring. About 30 percent of the time bronchiectasis is bilateral in manifestion, affecting the lower lobes, usually the right more than the left. Daily hydration is essential for assisting with the thinning of secretions (Callow, 1995).

## Cystic Fibrosis

*Cystic fibrosis* (CF) is the most common life-threatening genetic disease in the United States today (Cystic Fibrosis Foundation [CFF], 1997). It occurs more commonly in whites than in any other ethnic group and tends to be more prevalent among those persons who are of northern or central European descent (Doershuk & Boat, 1983). At the present time, literature regarding the prevalence of CF is mixed; reported incidence ranges from 1 in every 3300 live births to 1 in every 2500 newborns (Collins, 1992; CFF, 1997).

CF is a disease that impacts many of the body's systems and subsequently many of the occupational performance areas of childhood and adolescence. The chief characteristics of CF are chronic airway obstruction and difficulties with the digestive process. Both the pancreas and the liver may also be impacted by this disease (Doershuk & Boat, 1983). CF causes the body to produce thick mucus. This abnormally sticky mucus clogs the lungs and causes infections. The secretions also obstruct the pancreatic ducts and prevent normal digestion. The enzymes produced by the pancreas are unable to reach the intestines to aid in food digestion (CFF, 1997).

Symptoms of CF include a persistent cough or wheezing; pneumonia; poor weight gain despite appropriate food intake; and greasy, bulky stools caused by poor functioning of the digestive system. The current diagnostic test for CF is known as the "sweat test." In this laboratory test a child's sweat is analyzed for excessive chloride, an indicator of CF (Doershuk & Boat, 1983).

Major progress has been made in both the treatment of CF and in increasing life expectancy of youths with CF. The median life expectancy 30 years ago was 8 years of age. Today the figure is approaching 30+ years, depending on the sources reviewed (Cystic Fibrosis Web [CF Web], 1997; CFF, 1997). A major breakthrough in CF research was made in 1989 when scientists discovered which gene, when defective, causes CF. The gene's defective protein has also been identified and gene therapy research is being pursued vigorously (CF Web, 1997; Collins, 1992).

The major areas for intervention include those directed at the pulmonary system and those targeted at children's digestive system functioning. Medical interventions include antibiotic therapy to decrease lung infections, and mist inhalation to help unclog obstructed airways. Allied health personnel are also involved in "front-line" interventions. Nutritionists assist children and their families with diet adjustments and vitamin and enzyme replacements. Physical therapists are often involved in chest physical therapy (CPT), which is also known as *postural drainage.* OTs are involved with enhancing occupational performance by using: (1) pulmonary compensation techniques; (2) adaptive techniques and equipment for activities of daily living, school, and play; and (3) family and caregiver support and education.

---

■ *THERAPEDS POINTER*

Postural drainage is a technique used to loosen the thick mucus in the lungs. The child is positioned in a prone position and a therapist or other trained person uses vigorous percussive movements on the child's back (CFF, 1997). This process may require 20 to 30 minutes per day. It is important to be consistent about this intervention because it encourages health stability in the child. Parents often need encouragement and strategies for ways to make this a routine activity for their children (Doershuk & Boat, 1983).

---

## RESTRICTIVE LUNG DISEASE

Restrictive lung disease is characterized by a decrease in chest wall compliance. *Restrictive impairments,* such as respiratory distress syndrome (RDS) of infants, are characterized by reduced pulmonary ventilation due to decreased lung expansion and, therefore, diminished airflow. In this case, there is increased resistance to lung expansion with increased pressure needed to maintain lung expansion and ventilation. The work of breathing is, therefore, increased. As a result, the respiratory rate has to increase (tachypnea), and the respiratory muscles work harder to make this happen. Increased oxygen expenditure occurs at a rate 25 percent greater than in a person with normal lung function, and hypoxemia occurs. Shortness of breath then results. Rales (crackles that sound like pieces of Velcro being pulled apart) can be heard through a stethoscope and cyanosis may be observed. Severe symptoms include clubbing of the tips of the fingers. Bronchopulmonary dysplasia is an example of restrictive lung diseases (Swanson & Brown, 1992).

## *Bronchopulmonary Dysplasia*

*Bronchopulmonary dysplasia* (BPD) is a chronic lung disease that is present in an infant (more than 28 days of age) who has received mechanical ventilation during the first 3 days of life (Swanson & Brown, 1992). This condition develops from the treatment of RDS in premature infants or treatment of meconium aspiration, persistent fetal circulation, or neonatal pneumonia in full-term children. It occurs in 10 to 20 percent of infants who require prolonged ventilation and high oxygen concentrations for treatment of RDS (Wasserman et al., 1987). This treatment can be with extracorporeal membranous oxygenation (ECMO), mechanical ventilation, and medications.

The progression of BPD is fairly predictable. It is outlined here (McFadden, 1988).

| Stage | Characteristics of Stage |
|---|---|
| Birth | • Presence of hyaline membrane disease (RDS) |
| | • Decreased amounts of surfactant leading to atelectasis of the lung |
| Postnatal period | • Repair and regeneration of damaged tissue with granulated tissue |
| | • Small and medium-sized bronchi become narrowed or blocked |
| 10–20 days of life | • Transition to a chronic disease |
| | • Mucus production increases and restrictive changes are present |
| 1 month to 2–3 years | • Chronic disease phase of BPD |
| | • Smooth muscle hypertrophy, hyperinflation, and subepithelial fibrosis |
| | • Pulmonary artery thickening; right ventricle hypertrophy |
| | • Alveolar hypoplasia |
| | • Barotrauma from high ventilatory pressures |
| | • Pulmonary interstitial edema; infectious diseases |

The severity of BPD varies. A child with a mild case of BPD may exhibit occasional tachypnea or cyanosis with feeding or crying. The child with severe BPD will exhibit increased tachypnea, cyanosis (if allowed to breathe room air), rib retractions, nasal flaring, and grunts or snorts. These are signs that the child is "air hungry" and working hard at breathing. Desaturation may occur and remain at a lower rate for longer. The child with a nasogastric tube is at greater risk for desaturation events (Moller et al., 1988). Some children with BPD may have frequent rehospitalizations for pneumonia and bronchiolitis (Northway et al., 1967). BPD can and does improve with growth unless there are persistent circulatory problems such as cor pulmonale. Since BPD is a relatively new phenomenon, the oldest survivors of BPD are now in their twenties with their lung function still being studied. Among these survivors, abnormalities of the lungs have persisted to age 10 (Garritan, 1994).

Again because of the risks associated with decreased blood oxygenation or decreased blood flow, and with prematurity in general, children with BPD are also at high risk for CNS and developmental dysfunctions. OTs can play an important role in the identification and management of such conditions. Refer to Chapter 10 for a more detailed description of the role of occupational therapy with children who have received newborn intensive care.

Some children with BPD may remain ventilator-dependent (via tracheostomy) for the first few years of life. With good nursing care and support, these children can be managed well at home. Because of their risk for growth retardation and developmental delay, they should be carefully monitored. The need to minimize the work of breathing *will always be a priority* even before choosing to eat or play.

Feeding can be difficult for the child with BPD. If conditioned dysphagia results, feeding may not progress past the pureed food state (Wedig et al., 1984). Nonnutritive sucking experiences may serve to shorten breathing pauses, normalize heart rate, and shorten desaturation events. External pacing of prolonged sucking bursts will also help normalize $O_2$ saturation durations.

For children who are being weaned from ventilator support, activity restrictions will be necessary during a trial to challenge, but not exhaust, the work of breathing. Vital signs are closely monitored during weaning. Weaning may occur in stages, first to a lower setting, then to $O_2$ nasal cannula or to pulmonary assistance at night only. Anxiety related to difficulty getting a breath may accompany periods of ventilation weaning or may signal illness.

Play will progress fairly typically, especially in the area of fine-motor skills. Limitations may be seen in trunk rotation, bilateral integration, and gross-motor function. Children with BPD generally have only minimal opportunities to be in the prone position because of the possibility for lung compression. They typically spend much of the day in supported sitting in order to maintain good respiratory function. Further, for children tethered to a ventilator, there may be limited opportunities to pull to stand, ambulate, and explore the environment. Isolation from playmates and play experiences can be difficult for the child with BPD. It is important to consider ways to provide developmental and play opportunities within each child's particular constraints.

## THE IMPACT OF RESPIRATORY DISEASE ON CHILD HEALTH AND DEVELOPMENT

To preserve energy, the child with pulmonary dysfunction may be moderately to maximally dependent on caregivers for basic self-care. These children can learn to dress themselves and perform other self-care tasks, but skills are delayed as long as respiratory dysfunction is significant. Proximal muscle weakness may also be a significant factor. Speech may be limited in production to save energy for breathing. Sometimes words are mouthed or augmentative-assistive methods may be used.

Children with pulmonary dysfunction may have respiratory instability with sleep. Sleep-related apnea may occur. Interruptions in sleep caused by high levels of arousal or alarms may leave the child sleep deprived (Hislop, 1997). Sleep may be limited to one or two positions.

Although medical progress and new drug and surgery interventions have arrived on the scene for youth with respiratory disease, the daily "nitty-gritty" of life is handled by families and their local support systems. As Goldman (1994, p. 28) notes, "the responsibility and commitment for the time-consuming, unremitting, practical day-to-day care falls on the parents." . OTs must continually assess how their interventions may impact the family (as a system) as well as the child.

The role of the OT in working with youth with respiratory disease will continue to change as the progress in medicine increases life-expectancy statistics. What will not change is the need to consider the individual, the life tasks of youth, and the individual's motivation to pursue specific choice-driven occupations. Play, self-care, and school and work areas all provide opportunities for therapists to support children with respiratory disease and their families as they pursue life goals. The table below offers some areas of intervention and occupation therapy–related tasks.

| Area of Occupation | Issues and Concerns | Possible Strategy or Solution |
| --- | --- | --- |
| Play and leisure | Postural drainage sessions interfere with play time. | • Let child help choose time to do this activity each day (similar to "homework" time required for school). <br> • Help parents generate activities to do during these sessions such as counting or alphabet games; story-telling sessions; or guessing games. |
| | Exercise tolerance for activities of play may need to be monitored. | • Collaborate with physical therapists (PTs) and physicians (MDs) regarding levels of optimal activity to promote increased endurance in play. <br> • With input from PT and MD, help family develop daily plans of activity that meet family needs for time management and child's needs for exercise and physical activity. |
| Self-care, ADL | Efforts for dressing are taxing for child or youth in morning preparation for school. | • Discussion with child and family on ways to conserve energy in these dressing tasks or reconsider importance |

| | | of this as an independent area in the "grand scheme" of life for this child. |
|---|---|---|
| | Mealtime choices of teenager with respiratory disease become family stressor regarding healthy eating. | • Collaborate with nutritionist regarding mealtime activities to increase teen control, i.e., shopping with parent, meal planning to incorporate healthy choices, cooking new recipes as the teen "chef." |
| School and work | High school student with CF is looking toward vocation after school. | • Collaborate with student and counselor regarding student's interests, skills, and the possible needs for work and school adaptations in the future<br>• Make student aware of Americans with Disabilities Act (ADA) information (as appropriate) to teach self-advocacy. |

*Source:* Adapted from Doershuk & Boat, 1983; Gordon et al., 1996; Kidd, 1997.

# WRAPPING IT UP

The heart and the lungs are essential to life. Disease or impairment in these organs can create significant dysfunction and disability. Cardiac or pulmonary disease may be congenital or acquired. It may occur with other disabling conditions, or it may cause dysfunction in other systems, such as the CNS damage that may result from anoxia.

The role of the OT in cardiopulmonary disease depends on a number of factors, including type and severity of disease, age, developmental level of child, setting of care (hospital, school, home, community), and, of course, the impact on occupation and function. Specialized knowledge and expertise is required to best help children with this type of disorder. Collaboration with other health-care professionals and families will enhance the impact of occupational therapy services. This chapter provides an overview of some unique aspects of cardiopulmonary disease. It is the authors' hope that you will continue to develop knowledge and understanding in this area. The health of children's hearts and lungs is essential to their function. OTs can make an important contribution to maintaining health and promoting optimal function.

Seth was born at 37 weeks gestation. Delivery was by cesarean section secondary to an abruptio placentae. His Apgar scores were 2 at 1 min and 5 at 5 min due to respiratory distress. He was stabilized and admitted to the neonatal intensive care unit (NICU). There, he found to have a ventricular septal defect (VSD). Two weeks later, surgery to close the VSD and to repair an inguinal hernia sent him into acute respiratory distress. He was placed on mechanical ventilation. After another month, multiple trials to wean him from the ventilator failed. He was also experiencing feeding difficulties and gastroesophageal reflux. At the age of 2½ months, he received a tracheostomy, a gastrostomy tube with fundoplication of the stomach, and a Broviac placement. Ventilator weans were now well tolerated, and his stomach could tolerate full-strength, high-calorie formula. He showed slow, progressive growth. At 4 months of age, still in the hospital during February, he contracted respiratory syncytial virus (RSV) and *Candida* sepsis. This illness sent him back onto full ventilator support and IV antibiotic therapy with decreased tolerance for feeding. He was gravely ill at this time. A month later, with illness resolving, he began ventilator weaning, again with bradycardia. He was showing evidence of moderate bronchopulmonary dysplasia (BPD) with copious secretions.

At 5 months of age, he was still in NICU. He had not yet achieved head control or an efficient nonnutritive suck. He rejected tastes of food in his mouth as noxious stimuli. He could bring a hand to his mouth and enjoyed resting his hand at midline on his ventilator tubing. He had poor antigravity movements at his shoulders because of muscle wasting and mild atrophy. He was found at that time to have a hearing loss, in part as a result of medications. He began to have problems with his skin integrity over his bony prominences, with frequently excoriated buttocks requiring cream and heat lamp therapy. As a result, he was positioned side to side, and was not allowed to be upright and weight-bearing for a month. He could be held for brief periods in a vertical position if his buttocks were not touched. He tolerated handling poorly. He was beginning to demonstrate a thoracic scoliosis.

Occupational therapy goals, developed in collaboration with the NICU team and the family, included:

1. Normalize arousal to day and night schedule.
2. Decrease tactile defensiveness to light touch or pain.
3. Decrease oral defensiveness to touch, flavor, and smell.
4. Improve nonnutritive suck to improve oral organization for state regulation.
5. Evaluation of swallow function with three-phase swallow study as tolerated.
6. Increase visual awareness of environment.
7. Increase reach and grasp of ½-in cylindrical objects.
8. Improve strength for antigravity reach from the shoulder from supine.
9. Support and educate parents and actively involve them in their child's care.

At 7 months of age, Seth was hemodynamically and neurologically stable, but still living in a hospital. A case conference was convened to formulate a discharge plan. It was attended by 15 team members (his parents, primary and specialist physicians, nurses, respiratory therapist, physical therapist, occupational therapist, speech pathologist, early intervention coordinator, discharge coordination, social worker, home care nurse).

A care plan, including 24-hour in-home respiratory nursing care and early intervention, was drawn up. Follow-up physician services were scheduled. He was discharged to his home at 8 months of age.

Rehospitalization occurred 6 weeks later for respiratory distress and pneumonia. He spent 21 days as an inpatient. He lost oral motor skill and a repeat swallow study was done that revealed risks of aspiration. He was only given nonnutritive oral motor stimulation. He continued to require a ventilator about 18 hours a day. At home again, he continued to grow slowly. Small gains in sitting, fine-motor skills, and tolerance of bolus feeds were observed.

At 2 years of age, he could roll, sit, and try to pull to stand. He was taking small quantities of pureed baby food with moderate oral defensiveness. He continued with a tracheotomy and nighttime ventilator assistance because of bradycardia and apnea. He had 8 hours of overnight nursing care in his home so that his mother could sleep. He was rehospitalized six times that year for pneumonia and revisions of his tracheotomy and gastrostomy tube. His mother had since had another child who had no apparent special needs. Seth enjoyed his baby sister Sara.

At age 4, he continued with a partially plugged tracheotomy, he could walk short distances, and was beginning to tolerate soft chunk foods. His primary nutrition remained gastrostomy tube feedings of Pediasure. He was able to remove his clothing independently and use a sipper cup to drink. As his respiratory status permitted, he attended a preschool program that included occupational therapy services. He returned to the hospital as an outpatient for 12 visits to address his oral sensitivities and feeding impairments. He was hospitalized twice that year, for less than 2 weeks, for respiratory infections. In-home nursing care had been discontinued at age 3. He continued his own upward growth and development progression.

1. At this point, if you were Seth's OT what suggestions would you make?

| | **To his mother** | **To his teacher** |
|---|---|---|
| Play | | |
| Dressing | | |
| Feeding | | |
| Gross motor | | |

Fine motor

Other

2. What issues or concerns might be present for Seth's sister Sara?
3. How would you address your own and Seth's family's fear that he may die?

## CASE STORY 2

You are a hospital-based therapist and you have on your caseload Amy, a 5½-year-old girl with respiratory compromise. This is her story. She was born several weeks early with a left congenital diaphragmatic hernia. A congenital diaphragmatic hernia is an abnormal opening of the diaphragm in which contents of the abdominal cavity protrude upward, restricting lung growth.

Amy required 12 days of extracorporeal membrane oxygenation (ECMO) after the hernia repair and ventilator assistance to maintain an airway. ECMO is a machine used as a lung bypass to relieve the lung of its work so that physiological stability can be achieved and healing can occur. Superior vena cava syndrome resulted from the ECMO. She had a congenital bronchomalacia, a deficiency in the wall of the trachea, that caused obstruction and could lead to atelectasis of the lung. A tracheostomy was placed several weeks later to assist in managing her ventilator dependence. The difficulties with the diaphragm affected her distal esophagus and caused problems with vomiting (reflux) of stomach contents back upward, putting her at risk for aspiration. A computed tomography (CT) scan at this time revealed mild bilateral brain dysfunction consistent with a hypoxic insult.

During this time she began to gag to items placed into her mouth as part of her nursing care and eventually to a pacifier.

Occupational therapy goals for Amy:

1. Decrease oral-facial hypersensitivity to caregiving tasks.
2. Increase tongue protrusion, lateralization, and lip closure.
3. Increase duration of her hand-to-mouth exploratory play and modulation of arousal.
4. Increase tolerance to drops of liquid introduced to the lips.
5. Initiate a suck to therapist's finger or drops of liquid.

After 7 months in the hospital Amy was discharged home with specialized nursing care because of her continuing ventilator dependence. A gastrostomy tube was placed for nonoral nutrition. A swallow study was performed at 10 months of age, with findings of poor oral-motor skills, hypersensitive gag, oral-pharyngeal residue, and no aspiration into the lungs.

Occupational therapy goals for Amy:

1. Position upright 70 to 90 degrees for oral feeding and at least 20 min after to maximize feeding experience.
2. Decrease oral hypersensitivity around and within the mouth.
3. Presentation of thick liquid to puree consistency to the lateral borders of the oral cavity to minimize gag in a 5-mm bolus (dab) from swab or infant spoon.
4. Minimize tactile defensiveness of food contact to hands.

At 18 months of age she continued to require the tracheostomy, but she had been weaned from assisted ventilation. She had several large adhered surgical scars on her thorax. She had improved mobility of the tongue for control of pureed foods. Her hypersensitive gag had decreased to purees but remained for textures. The harder textures encountering her palate could trigger a gag. Her swallow response was more immediate. She was experiencing pleasurable nonfeeding oral experiences to a variety of toys. Early-intervention occupational therapy services provided by her local community began in this period, with more of a focus on play-based activities and fine-motor-skill development.

Occupational therapy goals for Amy:

1. Increase Amy's tolerance for varied sensory qualities of tastes and texture in foods.
2. Improve control of a soft-mass bolus within the oral cavity.
3. Increase the quantity of food per feeding.

At age 2, she was tolerating liquid in her mouth from a two-hole sip cup placed to her mouth. If she brought it to her mouth, the bolus was frequently too large and was occasionally coughed. Drinking 2 ounces of liquid by cup could take her 30 minutes. Most liquid was still given by gastrostomy tube. Her lingual control of a soft bolus was now within normal limits. Her chewing pattern was primarily a munch (up-down). It was evident that with her history of limited oral feeding and primary nonoral tube feedings that she had minimal association of hunger with feeding. Her tube feedings were reduced to 75 percent of her total daily calorie needs and given primarily while she slept to improve her hunger sensations during the day. Her brother Andrew, 2 years older, served as a good role model for typical oral feeding.

Occupational therapy goals for Amy:

1. Improve lip closure around a cup with minimal liquid loss.
2. Advance diet from mashed table foods to more minced table food with tiny particles, without gagging.
3. Begin self-feeding experiences with softened finger foods, such as cereals in milk, for bite and chew experience.
4. Increase tastes of a variety of foods, allowing her to control introduction into her mouth.

At age 3, she was accepting tastes of a wide variety of foods, if she could lick them from her finger or hand first. If the initial texture was too aversive to the hand, it would not be placed into the mouth. She still had an aversion to rubber toys and nipples. She preferred cloths or clothing cuffs and collars in her mouth for oral exploration and organization. She was expanding her range of feeding skill with generalization to other places such as restaurants.

Occupational therapy goals for Amy:

1. Increase oral feedings to three meals (with family) a day with decreasing reliance on gastrostomy feedings.
2. Increase self-feeding with a 2- to 3-hole cup, 2 to 3 ounces in 20 minutes.
3. Increase self-feeding of mashed table foods with a bent-angle spoon.
4. Increase texture of food to coarse mince with some adhesion.
5. Diminish oral stasis of food toward end of feeding.
6. Diminish distractions during feeding to lengthen quality time.
7. Provide more flavors of foods (spicy, garlic, vinegar, salty, etc.) to improve taste perception.

At age 4, intervention shifted to areas other than solely feeding. She had moved forward in her speech and language skills and had the ability to ambulate independently although her gait was wide-based and postural insecurity was noted. She was found to have a visual impairment requiring glasses, with some visual-perceptual dysfunction. She had mild hypotonia. She had had very limited sensorimotor experiences. She had not mastered stair climbing. She did not enjoy riding toys or swings unless a foot stayed on the ground. She was unable to balance on one foot or jump forward. Hand dominance was still not easily identified.

Occupational therapy goals for Amy:

1. Increase linear vestibular stimulation to 10 sustained minutes.
2. Increase oral-motor and respiratory power through play with mouth toys for 3 to 5 minutes before becoming dusky cyanotic.
3. Improve prone extension posture to both feet off of the ground for 20 seconds.
4. Improve upper-extremity reach to obtain a toy located across the midline in seated play.
5. Improve weight bearing upon an open palm while shifting her weight across the extremity.
6. Improve cylindrical grasp around an object for a minimum of 30 seconds and demonstrate action with that object.

At age 5, her tracheostomy and gastrostomy tubes had been removed. She was able to maintain her airway even in the presence of infections. She was consistently maintaining her weight with a slow, progressive weight gain. Her diet remained soft chunks with minimal particulates. She did not gag to defensive texture, rather she spit it out or refused to eat any more. Hand function was delayed at the 3½-year level with hypermobility at the proximal thumb joint. Her cylindrical grasp of an object frequently neglected the thumb. Visual-perceptual dysfunction was evident for prewriting and drawing activities, dressing sequences, ambulation across changing surfaces, and play with manipulatives. She was highly visually distractible. Her mother was becoming comfortable with the idea of enrolling her in a preschool for several partial days.

Occupational therapy goals for Amy:

1. Use both feet simultaneously to jump forward 10 inches, jump off a 6-inch step, and jump over a 2-inch-wide line without stumbling.
2. Maintain a prone extension posture for 20 seconds.
3. Accurately reproduce a vertical and horizontal line, cross, and circle in response to a verbal prompt.
4. Use a dynamic tripod grasp upon a writing tool.
5. Independently dress self with pull-on clothing (no fasteners) using a sequential dressing technique.

At age 5 years, 5 months, Amy is medically stable. She has gotten through a winter without pneumonia or a hospitalization. Her endurance has increased, she is taller, and she is gaining weight. She enjoys preschool three mornings a week, but her mother sees her lagging behind the other children. She is showing evidence of delayed visual-perceptual development and the fine-motor development that are necessary for school readiness. Her sensorimotor integration and proximal stability is incomplete. Her *Test of Visual Motor Integration* score is at the level of 4 years. Her *Peabody Developmental Motor Scale* age equivalent for gross motor is 4 years, 8 months, and 3 years, 8 months for the fine-motor portion. Attentional difficulties and diminished inhibition are obvious in a group situation. She is at risk for delays in academic achievement unless she receives support services.

Her mother has asked for your recommendations about further needs for the next year or so for the purpose of program planning for Amy. Her insurance will give her 20 visits for occupational therapy a year. Amy's school program has stated that they will offer her 20 minutes a week within her classroom to address fine-motor and visual-perceptual delays, as well as weekly consultation by the classroom teacher. Mother is concerned because she knows Amy had several hypoxic events as an infant and wonders if she had brain damage that will lead to learning disabilities.

If you were Amy's occupational therapist, what recommendations would you make to her mother?

Here are some ideas:

| Area | Intervention |
|------|-------------|
| Medical | 1. Discuss with Amy's pediatrician your findings and her mother's concerns. |
| | 2. Suggest the possibility of neuropsychological evaluation to look for potential learning disabilities. |
| | 3. Have current hearing and vision exams. |

<table>
<tr><td></td><td>4. Identify her exercise tolerance and safety for inclusion in such activities as bicycle riding, TeeBall, soccer, and exploratory gymnastics.</td></tr>
</table>

|  |  |
|---|---|
| Educational | 1. Collaborate with the school OT and teacher to identify fine-motorand visual-perceptual areas in which you should concentrate. |
| | 2. Determine a handwriting program that everyone working with Amy will follow. |
| | 3. Work with the school OT and the physical education teacher to define her respiratory endurance parameters and then with the school OT and the classroom teacher to define Amy's daily activity schedule. |
| | 4. Identify what additional assistance Amy can receive. Is there an aide, tutor, retired volunteer, etc., who can give Amy additional help? |
| Play and Leisure | 1. Amy has been medically cleared for a moderate activity level that does not compress or bang her chest in any way (superior vena cava syndrome). |
| | 2. Help her parents define Amy's day in terms of activity and energy conservation. |
| | 3. Amy would like to play TeeBall and soccer like her brother does. Recommend that she wear chest protection such as a catcher would wear. She needs to learn to determine her respiratory endurance level and be taken out just prior to when she might turn dusky cyanotic. |
| Self-Care | 1. Continue to work toward improvements in shoe tying, zipper use, and use of other fasteners on clothing. |
| | 2. Identify a backpack she can independently open or adapt the fastener for increased independence at school. |
| | 3. Continue the use of a shampoo hat (Lillian Vernon catalog) to have her shampoo her hair. Add a hand held shower to improve rinsing independence. |
| | 4. Continue with the dressing sequence of clothes laid out the night before in sequential order, in a trail toward the door of her room. |
| | 5. Work with her mother on hair care ideas to increase Amy's independence for brushing and use of clips/barrettes. |
| Hand Function | 1. Improve dynamic tripod grasp with a variety of writing tools. |
| | 2. Improve precision of release into a ½-inch opening. |

3. Improve integration of dominant hand–assistive hand skills for self-care, e.g., buckling belt and shoe, joining coat zipper, and fine-motor tasks such as scissors skills and opening containers.

4. Improve in-hand manipulation skill for carrying items in a hand, cupped object transfers, shoe tying, etc.

Sensori-motor Skills

1. Improve neuromuscular performance for fine-motor coordination, strengthening of proximal muscle groups, and endurance.

2. Improve sensory integration of proprioceptive, vestibular, and tactile awareness; bilateral integration, visual spatial awareness.

Feeding

1. Continue to advance her diet into food with a greater variety of flavors and textures. Raise her awareness to what and how others eat so that she can cognitively process the attributes of foods that she may otherwise be tempted to refuse.

What additional issues, concerns, or recommendations might you have? How many visits would you recommend to her doctor for the coming year? What resources can you access for this child and family?

## Real-Life Lab

1. You are an OT serving children in an early-intervention (0–3) program in a primarily rural midwestern county. The largest city has a population of 20,000 with a community hospital approximately 100 miles from a major medical center. You are told to expect an extremely premature child who has spent the first 7 months of life in the hospital. This child has chronic lung disease with tracheostomy and a portable ventilator, feeding problems, and developmental delays. The child will have 24-hour nursing care in home for 3 months, then the need will be reassessed. Your team has not yet encountered a child this medically fragile.

a. What resources can you access?

b. What personal fears can you identify?

c. What additional information do you need to be able to plan appropriate interventions?

d. How could your colleagues in the following disciplines be helpful to you:

| | | |
|---|---|---|
| Nursing and Medicine | Physical Therapy | Education |
| Nutrition | Speech | Social Service |

e. What information do you hope to obtain from the parents?

f. What might your unique contribution to interdisciplinary care plan be?

# References

Alexander, R., Boehme, R., & Cupps, B. (1993). *Normal acquisition of functional motor skills.* Tucson: Therapy Skill Builders.

American Heart Association. (1971). Resources of optimal long-term care of congenital heart disease (A-208–9). New York: Author.

Bader, D., Ramos, A. D., Lew, C. D., et al. (1987). Childhood sequelae of infant lung disease: Exercise and pulmonary function abnormalities after BPD. *Journal of Pediatrics, 110,* 693–699.

Balfour, I. A., Drimmer, A. M., Nouri, S., Pennington, D. G., Hemkens, C. L., & Harvey, L. L. (1991). Pediatric cardiac rehabilitation, *American Journal of Diseases of Children, 145,* 627–630.

Barton, J. S., Hindmarsh, P. C., Scrimgeour, C. M., Rennie, M. J., & Preece, M. A. (1994). Energy expenditure in congenital heart disease. *Archives of Disease in Childhood, 70,* 5–9.

Batshaw, M. L., & Perret, Y. M. (1992). *Children with disabilities: A medical primer.* Baltimore: Brookes.

Bernbaum, J. C., Pereira, G. R., Watkins, J. B., & Peckham, G. J. (1983). Nonnutritive sucking during gavage feeding enhances growth and maturation in premature infants. *Pediatrics, 71*(1), 41–45.

Bowen, J. (1985). Helping children and their families cope with congenital heart disease. *Critical Care Quarterly, 8*(3), 65–74.

Braun, M. A., & Palmer, M. M. (1985). A pilot study of oral motor dysfunction in "at-risk" infants. *Physical and Occupational Therapy in Pediatrics, 5*(4), 13–25.

Brown, M. A., & Swanson, C. (1993). Understanding children with chronic lung disease: Part II: Respiratory supports and treatments. *Infants and Young Children, 6*(2), 57–66.

Callow, L. (1995) *HLHS: Frequently asked questions.* Ann Arbor: University of Michigan Medical Center.

Callow, L. B., & Wild, L. (1990). *Cardiac resource manual.* Ann Arbor: University of Michigan, C. S. Mott Children's Hospital.

Casaer, P., Daniels, H., Devleiger, H., DeCock, P., & Eggermont, E. (1982). Feeding behaviour in preterm nenates. *Early Human Development, 7,* 331–346.

Case-Smith, J. (1988). An efficacy study of occupational therapy with high risk neonates. *American Journal of Occupational Therapy, 42,* 499–506.

Case-Smith, J., Cooper, J., & Scala, V. (1989). Feeding efficiency of premature neonates. *American Journal of Occupational Therapy, 43,* 245–250.

Collins, F. S. (1992). Cystic fibrosis: Molecular biology and therapeutic implications. *Science, 256*(5058), 774–779.

Criteria Committee, New York Heart Association, Inc. (1964). *Diseases of the heart and blood vessels. Nomenclature and criteria for diagnosis* (6th ed.), Boston: Little, Brown.

Cystic Fibrosis Foundation (1997). *Facts about cystic fibrosis* [WWW document]. URL http://208.196.156.141/factsabo.htm.

Cystic Fibrosis Web (1997). *About cystic fibrosis* [WWW document]. URL http://cf-web.mit.edu/what-is-cf.html

D'Antonio, I. G. (1979). Cardiac infant's feeding difficulties. *Western Journal of Nursing Research, 1*(1), 53–55.

DiScipio, W. J., Kaslon, K., Ruben, R. J. (1978). Traumatically acquired conditioned dysphagia in children. *Annals of Otolaryngology, 87,* 509.

Doershuk, C. F., & Boat, T. F. (1983). Cystic fibrosis. In R. E. Behrman & V. C. Vaughan (Eds.), *Nelson textbook of pediatrics* (12th ed, pp. 1086–1099). Philadelphia: W. B. Saunders.

Garritan, S. L. (1994). Chronic obstructive pulmonary diseases. In Hillegass, E. A., & Sadowsky, H. S. *Essentials of cardiopulmonary physical therapy.* (pp. 257–284). Philadelphia: W. B. Saunders.

Gaultier, C. (1995). Cardiorespiratory adaptation during sleep in infants and children. *Pediatric Pulmonology, 19,* 105–117.

Goldman, A. (Ed.). (1994). *Care of the dying child.* New York: Oxford University Press.

Gordon, C. Y., Schanzenbacher, K., Case-Smith, J., & Carrasco, R. (1996). Diagnostic problems in pediatrics. In J. Case-Smith, A. Allen, & P. N. Pratt (Eds.), *Occupational therapy for children* (pp. 113–162). St. Louis: Mosby.

Gryboski, J. (1969). Suck and swallow in the premature infant. *Pediatrics, 43,* 96–102.

Harris, M. (1986). Oral-motor management of the high risk neonate. *Physical and Occupational Therapy in Pediatrics, 6,* 231–253.

Higgins, S. S., Kayser-Jones, J., & Savedra, M. (1996). Parental understanding of consequences of pediatric heart transplant. *Progress in Cardiovascular Nursing, 11* (3), 10–16.

Hislop, A. A. (1997). Bronchopulmonary

dysplasia: Pre- and postnatal influences and outcome. *Pediatric Pulmonology, 23,* 71–75.

Jackson, M., & Poskitt, E. M. E. (1991). The effects of high-energy feeding on energy balance and growth in infants with congenital heart disease and failure to thrive. *British Journal of Nutrition, 65,* 131–143.

Kidd, C. (1997). *Physical therapy and cystic fibrosis* [WWW document]. URL http://gcedunet.gac.peachnet.edu/~chris/cf/physical1.html

Kinnear, M. D., & Beachy, P. (1994). Nipple feeding premature infants in the NICU: Factors and decisions. *Journal of GNN, 23*(2), 105–112.

Krementz, J. (1991). *How it feels to fight for your life: The inspiring stories of fourteen children who are living with chronic illness.* New York: Simon and Schuster.

Leaf, J. P., & Gisell, E. G. (1986). Neonatal sucking behavior: A quick method of evaluation through structured visual observation. *Physical and Occupational Therapy in Pediatrics, 6*(20), 27–37.

Levin, S. R., Walker, L. M., Gorga, D. I., O'Loughlin, J. E., & Nagler, W. (1988). A rehabilitation approach to improving feeding behavior in infants with symptomatic congenital heart disease. *Archives of Physical Medicine, and Rehabilitation,* 69:744.

Linde, L. M. (1982). Psychiatric aspects of congenital heart disease. *Psychiatric Clinics of North America, 5*(2), 399–406.

Lobo, M. (1992). Parent-infant interaction during feeding when the infant has congenital heart disease. *Journal of Pediatric Nursing, 7*(2), 97–105.

Lowery, G. H. (1973). *Growth and development of children,* (6th ed.), Chicago: Yearbook.

McFadden, E. R. (1988). Asthma: General features, pathogenesis, and pathophysiology. In Fishman, A. P. (Ed.), *Pulmonary diseases and disorders* (Vol. 2) (2d ed., pp. 1297–1310). New York: McGraw-Hill.

Meert, K., Heidemann, S., Lieh-lai, M., & Sarnail, A. P. (1989). Respiratory syncitial virus with BPD or CHD. *Pediatric Pulmonology, 7,* 176–170.

Mendoza, J. C., Wilkerson, S. A., & Reese, A. H. (1991). Followup of patients who underwent arterial switch repair for transposition of the great arteries. *American Journal of Diseases of Children, 145,* 40–43.

Menon, G., & Poskitt, E. M. E. (1985). Why does congenital heart disease cause failure to thrive? *Archives of Disease in Childhood, 60,* 1134–1139.

Mintzer, D., Als, H., Tronick, E. Z., et al. (1984). Parenting an infant with a birth defect. The regulation of self esteem. *Psychoanalytical Studies of Children, 39,* 561–589.

Moller, J. H., Neal, W. A., & Hoffman, W. R. (1988). *A parent's guide to heart disorders.* Minneapolis: University of Minnesota Press.

Morris, S. E. (1982). *Normal acquisition of oral feeding skills: implications for assessment and treatment.* New York: Therapeutic Media.

Morris, S. E. (1996). *Development of oral motor skills in children receiving non-oral feedings.* Faber, VA: New Visions.

Morris, S. E., & Klein, M. D. (1987). *Prefeeding skills,* Tucson: Therapy Skill Builders.

Mullins, C. E., & Mayer, D. C. (1988). *Congenital heart disease: A diagrammatic atlas.* New York: A. R. Liss, Inc.

Northway, W. H., Rosan, R. C., & Porter, D. Y. (1967) Pulmonary disease following respiratory therapy of hyaline membrane disease: Bronchopulmonary dysplasia. *New England Journal of Medicine, 276,* 357–368.

Rybski, D. A., & Gisel, E. G. (1984). Optimal and suboptimal feeding behaviors in neonates. *Physical and Occupational Therapy in Pediatrics, 4,* 37–48.

Sade, R. M., Cosgrove, D. M., & Castenada, A. R. (1977). *Infant and child care in heart surgery.* Chicago: Yearbook.

Shaker, C. S. (1990). Nipple feeding premature infants; a different perspective. *Neonatal Network, 8*(5), 9–15.

Shiao, S. P. K., Brooker, J., & Fiore, T. (1996). Desaturation events during oral feedings with and without nasogastric tube in very low birth weight infants. *Heart & Lung, 25*(3), 236–245.

Sparacino, P. S. A., Tong, E. M., Messias, D. K. H., Foot, D., Chesla, C. A., & Gilliss, C. L. (1997). The dilemmas of parents of adolescents and young adults with congenital heart disease. *Heart & Lung, 26*(3), 187–195.

Swanson, C., & Brown, M. A. (1992). Understanding children with chronic lung disease. Part I: Lung function. *Infants and Young Children, 5*(2), 68–77.

Swartz, M. N. (1988). Bronchiectasis. In Fishman, A. P. (Ed.), *Pulmonary diseases and disorders* (Vol. 2) (2nd ed., pp. 1553–1581). New York: McGraw-Hill.

*Taber's cyclopedic medical dictionary* (18th ed.). (1997). Philadelphia: F. A. Davis.

Thommesson, M., Heiberg, A., & Kase, B. F.

(1992). Feeding problems in children with congenital heart disease: The impact on energy intake and growth outcome. *European Journal of Clinical Nutrition, 46,* 457–464.

Wasserman, K., Hansen, J. E., Sue, D. Y., & Whipp, B. J. (1987). *Principles of exercise testing and interpretation.* Philadelphia: Lea & Febiger.

Wedig, K. E., Bruce, M. C., Martin, R. J., & Fanaroff, A. A. (1984). Bronchopulmonary dysplasia. In Nussbaum, E., Galant, S. (Eds.), *Pediatric respiratory disorders: Clinical approaches* (pp. 83–90). Orlando: Grune & Stratton.

Wolf, L. S., & Glass, R. P. (1992). *Feeding and swallowing disorders in infants.* Tucson: Therapy Skill Builders.

Yahav, J., Avigad, S., Frand, M., Shem-Tov, A., Barzilay, Z., Linn, S. & Jonas., A. (1985). Assessment of intestinal and cardiorespiratory function in children with congenital heart disease on high-calorie formulas. *Journal of Pediatric Gastroenterology and Nutrition 4,* 778–785.

# *Appendix 4-1*

## OCCUPATIONAL THERAPY FEEDING SCREENING

| Question to Caregiver | Possible Concerns |
| --- | --- |
| 1. How long does it take to feed your child? | Decreased coordination and endurance parental tolerance |
| 2. How do you feed your child (position, equipment, general environment)? | Inadequate positioning<br>Poor match of feeding device (i.e., nipple) to oral cavity or coordination<br>Understimulated or overstimulated child |
| 3. What have you tried? What has worked and who has helped you? | Caregiver perceptions of feeding experience<br>Problem-solving strategies of caregiver<br>Length of time problem has existed<br>Whether multiple feeding devices (i.e., nipples) have been tried (which ones?)<br>Source(s) of advice and assistance |
| 4. Does the child resist eating? If so, in what ways? | Arching body, turning head or body, holding mouth closed<br>Spitting, gagging<br>Resist being held or seated |
| 5. What does your child like to eat? What have you tried that your child does not like to eat? | Tolerance for flavors, textures, temperatures |
| 6. Does your child have frequent coughing with feeding? Does he or she have frequent respiratory infections or pneumonias? | Aspiration risks |

# Appendix 4–2

## SPECIAL CONSIDERATIONS FOR FEEDING THE CHILD WITH HEART OR LUNG DISEASE

To achieve success with feeding children with heart or lung disease, it is essential to understand the relationship of the cardiac and respiratory function to the feeding process. It is helpful to know that children with cardiac or pulmonary disease tend to follow their own growth curve; they may experience some "catch-up" growth after surgical repairs, depending on the type and severity of the heart defect (Callow & Wild, 1990).

Here are some specific strategies to maximize the feeding experience for children with heart or lung disease:

**1. Carefully monitor heart rate, respiratory rate, and oxygen saturation of the child during feeding. This is done initially with telemetry and then with training by visual observation.** Changes in cardiac and respiratory rate indicate that the heart is having difficulty functioning. Feeding presents multiple demands on the heart, necessitating careful monitoring of these indicators.

The *physical environment* during feeding should be monitored for appropriate light and noise levels. A temperature of 74 to 78°F is most desirable. Extremes in noise, light, temperature, and other factors may also exacerbate cardiac symptoms.

Another indicator of function is the oxygen saturation rate ($O_2$ sat). This reflects the extent to which the blood is *actually* oxygenated compared to the amount it is *capable* of being oxygenated. A normative $O_2$ sat level is 95% or above. Many children, however, can be safely fed if their level is 90% (Shiao, Brooker, & Fiore, 1996). Because of individual variability, each child's baseline heart, respiratory, and $O_2$ sat rates should be determined.

The therapist uses these indicators to determine the quality of a feeding intervention. For example, if a child is unable to maintain an $O_2$ sat level in the normative range during feeding, then oxygen may need to be provided. Or, if a child repeatedly desaturates, feeding should be ended until a specific cause can be found. Such causes may include the need for suctioning, bradycardia, or feeding-related apnea.

**2. Use positioning to improve cardiopulmonary function and maximize feeding interaction.** For infants, the position of approximately 30 degrees upright is generally selected to maximize the gravity-assisted movement of the food bolus from the mouth to the stomach, and to minimize reflux (Shiao, Brooker, & Fiore, 1996). A knee-chest position is also frequently used because it helps the infant sustain a stronger suck with greater volume (Swanson & Brown, 1992; D'Antonio, 1979). This position decreases hypoxia, increases pulmonary blood flow, and increases $O_2$ sat by producing systemic vascular resistance, especially in the lower extremities.

In order to accomplish this desired feeding position, the child is held on the lap with his or her left side facing down and away from the feeder. The feeder places the infant's head onto his or her left arm, over the neck, and across the chest to maintain the knees in flexion across the infant's abdomen. The right arm assists with maintaining the legs and holds the bottle for feeding.

A variation of this is to place the seated feeder's legs into flexion such as upon a 10-inch stool with a pillow on the lap and position the child supine, facing the feeder, with the child's knees flexed into the abdomen. The child can be slightly (45 degrees) rotated to the left.

This special feeding position can decrease coughing and sputtering of liquid to fast flow or poor control of bolus. The baby can also be easily brought to upright with a quick change of the feeder's knees. Gentle passive movement of the left knee into the abdomen can produce a burp.

For children, an upright position with good support is suggested, again in order to maximize the gravity-assisted movement of food and to minimize the risk of reflux or aspiration.

**3. Provide formula or foods with high caloric density to afford the maximum calories for the minimum effort.** Jackson and Poskitt (1991) found that children with CHD begin with leaner body mass and require energy intake at 120 percent of that normally recommended for body and brain growth and catch-up.

For infants, early initiation of high-calorie formula is recommended. Use of a high-calorie formula increases the mean caloric intake 41 percent over standard infant formula given by mouth. Given by supplemental tube feedings, there is a 92 percent increase over standard normal food intake (Yahav et al., 1985). With the use of high-calorie formula, a decrease in metabolic demands and improved absorption can be achieved to produce weight gain. Continuous or nighttime enteral tube feedings can also facilitate weight gain.

For children, diet continues to be an important consideration. A difficult balance must be achieved, as many high-calorie foods have high fat and cholesterol content, which may be contraindicated. Professional nutrition counseling can be helpful.

**4. Minimize energy expenditure during feeding.** Children with heart or lung disease often have an imbalance between their food quotient and their respiratory quotient. Factors such as tachypnea, use of diuretics to reduce edema, stooling, and excessive sweating typically contribute to increased resting energy expenditure. Extra respiratory work combined with cardiac inefficiency many account for increased oxygen consumption. This in turn results in poor weight gain (Barton et al., 1994; Menon & Poskitt, 1985).

In the first six months of life, Barton et al. state that total energy expenditure increases each day by almost 100 percent. This corresponds directly to an infant's increase in motor activity from random movements of all extremities, to rolling and sitting. Conservation of energy, therefore, is a critical goal of therapeutic feeding. Energy intake is the critical factor in weight gain and growth for the child with CHD.

Although the growth curve stabilizes in childhood, energy conservation in all functional activities, including feeding, remains a priority for children with heart or lung disease. Adaptive equipment and techniques, especially energy conservation strategies, can be incorporated into daily routines to address this concern; meal and snack time should be pleasurable, satisfying experiences for all children, so a balance between energy expenditure and energy (caloric) intake is a meaningful goal of therapy.

# Appendix 4–3

## FAILURE TO THRIVE: A SPECIAL RISK FOR CHILDREN WITH HEART OR LUNG DISEASE

"Failure to thrive" is a failure to grow at least to the 5th percentile of expected growth rate for age. Its causes may be organic or inorganic. Jackson & Poskitt (1991) found that failure to thrive may be associated with high resting metabolic rates in children with *congestive heart failure* and *pulmonary hypertension.* An increased metabolic rate may mean that energy intake is insufficient for normal growth and development (Jackson & Poskitt, 1991). Menon & Poskitt (1985) gave *hypoxia* and *breathlessness* leading to feeding problems, *anoxia* and *venous congestion of the bowel* leading to malabsorption, *peripheral anoxia* and *acidosis* leading to inefficient use of nutrients and an increased metabolic rate. *Because of the nature of the cardiopulmonary problems and growth, feeding takes on special significance. The need to watch intake and count calories becomes paramount, and the feeding process may be difficult.*

# *Appendix 4–4*

## RED FLAGS FOR POTENTIAL FEEDING DIFFICULTIES:

Slow feeding progression
Respiratory difficulties
Spits out food
Oral touch sensitive
Coughs frequently
Hypersensitive gag (stimuli)

Tube feeding beyond 2 months
Persistent reflexes
Jaw moves excessively
Abnormal muscle tone
Color change with feeding
Poor transition to solids

## RED FLAGS FOR SWALLOWING DIFFICULTIES:

History of respiratory difficulties
Pneumonias
Muscle tone abnormalities
Anoxic events
Traumatic brain injury
Ventilator dependence
Gulping during feeding

Apnea
Stridor
Color changes
Coughing during or after
    feeding
Poor handling of secretions
Noisiness of audible residue
Slow growth pattern

# Appendix 4–5

**For Parents:**

**Oral feeding of your child may be possible if,**

Your child can swallow his or her own saliva.
Fluid overload is not a concern for your child.
Your child's respiratory rate is stable.
Your child is not fatigued with feeding.
Your child is not irritable with handling.

**Perhaps you have been feeding your child and have not found it to be as successful as you hoped. Review the following statements. If _any_ of these are true in your situation, please let your health-care provider know so that a special program can be developed to help you and your child have a more enjoyable mealtime experience.**

It takes longer than 20 minutes for my child to take an ounce of fluid.
I've tried a lot of different nipples with my child and nothing seems to work!
My mother/grandmother thinks I should do _____ to help my child feed better, but I am not sure because of the heart problem.
My child resists eating by pulling away, gagging or spitting, etc. What should I do?
My child likes to drink but will not take food from a spoon.
My child is more than year old now and is still unable to take food from a spoon.
My child will take smooth baby foods, but gags on or refuses anything with more texture
My child frequently coughs with feeding.
My child has:
- a lot of respiratory infections and pneumonias
- medical instability
- factors complicating discharge to home
- abnormal living conditions and family stresses

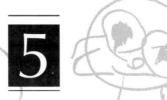

# 5

# *The Nervous System*

Scott D. Tomchek, MS, OTR/L

*Problems do not go away. They must be worked through or else they remain, forever a barrier to the growth and development of the spirit.*
—M. Scott Peck, MD

## KEY POINTS

- Cerebral palsy (CP) is an umbrella term referring to nonprogressive disorders of movement and posture.
- CP can be classified physiologically (pyramidal, extrapyramidal, or mixed types) and topographically by the level of limb involvement.
- The most common associated disabilities affiliated with CP are seizure disorders, mental retardation (MR), sensory deficits (hearing or vision), and speech-language disorders.
- Seizures are one of the most common of the neurological disorders that occur in children.
- Seizures are caused by any factor that can alter or disturb brain function, which may include developmental brain abnormalities, anoxia, metabolic errors, trauma, and/or infections.
- Together, the history, electroencephalograph (EEG) findings, and neuroimaging results attempt to classify the seizure type and determine the most appropriate pharmacological management.
- Neural tube defects (NTDs) refer to a group of congenital malformations of the vertebrae and spinal cord. Spina bifida is the most common form of NTD.
- The cause of spina bifida is many times unknown. These disorders are believed to be multifactoral in origin with both environmental and genetic influences.

- Spina bifida is referred to as being open (operata) or closed (occulta). An open defect is either completely open or covered by a very thin membrane. Closed deficits are covered with thick skin or membrane.
- The higher the lesion in spina bifida, the greater the impairment's effect on ambulation, motor function, and childhood occupation.
- Meningitis is an acute, potentially life-threatening illness describing inflammation of the meninges (lining of the brain).
- Encephalitis is an infection or inflammation of the brain tissue manifested by altered consciousness, fever, headache, and/or focal neurological signs.
- Guillain-Barré syndrome is a neurological disorder affecting the peripheral nerves and is manifested by a rapidly progressing symmetrical paralysis.
- Rett's syndrome is an X-linked dominant disorder occurring only in girls, characterized by a development regression consisting of loss of language, decreased functional use of the hands, gait ataxia, truncal apraxia or ataxia, and autistic behaviors.
- The clinical course of MS involves exacerbation and remissions, with disturbances in motor function, weakness, and incoordination or ataxia most commonly noted.
- No cure or prevention is available for MS and, therefore, conservative supportive treatment programs are encouraged.

# BEGINNINGS

This chapter explores neurological diseases of children. Specifically, cerebral palsy, neural tube defects, and seizure disorders will be discussed. Additionally, several infectious and degenerative diseases of childhood will be presented. The importance of an intact central nervous system (CNS) cannot be understated. Neurological disorders often have long-term effects on the child's physical and occupational status, and oftentimes carry no functional cure. However, much can be done for these children and their families to help them accommodate and adjust to these residual effects. OTs play a vital role in this intervention process. Not only do we work directly with the child, but our interventions may also be focused on family support and education or environmental adaptation in a number of settings. In these situations, we work with other allied health professionals. Together, the facilitation of childhood occupation is the goal.

# CEREBRAL PALSY

## THE CLINICAL PICTURE

Cerebral palsy (CP) is an umbrella term referring to nonprogressive disorders of movement and posture (Capute & Accardo, 1996; DeLuca, 1996; Kurtz, 1992;

Moe & Seay, 1995). It is caused by a brain insult or injury occurring before birth, at birth, or within the first year of life. CP types vary widely in their causes, manifestations, and prognosis. Consistent with all types, however, is the impairment of voluntary muscle function. In the United States, CP affects approximately 0.2 percent (or 2 per 1000) of neonatal survivors (Moe & Seay, 1995).

Many conditions may cause a cerebral insult or injury and cause CP. These conditions are often defined by the period of insult occurrence as prenatal, perinatal, or postnatal. The most common causes are listed in Table 5–1. Initially, it was thought that the most common cause of CP was birth trauma. A change in thinking over the last two decades has placed less of the blame on obstetric risk factors in the etiology of CP (Nelson, 1988; Nelson & Ellenberg, 1986). Currently, it is believed that prenatal etiology can account for the majority of known causes of CP, even in cases of multiple minor malformations (Coorssen, Msall, & Duffy, 1991).

Prenatally, many of the conditions that correlate with CP occur in the first trimester—a period of fetal development in which a mother may not know she is even pregnant. Radiation and teratogen exposure are risk factors that can be controlled. Genetic syndromes and congenital brain malformations are uncontrollable factors. Twin pregnancies have been shown to carry a twelvefold risk for developing CP, and the death of one twin has been shown to increase the risk for CP in the surviving twin by more than 100 times (DeLuca, 1996). Intrauterine infections, placenta previa, and placental functioning problems often occur later in pregnancy and also place a child as a higher risk of CP.

The combination of prematurity and related low birth weight is thought to be the leading cause of CP (Nelson & Ellenberg, 1986). Many of the other perinatal risk factors are associated with prematurity. Often sepsis and/or CNS infection are seen at birth in a prematurely born child. Anoxia or

Table 5–1 **Causes of Cerebral Palsy**

| Period of Brain Development | Cause |
| --- | --- |
| Prenatal | Viral infections |
| | Radiation exposure |
| | Teratogen exposure relating to maternal use |
| | Congenital brain malformations |
| | Genetic syndromes or chromosomal abnormalities |
| | Twin pregnancies |
| | Problems with fetal or placental functioning |
| Perinatal | Pre-eclampsia |
| | Asphyxia or anoxia |
| | Perinatal trauma |
| | Intraventricular hemorrhage |
| | Respiratory disorders of prematurity |
| | Sepsis or CNS infection |
| Postnatal | Traumatic head injury |
| | Viral and bacterial meningitis |
| | Anoxia |
| | Toxins |

asphyxia can occur during a traumatic delivery, as in the birth of a child with a prolapsed cord, placenta previa, and/or shoulder dystocia. Perinatal trauma can cause a hemorrhage in the immature brain, also resulting in CP. Notably, recent advances in obstetric and neonatal care have resulted in higher survival rates of very small infants who have increased risk of neurological deficits (Hagberg, Hagberg, & Zetterstrom, 1989).

Several postnatal events occurring prior to the age of 2 are also risk factors for CP. Viral and bacterial meningitis are risk factors and will be discussed later in this chapter. Traumatic head injury following a motor vehicle accident, a fall, or abuse can also produce CP. Postnatal anoxia, as a result of near-drowning, cerebrovascular accidents, tumors, radiation, or surgery, is also associated with CP.

Whether prenatal, perinatal, or postnatal, the previous are risk factors associated with causing CP. The clinician must realize that these risk factors occur frequently; however, in a significant number of children presenting with CP, they may not be present (DeLuca, 1996).

Classification of CP is often done using a combination of physiological and topographical types. Under the physiological classification are pyramidal, extrapyramidal, or mixed types. Pyramidal CP indicates damage to the motor cortex or to the pyramidal tract of the brain. It accounts for 75 percent of CP cases (Moe & Seay, 1995). Damage occurring in the motor strip of the frontal lobe, or in the pyramidal tracts passing signals to the spinal cord from the motor strip, results in a spastic presentation. Therefore, pyramidal CP is also known as spastic CP. These children demonstrate hyperreflexia, with "clasp-knife" type of hypertonia. When an arm or leg is moved, the initial resistance is strong, but it releases very quickly (as in closing a pocket knife). Given the resultant spastic musculature, the child with pyramidal CP is prone to contracture development as she or he grows. Because of the neuromuscular presentation, these children also often have difficulty initiating movement (Kurtz, 1992).

In extrapyramidal CP, the brain injury occurs outside of the pyramidal tract. Damage may occur in the basal ganglia or cerebellum and result in a movement disorder. One type of extrapyramidal CP is choreoathetoid. In choreoathetoid CP involuntary movements of the extremities are noted. Ataxic CP is another form of extrapyramidal CP and is characterized by incoordinated movements of voluntary muscles. In extrapyramidal CP, children have difficulty controlling movements and maintaining posture. Unlike clasp-knife spasticity in pyramidal CP, children with extrapyramidal CP typically present with "lead-pipe" rigidity. In lead-pipe rigidity, the limb appears rigid, although it can be ranged with constant tension. Rigid CP and atonic CP are other forms of extrapyramidal CP. In rigid CP lead-pipe rigidity persists, whereas atonic CP is characterized by low or floppy muscle tone. Both of these types are absent of choreoathetoid movements.

Mixed-type CP involves a combination of both pyramidal and extrapyramidal CP. For instance, a child may present with generalized choreoathetoid movements in conjunction with spasticity in the extremities. In these cases considerable brain damage will likely be noted.

Topographical classification of CP describes the level of limb involvement. *Hemiplegic* CP involves one side of the body (upper and lower extremity), with the upper extremity usually more involved than the lower extremity (DeLuca, 1996). Bilateral involvement denotes *diplegic* CP, with the lower extremities usually more involved than the upper extremities. *Paraplegia* indicates only lower-extremity involvement. Total body involvement indicates *quadriplegic* CP, which is often seen as most severe and in conjunction with mental retardation. In contrast to quadriplegic CP, in *bilateral hemiplegic* CP all limbs are involved; however, more involvement is noted in the upper extremities. *Monoplegic* CP involves only one limb, whereas *triplegic* CP leaves one limb unaffected.

Together, physiological and topographical classifications of CP provide descriptive information about the type and level of involvement. For instance, in pyramidal (spastic) quadriplegic CP you can expect spasticity in all four limbs, whereas in right pyramidal hemiplegia you can expect involvement of both the right lower and upper extremity. In some cases, the type of CP (both physiological and topographical) provides information as to the source of the brain insult or injury (Capute & Accardo, 1996). Some examples are found in Table 5–2.

The type of CP also provides a predictive measure of associated deficits that may be present. The most common associated disabilities affiliated with CP include seizure disorders, mental retardation (MR), sensory deficits (hearing or vision), and speech-language disorders. Seizures are seen in 50 percent of all children with CP (Moe & Seay, 1995), with the more severe pyramidal palsies carrying the highest incidence. Although an accurate estimate of intelligence is difficult to obtain given the degree of motor impairment, at least 50 percent of children with CP are thought to have some degree of MR. Among the children with CP and MR, 15 percent have mild MR, 35 percent have moderate MR, and 50 percent have severe and profound MR. The incidence correlates directly with the severity of the CP, with MR usually noted in the more severe forms of CP (pyramidal quadriplegia, extrapyramidal, and mixed types). Vision problems are also often present in CP. Strabismus is frequently seen. Homonymous hemianopsia (visual field cut) is also frequently seen, especially in children with hemiplegic forms of CP. Nystagmus may also be noted in children, especially in ataxic forms. Visual perceptual deficits may also be noted with and without normal intelligence. Hearing deficits are also common. Related speech and language deficits are also frequently noted and relate to impairments in the control of the fine-motor movements required of the oral musculature. These coordination deficits also commonly impair the child's feeding status. As can be seen, children with CP not only have neuromuscular abnormalities, but often also present with associated disabilities that cause further difficulty in daily living performance.

Table 5–2 **Cerebral Palsy Type and Suspected Etiology**

| Type of Cerebral Palsy | Etiology |
| --- | --- |
| Spastic diplegia | Prematurity |
| | Hydrocephalus |
| Choreoathetosis | Severe asphyxia |
| | Bilirubin encephalopathy |
| Spastic hemiplegia | Postnatal brain damage |
| Ataxic | Hydrocephalus |

No one test can be used for diagnosis. Instead, diagnosis is based primarily upon a thorough patient history and clinical findings. Often, children present with developmental milestone delays or a movement disorder. The child's parents may report that he or she was a floppy baby or conversely was stiff and frequently arched when laying on the floor. The child may have been a poor feeder with a weak suck. Hand fisting and cortical thumbing early in life and specific hand preference prior to 12 months of age may also be reported. Behaviorally, the child may be described as irritable and as having a weak cry. Parents may describe the child as showing little interest in his or her environment and report a general decrease in motor activity. These findings are all suggestive of CP, especially in the presence of previously noted etiological factors.

Upon physical exam, the child often presents with overt developmental delays relating to skill acquisition or quality of movement. Tonal abnormalities may be detected upon muscle palpation. Hypotonia, hypertonia (clasp-knife or lead-pipe) or variable tone may be noted. If tone can be sufficiently relaxed, deep tendon reflexes may be hyperactive. Tremors and/or clonus may also be present. Plantar responses are often extensor. Toe walking may also be noted during ambulation, as may associated foot deformities (varus or pes planovalgus). During voluntary movement, control is impaired, with increased associated and overflow movements often present. Within these movements, ataxia may be difficult to differentiate in the presence of tone. Nonintegration of primitive reflexes may also be noted. Primitive reflexes usually integrate during 6 and 12 months of age. In children with CP these reflexes often persist, which impairs development of postural responses (righting and equilibrium reactions).

Together, past medical history, parent report, and physical exam findings serve as the foundation for diagnosis of CP. With the diagnosis, further testing may assist in defining the child's disability. Hip radiographs may be conducted to rule out hip dislocation in the presence of spasticity. MRI or CT scans may assist in determining the cause, or at least the timing of the neurological insult. An EEG may also be indicated to rule out seizure activity.

After diagnosis, the process of management begins, often under the direction of the primary physician or developmental pediatrician. Early intervention is often the first step in the management process. Therapeutic intervention is both an independent and adjunct component in the management of CP. Independently, direct intervention by occupational, physical, and speech-language therapies is usually requested by the physician. Occupational therapy will be addressed later in this section. Physical therapists typically address neuromuscular concerns in conjunction with occupational therapy, as well as improve gross motor development. Speech and language intervention addresses feeding concerns (often in conjunction with occupational therapy) and language development. As an adjunct, therapeutic intervention is used to assist following other procedures. For instance, following orthopedic surgery or neurosurgery, range-of-motion (ROM) and splinting programs are often essential and conducted by occupational and physical therapists. Orthopedic surgery and neurosurgery will also be discussed later in this section.

Medications can be used to control or improve muscle tone. No medications, however, have been proved to be effective in the treatment of choreoathetosis (Kurtz, 1992). Diazepam (Valium) and baclofen are CNS inhibitors, meaning they act directly on the brain to control tone. Side effects to these medications include drowsiness, drooling, and nausea. In contrast to diazepam and baclofen, dantrolene affects the muscle cells directly to control tone by inhibiting contraction of the muscle. Side effects of dantrolene also include drowsiness and drooling, while also including muscle weakness. These medications do not eliminate spasticity, nor are they effective in all children. All have side effects. Therefore, the effectiveness and continued use of these medications is often weighed against the extent of the side effects.

Given the tonal abnormalities in CP and their effects on neuromuscular development, orthopedic management is integral. In attempting to maintain ROM and prevent contracture formation, orthopedic management may include use of orthotics or splints, orthopedic surgery, and/or neurosurgery. Orthotics and splints are often used in conjunction with active therapy. In the upper extremity, resting hand splints are used to prevent flexor contractures in the hand by maintaining it in a neutral position. Thumb spica splints are also frequently used in the presence of cortical thumbing. In the lower extremity, an ankle-foot orthosis (AFO) is used in an attempt to maintain or increase heel cord ROM. The AFO may or may not be hinged to allow for dorsiflexion while continuing to limit plantar flexion. In doing so, toe walking is limited or eliminated. By decreasing the amount of plantar flexion, tonal differences are also noted in the knees and hips. Secondary to these changes there may be a decreased need for splint or orthotic use at the knees and hips. In cases where splints are used, knee immobilizers can prevent flexor contractures of the knee flexors. Hip abduction orthoses are used to prevent subluxation of the hips and prevent contracture formation secondary to hip adductor spasticity.

Casting can also be used in the management of spasticity for a number of purposes. Inhibitive casting can be used to allow for weight bearing or for immobilization, and in doing so reduce the tone. Casting can be used for both the upper and lower extremities and places the spastic muscle in an elongated position to provide prolonged stretch. Use of casting in this fashion has demonstrated short-term reduction of both tone and contractures (Hanson & Jones, 1989), although long-term effects have not been demonstrated (Hinderer, Harris, Purdey, et al., 1988). Serial casting may be used to reduce contractures by gradually increasing joint ROM. After maximal ROM has been achieved, the cast will be worn periodically to maintain the newly achieved ROM. Serial casting can restore ROM to functional levels, and may be used as the child grows and joints contract or recontract (DeLuca, 1996). Serial casting is commonly used at the elbow, wrist, ankle, and knee. Failure to regain ROM is one indication to proceed with surgical management.

Orthopedic surgery is indicated in cases of contracture formation that have not responded to pharmacological, orthotic or splint, and/or casting management attempts. The goal of orthopedic surgery is to increase ROM through release, lengthening, or transfer of the affected muscles and tendons (Kurtz, 1992). Hip adductor, hamstring, and Achilles tendon releases are some of the most common surgical procedures performed. Release of the hip adductor can be effective in preventing complete hip dislocation when hip subluxation is noted. Casting and/or splinting usually follows these procedures to maintain the newly gained ROM. In cases that do not respond effectively to the above interventions, hip dislocation(s) may develop. These require surgical intervention to replace the humeral head back into socket and improve hip stability. Orthopedic surgery may also be involved in cases where a scoliosis develops (see Chapter 6).

Neurosurgery management may include selective posterior rhizotomy. This procedure involves isolating the posterior roots of the second lumbar to the first sacral spinal nerves and providing selective electrical stimulation to discover which rootlets make the greatest contribution to the spasticity (Kurtz, 1992). Once identified, these rootlets are then cut. This procedure has been shown to reduce tone while preserving sensation (DeLuca, 1996; Hinderer, Harris, Purdy, et al., 1988; Phillips & Audet, 1990). Functionally, improvements have been noted for stability during sitting and standing, and dynamically for ambulation (Arens, Peacock, & Peter, 1989; Berman, Vaughn, & Peacock, 1990).

Adaptive equipment is often needed to assist children with CP to maintain their childhood occupations. Positioning devices are used to prevent abnormal posture development in the presence of muscle tone differences. Splinting needs are discussed above. Prone and supine standers, sidelyers, and seating systems are used to position the child in normal postures. These devices also provide the child with a stable foundation from which more skilled movement of the upper extremities can be accomplished. Additionally, these devices build the stability that is a stepping stone for mobility. Mobility aids assist families in transporting the child with CP who has limited mobility. Wheelchairs and/or strollers are often used. Many configurations can be made to the wheelchair, depending on the child's neuromuscular status. Head and thoracic supports can provide stability in the trunk. An abductor pad can counter hip adductor tightness. For the child who has more mobility, walkers, crutches, and/or gait trainers may be used to further develop skill or to provide stability during movement interactions.

## THE OCCUPATIONAL THERAPY PERSPECTIVE

### Evaluation

CP interferes with role function in the presence of developmental delay and tonal abnormalities. Therefore, a child will likely be evaluated to determine etiology and, if applicable, diagnosis. OTs may be involved in this diagnostic evaluation process or may see the child following diagnosis for intervention planning. In either case, the evaluation process begins by reviewing the child's medical and developmental histories. Parental report of childhood occupations also often initiates the evaluation process. The parents may report that the child sleeps excessively or is irritable when awake. They may describe their child as having a weak cry and poor suck. Further, decreased environmental awareness may be noted. In many instances the concerns parents express regarding their child's development relate to the impact the developmental difficulties have on occupational performance.

A comprehensive neuromuscular assessment often initiates the physical evaluation. Overall active and passive ROM measurements are obtained. Proximal and distal muscle tone is also evaluated. Joint involvement is documented to determine the presence of asymmetries or distribution variations between the upper and lower body. Strength is often assessed through observation of antigravity postures and movements because specific muscle testing is difficult in the presence of tone.

To supplement neuromuscular findings, a neurodevelopmental assessment will likely be conducted next. The neurodevelopmental assessment should include two groups of automated responses as markers for motor dysfunction (Capute & Accardo, 1996). The first group of automated responses to be evaluated are the primitive reflexes. These reflexes appear during the late gestational period, are present at birth, and normally are suppressed by higher cortical function by approximately 6 months (Capute & Accardo, 1996). In CP, these reflexes often persist and are not suppressed in an age-appropriate manner and therefore continue to cause changes in tone and movement of the limbs.

---

■ *THERAPEDS POINTER*

Nonintegrated primitive reflexes cause tone and movement changes in the limbs. The following are examples:

*Asymmetrical tonic neck reflex (ATNR).* As the child turns his or her head, the arm and leg on the side to which the child is looking will extend, while the contralateral arm and leg become more flexed. Failure to integrate this reflex may lead to difficulties with rolling as the extended arm blocks the roll. Further, the child's fine-motor skills will also be affected and may inhibit self-feeding, play, and bilateral hand skill.

*Positive support reaction (PSR).* As the child is bounced and the balls of his or her feet come in contact with a firm surface, the legs extend. Failure to integrate this reflex leads to rigid extension in the legs. This marked extension often inhibits walking.

*Tonic labyrinthine response (TLR).* As the child extends his or her neck, the shoulders retract, the upper extremities flex, and the lower extremities extend; as the child flexes his or her neck, the shoulders protract, and the lower extremities flex. Failure to integrate this reflex leads to delayed development of equilibrium reactions. Therefore, a strong TLR will cause patterns of flexion and extension in the body and a child will be unable to maintain an upright position for sitting.

---

Following evaluation of the primitive reflexes, the second group of automated responses to be evaluated are the postural reactions. These reactions normally appear by 6 months of age following suppression of the primitive reflexes. Righting, equilibrium, and protective reactions must be evaluated. These reactions are especially prominent just prior to the appearance of motor milestones, and thus can be useful in evaluating readiness for and predicting motor function (Capute & Accardo, 1996). In children with CP, the delayed integration of primitive reflexes often inhibits the emergence of these postural reactions.

The child's neuromuscular and neurodevelopmental status has significant impact on his or her movement patterns. Often, the pattern of movement reflects the nature of CP. For instance, observing a child crawling with one arm tucked under while propelling with the other arm will identify hemiplegia. Similarly, in diplegia the child often "commando-crawls," with legs extended and pulling his or her body forward with the arms. Also in diplegia, sitting is difficult secondary to hamstring spasticity that extends the hips. Therefore, the child may W-sit for stability. During manipulation, the child may exhibit early hand dominance and persist in using full-hand-grasp patterns. Since the movement quality and patterns of movement are very important in the evaluation of the child with CP, using an assessment tool that addresses these areas is crucial. Many tests can be used. Examples include the *Bayley Infant Neurodevelopmental Screen (BINS)* (Aylward, 1994), *Movement Assessment of Infants (MAI)* (Chandler, Andrews, & Swanson, 1980), *Toddler and Infant Motor Evaluation (T.I.M.E.)* (Miller & Roid, 1994), *the Milani-Comparetti-Gidoni Motor Development Screening Test* (Milani-Comparetti & Gidoni, 1992), and the *Infant Motor Screen* (Nickel, 1987). To determine developmental ages for gross- and fine-motor skill the *Peabody Developmental Motor Scales (PDMS)* (Folio & Fewell, 1983) may be used, as may any of a number of other criterion-referenced evaluations.

Evaluation of self-help and adaptive living skill is a specific area of emphasis for occupational therapy. Difficulties in these areas are often of primary concern to parents. Tonal abnormalities may interfere with the child's feeding status and make diaper changes more difficult. The reflexive movement and motor skill delays will often challenge safety during bathing. Play and social interaction limitations are also frequently noted. Several independence measures are available to assess these areas. *The Vineland Adaptive Behavior Scales* (Sparrow, Balla, & Cicchetti, 1984) measures communication, daily living, socialization and motor skill status. These domains, as well as cognition, can be assessed using the *Batelle Developmental Inventory (BDI)* (Newborg, Stock, & Wnek, 1984). Similarly, independence levels within physical, self-help, social, academic, and communication areas can be obtained by using the *Developmental Profile II (DPII)* (Alpren, Boll, & Shearer, 1984). The *Wee Functional Independence (WeeFIM)* (Uniform Data Systems, 1993) can be used as a measure of independence in self-care, sphincter control, transfer, locomotion, communication, and social cognition areas. All of the above assessment tools are completed primarily as parent report measures.

## Intervention

Following formal evaluation and the establishment of the child's developmental status, the process of intervention begins. The intervention plan for the child with CP often involves an interdisciplinary team of allied health professionals and is habilitative in nature. The team will likely include occupational, physical, and speech-language therapy, audiology, nutrition, psychology, social work, and special education. The team can also include a developmental pediatrician or pediatric psychiatrist to coordinate neurology and neurosurgery, orthopedics and orthopedic surgery, ophthalmology, and orthotic needs. Together, this team attempts to enhance overall development and allow for acquisition of childhood occupations, with each discipline focusing on specific aspects of development. Often, integration and carryover to the home are the role of the family of the child with CP and therefore the family members are among the most important members of the interdisciplinary team.

The OT will often address motor development and stability concerns in conjunction with physical therapy. This therapy may be done in cotreatment. A neurodevelopmental treatment (NDT) approach is the primary method of intervention to address these motor areas for the child with CP (Capute & Accardo, 1996; Kurtz, 1992; Perin, 1989). NDT is based on the concept that antigravity postural control is significantly compromised by cerebral damage (Bobath, 1980; Capute & Accardo, 1996); therefore, treatment attempts to normalize tone and/or minimize its effects on postural control. Positioning (for rest and play), neurodevelopmental handling, and play foster the development of normal movement patterns. Sensory integrative intervention may be used to promote increased vestibular processing through tactile and proprioceptive inputs to the trunk (Capute & Accardo, 1996). Other interventions may include the Rood method, in which cold and heat modalities are used to reduce tone in the spastic musculature through inhibition or facilitation of the antagonist muscle.

Inherent in these treatment approaches are motor control and motor learning assumptions regarding normal and abnormal motor control. Therefore, clinical practices have been developed based on these assumptions regarding the nature and cause of normal motor control, abnormal motor control, and the recovery of function (Shumway-Cook & Woolacott, 1995). It is assumed that reflexes are the basis for normal motor control. This approach suggests that normal movement probably results from a sequencing of reflexes organized in top-down fashion within the CNS. Thus, normal movement requires that the cortex (the highest level) be in control of both the brainstem and spinal cord. Conversely, it is assumed that disruption of normal reflex mechanisms underlies abnormal motor control (Shumway-Cook & Woolacott, 1995). Based on these concepts, therapeutic intervention has focused on training motor control through techniques designed to facilitate and/or inhibit different movement patterns. In doing so, two key assumptions are that: (1) functional skills will automatically develop/return one abnormal movement patterns are inhibited and normal movement patterns facilitated; and (2) repetition of these normal movement patterns will automatically transfer to functional tasks (Shumway-Cook & Woolacott, 1995).

Research studies have had difficulty establishing positive qualitative and/or quantitative treatment effects in early intervention with CP (Ottenbacher, Biocca, DeCremer, et al., 1986; Palmer, Shapiro, Wachtel, et al., 1988; Turnbull, 1993). Other studies, however, have shown that early intervention with NDT increases the rate and quality of motor development in children with CP (Bower & McLellan, 1992; Kanda, Yoge, Yamori, et al., 1984). Failure to demonstrate positive findings is often the result of methodological error. Nonetheless, current thinking is that the optimal form of management for the motor involvement of cerebral palsy appears to be a combination of home therapeutic intervention with ongoing orthopedic observation (Capute & Accardo, 1996).

The child's fine-motor and visual-perceptual development and how they impact on play, self-feeding, and occupational performance are also areas of concentration for the OT. Oral-motor and feeding difficulties may be addressed in conjunction with a speech-language pathologist.

OTs often assist their patients and families to obtain necessary adaptive equipment, splints, and/or orthotics. Adaptive aids can promote increased self-care independence and improve play performance. Splinting and equipment needs are often coordinated with physical therapy.

**The child.** Therapeutic intervention attempts to facilitate normal development and occupational performance by minimizing the effects of tonal and movement control abnormalities. Adaptive equipment is often a vital component in this intervention process. OTs often work in conjunction with other allied health professionals to accomplish team goals.

| Child Characteristic | Seen As | In | Possible Strategy or Solution |
|---|---|---|---|
| 3-year-old with athetoid CP | Decreased upper-extremity control | Self-feeding | 1. Weighted utensils<br>2. Small wrist weights |
| 9-year-old with spastic diplegia CP of the lower extremities | Anxiety regarding decreased gross-motor skill | Play and recreational activities | 1. Engage the child in play situations in which he or she can be successful.<br>2. Teach the child relaxation.<br>3. Use art media to work out anxiety, aggression, and/or anger. |
| 12-month-old with spastic quadriplegia CP | Fisted hand posture with loss of ROM | At rest | 4. Teach the parent(s) passive ROM exercises.<br>5. Evaluate soft tissue integrity for splinting needs. |

**The parent.** Often of primary concern to the parents of a child with CP are the motor delays. These delays impact all areas of development. Initially, feeding difficulties may be noted. Tonal abnormalities will also impact positioning and dressing. As the child grows and matures, other skill deficits will likely arise. Assisting parents through these challenges is often the role of occupational therapy.

## ▮▮▮ FROM THE BOOKSHELF

A good book for early school-aged children with cerebral palsy to read independently or with a friend:

Grimm, E. (1992). *Walk with me.* United Cerebral Palsy Association, Frederick, MD.

| Parent Characteristic | Seen As | Possible Strategy or Solution |
|---|---|---|
| 8-year-old with hemiplegia wants to participate in extracurricular activities | Parents have anxiety because they fear the child may not be able to keep up with the other children. | Parents can encourage participation in non-competitive activities. |
| 7-month-old with spastic quadriplegia CP | Parents report positioning difficulties. | 1. Assist the parents in obtaining positioning aids from the local early intervention system loan closet. 2. Explore positioning needs for bathing and feeding. |
| 2-year-old with spastic quadriplegia CP | Parents have increased difficulty with mobility of the child. | Discuss with physical therapy the need for obtaining a wheelchair or stroller. |

## ▟▐▌ FROM THE BOOKSHELF

A couple of good resources for parents of children with cerebral palsy:

Geralis, E. (1991). *Children with cerebral palsy: A parent's guide.* United Cerebral Palsy Association, Frederick, MD.

Weiss, S., & Hunt, M. (1993). *Each of us remembers: Parents of children with cerebral palsy answer your questions.* United Cerebral Palsy Association, Frederick, MD.

**The environment.** Adaptive equipment will assist in promoting independence and childhood occupation. The equipment can be used directly by the child or the environment can be adapted to allow for improved skill. Determining the most beneficial adaptive aids, providing guidance to obtain them, and providing the needed training is often a role of the occupational therapist.

| Characteristic | Seen As | Possible Strategy/Solution |
|---|---|---|
| 12-month-old with athetoid CP | Child has cause-and-effect relation skill, but has difficulty with fine motor skill for toy exploration | 1. Adapted toys or switches to allow for less-skilled use 2. Recommend toys that make noise just by banging or hitting |
| 30-month-old child with lower body spastic diplegia | Child has difficulty sitting in circle time on the floor | 1. Allow the child to sit on an air cushion or bean-bag chair. 2. Obtain a seating system for the child to use in the preschool program. |

| Characteristic | Seen As | Possible Strategy/Solution |
|---|---|---|
| | | 3. If the child has a wheel-chair, be sure he or she comes to the program in it. |
| 9-year-old child with spastic quadriplegia | Child has difficulty with fine motor skill to interface with an augmentative communication system | Explore computer access for:<br>1. head master interfaces<br>2. scanning programs and systems<br>3. sip and puff interfaces |

## ▰▰▰ FROM THE BOOKSHELF

A comprehensive text on early diagnosis and intervention of children with cerebral palsy:

Scherzer, A. L., & Tscharnuter, I. (1990). *Early diagnosis and therapy in cerebral palsy: A primer on infant developmental problems.* New York: Dekker.

---

## ▰ *THERAPEDS POINTER*

Further information on cerebral palsy can be obtained from:

United Cerebral Palsy Association
1660 L Street, NW, Suite 700
Washington, DC 20036-5602
1-800-USA-5UCP
202-776-0414 (FAX)

# SEIZURE DISORDERS

## THE CLINICAL PICTURE

Seizures are one of the most common of the neurological disorders that occur in children, with prevalence rates of 4 to 10 in 1000 in children (Noronha, 1995). In general, boys are at greater risk for seizures that girls. A seizure can be defined as a sudden, involuntary, time-limited alteration in neurological function secondary to an abnormal discharge of neurons in the CNS (Holmes, 1992; Noronha, 1995). A seizure can be manifested by involuntary motor, sensory, or autonomic events, alone or in any combination, often accompanied by alteration or loss of consciousness (Moe & Seay, 1995). A seizure may occur after a transient metabolic, traumatic, anoxic, or infectious insult to the brain. Epilepsy is the condition in which seizures reoccur without evident time-limited cause.

Seizures are caused by any factor that can alter or disturb brain function, which may include developmental brain abnormalities, anoxia, metabolic errors, trauma, and/or infections. Seizures are often classified as symptomatic or idiopathic, with causes more likely identified in younger children. Once a child has a seizure disorder, a seizure can reoccur at any time. It does appear, however, that seizures are more likely to reoccur in the presence of head injury, fevers, emotional excitement, and/or fatigue. The chance of having a second seizure after an initial unprovoked episode is 30 percent (Noronha, 1995).

The most widely accepted classification of seizures is the International Classification of Epileptic Seizures, which was established in 1981 by the Commission of Classification and Terminology of the International League Against Epilepsy (ILAE). This classification is used to describe individual epileptic seizures and is based on three main factors: (1) clinical manifestations, (2) during-seizure encephalographic (EEG) patterns, and (3) between-seizure EEG patterns. Additionally, there is a category of syndromes in which seizures play a principle role. For the purpose of this chapter, the type of seizure will be the focus.

There are two basic types of seizures: generalized and partial (Dreifuss, 1989; Holmes, 1992). Generalized seizures involve both sides of the brain, whereas partial seizures are more localized and involve only one side of the brain. Notably, partial seizure may spread to develop into a generalized seizure. A child also may have both types of seizures, known as mixed-seizure disorder. Therefore, the ILAE (1981) classification denotes these three as the main categories, each with subtypes:

Partial seizures
    Simple partial seizure
    Complex partial seizure
Generalized seizures
    Absence seizure
    Tonic-clonic seizure
    Myoclonic seizure
    Atonic seizure
Mixed seizures

---

■ *THERAPEDS POINTER*

An understanding of the phases of seizures and their names will assist in discussing the types of seizures:

*Aura:* Unusual feelings a child may have that precede and predict
    a seizure
*Ictal:* Events during the seizure
*Postictal:* Events after the seizure

---

*Partial seizures* account for 60 percent of all seizures. There are two main types of partial seizures: simple and complex. Although in simple partial seizures there is no loss of consciousness, there is an alteration of consciousness in complex partial seizures. In 75 percent of children with partial seizures, there is a documented abnormality or lesion of the brain.

*Simple partial seizures* often occur between the ages of 4 and 12 years. The clinical signs of simple partial seizures are dependent on the area of focus (brain region in which the seizure is initiated). For example, if the focus is in the occipital region, visual manifestations are expected. Simple partial seizures are further classified into those with motor, somatosensory or special sensory, autonomic, or psychic symptoms. Given these symptoms, simple partial seizures are often also referred to as an aura.

In simple partial seizures with motor symptoms, the manifestations are dependent on the area of the motor cortex involved. The seizure may involve only a small muscle group (finger, tongue) or larger muscle groups. Following partial motor seizures, there may be paralysis of the involved muscle groups, known as Todd's paralysis. This paralysis can last from minutes to hours. Autonomic symptoms in simple partial seizures may include abdominal pain, tachycardia, pupil dilation, and flushing. Somatosensory symptoms often involve sensory functions, with the symptoms varying depending on region and level of cortex involvement. Typically, children report numbness in an extremity. Olfactory manifestations may include unpleasant odors. Foods may taste metallic. Vestibular processing symptoms may include sensations of falling or floating in space. Psychic features in simple partial seizures may include illusions, delusions, hallucinations, and/or paranoia. It is believed that the etiology of simple partial seizures relates to early birth trauma, subarachnoid hemorrhage, brain tumor, or encephalitis.

*Complex partial seizures* were once called psychomotor or temporal lobe seizures. They resemble absence seizures, which will also be discussed in this section. Of the children who have this type of seizure, 50 percent are thought to have an aura that precedes the onset of the main seizure. Most complex partial seizures have a temporal lobe focus and therefore a variety of manifestations may be noted. Aura may include a sensation of fear, upset stomach, odd smell or taste, or hallucination. The aura is often consistent for each child over time. The main seizure (ictal) involves involuntary motor responses or activity during a period of altered consciousness. This unconsciousness may be ictal and/or postictal. The motor manifestations may include eye blinking, staring, lip smacking, chewing, swallowing, hand gestures, crying, laughing, or repeating a word or phrase. Unlike absence seizures, complex partial seizures tend to occur in clusters and last for a longer time period (30 s to 5 min). Postictal amnesia, confusion, and fatigue are often present. Temporal lobe insults, asphyxia, head injury, tumor, or infections are felt to be the etiological factors.

In *generalized seizures* both sides of the brain are involved. They account for 40 percent of all seizures. Four types will be discussed here: absence, tonic-clonic, myoclonic, and atonic.

*Absence seizures*, also known as petit mal seizures, account for about 5 percent of all seizure disorders. These seizures typically have an onset from 3 to 15 years of age. An aura never precedes absence seizures. Instead, these seizures are characterized by lapses in consciousness or blank stares lasting about 10 s. These seizures cannot be interrupted by talking to or touching the child, and therefore can be differentiated from just daydreaming. Involuntary movements may also be present and can include lip licking, chewing, smiling, or scratching. After the seizure, the child recovers rapidly without confusion or fatigue. The child is often unaware that the seizure occurred and, therefore, frequent absence seizures will lead to poor school performance in that the child may frequently miss directions.

*Tonic-clonic seizures* are the most common type of generalized seizure. They are also the most dramatic and can occur at any age. Tonic-clonic seizures were formally known as grand mal seizures. In tonic-clonic seizures there is typically a vague aura or cry. The main seizure begins with a loss of consciousness and the child falling to the floor. The tonic phase is characterized by sudden rigid extension of the arms and legs. This phase may last 30 seconds to 1 minute and may be accompanied with apnea. The child may also bite his or her tongue during the seizure. The clonic phase follows and is characterized by alternating periods of muscle relaxation and contraction resulting in rhythmic body jerks. Following the last clonic jerk, the bladder sphincter is relaxed and incontinence may occur. This clonic phase may last several minutes. Postictal sleep and lethargy are common. The extent of postictal impairments relates to the duration of the seizure. The specific etiology of tonic-clonic seizures is often unknown. They may be seen in the presence of metabolic disturbance, trauma, infection, degenerative disorders, brain tumors, intoxication, or other disorders.

*Myoclonic seizures* usually present between the ages of 2 and 7 years. They are characterized by abrupt jerking in muscles of one or more muscle groups. These movements are brief and involuntary, and may range from an arm fling in a single muscle group, to full body movements forward, backward, or to the side in multiple muscle groups. Consciousness is only briefly altered if at all.

*Atonic seizures* also present between 2 and 7 years of age and are thought of as the opposite of myoclonic seizures. In atonic seizures, there is a sudden loss of muscle tone followed by a fall to the floor and loss of consciousness.

In addition to the above specific types of seizures, there are also several syndromes in which seizures have a principal role. These syndromes are often associated with MR and in many instances are difficult to control. Several are presented in Table 5–3.

A seizure is a clinical phenomenon (Moe & Seay, 1995). Therefore, history and neurological examination serve as the foundation for diagnosis in seizure disorders. An EEG helps localize the focus area of the seizure to allow for classification. Neuroimaging studies may also be used in the diagnostic evaluation. Together, this information is used to classify the seizure type to aid in diagnosis and treatment, as well as to understand the child's prognosis.

The key to a diagnosis of a seizure disorder is often an accurate history. All events prior to, during, or after the seizure can help classification. It is important to note the presence of an aura and its components. During the ictal period: Did the child become pale? Did she or he fall stiffly or gradually slump to the floor? Was there an injury? Was there an alteration in consciousness? How long did the stiffening or motor jerking last? What body parts were involved? Postictal, was the child confused or lethargic? Did the child fall asleep, and if so how long after the seizures did he or she sleep? Was the child's speech altered? Together, the aura and ictal and postictal characteristics often are the integral components in classifying the seizure type.

Table 5–3 **Common Epileptic Syndrome**

| Syndrome | Onset Age | Incidence | Characteristics | Related Condition |
|---|---|---|---|---|
| West's (infantile spasms) | 6–24 months | 1:6000 children | Myoclonic seizures with forward and backward extension of the body 5–10 times in a row | MR; neurodevelopment is halted with seizure onset; often develops into Lennox-Gastaut |
| Lennox-Gastaut | 1–8 years | 1:6000 children | Mixed seizure pattern including tonic-clonic, myoclonic, and atonic | 90% have moderate to severe MR |
| Aicardi | | girls only | Infantile spasm associated with absence of the corpus callosum and eye problems | MR, visual deficits |
| Febrile convulsions | 6 months–5 years | 1:200 children | Typically tonic-clonic seizures associated with a high fever | Full recovery if treated |

In any case of a suspected seizure disorder, an EEG should be obtained. An EEG measures electrical activity in the child's brain through electrodes placed all over the head. Information obtained from the EEG may confirm or extend the clinical diagnosis, but does not make the diagnosis. Therefore, the greatest value of the EEG is to assist in classifying seizure types, especially in mixed seizure patterns.

Neuroimaging studies (CT and MRI) are also a component of a diagnostic evaluation. These studies often produce abnormal findings in children with partial seizures. Although these findings rarely alter the clinical management of the seizure(s), they may offer important information as to its etiology. These studies also often ease both physician and parent anxiety because they often rule out tumors and vascular disease. These studies may also be used if there is difficulty in controlling the seizures or if the child's neurological status deteriorates.

Together, the history, EEG findings, and neuroimaging results attempt to classify the seizure type. With the seizure type identified, the process of treatment can be initiated. This process often begins with pharmacological management. Anticonvulsants are the line of medications used to control seizures. A medication is chosen based on the seizure type and treatment is initiated. The child is not, however, immediately protected against seizures, in that it may take up to 2 weeks for the medication to be at a steady level in the body. Therefore, the dosage is adjusted to control the seizure and minimize the side effects. This level is known as the therapeutic level and can be measured in the blood. The most commonly used anticonvulsant medications, dosage, effective blood level (therapeutic level), and side effects are listed in Table 5–4. Medications that are effective in the specific seizure types are noted in Table 5–5.

Anticonvulsants are often discontinued after 2 to 4 seizure-free years. In these situations, it is recommended that the medication be withdrawn slowly (over months). The risk of relapse is approximately 20 to 25 percent (Noronha, 1995).

Another approach in the treatment of seizures is the ketogenic diet. This diet is high in fats and low in carbohydrates, with sufficient protein for body growth and maintenance. The body is forced to break down fats because of the carbohydrate deficiency, resulting in ketosis. Ketosis raises the threshold for seizures and therefore decreases seizure activity in about half of the children on the diet. The diet is thought to be most effective in young children, especially those with infantile spasms, tonic-clonic seizures, and Lennox-Gastaut syndrome.

Table 5–4 **Common Anticonvulsants**

| Anticonvulsant | Dosage (mg/kg/day) | Therapeutic Level (μg/mL) | Side Effects |
|---|---|---|---|
| Carbamazepine (Tegretol) | 15–25 | 4–12 | Dizziness, ataxia, rash, lethargy |
| Clonazepam (Klonopin) | 0.03–0.1 | 15–80 | Drowsiness, slurred speech, ataxia, salivation |
| Ethosuximide (Zarontin) | 10–70 | 40–100 | Nausea, sedation, dizziness, liver damage |
| Phenobarbital | 1–5 | 15–40 | Hyperactivity, rash, decreased cognitive ability, drowsiness |
| Phenytoin (Dilantin) | 4–12 | 5–20 | Ataxia, gum swelling, nausea, nystagmus, diplopia |
| Primidone (Mysoline) | 10–20 | 4–12 | Drowsiness, ataxia, vertigo, nausea, rash |
| Valproic acid (Depakene, Depakote) | 50–120 | 10–70 | Lethargy, hair loss, nausea |

Table 5–5 **Recommended Anticonvulsants by Seizure Type**

| Anticonvulsant | Absence | Generalized Tonic-Clonic | Infantile Spasms | Simple/Complex Partial |
|---|---|---|---|---|
| Carbamazepine (Tegretol) | − | + | − | + |
| Clonazepam (Klonopin) | + | ± | + | ± |
| Ethosuximide (Zarontin) | + | − | − | − |
| Phenobarbital | − | + | − | + |
| Phenytoin (Dilantin) | − | + | − | + |
| Primidone (Mysoline) | − | + | − | + |
| Valproic acid (Depakene, Depakote) | + | + | ± | ± |

*Note:* − = ineffective; ± = partially effective/second line; + = effective/first line.

For seizures that are unresponsive to anticonvulsant medications, surgical management may be considered. Focal excision, removal of the seizure focus, is performed in cases of partial seizures that can be localized in one brain region. In a callosotomy, the corpus callosum is severed to prevent the spread of a seizure discharge in cases of poorly controlled generalized seizures and partial seizures with secondary generalization (Batshaw & Perret, 1992). In a more radical procedure, a hemispherectomy, almost all of one cerebral hemisphere is removed to stop the most severe uncontrollable seizures. In addition to the above medical interventions, education plays an important role in the therapeutic process. Assisting children and their parent(s) to understand the principles of seizures is helpful in management.

Encouraging normal living and childhood occupation is also a focus in the intervention process. How to accomplish this goal will be discussed in the occupational therapy perspective component of this section.

---

■ *THERAPEDS POINTER*

In the event of a seizure, precautionary management may prevent further injury to the child. During a seizure the child may fall to the floor and sustain an injury. To prevent further injury the child should be laid on the floor with a pillow under his or her head. The child should also be turned on his or her side to prevent aspiration if she or he vomits. Beyond that, no specific intervention is needed. A spoon or finger should not be placed in the child's mouth, nor should the child be restrained. Doing so may cause worse injuries than a bitten tongue or bruised limbs. As the child becomes awake and alert, comforting will assist him or her through the postictal process of recovery.

---

## THE OCCUPATIONAL THERAPY PERSPECTIVE

### *Evaluation*

The child with a seizure disorder is often seen by occupational therapy after the diagnosis has been made. The seizure disorder may be associated with another disability or may be seen independently and causing developmental delay. Therefore, the early onset of seizures leads to early intervention to remediate the developmental difficulties. The intervention process is initiated by establishing the child's current developmental and occupational status. Past medical and occupational histories are obtained initially. Here it is important to differentiate whether the intervention process will be rehabilitative or habilitative in nature, because the history obtained for a seizure disorder causing developmental delay will be different from the history obtained when a seizure disorder is seen with a medical condition that has caused skill regression. Obtaining histories to reflect this difference is important in determining the level of disability and long-term goal plans.

Integral in the history is to obtain information specific to the child's seizures. More specifically, information on the type of seizure, how it manifests, any precipitating events or activities, and/or the typical duration can be helpful in planning ahead in the case of a seizure during treatment.

Because a ROM and tonal abnormalities can impact on a wide range of occupations, a comprehensive neuromuscular assessment often initiates the physical evaluation. Active and passive ROM measurements are obtained. Proximal and distal muscle tone is also evaluated. Joint involvement is documented to determine the presence of asymmetries or distribution variations between the upper and lower body. Strength is often assessed through observation of antigravity postures and movements as specific muscle testing is difficult if tone is present. Balance reaction development, as well as overall balance should also be evaluated.

The child's neuromuscular status often serves as the foundation for motor skill development. To evaluate motor skill development in younger children, the *MAI* (Chandler, Andrews, & Swanson, 1980), *T.I.M.E.* (Miller & Roid, 1994), or *PDMS* (Folio & Fewell, 1983) can be used. A number of other criterion-referenced evaluations may also be used to determine approximate developmental ages. In older children the *Bruininks-Oseretsky Test of Motor Proficiency (BOTMP)* (Bruininks, 1978) can be used to obtain standardized measures of these areas.

Also in school-aged children, visual-perceptual and visual-motor skill development will need to be evaluated. Difficulties in these areas can have significant impact on academic performance. The *Motor-Free Visual Perception Test-Revised (MVPT-R)* (Colarusso & Hammill, 1996) or the *Test of Visual-Perceptual Skills (TVPS)* (Gardner, 1982) are both nonmotor evaluations that could be used to evaluate the child's current visual-perceptual status. Visual-motor skill development can be evaluated using the *Test of Visual-Motor Skills-Revised (TVMS-R)* (Gardner, 1996) or the *Developmental Test of Visual Motor Integration (VMI)* (Beery, 1989).

Evaluation of self-help and adaptive living skill is a specific area of emphasis for occupational therapy. Difficulties in these areas are often of primary concern to parents. Several independence measures are available to assess these areas. The *Vineland* (Sparrow, Balla & Cicchetti, 1984) measures communication, daily living, socialization, and motor skill status. These domains, as well as cognition, can be assessed using the *BDI* (Newborg, Stock, & Wnek, 1984). Similarly, independence levels within physical, self-help, social, academic, and communication areas can be obtained by using the *DPII* (Alpren, Boll, & Shearer, 1984). The *WeeFIM* (Uniform Data Systems, 1993) can be used as a measure of independence in self-care, sphincter control, transfer, locomotion, communication, and social cognition. All of the above assessment tools are completed primarily as parent report measures. To assess independence in the academic setting, the *School Assessment of Motor and Process Skill (SAMPS)* (Fischer, Bryze, & Magalhaes, 1998) is currently being developed and will assess 16 motor and 20 process behaviors at the level of dysfunction for standardized academic activities.

## *Intervention*

Based on the evaluation findings, an intervention plan is developed. The identified problem areas may be motor, educational, or psychosocial in nature, and likely will be interfering with occupational performance. Many of the psychosocial issues can be addressed through family education in conjunction with the child's neurologist. The family may have questions regarding activity restrictions or precautions. As the child ages, these issues become more difficult, especially in adolescence, because of driving and exposure to alcohol. Improving skill development, minimizing the effects of the seizures, and promoting normal living within sensible confines are often the goals of intervention. To accomplish these goals, close collaboration between the interdisciplinary team of health-care professionals is essential. Often, the child's neurologist will direct the team and advise the members as to precautions.

**The child.** The promotion of normal skill development and occupational performance is often the focus of intervention for the OT. This process may be habilitative or rehabilitative in nature. As the child ages, identifying and addressing the psychosocial difficulties of living with a seizure disorder is integral to the intervention process.

| Child Characteristic | Seen As | In | Possible Strategy or Solution |
|---|---|---|---|
| 9-year-old status post hemispherectomy | Decreased right strength and coordination | Self-care skills | 1. Teach the child hemi dressing techniques presurgery to allow for practice. 2. Work to improve hemi skills postsurgery. 3. Adapt clothing to simplify dressing. |
| 10-year-old with simple partial seizures | Child wants to engage in sports | School | 1. Sports and recreational activities that are age– and social group–appropriate are usually encouraged. 2. Check with the neurologist to identify activity precautions prior to initiation. |

**The parent or caregiver.** Helping parents and family members understand the seizure disorder and its impact on development is often an initial focus of intervention. Additionally, occupational therapy fosters developmentally appropriate occupational performance through direct intervention with the child. For this process to be successful, carryover in the home is essential. As the child ages, occupational therapy can assist in problem solving with the family through many of the psychosocial issues.

| Parent Characteristic | Seen As | Possible Solution or Strategy |
| --- | --- | --- |
| 16-year-old who has been seizure-free for 1.5 years | He wants to get his learner's permit to drive. | 1. Discuss with neurology. 2. Check state laws. |
| 9-year-old with infrequent simple partial seizure disorder | Parents feel the child's academic performance and function are suffering because of medications. | 1. Discuss with neurology whether it is better to have an occasional seizure and stop meds to improve function. 2. Teach energy conservation techniques. |
| 7-year-old with absence seizure disorder who wants to swim with friends | Parents have anxiety about safety in the water. | 1. Restrict swimming only to pools with adequate lifeguard coverage. 2. Buddy system for swimming. 3. Restrict high diving. |

**The environment.** Environmental adaptation is often necessary for children with seizure disorders. This adaptation may be physical in nature or it may entail adapting how a task is completed. Providing these supports and education within the child's surroundings is important not only for their safety in the event of a seizure, but they help others understand the process of living with a seizure disorder.

| Characteristic | Seen As | Possible Solution or Strategy |
| --- | --- | --- |
| Fourth-grade student with tonic-clonic seizures | Teacher has anxiety about having the student in class. | Educate the class regarding seizures and what to do in the event of a seizure. |
| Fifth-grade student with absence seizures | Academic performance is diminishing. | Teacher should alert the parent(s) because the child may be having more seizures or the medication level may be too high. |
| 7-year-old with uncontrolled tonic-clonic seizures | Frequent falls with blows to the head | Have the child wear a helmet during antigravity tasks. |

■ *THERAPEDS POINTER*

Further information on epilepsy can be obtained from:

Epilepsy Foundation of America
    4351 Garden City Dr., Suite 406
    Landover, MD 20785
    1-800-332-1000

# NEURAL TUBE DEFECTS

## CLINICAL PICTURE

Neural tube defects (NTDs) are a group of congenital malformations of the vertebrae and spinal cord. Spina bifida is the most common form of NTD and will be the focus of discussion here. Spina bifida is the failure of fusion of the vertebral arches (bones that make up the spinal column) (Charney, 1992; Haller, 1992). Spina bifida occurs in the first month of pregnancy when the fetus's CNS is developing. At the end of the first month of pregnancy, the baby is a flat layer of cells. This plate then rolls up to form the hollow neural tube, with the top portion forming the brain and the lower portion forming the spinal cord. The tube is supposed to close up like a zipper and form a solid tube. If the bones comprising the spine do not form properly, an opening will result and is referred to as an NTD (Tenenholz, 1993).

Spina bifida occurs in about 1 in 1000 births in the United States (Leggate & St. Clair Forbes, 1995; Sarwark, 1996; Tenenholz, 1993). Its incidence is thought to be four times greater in parts of Ireland (Leggate & St. Clair Forbes, 1995; Sarwark, 1996). Girls are more frequently affected than boys.

The cause of spina bifida is often unknown. These disorders are believed to be multifactoral in origin with both environmental and genetic influences (Charney, 1992; Teneholz, 1993). It is thought that approximately 50 percent of the cases are related to a nutritionally based deficiency of folate (folic acid, B vitamin) (Medical Research Council [MRC], 1991). Studies have demonstrated a significant decrease in NTD reoccurrence in women with a previous NTD birth who were given supplemental folic acid (MRC, 1991; Smithells, Nevin, Seller, et al., 1983). The reduction risk has ranged from 86 percent (Smithells, et al., 1938) to 72 percent (MRC, 1991). Maternal alcoholism, diabetes, and treatment with certain anticonvulsant medications are also thought to increase the risk of spina bifida.

Spina bifida is referred to as being open (operata) or closed (occulta). An open defect is either completely open or covered by a very thin membrane. Closed deficits are covered with thick skin or membrane. Approximately 80 percent of children with spina bifida will have an open defect, with the remaining 20 percent having a closed defect.

Two main forms of open defects are noted: meningocele and myelomeningocele. Many babies with spina bifida will be born with a meningeal fluid-filled sac on their back. Myelomeningocele describes a fluid-filled sac that protrudes from the defective spine and contains the malformed spinal cord (Charney, 1992). In myelomeningocele defects part of the spinal cord is visible at birth. The nerves below that opening fail to develop, resulting in paralysis and sensory loss. In meningocele there is a protruding sac that surrounds a normal spinal cord. Therefore, there are no neurological deficits. Typically, 75 percent of myelomeningoceles and meningoceles are found in the thoracolumbar and sacral region, with 10 percent in the thoracic region and 5 percent in the cervical region.

Closed defects, referred to as spina bifida occulta, can exist without any deficit or manifested only by a thin discolored area of skin, patch of hair, or palpable mass (Haller, 1992). Late-onset clinical features include progressive lower-extremity weakness and persistent enuresis. There are two main types of closed defects: ones that compress the spinal cord and ones that cause the spinal cord to stretch (tethered cord).

If the spinal defect is leaking or open at birth, major concerns relate to infection and drying of the nerve roots. To prevent these from occurring, and thus preventing further loss of function, surgical closure of the defect is usually performed within the first few days of life (Charney, 1992; Stewart, Manchester, & Sujansky, 1996). Although surgical closure may prevent an infection, it has no bearing on the neurological function of the infant. The extent of associated abnormalities is dependent on the level of spinal cord lesions, with all function below that level impaired somewhat. Some of the most significant deficits are in the infant's neurological status and bowel and bladder function. Hydrocephalus may be apparent at birth, but most often there is an increased head circumferences, irritability, and poor feeding shortly after the closure is performed. With a sacral defect, the infant may have only mild weakness at the ankles or toes. Bladder and anal sphincters remain intact. Infants with low lumbar (L4, L5) lesions can flex their hips and extend at the knees, but often have weak plantar flexion and hip extension. Midlumbar (L3) defects result in the ability to flex at the hips and extend at the knees, but paralysis at the ankles and toes is noted. High lumbar (L1, L2) and thoracic lesions will cause variable weakness throughout the lower extremities. Any lumbar or thoracic lesion will affect bladder and anal sphincters and musculature. In all levels of defect, over time neuromuscular factors diminish to some degree.

As can be seen, the higher the lesion, the greater impairment on ambulation and motor function. Most children with myelomeningocele have delayed motor skill development from the beginning. Rolling and sitting are delayed. The child's first mode of mobility is to commando crawl. The child's ability to walk varies according to the level of lesion. Children with sacral and low lumbar defects will walk with minimal support (bracing) or adaptive devices. Those with midlumbar or high lumbar lesions may walk, but often require extensive bracing and/or adaptive equipment. It is thought that the children with higher-level lesions who walk are generally the children who do not have MR (Charney, 1992).

Sensory impairments also often correlate to motor function. In areas of anesthesia, skin break down is a threat, especially at the foot and perineal region. Therefore, prevention is an integral component of management. Wheelchairs must be cushioned properly and special attention must be paid to pressure areas as splints are fabricated.

With partial or total paralysis, muscle imbalances often develop and may lead to deformities. A variety of foot deformities, flexion contractures, dislocated hips, or totally flaccid hips can be noted. These musculoskeletal deformities often require bracing and/or surgical correction. Additionally, spinal curvatures and humps are often seen in children with myelomeningocele. The child may develop scoliosis, kyphosis (spinal hump), or kyphoscoliosis (combination of both) (Charney, 1992). These conditions also often require bracing and/or surgical management (see Chapter 6).

There is a wide range of intellectual and cognitive functioning in children with spina bifida. Most children function in the borderline to low-normal range (Stewart et al., 1996). Factors that aid in predicting cognitive ability relate to neurological complications. Although a hydrocephalus and spina bifida combination does not significantly alter a child's testable IQ, shunting complications, seizures, anoxia, and CNS infections do (Mapstone et al., 1984). Seizures are noted in approximately 15 percent of the children with myelomeningocele. These seizures are often of tonic-clonic type and respond well to anticonvulsant medications (see seizure disorders component of this chapter).

Given the above-described associated disabilities, children with spina bifida often are challenged with day-to-day activities and childhood occupations. Regarding school performance, most children are now mainstreamed, but have a higher incidence of visual-perceptual and fine-motor problems (Stewart et al., 1996). Decreased self-care independence is also noted and often relates to the previously noted motor difficulties.

Spina bifida and other NTDs are often diagnosed prenatally using several techniques. Initially, an NTD may be suspected following an initial ultrasound examination. In these suspected cases, an amniocentesis is often recommended. Amniocentesis involves removing for analysis some of the amniotic fluid that surrounds the fetus. The fluid contains a protein made by the fetus called alpha fetoprotein (AFP). When a fetus has an NTD, excess amounts of AFP spill into the amniotic fluid though the opening (Tenenholz, 1993). AFP levels will be significantly elevated in 95 percent of fetuses with open-tube defects (Charney, 1992). Acetylcholinesterase (AChE) levels are also evaluated. AChE is present around nerve cells, and therefore in spina bifida excess amounts are noted in the presence of the exposed nerves. Documenting significantly elevated AFP and AChE levels in the amniotic fluid will confirm the diagnosis of spina bifida (Tenenholz, 1993). Repeat ultrasounds may be used to identify the location of the opening in the spine and its size. Information about growth of the fetus will also be obtained. Additionally, serial sonograms will also be used to screen for hydrocephalus and other congenital anomalies.

With prenatal diagnosis, the intervention and management process for spina bifida begins at birth. The place of birth is often prearranged to allow specialists to be available at or shortly after birth. Usually within 24 hours of birth, the baby is taken to surgery for surgical closure of the opening on the back to prevent infection and further nerve damage. If hydrocephalus is also present at birth, a shunt will be placed. A shunt is a small plastic tube with one end inserted in the ventricles of the brain and the other in the abdomen. This tube will drain the excess fluid in the brain into the abdomen. As the child grows, a shunt revision will likely be performed to make it longer. If a shunt gets blocked, it will likely cause the baby or child to have seizures and will need to be replaced.

Prior to leaving the hospital, the parent(s) of a child with spina bifida (especially those with higher-level defects) need extensive education. Information about the shunt will need to be provided and the parent(s) will need to be taught what to look for if the shunt is not functioning properly. The parent(s) will also need to be taught how to use a urinary catheter to extract all the urine from the baby's bladder, because the baby will likely be unable to rid the body of urine independently, and failure to do so may lead to kidney problems. The parent(s) will also have to be taught scar management for the baby's back to prevent infection and promote healing. In the presence of foot deformities (i.e., club foot), splinting may be implemented prior to discharge from the hospital, and therefore an application schedule will need to be discussed, as will pressure area identification.

Once the child recovers from surgery and is discharged from the hospital, the early intervention process begins. Because of the vast associated anomalies in spina bifida, management is usually accomplished by a team of medical, allied health, and educational professionals. Together, this team attempts to facilitate optimal motor, self-help, and occupational performance. A physician will often coordinate the care of the child and refer the child for appropriate services. Orthopedics may be involved early on to manage foot deformities. OTs and physical therapists will also often be involved early to facilitate motor milestone attainment to allow for successful acquisition childhood occupations.

As the child ages, orthopedic and neurosurgery may be called upon to manage hip deformities. Many of these, as well as their surgical intervention, have been previously discussed in the CP section of this chapter. These disciplines may also be involved in the care of spinal deformities (see Chapter 6). Following these surgical interventions, OTs and physical therapists often have a rehabilitative role in restoring motor functioning and occupational performance to presurgical levels.

Throughout the intervention process, adaptive equipment has an integral role. Splinting, bracing, or casting will often be used in the management of skeletal deformities. Adaptive equipment is also used during motor interventions. Standing frames and specialized seating systems will frequently be used early in development to help build stability. As the child is more stable, walkers, crutches, and/or braces will likely be used to gain skilled mobility. For those children for whom ambulation is not a goal, a wheelchair may be required for mobility. Adaptive equipment will also likely be used by OTs to promote self-care independence.

Prognosis for the child with spina bifida is often dependent on the type and level. Prognosis is good for children with spina bifida occulta or meningocele. For children with myelomeningocele, the higher the level, the less mobility and therefore the more difficulty with independent living. For children whose condition is complicated by hydrocephalus with shunt difficulties and cognitive deficits, independent living is less likely.

## THE OCCUPATIONAL THERAPY PERSPECTIVE

### *Evaluation*

As previously implied, evaluation of spina bifida is often conducted by a team of professionals at a tertiary care center by an interdisciplinary team of professionals with expertise in NTDs. Secondary to research data suggestive of varying cognitive ability and its impact on developmental outcome, the physician may wish to have the child's overall cognitive ability formally assessed by a psychologist. The psychologist may administer one of a number of psychological tests assessing intelligence (see Chapter 9). Also, as part of a comprehensive workup, the physician will typically request occupational and physical therapy services to conduct formalized evaluations. Evaluation consists largely of formalized testing of the child's overall ROM and muscle strength because deficits in these performance components often compromise life role function (occupation). OTs may be involved in this diagnostic evaluation process or may see the child following diagnosis for intervention planning. In either case, the evaluation process begins by reviewing the child's past medical and developmental histories. Parental report of childhood occupations also often initiates the evaluation process. The parents may report that the child sleeps excessively, is irritable, or has difficulty feeding. In many instances the occupational performance difficulties that parents report will relate to their developmental difficulties.

A comprehensive neuromuscular assessment often initiates the physical evaluation. Overall active and passive ROM measurements are obtained. Proximal and distal muscle tone is also evaluated. Joint involvement is documented to determine the presence of asymmetries or distribution variations between the upper and lower body. Strength is often assessed through observation of antigravity postures and movements because specific muscle testing is difficult in this age group and in the presence of tone.

To supplement these neuromuscular findings, a neurodevelopmental assessment is also conducted. Here, the child's balance reactions and movement patterns are formally assessed to determine the level and impact of paralysis. Additionally, standardized testing will often be conducted by both occupational and physical therapy services to assess motor skill development (both gross and fine). Since the movement quality and patterns of movement are very important in the evaluation of the child with spina bifida, using an assessment tool that addresses these areas is crucial. As previously noted, the therapist may wish to use the *MAI* (Chandler, Andrews, & Swanson, 1980) or the *T.I.M.E.* (Miller & Roid, 1994). To determine developmental ages for gross and fine motor skill acquisition, the *PDMS* (Folio & Fewell, 1983) may be used, as may a number of other criterion-referenced evaluations.

Older children, especially in the presence of visual-perceptual and fine-motor deficits, often require more specialized testing. Occupational therapy will usually specifically assess visual perception and fine- and visual-motor integration using any of a number of assessment tools.

---

■ *THERAPEDS POINTER*

Evaluation of motor skill, visual perception and visual motor integration in older children is often the role of the OT on the interdisciplinary team. Possible tools that could be used:

**Motor Skill**

*Tests and Ages:*
- *Bruininks-Oseretsky Test of Motor Proficiency* (BOTMP) (Bruininks, 1978); 4.5–14.5 yr
- *The Miller Assessment for Preschools (MAP)* (Miller, 1988); 2.9–5.8 yr
- *School Assessment of Motor and Process Skill* (SAMPS) (Fischer, Bryze, & Magalhaes, 1988)

*Skills Assessed:* The *BOTMP* can be used as measures of gross and fine motor abilities. The *MAP* may also be used to assess preacademic skill development in the preschool-aged child. The *MAP* will provide some information on a child's sensory and motor abilities, while also opening a window to verbal and nonverbal abilities. The *SAMPS* is currently being developed. It will measure 16 motor and 20 process behaviors at the level of dysfunction for standardized academic activities.

### Visual Perception
*Tests and Ages:*

- *Motor-Free Visual Perception Test-Revised (MVPT-R)* (Colarusso & Hammill, 1996); 4–11 yr
- *Test of Visual Perceptual Skills (TVPS)* (Gardner, 1982); 4–12.11 yr

*Skills Assessed:* Both tools assess visual discrimination, visual-spatial relationships, visual memory, visual figure-ground, and visual closure, while the *TVPS* also assesses visual form constancy and visual sequential memory. Both tools are nonmotor.

### Visual-Motor Integration
*Tests and Ages:*

- *Test of Visual-Motor Skills-Revised (TVMS-R)* (Gardner, 1995); 3–13.11 yr
- *Developmental Test of Visual-Motor Integration (VMI)* (Beery, 1989); 2–15 yr

*Skills Assessed:* Both assessments are made up of design copying items of increasing difficulty and assess the child's ability or inability to translate with his or her hand what he or she visually perceives.

---

The child's self-help and adaptive living status is a vital area of emphasis specifically addressed by occupational therapy during the evaluation process. Several independence measures are available to assess these areas. *The Vineland* (Sparrow, Balla, & Cicchetti, 1984), *BDI* (Newborg, Stock, & Wnek, 1984), *DPII* (Alpren, Boll, & Shearer, 1984), or the *WeeFIM* (Uniform Data Systems, 1993) could be used to assess independence in these areas. All of the above self-care assessments can be completed primarily as parent report measures.

## *Intervention*

Following formal evaluation and the establishment of the child's developmental status, the process of intervention begins. As in evaluation, the intervention process for the child with spina bifida often involves an interdisciplinary team of allied health professionals. This process is habilitative in nature. Together, this team attempts to foster normalized overall development to allow for childhood occupations, with each discipline focusing on specific aspects of development. Often, integration and carryover to the home are accomplished by the family if the direct interventions are not accomplished within the home.

The OT will often address motor development and stability concerns in conjunction with physical therapy. This therapy may be done in cotreatment. A neurodevelopmental treatment (NDT) approach may be used as a method of intervention for the child with spina bifida to address these motor areas. Positioning (for rest and play), neurodevelopmental handling, and play foster the development of normal movement patterns. Sensory integrative intervention may be used to promote increased vestibular processing through tactile and proprioceptive inputs to the trunk and hips.

The child's fine-motor and visual-perceptual development and how they impact on play, self-care, and academic and occupational performance are also areas of concentration for the OT. Alleviating or compensating for deficits in these areas may be done in the home, preschool program, and/or school. OTs also often assist their patients and families to obtain necessary adaptive equipment, splints, and/or orthotics. Adaptive aids can promote increased self-care independence and improve play performance. Splinting and equipment needs are often coordinated with physical therapy.

**The child.** Child-based interventions attempt to facilitate normal developmental milestones by minimizing the effects of neuromuscular and motor deficits. Adaptive equipment (splints, mobility aids, self-help aids, etc.) is integral in this habilitative process. Occupational therapy often works closely with and builds upon other allied health team interventions to attain team goals.

| Child Characteristic | Seen As | In | Possible Solution or Strategy |
|---|---|---|---|
| 7-year-old with high-lumbar defect | Lower-extremity weakness | Dressing | 1. Having the child use adaptive equipment for dressing (i.e., reacher, long-handled shoe horn).<br>2. Adapt clothing (i.e., elastic shoelaces). |
| 7-year-old with midlumbar defect | Bladder incontinence | School | 1. Have child wear pullups to school.<br>2. Allow the child to self-catheter his or her bladder periodically throughout the day<br>3. Educate the other students on the child's condition to prevent them from teasing. |
| 11-year-old with myelomeningocele | Decreased fine- and visual-motor control | Writing tasks | 1. Allow more time for written work.<br>2. De-emphasize written work and allow for more oral experiences.<br>3. Allow a trial with key boarding. |

**The parent.** Early education and support to the family provides a means to care for the specialized demands of the child with spina bifida. Helping the child and family with ongoing self-help, academic, and psychosocial difficulties are goal areas for occupational therapy. OTs solve problems with the parents and enable them to play, interact, and work freely with their child.

| Characteristic | Seen As | Possible Strategy or Solution |
|---|---|---|
| 12-month-old with spina bifida myelomeningocele | Parents have a difficult time positioning the child for prolonged periods without holding him or her | 1. Continue active occupational and physical therapy to improve proximal stability. 2. Check local early intervention to see if adapted seating is available from the loan closet. |
| 7-year-old with spina bifida meningocele wants to enroll in after school activities with friends | Parents have anxiety about activities because the child may not be able to keep up with the others. | 1. Parents can encourage participation in non-competitive activities. 2. Have the child join recreational clubs (Boy or Girl Scouts, 4 H, etc.). |
| 16-year-old with spina bifida myelomeningocele | Parents feel the child is depressed and socially withdrawing. | 1. Enroll the child in a spina bifida support group. 2. Facilitate peer interactions by organizing activities. 3. Explore the need for professional counseling. |

**The environment.** Adaptive equipment often assists in promoting independence and childhood occupation. To improve skill the equipment can be used directly by the child or the environment itself can be adapted. Additionally, environmental adaptation and task adaptation often allow for increased independence as skill development is progressing

| Characteristic | Seen As | Possible Strategy or Solution |
|---|---|---|
| 10-year-old with midlumbar myelomeningocele ambulates with braces | Slow ambulation and difficulty transitioning from class to class | 1. Allow the child to leave early to get to the next class. 2. Have the child use a wheelchair to change classes. 3. Allow the child to be a few minutes late to class. |
| 24-month-old child with thoracic myelomeningocele | Child has difficulty sitting in circle time on the floor. | 1. Allow the child to sit on an air cushion or bean bag chair. |

| Characteristic | Seen As | Possible Strategy or Solution |
|---|---|---|
| | | 2. Obtain a seating system for the child to use in the preschool program. |
| | | 3. If the child has a wheelchair, be sure she or he comes to the program in it. |

■ *THERAPEDS POINTER*

Further information on spinal bifida can be obtained from:

Spina Bifida Association of America
  1700 Rockville Pike, Suite 250
  Rockville, MD 20852-1654
  1-800-621-3141

## ▰▰ FROM THE BOOKSHELF

Further information on assistive technology can be found within:
  Angelo, J. (1996). *Assistive technology for rehabilitation therapists.*
Philadelphia: F. A. Davis.

# CHILDHOOD INFECTIOUS DISEASE

## MENINGITIS

Meningitis is an acute, potentially life-threatening illness that requires rapid diagnosis and treatment. Meningitis, stated basically, is inflammation of the meninges (lining of the brain) (Aronoff, Corder, Ferrari, et al., 1994; Moe & Seay, 1995). The clinical picture of meningitis is quite variable and is dependent on the age of the child and the duration of the illness prior to diagnosis. In neonates, early symptoms include irritability, poor feeding, and vomiting. Lethargy, seizures, a bulging anterior fontanelle, and poor tone are later findings. Older children usually have a fever. Symptoms may also include nausea, vomiting, lethargy, headache, confusion, and light sensitivity. Focal neurological signs (paresis, ataxia, hearing deficit) may also be present. Kernig's and Brudzinski's signs are classic signs of neck stiffness reflecting meningeal irritation (Aronoff et al., 1994; Fishman, 1992).

■ *THERAPEDS POINTER*

*Kernig's sign* is elicited by flexing the hip and knee, and then
  extending the knee with the hip still flexed. Report of pain or

resistance of knee extension by the child suggests meningeal irritation.

*Brudzinski's sign* is elicited by passively flexing the neck. If knee and hip flexion result, this too is a sign of meningeal irritation.

---

Meningitis may be classified according to CSF findings that indicate bacterial or viral infection. The CSF is acquired by lumbar puncture. These laboratory studies of CSF, along with blood cultures, are key components of the diagnostic evaluation for meningitis. The studies can identify the bacteria, virus, or fungus that is causing irritation in the meninges. Imaging studies (CT or MRI) are also frequently used to detect complications and possible causes in meningitis. In cases where the child has a fever and the neurological exam reveals focal neurological signs, these imaging studies should be performed prior to doing the lumbar puncture.

Together, the laboratory and imaging findings guide appropriate medical management and prognostic statements. Medical management usually initiates with pharmacological therapy. The child is often initially treated with broad-spectrum medication(s) geared toward the pathogens that usually affect the child's age group. As culture and laboratory findings become more complete, the therapy is adjusted to target the known pathogen (bacterial, fungal, or viral). During this period the child needs close monitoring for physical and/or neurological and complications.

Long-term sequelae of meningitis result from brain cell destruction secondary to edema and/or vascular disease. These sequelae may include hearing deficit, seizures, language disorders, MR, motor abnormalities, visual impairment, behavior and learning disorders, attention deficits, and lower intelligence quotients (Aronoff et al., 1995; Moe & Seay, 1995). These resultant developmental difficulties often have significant impact on occupational performance. Here is where OTs foster independence in childhood occupations.

## ENCEPHALITIS

Encephalitis is an infection or inflammation of the brain tissue manifested by altered consciousness, fever, headache, and/or focal neurological signs (Aronoff et al., 1994; Clarke & St. Clair Forbes, 1995; Fishman, 1992). There is usually a generalized viral infection that precedes the neurological syndrome. These may include upper respiratory symptoms, nausea, vomiting, or headache. Lethargy or drowsiness, which may lead to coma, often indicates brain involvement. Confusion, hallucinations, and disorientation may be noted if consciousness is less significantly altered. Seizures, hemiplegia, ataxia, dysarthria, dysphagia, and hemianopsia may also be noted. These signs and symptoms are often beneficial in detecting the location(s) of CNS inflammation. For instance, ataxia tremor and coordination deficits often trigger cerebellar involvement, whereas spinal cord involvement usually results in paraplegia, sensory level alterations, and bowel and bladder control difficulties.

As in meningitis, laboratory studies of CSF, blood cultures, and radiographic results serve as key components of the diagnostic evaluation for encephalitis. Although most cases of encephalitis are viral in origin, these studies can also identify bacterial or fungal pathogens. MRI has proved to be more sensitive than CT in early detection of viral encephalitis. EEG studies are also usually abnormal.

The diagnosis of encephalitis is based on the above findings, although the only definitive method of diagnosis is brain biopsy with tissue cultures (Fenichel, 1993). However, this is not commonly done. Instead, pharmacological treatment is initiated based on the history of present illness and available test results. As with meningitis, occupational therapy's role in cases of encephalitis is in the management of residual neurological dysfunction.

## GUILLAIN-BARRÉ SYNDROME

Guillain-Barré syndrome (GBS) is a neurological disorder affecting the peripheral nerves (Batshaw & Perret, 1992; Soueidan, 1992). Patients present with a rapidly progressing symmetric paralysis. The paralysis usually begins in the lower extremities and moves upward. Proximal muscles are occasionally weaker than distal muscles. Given these characteristics, it should be noted that the diaphragm and upper extremities are often involved. Therefore, breathing may be impaired and mechanical ventilation may be required. Some degree of sensory loss is also often present. This degenerative process can last for 3 weeks or more.

The onset of the muscle weakness is usually preceded by a viral illness 1 to 2 weeks prior. This virus is usually upper respiratory or gastrointestinal in nature. It is thought that GBS results from an autoimmune response to this viral infection. In other words, the child's immune system is too aggressive in its fight of an infection and mistakenly destroys parts of the body. In GBS peripheral nerves are affected. Specifically, demyelination of the nerve roots occurs and thus nerve conduction is affected.

Diagnosis of GBS is based on the above clinical course and adjunct studies. Analysis of CSF will show elevated protein levels, while electromyographic (EMG) studies will show a slowing of nerve conduction, reflecting the demyelination and axonal damage.

Since GBS is believed to be an autoimmune disease, one of the management principles attempts to alter this response. Plasmapheresis (exchanging plasma) is often instituted before the child's weakness plateaus. Improved outcome has been correlated with this procedure (Epstein & Sladky, 1990; Soueidan, 1992). When the patient is medically stable, OTs are integral in the rehabilitation process to restore function. Prognosis is good for children with GBS; most children make close to a full recovery. Some children do, however, have persistent facial and/or lower-extremity weakness.

---

■ *THERAPEDS POINTER*

Further information on GBS can be obtained from:

Guillain-Barré Syndrome Foundation, International
    P.O. Box 262
    Wynnewood, PA 19096
    (215) 667-0131

---

# THE OCCUPATIONAL THERAPY PERSPECTIVE

## *Evaluation*

When medically stable, the child will frequently be seen by an OT as part of the rehabilitative process. Together, the rehab team will try to restore function and occupational performance to preillness levels. The intervention process is initiated by establishing the child's current developmental and occupational status. Past medical and occupational histories are obtained initially.

A comprehensive neuromuscular assessment often initiates the physical evaluation. Active and passive ROM measurements are obtained. Proximal and distal muscle tone is also evaluated. Joint involvement is documented to determine the presence of asymmetries or distribution variations between the upper and lower body. Strength is often assessed through observation of antigravity postures and movements. Specific manual muscle testing may be possible with older children. Balance reaction development, overall balance, and stability should also be evaluated.

The child's neuromuscular status often serves as the foundation for motor skill development. To evaluate motor skill development in younger children, the *MAI* (Chandler, Andrews, & Swanson, 1980), *T.I.M.E.* (Miller & Roid, 1994) or *PDMS* (Folio & Fewell, 1983) may be used. A number of other criterion-referenced evaluations may also be used to determine approximate developmental ages. In older children the *BOTMP* (Bruininks, 1978) may be used to obtain standardized measures of these areas.

Also in schoolaged children, visual-perceptual and visual-motor skill development may need to be evaluated. Difficulties in these areas can have significant impact on academic performance. The *Motor-Free Visual Perception Test—Revised (MVPT-R)* (Colarusso & Hammill, 1996) or the *Test of Visual-Perceptual Skills (TVPS)* (Gardner, 1982) are both nonmotor evaluations that could be used to evaluate the child's current visual-perceptual status. Visual-motor skill development can be evaluated using the *Test of Visual-Motor Skills—Revised (TVMS-R)* (Gardner, 1996) or the *Developmental Test of Visual Motor Integration (VMI)* (Beery, 1989).

Evaluation of self-help and adaptive living skill is a specific area of emphasis for occupational therapy. Difficulties in these areas are often of primary concern to parents. Several independence measures are available to assess these areas and have been previously discussed.

## *Intervention*

The intervention process in these infectious diseases varies depending on the stage of disease. During the infectious process, an alteration in consciousness is often noted in all of these diseases. During this disease process, the role of the OT is often preventive in nature. Promoting maintenance of ROM and prevention of contracture is the focus of treatment. In cases of prolonged coma during the infectious process, a sensory stimulation and orientation program may be implemented by the OT. In the presence of tonal abnormalities, splints may also need to be fabricated.

After the child has stabilized medically, the intervention process is focused on rehabilitation. As previously noted, with all of these infectious diseases, focal neurological signs and/or muscle weakness are likely noted. With these limitations occupational performance limitations will also likely be noted. As part of a rehabilitative process, the OT will work jointly with other allied health professionals to improve strength and stability. Endurance will likely be decreased and need to be rebuilt. Increasing the child's awareness of, and compensating for, residual sensory deficits will also be an occupational therapy function. Residual effects may also have impact on school functioning and occupational performance, and therefore occupational therapy attempts to minimize these effects. Until skill is regained, initial compensation may be necessary.

**The child.** Intervention with the child is often focused on rehabilitation of lost skill and occupational roles. These may include neuromuscular, motor, visual-motor, and/or occupational skills. The intervention process is often a team effort with the OT working jointly with other allied health professionals and the family. Improving these skills to optimal levels (as close to predisease levels as possible) is often the goal of occupational therapy intervention.

| Child Characteristic | Seen As | In | Possible Solution or Strategy |
|---|---|---|---|
| 9-year-old, status post viral encephalitis | Decreased balance in sit and stand | Self-help tasks | 1. Have the child sit in a chair or on the bed to dress. 2. Have the child sit in a chair at the sink to bathe and brush teeth. 3. Make sure supervision is present when out of bed. |
| 10-year-old, status post bacterial meningitis | Ataxia in bilateral upper extremity | Feeding | 1. Wrist weights for arms. 2. Use weighted utensils. |
| 11-year-old recovering from GBS | Lower-extremity weakness | Dressing | 1. Continue strength and endurance intervention. 2. Use adaptive equipment to compensate for these deficits while strength is built. |

**The parent or caregiver.** The infectious process is quite frightening for the parents of the child, especially the speed with which the regression occurs. Assisting parents to feel comfortable with the rehabilitative process and defining the parents' role on the team are important first steps. Occupational performance concerns are often of greatest magnitude for the parents.

| Characteristic | Seen As | Possible Solution or Strategy |
|---|---|---|
| Child with vision loss in left eye with left neglect following viral encephalitis secondary to residual optic neuritis | Parents are concerned because the child keeps bumping his head and left eye. | 1. Work on left orientation activities. 2. Have the child wear protective acrylic glasses. |

**The environment.** In many cases, either during or following these infectious disease processes, adaptive equipment will be used to maintain or regain function. Following the disease process, environmental adaptation promotes skill recovery during the rehabilitation of strength and endurance.

| Characteristic | Seen As | Possible Solution or Strategy |
|---|---|---|
| 11-year-old in coma secondary to GBS | Tightening in the hands | 1. Resting hand splints. 2. Teach the parents to do PROM 1–2 times a day. |
| 5-year-old, status postviral encephalitis, on phenobarbital to control seizures | Hyperactivity in kindergarten | 1. Allow periodic breaks during the day. 2. Allow the child to sit on a rocker board or air cushion to regulate movement need. 3. Incorporate a feel-good box in the classroom to allow the child to regulate himself or herself through the tactile and proprioceptive systems. |

# CHILDHOOD DEGENERATIVE DISORDERS

## RETT'S SYNDROME

Rett's syndrome is an X-linked dominant disorder occurring only in girls. Typically, these girls develop normally the first year of life. The halting of development usually begins around 12 months of age, but may appear as early as 6 months or as late as 18 months. Within a few months, developmental skills are lost and a plateauing of developmental progress follows. This developmental regression is characterized by a loss of language, decreased functional use of the hands, gait ataxia, truncal apraxia or ataxia, and autistic behaviors (Fenichel, 1993; Newton, 1995). Head growth is arrested with eventual microcephaly noted. A characteristic feature of the syndrome is the loss of purposeful hand function. The hands are often held at the level of the mouth. Repetitive movements develop and may include hand wringing, hand flapping, and/or flicking of the lower lip (Newton, 1995). Socially, the girls lose the ability to orient to their environment. When stimulated or approached, a sterotypic reaction consisting of jerky movements of the trunk and limbs often follows. During these episodes breathing irregularities and apnea may be noted followed by hyperventilation. Seizure activity is often noted during sleep. There is also a gradual decline in neurological status. Spasticity develops that often leaves the girls nonambulatory and nonverbal. Scoliosis is also often present.

No one test is available to diagnose Rett's syndrome. Instead, the diagnosis is based on the observation of clinical signs. The Rett's Syndrome Diagnostic Criteria Work Group (1988) established the diagnostic criteria (Table 5–6). Additional studies may be useful in managing Rett's syndrome. An EEG can document seizure activity to assist in controlling them with appropriate anticonvulsants.

The degenerative nature of this disorder makes management quite difficult. Although seizures are reported to be controlled by conventional anticonvulsant medications (Fenichel, 1993), other studies report that seizures are difficult to control (Swaiman & Dyken,1994). Orthopedic management is often needed to prevent pain related to contracture formation and scoliosis. One study (Aron, 1990) has reported elbow extension splints to be effective in inhibiting aberrant upper-extremity movement and preventing hand injury. In this study, the girls demonstrated less hand-to-mouth and hand-wringing behaviors and were also reported to be more social and to have increased environmental interaction.

Table 5–6 **Rett's Syndrome Diagnostic Criteria**

### NECESSARY CRITERIA

1. Apparently normal prenatal and perinatal period and development in first 6 months
2. Normal head circumference at birth and deceleration of head growth between 5 month and 4 years
3. Loss of acquired purposeful hand movements between 6 and 30 months
4. Development of stereotyped hand movements
5. Severe progressive dementia
6. Appearance of gait apraxia and truncal apraxia and ataxia between 1 and 4 year of age

### SUPPORTIVE CRITERIA

1. Breathing dysfunction
2. EEG abnormalities and seizures
3. Growth retardation and hypotrophic small feet
4. Spasticity and dystonia
5. Peripheral vasomotor disturbances
6. Scoliosis

---

■*THERAPEDS POINTER*

Further information on Rett's syndrome can be obtained from:

International Rett Syndrome Association
  9121 Piscataway Rd, Suite 2B
  Clinton, MD 20735

---

## MULTIPLE SCLEROSIS

Though typically thought to be a disease of young adults, multiple sclerosis (MS) has been diagnosed in children as young as 24 months. Neurological symptoms usually develop in children between 10 and 15 years of age, although 20 percent have onset of symptoms prior to age 10 (Fishman, 1994). The female-to-male ratio varies, although it is thought to range from 2:1 to 4:1 (Fenichel, 1993).

The clinical course of MS involves exacerbations and remissions, but a chronic progressive course is not unusual. Ataxia is the most common initial feature in children. Encephalopathy, hemiparesis, or seizures are alternative initial manifestations (Fenichel, 1993). This acute period is followed by a period of remission, and then by a subsequent episode. This exacerbation will involve a different region of the brain. These episodes represent repeated episodes of CNS demyelination. Each episode is characterized by weeks of focal neurological signs separated by months or years of remission. These episodes are often associated with febrile episodes and/or illness. In the periods of remission, the child has partial or complete recovery. Over time, there will likely be less recovery after an exacerbation and therefore greater degrees of dysfunction persist (Fishman, 1994). The disease eventually enters a chronic phase and becomes progressive over years. Death most often is related to respiratory problems or infection.

Disturbances in motor function, weakness, and incoordination and ataxia are common. The extent and distribution of deficits is dependent on the location of the white matter lesion. Somatosensory deficits may also accompany the motor dysfunction. Visual disturbances are frequently noted and are often associated with optic neuritis (inflammation of the optic nerves). Headaches and vertigo may also be reported.

MS may be suspected at the time of first attack, but definitive diagnosis requires recurrence to establish the multiphasic course. Additional studies may be beneficial in diagnosing MS. CSF abnormalities are noted in most cases. CT and MRI studies can detect the location and extent of the white matter lesions. These studies may reveal multiple lesions that may or may not relate to the clinical findings. Electrophysiological studies may be used to detect auditory, visual, and somatosensory pathway abnormalities through examination of evoked potentials. This information assists in establishing the involvement and extent of multiple brain regions.

No cure or preventive measure is available for MS. Conservative supportive treatment programs are encouraged (Allen, 1992). A course of adrenocorticotropic hormones or corticosteroids may be used in an acute exacerbation to shorten its duration, although these medications are not believed to alter the course of the disease (Fishman, 1993). Other management techniques, and the primary roles of occupational therapy, involve the management of spasticity and the promotion of independence following an exacerbation.

## THE OCCUPATIONAL THERAPY PERSPECTIVE

### Evaluation

In degenerative disease, the evaluation process is very important in establishing an accurate baseline. This baseline often establishes the skill levels at which intervention attempts to maintain the child. As usual, the evaluation is initiated by obtaining pertinent medical and occupational history for the child. For MS, obtaining information regarding length of exacerbation and prior levels of functioning is important in establishing the progression of the disease. Additionally, the parent's overall level of understanding and acceptance of the disease should be explored to determine further educational and/or intervention needs. The physical evaluation is often initiated with a neuromuscular assessment. Active and passive ROM and overall muscle tone are assessed. Strength is often assessed through observation of antigravity postures and movements in younger children. In older children with MS, manual muscle testing may be accomplished. Tonal abnormalities with ROM limitations may warrant splinting to prevent contractures. Balance reaction development, as well as overall balance, should also be evaluated.

In school-aged children with MS, visual-perceptual and visual-motor skill development may need to be evaluated. Difficulties in these areas can have significant impact on academic performance. The *MVPT-R* (Colarusso & Hammill, 1996) or the *TVPS* (Gardner, 1982) are both nonmotor evaluations that could be used to evaluate the child's current visual-perceptual status. Visual-motor skill development can be evaluated using *TVMS-R* (Gardner, 1996) or *VMI* (Beery, 1989).

Evaluation of self-help and occupational performance is an area of emphasis for occupational therapy, as well as an area of concern for parents. As previously discussed, several independent measures are available to assess these areas. The *Vineland* (Sparrow, Balla, & Cicchetti, 1984), *BDI* (Newborg, Stock, & Wnek, 1984), *DPII* (Alpren, Boll, & Shearer, 1984), or the *WeeFIM* (Uniform Data Systems, 1993) can be used as a measure of independence in self-care. All of the above assessment tools are completed primarily as parent report measures. Independence in school can be assessed using the *SAMPS* (Fischer, Bryze, & Magalhaes, 1998).

### Intervention

As previously noted, the evaluation often establishes a developmental baseline. This baseline also often serves as the level at which the intervention plan attempts to maintain the child. With degenerative disease, the goal of intervention is to prolong independence and skill as long as possible. This process often requires more support of families given the degenerative nature of the disease.

Direct intervention for *the child* attempts to maintain independence. After an exacerbation in MS this process is often rehabilitative, because the focus of treatment is to regain independence. In Rett's syndrome, the process is more preventive in nature as treatment attempts to prevent skill loss. In both cases, promoting neuromuscular (ROM and strength) maintenance is important. Therapeutic and occupational activity attempt to preserve ROM and limit spasticity. As these factors deteriorate, tasks are often adapted to prolong independence. Tasks are often simplified and/or adaptive equipment is used.

**Parents and caregivers.** Parents often need increased support in degenerative disease, because it is difficult to see a child regress developmentally. This skill regression is a constant reminder of the continued care and support their child will need. Assisting the emotional status of the parent or caregiver may be one role of occupational therapy that may include recommending a support group, providing educational materials, and/or improving the quality of life of the child. Problem solving through the day-to-day self-care difficulties to ease the parent's load may also be a goal of intervention.

Adaptations to *the environment* are often integral parts of the intervention process. These adaptations will hopefully allow for prolonged independence. Splinting is often required to prevent contracture formation in the presence of spasticity. Also, as previously noted, elbow splints are frequently used in the treatment of Rett's syndrome to limit the repetitive hand movements. As the child ages, additional equipment may be required for mobility (wheelchair).

# WRAPPING IT UP

As can be seen in the preceding discussions, there is no cure for these conditions, only management. Additionally, all of these conditions will likely have long-term effects on the child's physical and occupational status. Minimizing these effects within all systems the child functions in is often the goal of occupational therapy intervention. However, we cannot do it alone. Working collaboratively with the family and medical and allied health team members is essential for goal attainment. This process can be preventive, habilitative, or rehabilitative in nature and often requires direct intervention, family education, and environmental adaptation. Prognosis is variable for these conditions, although OTs can positively affect outcome with appropriate therapeutic intervention.

## CASE STORY

Julie is a 3-year, 1-month-old white female child. She is the full-term product of a 36-week pregnancy. She has been previously diagnosed with myelomeningocele spina bifida. By history, she had a high-lumbar defect that was surgically repaired on day 1 of life. She endured a prolonged neonatal course in the intensive care nursery of 34 days secondary to feeding difficulties. She was discharged home to the care of her mother. Julie also has two older brothers in the home, David, 6, and Tim, 8. Upon discharge home, Julie was also enrolled in the local early-intervention program. She has received the benefit of occupational, physical, and speech-language therapy services in the home since this time.

Currently, Julie has been transitioned into the local school system. She has been enrolled in a developmental preschool program in which you provide occupational therapy services. Motorically, you have been told that Julie is now crawling and sits independently in a chair. She has increased difficulty, however, sitting on the floor. Regarding fine-motor development, her skills are described as delayed, especially for visual-motor and functional application to self-help (dressing, feeding). Specifically, Julie is unable to doff clothing at this time and continues to exclusively finger-feed. Further, she will only eat rougher textures of foods. Previous testing has also revealed delayed cognitive skills in the borderline range. Although speech and language development are reported to be low average to slightly delayed, significant difficulty is noted for social interaction development. Julie is described as interacting freely and appropriately with adults, although reportedly has difficulty with peer interaction.

1. What adaptations to the classroom may need to be made at circle time, given Julie's difficulty sitting on the floor?
2. What would your primary focus be for treatment?
3. Julie's mother seeks some recommendations on how to foster play with her older brother. Any suggestions?
4. What suggestions would you make to facilitate peer interaction?

## Real-Life Lab

As stated above, Julie is 3 and is going to attend a developmental preschool program. This program is located within the same school her brothers attend. Therefore, Julie will ride the bus along with her brothers. You have been asked to consult on a seating system for Julie to be used for mobility and positioning during the day at preschool. Given the level of spinal defect, what type of seat pad and supports may be needed for this wheelchair?

# References

Allen, R. J. (1992). Neuroimmunologic disorders. In David, R. B. (Ed.), *Pediatric neurology for the clinician*. Norwalk, CT: Appleton & Lange.

Alpren, G. D., Boll, T. J., & Shearer, M. S. (1984). *Developmental profile II*. Los Angeles: Western Psychological Services.

Arens, I. J., Peacock, W. J., & Peter, J. (1989). Selective posterior rhizotomy: A long-term follow-up study. *Child's Nervous System, 5*, 148.

Aron, M. (1990). The use and effectiveness of elbow splints in the Rett syndrome. *Brain Development, 12*, 162.

Aronoff, S. R., Corder, W. T., Ferrari, ND, III, Kamei, R. K., Rosas, A., Rosas, F., & Uba, A. K. (1994). Infectious diseases. In Rudolph, A. M., & Kamei, R. K. (Eds.), *Rudolph's fundamentals of pediatrics*. Norwalk, CT: Appleton & Lange.

Aylward, G. P. (1994). *Bayley infant development screen manual*. San Antonio: Psycorp.

Batshaw, M. L., & Perret, Y. M. (1992). Seizure disorders. In *Children with disabilities: A medical primer* (3d ed.). Baltimore: Brookes.

Beery, K. E. (1989). *Developmental test of visual motor integration: Administration and scoring manual*. Chicago: Follette.

Berman, B., Vaughan, C. L. & Peacock, W. J. (1990). The effect of rhizotomy on movement in patients with cerebral palsy. *American Journal of Occupational Therapy, 44*, 511–516.

Bobath, K. (1980). A neurophysiological basis for the treatment of cerebral palsy. *Clinics in Developmental Medicine 75*, 77.

Bower, E., & McLellan, D. I. (1992). Effect of increased exposure to physiotherapy on skill acquisition of children with cerebral palsy. *Developmental Medicine and Child Neurology, 34*, 25.

Bruininks, R. H. (1978). *Bruininks-Oseretsky test of motor proficiency examiner's manual*. Circle Pines: American Guidance Service.

Capute, A. J., & Accardo, P. J. (1996). Cerebral palsy: The spectrum of motor dysfunction. In Capute, A. J., & Accardo, P. J. (Eds.), *Developmental disabilities in infancy and childhood*. (2d ed.). Baltimore: Brookes.

Chandler, L., Andrews, M., & Swanson, M. (1980). *The movement assessment of infants*. Rolling Bay, WA: MAI.

Charney, E. B. (1992). Neural tube defects. In Bratshaw, M. L., & Perret, Y. M. (1992). *Children with disabilities: A medical primer* (3d ed.). Baltimore: Brookes.

Clarke, M. A., & St. Clair Forbes, W. (1995). Encephalitis and encephalopathy. In Newton, R., *Color atlas of pediatric neurology*. London: Mosby-Wolfe.

Colarusso, R. P., & Hammill, D. P.: *Motor-free visual perception test—Revised manual*. Novato, CA: Academic Therapy Publications.

Coorssen, E. A., Msall, M. E., & Duffy, L. C. (1991). Multiple minor malformations as a marker of prenatal etiology of cerebral palsy. *Developmental Medicine and Child Neurology, 33*, 730.

DeLuca, P. A. (1996). The musculoskeletal management of children with cerebral palsy. *Pediatric Clinics of North America, 43*, 1135.

Dreifuss, F. E. (1990). Classification of epileptic seizures and the epilepsies. *Pediatric Clinics of North America, 36*, 265.

Epstein, M. A., & Sladky, J. T. (1990). The role of plasmapheresis in childhood Guillain-Barré syndrome. *Annals of Neurology, 28*, 68.

Fenichel, G. M. (1993). *Clinical pediatric neurology: A signs and symptoms approach* (2d ed.). Philadelphia: Saunders.

Fischer, A., Bryze, K., & Magalhaes, L. (1998). *School assessment of motor and process skill: Research edition*. Fort Collins: Colorado State University.

Fishman, M. (1994). Infectious diseases. In David, R. B. *Pediatric neurology for the clinician*. Norwalk, CT: Appleton & Lange.

Folio, M. R., & Fewell, R. R. (1983). *Peabody developmental motor scales and activity cards manual*. Chicago: Riverside.

Gardner, M. F. (1982). *Test of visual-perceptual skills (non-motor) manual*. Los Angeles: Western Psychological Services.

Gardner, M. F. (1995). *Test of visual-motor skills—Revised manual*. Los Angeles: Western Psychological Services.

Hagberg, B., Hagberg, G., & Zetterstrom, R. (1989). Decreasing perinatal mortality—Increase in cerebral palsy morbidity. *Acta Paediatrica Scandinavica, 78*, 664.

Haller, J. S. (1992). Congenital malformations of the central nervous system. In David, R. B. *Pediatric neurology for the clinician*. Norwalk, Appleton & Lange.

Hanson, C. J., & Jones, L. J. (1989). Gait abnormalities and inhibitive casts in cerebral palsy. *Journal of the American Podiatric Medical Association, 79*, 53.

Hinderer, K. A., Harris, S. R., Purdy, A. H., et al. (1988). Effects of "tone reducing" vs.

standard plaster-casts on gait improvement of children with cerebral palsy. *Developmental Medicine and Child Neurology, 30,* 370.

Holmes, G. (1992). Use of EEG in management of childhood epilepsy. *International Pediatrics, 7,* 223.

International League Against Epilepsy. (1991). Proposal for revised clinical and electroencephalographic classification of epileptic seizures. *Epilepsia, 22,* 489.

Kanda, T., Yuge, M., Yamori, Y., et al. (1984). Early physiotherapy in the treatment of spastic diplegia. *Developmental Medicine and Child Neurology, 26,* 438.

Kurtz, L. A. (1992). Cerebral palsy. In Bratshaw, M. L., & Perret, Y. M. *Children with disabilities: A medical primer* (3rd ed.). Baltimore: Brookes.

Leggate, J., & St. Clair Forbes, W. (1995). Hydrocephalus and spina bifida. In Newton, R. W. *Color atlas of pediatric neurology.* London: Mosby-Wolfe.

Mapstone, T. B., Rekat, H. L., Nulsen, F. E. Dixon, M. S., Jr., Glaser, N., & Jaffe, M. (1984). Relationship of CSF shunting and IQ in children with myelomeningocele: A retrospective analysis. *Child's Brain, 11,* 112–118.

Medical Research Council. (1991). Prevention of neural tube defects: Results of the Medical Research Council Vitamin Study. *Lancet, 338,* 131.

Milani-Comparetti, A., & Gidoni, E. A. (1992). *Milani-Comparetti motor development screening test.* Omaha, NE: Meyer Children's Rehabilitation Institute.

Miller, L. J. (1988). *Miller assessment for preschoolers—Revised edition.* San Antonio: The Psychological Corporation.

Miller, L. J., & Roid, G. H. (1994). The T.I.M.E.: Toddler and Infant Motor Evaluation. Tucson: Therapy Skill Builders.

Moe, P. G., & Seay, A. R. (1995). Neurologica and muscular disorders. In Hay, W.W., Groothius, J. R., Hayward, A. R., and Levin, M. J. *Current pediatric diagnosis and treatment* (12th ed.). Norwalk, CT: Appleton & Lange.

Nelson, K. B. (1988). What proportion of cerebral palsy is related to birth asphyxia? *Journal of Pediatrics, 112,* 574.

Nelson, K. B., & Ellenberg, J. H. (1986). Antecedents of cerebral palsy, II: Multivariate analysis of risk. *New England Journal of Medicine, 315,* 81.

Newborg, J., Stock, J. R., & Wnek, L. (1984). *Battelle developmental inventory examiner's manual.* Allen, TX: DLM Teaching Resources.

Newton, R. W. (1995). The child with special needs. In Newton, R.W. *Color atlas of pediatric neurology.* London: Mosby-Wolfe.

Nickel, R. E. (1987). *The infant motor screen.* Portland: Crippled Children's Foundation OHSU.

Noronha, M. J. (1995). Epilepsy. In Newton, R. W. *Color atlas of pediatric neurology.* London: Mosby-Wolfe.

Ottenbacher, K. J., Biocca, Z., Decremer, G., et al. (1986). Quantitative analysis of the effectiveness of pediatric therapy. Emphasis on the neurodevelopmental treatment approach. *Physical Therapy, 66:*1095.

Palmer, F. B., Shapiro, B. K., Wachtel, R. C., et al. (1988). The effects of physical therapy on cerebral palsy. A controlled trial with infants with spastic diplegia. *New England Journal of Medicine, 318,* 803.

Perin, B. (1989). Physical therapy for the child with cerebral palsy. In Teckli, J. S. *Pediatric physical therapy.* Philadelphia: Lippincott.

Phillips, W. E., & Audet, M. (1990). Use of serial casting in the management of knee joint contractures in an adolescent with cerebral palsy. *Physical Therapy, 70,* 521.

Rett's Syndrome Diagnostic Criteria Work Group (1988). Diagnostic criteria for Rett's Syndrome. *Annals of Neurology, 23,* 425.

Sarwark, J. F. (1996). Spina bifida. *Pediatric Clinics of North America 43,* 1151.

Shumway-Cook, A., & Woolacott, M. H. (1995). A conceptual framework for clinical practice. In Shumway-Cook, A., & Woolacott, M. H. *Motor control: Theory and practical applications.* Baltimore: Williams & Wilkins.

Smithells, R. W., Nevin, N. C., Seller, M. J., et al. (1987). Further experience of vitamin supplementation for prevention of neural tube defect recurrences. *Lancet, 1,* 1027.

Soueidan, S. (1992). Neuromuscular diseases. In David, R. B. *Pediatric neurology for the clinician.* Norwalk, CT: Appleton & Lange.

Sparrow, S. S., Balla, D. A., & Cicchetti, D. V. (1984). *Vineland adaptive behavior scales.* Circle Pines, MN: American Guidance Service.

Stewart, J. M., Manchester, D. K., & Sujansky, E. (1995). Genetics and dysmorphology. In Hay, W. W.,

Groothusis, J. R., Hayward, A. R., & Levin, M. J. *Current pediatric diagnosis and treatment* (12th ed.). Norwalk, CT: Appleton & Lange.

Swaiman, K. E., & Dyken, P. R. (1994). Degenerative diseases primarily of gray matter. In Swaiman, K. F. *Pediatric neurology: Principles and practice* (2d ed.) St. Louis: Mosby.

Tenenholz, B. (1993). *Now that you've been told . . . Your baby has spina bifida.* Wallingford, CT: National Society of Genetic Counselors.

Turnbull, J. D. (1993). Early intervention of child with or at risk for cerebral palsy. *American Journal of Diseases in Children, 47,* 54.

Uniform Data Systems. (1993). *The Wee functional independence measure.* Buffalo: Author.

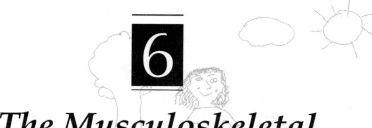

# The Musculoskeletal System

Scott D. Tomchek, MS, OTR/L

*Love,*
*Lorisa*
*age 9*

> *The child is like a soul in a dark dungeon striving to come out into the light, to be born, to grow, and which slowly but surely animates the sluggish flesh, calling to it with the voice of its will.*
>
> —Maria Montesorri

## KEY POINTS

- Muscular dystrophy (MD) is a group of inherited disorders characterized by progressive muscle weakness. Forms of MD differ by muscle involvement, severity, age of onset, and progression of the disease.

- Although there is no cure for MD, pharmacological and therapeutic intervention has been found to be beneficial in slowing the progression of the disease.

- Scoliosis types are classified by etiology, anatomical location, and direction of the curve.

- Prognosis and intervention strategies for scoliosis are based on the severity of the curve.

- Juvenile rheumatoid arthritis (JRA) is characterized by chronic synovial inflammation of unknown cause. There are three patterns of presentation in JRA that provide a mechanism to predict prognosis and sequelae of the disease.

- Intervention in JRA attempts to relieve symptoms (i.e., ease pain, reduce joint inflammation), maintain joint range of motion (ROM) and muscle strength, and maintain or restore optimal function to allow for participation in childhood occupations.

- JRA progressively diminishes with age and results in remission in 95 percent of cases by puberty.
- Osteogenesis imperfecta is a generalized disorder of genetic origin with at least four distinct forms characterized by the presence of brittle bones.
- Arthrogryposis describes a group of conditions characterized by the formation of multiple nonprogressive congenital contractures secondary to skeletal malformations.
- Limb amputations may be traumatic, pathological, or congenital in etiology.
- Intervention for these congenital conditions attempts to minimize the neuromuscular and developmental motor deficits to foster age-appropriate play and adaptive performance.

# BEGINNINGS

This chapter explores musculoskeletal diseases of children. Specifically, muscular dystrophy, scoliosis, juvenile rheumatoid arthritis, and congenital conditions (osteogenesis imperfecta, arthrogryposis, and limb amputations and deficiencies) are discussed. Not all of these conditions are progressive in nature, but as the affected child grows, their chronic nature impacts the development and acquisition of age-appropriate skills and childhood occupations. Understanding the etiology, presentation, and course of these conditions allows therapists to make more informed and effective intervention decisions. Occupational therapists (OTs) play a vital role in the intervention process. Occupational therapy intervention not only includes direct treatment of the child, but also collaborates with the family, school, and other systems involved with the child. The intervention process is quite dynamic, as status changes in the child often warrant corresponding intervention changes. Providing parent support and education is often another role of the therapist. This child-family-therapist team, along with other allied health professionals, works to facilitate childhood occupation.

# MUSCULAR DYSTROPHY

## THE CLINICAL PICTURE

The muscular dystrophies comprise a group of hereditary disorders characterized by progressive muscle weakness and wasting of the skeletal and/or voluntary muscles that control movement. The forms of muscular dystrophy (MD) differ in severity, age of onset, muscles first and most often affected, the rate at which symptoms progress, and the inheritable characteristics. There is no effective treatment for any of the muscular dystrophies (Emery, 1991).

The muscle cells are thought to be the primary site of disease in the muscular dystrophies (Muscular Dystrophy Association [MDA], 1995; Schanzenbacher, 1989). Each cell in our bodies contains tens of thousands of genes.

Each gene is a string of DNA and is the code for a protein. There are probably 3000 of these muscle proteins. Some muscle proteins are part of the structure of muscle fibers, whereas others influence the biochemical reactions within the muscle fibers. Errors in the muscle protein genes cause muscular dystrophies (Emery, 1991; MDA, 1995; Worton & Brooke, 1995). If the code for the muscular protein is incorrect, the protein is produced incorrectly—in the incorrect amount or sometimes not at all. These deficits cause biochemical and structural changes in the surface and internal membranes of the muscle cells, which in turn cause the progressive degeneration and weakness of various muscle groups. The particular defect in a muscle protein can influence the nature and severity of the muscle disease.

Identification of the gene errors and diagnosis of MD can be made through a combination of clinical and laboratory findings. Clinically, for any child who presents with muscle wasting and weakness for no apparent cause, and in whom there is no apparent evidence of central or peripheral nervous system damage, the possibility of MD should be entertained (Emery, 1991). A detailed medical history should be completed to obtain information about when weakness first appeared, its severity, and which muscles have been affected (MDA, 1995). On physical examination, the distribution of muscle wasting should be carefully charted, because this can be the key to determining the type of dystrophy. The affected muscles will be flaccid. Tendon reflexes will be depressed or even absent. The plantar responses will also likely be depressed and they will never be extensor.

Diagnostic testing is also often used to differentiate among forms of MD or between MD and other neuromuscular disorders. Essentially, three laboratory tests are useful in diagnosing MD: serum enzymes, electromyography (EMG), and muscle biopsy (Emery, 1991; Worton & Brooke, 1995). These diagnostic tests are only briefly discussed here. In MD, certain serum enzyme levels are raised. EMG reveals small action potentials of reduced amplitude and duration and an increase in the percentage of potentials with four phases ("polyphasic" potentials) (Emery, 1991). The most useful diagnostic tool in suspected cases of MD is muscle biopsy. The biopsy should be carried out on a muscle that is moderately affected to establish a firm diagnosis. Characteristic and diagnostic features of muscle cell structures in MD are variation of fiber size, fiber necrosis, and invasion by fibroblasts and macrophages (Emery, 1991). Ultimately, the muscle tissue is almost completely replaced by fat and connective tissue with only small islands of muscle fibers remaining.

MD types can be classified by their clinical features and mode of inheritance (Table 6–1).

Duchenne's dystrophy is the most common and most severe form of MD, occurring only in boys. Incidence of this form of MD is estimated at 1/3000 male births (Robinson & Linden, 1993). Symptoms usually occur between the ages of 2 and 6, and include emerging difficulty getting up from a sitting or lying position (Gower's sign or maneuver) (Fig. 6–1). Difficulty climbing stairs, unsteady gait, toe walking, low endurance, and frequent falls are also noted (Emery, 1991; MDA, 1995; Robinson & Linden, 1993; Schanzenbacher, 1989). The children often develop lordotic postures. Another distinctive feature of this form of MD is the enlargement of the calf muscles and sometimes of the forearm and thigh muscles. This results from an accumulation of fat and connective tissue in the muscle. Involvement begins in the

Table 6–1 **Muscular Dystrophy Characteristics by Type**

| Type | Onset Age | Inheritance/ Gender Affected | First Affected Muscles | Progression |
|------|-----------|------------------------------|------------------------|-------------|
| Myotonic | Early childhood to adulthood | Autosomal dominant/ males and females | Face, feet, hands, front of neck | Slow |
| Duchenne's | 2–6 years of age | X-linked/males | Pelvis, upper arms, upper legs | Slow, often with rapid spurts |
| Becker's | 2–16 years of age | X-linked/males | Pelvis, upper arms, upper legs | Slow |
| Limb-girdle | Teens to early adulthood | Autosomal recessive and dominant forms/males and females | Hips, shoulders | Usually slow |
| Fascio-scapulo-humeral | Teens to early adulthood | Autosomal dominant/ males and females | Face, shoulders | Slow, often with rapid spurts |
| Congenital | At birth | Autosomal recessive/males and females | Generalized | Slow |
| Oculopha-ryngeal | 40s–50s | Autosomal dominant/ males and females | Eyelids, throat | Slow |
| Distal | Adulthood | Autosomal recessive and dominant forms/males and females | Hands and lower legs | Variable |
| Emery-Dreifuss | Childhood to early teens | X-linked recessive/ males | Upper arms, lower legs | Slow |

*Source:* Adapted from Muscular Dystrophy Association. (1995). *Facts about muscular dystrophy.* Tucson: Muscular Dystrophy Association.

pelvic girdle and rapidly progresses to involve other skeletal muscles, with deterioration from proximal to distal. Children lose mobility quickly and are most often wheelchair-dependent by the ages of 9 to 12 years. About one-fourth of the boys affected are mentally retarded. In advanced stages, lordosis and kyphosis are common, as are contractures at various joints. Severe respiratory and heart problems mark the disease's final stages, usually in the teens or early twenties.

Interestingly, the signs, symptoms, and course of Duchenne's MD are very similar to those of Becker's MD. However, Becker's MD generally appears later and progresses more slowly. The incidence of Becker's dystrophy

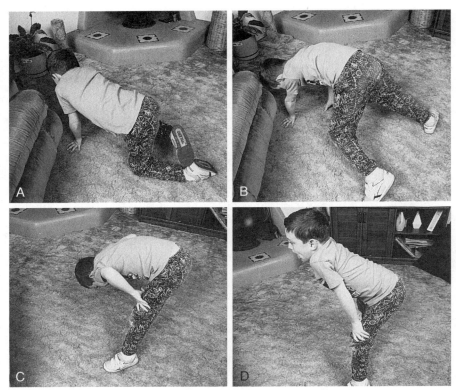

Figure 6–1 Gower's sign/maneuver. The child initially places hands on the floor for support (A); hips are raised (B); weight is shifted to the thighs (C); and trunk is raised by pushing on hands (D). (Photographs courtesy of MDA, Tucson, AZ.)

is more difficult to estimate because of its later age of onset, although it is thought to occur in approximately 3.3 to 5.5 per 100,000 births (MDA, 1995).

Medical management of MD may take a pharmacological course. Corticosteroids have been found to slow muscle destruction in some forms of MD but with serious side effects. Researchers are currently investigating new corticosteroids with fewer side effects. In addition, the value of drugs that inhibit proteases and stop the muscle tissue destruction in MD are also being investigated (Emery, 1991). Respiratory care and related medications are often also required in the later stages of MD.

Physical management of MD entails maintenance and preventive strategies (Emery, 1991; MDA, 1995). Exercise programs and specific therapeutic interventions minimize the development of contractures. Additionally, these programs may prevent or delay scoliosis development. A short period of bed rest often correlates with a marked decline in muscle function (Emery, 1991); therefore, maintaining mobility and independence as long as possible through therapeutic intervention is always recommended. Adaptive equipment (canes, walkers, power wheelchairs) is important in maintaining independent mobility. Occupational therapy plays a vital role in maintaining meaningful occupation and independent living and often uses adaptive equipment to meet such goals. Surgical procedures (primarily tenotomy) have been used to relieve contractures, although some researchers believe this treatment is unwarranted in MD management (Emery, 1991, 1987).

---

■ *THERAPEDS POINTER*

Surgical management of contractures in MD may include tenotomy. In a tenotomy, a transection or cross section of a tendon is performed to release the contracture(s), and in turn improve or maintain the patient's motor status. Tenotomies of the hip flexors, tensor fascia latae, Achilles tendon, and in some cases the posterior tibias are used to release contractures and assist with standing maintenance and walking (in long leg braces) (Smith, Green, Cole, Robison, & Fenichel, 1993). Refer to the following studies investigating the use of tenotomies in MD management:

- Goertzen, M., Baltzer, A., & Voit, T. (1995). Clinical results of early orthopedic management in Duchenne muscular dystrophy. *Neuropediatrics, 26,* 257.
- Smith, S. E., Green, N. E., Cole, R. J., Robison, J. D., and Fenichel, G. M. (1993). Prolongation of ambulation in children with Duchenne muscular dystrophy by subcutaneous lower limb tenotomy. *Journal of Pediatric Orthopedics, 13,* 336.

---

Just as the above treatment methods focus on maintenance of functional independence and prevention of muscular deformity, more global prevention is the overall approach to MD (Emery, 1991). Genetic counseling can identify MD carriers (dominant or recessive) and determine birth risks in prospective parents. Future advances in gene therapy may also be useful in providing more information on presence and severity of MD to expecting parents. This would allow them to make educated decisions about whether to carry the pregnancy to term. Exciting new investigations show promise in minimizing the effects of the disease. Research findings have shown that 50 percent of one of the flawed protein-producing genes in MD can be deleted, resulting in only very mild forms of MD (England, Nicholson, & Johnson, 1990). Future advances in gene therapy may allow for total replacement of the gene and thus prevention of MD or certain forms of it.

## THE OCCUPATIONAL THERAPY PERSPECTIVE

**Evaluation.** As previously implied, evaluation for diagnosis of MD is often conducted by a team of professionals. Typically, in suspected cases of MD, a child is referred by the primary pediatrician to a clinical geneticist with expertise in developmental pediatrics. After obtaining a medical history and conducting a physical examination with MD, the geneticist would likely refer the child for the related laboratory testing. Cytogenetic testing for chromosome, DNA, and gene analysis, as well as serum enzyme testing will be conducted. Additionally, the child would likely be seen by a pediatric neurologist for EMG and/or muscle biopsy studies. Together, these tests support a definitive diagnosis of MD or another neuromuscular disorder.

Secondary to research data suggestive of increased rates of mental retardation in MD, the geneticist may wish to have the child's overall cognitive ability formally assessed by a psychologist. The psychologist may administer one of a number of psychological tests assessing intelligence (see Chapter 9). Also as part of a comprehensive workup, the physician may want occupational and physical therapy services to conduct formalized evaluations. Often, an interdisciplinary or transdisciplinary evaluation is conducted to avoid duplication of procedures. Evaluation consists largely of formalized testing of the child's overall ROM and muscle strength because deficits in these areas often compromise life-role function (occupation). In addition, baseline data to monitor for skill level regression as muscular deterioration occurs are often obtained. Standardized testing will often be conducted by both occupational and physical therapy services. Often, occupational therapy will specifically assess visual perception and fine and visual motor integration using a myriad of assessment tools.

---

### ■ *THERAPEDS POINTER*

Evaluation of motor skill, visual perception and visual motor integration is often the role of the occupational therapist of the interdisciplinary team. Possible tools that could be used:

**Motor Skill:**
Tests and Ages:
  Peabody Developmental Motor Scales (PDMS) (Folio & Fewell, 1983); birth–83 months
  Bruininks-Oseretsky Test of Motor Proficiency (Bruininks, 1978); 4.5–14.5 years
  The Miller Assessment for Preschools (MAP) (Miller, 1988); 2.9–5.8 years
  School Assessment of Motor and Process Skill (SAMPS) (Fischer & Bryse)
Skills Assessed: The PDMS and BOTMP can be used as measures of gross and fine motor abilities. The MAP may also be used to assess preacademic skill development in the preschool-aged child. The MAP will provide some information on a child's sensory and motor abilities, while also opening a window to verbal and nonverbal abilities. The SAMPS is currently being developed. It will measure 16 motor and 20 process behaviors at the level of dysfunction for standardized academic activities.

**Visual Perception:**
Tests and Ages:
  Motor-Free Visual Perception Test-Revised (MVPT-R) (Colarusso & Hammill, 1996); 4 to 11 years
  Test of Visual Perceptual Skills (TVPS) (Gardner, 1982); 4 to 12.11 years

Skills Assessed: Both tools assess visual discrimination, visual-spatial relationships, visual memory, visual figure-ground, and visual closure, while the TVPS also assesses visual form constancy and visual sequential memory. Both tools are non-motor.

**Visual-Motor Integration:**
Tests and Ages:
Test of Visual-Motor Skills-Revised (TVMS-R) (Gardner, 1995); 3 to 13.11 years
Developmental Test of Visual-Motor Integration (VMI) (Beery, 1989); 2 to 15 years
Skills Assessed: Both assessments consist of design-copying items of increasing difficulty and assess the child's ability or inability to translate with his or her hands what is being visually perceived.

---

The child's self-help and adaptive living status is a vital area of emphasis specifically addressed by occupational therapy during the evaluation process. Several independence measures are available to assess these areas. *The Vineland Adaptive Behavior Scales* (Sparrow, Balla, & Cicchetti, 1984) is frequently used as a measure of communication, daily living, socialization, and motor skill. These domains, as well as a cognitive domain, can be measured using the *Battelle Developmental Inventory (BDI)* (Newborg, Stock, & Wnek, 1984). Similarly, independence levels within physical, self-help, social, academic, and communication areas can be obtained using the *Developmental Profile II (DPII)* (Alpren, Boll, & Shearer, 1984). The *Wee Functional Independence Measure (WeeFIM)* (Uniform Data Systems, 1993) can also be used to assess independence in self-care, sphincter control, transfer, locomotion, communication, and social cognition skill areas. All of the above self-care assessments are completed primarily as parent report measures.

**Intervention.** Based on findings from the above assessments, appropriate intervention programs are developed. Coupled with physical therapy intervention, occupational therapy intervention plays a vital role in the maintenance of motor skill and neuromuscular status by developing and fostering participation in an activity and exercise program. Maintaining optimal levels of potential muscle strength is a crucial component in slowing the rate of and in preventing skill loss. Once skill loss occurs and the child begins to lose functional independence, the OT may provide assistive devices and/or environmental adaptations to prolong independence. Technological advances are assisting many children in attaining this goal. As the children age, computer access allows for academic occupations. Environmental control units (ECUs) often assist the young adults' transition into independent living. ECUs can control most household functions, from answering the door to answering the phone.

*The child.* MD eventually causes skill loss in children. As a child is deprived of independence and can see himself or herself losing skills, the child often feels a loss of control. The role of the OT may be to enable the child to regain control through improvement of skill and reacquisition of independence.

| Child Characteristic | Seen as | In | Possible Strategy or Solution |
|---|---|---|---|
| 9-year-old at beginning of Becker's dystrophy | Lower-extremity weakness | Decreased dressing independence (especially for lower body) | Adaptive equipment can be used to enhance independence (i.e., reacher, elastic shoe laces, sock aid) |
| 12-year-old with progressing Duchenne's dystrophy | Distal upper-extremity strength and coordination deficit | Decreased ability to accommodate clothing fasteners | a) If the child's skill level is appropriate for adaptive devices, button hooks and zipper pulls may be attempted<br>b) Compensatory techniques to adapt clothing may be necessary (elastic waist band pants, pullover shirts |
| 5-year-old with Becker's dystrophy | Poor postural control and decreased anti-gravity strength | Poor sitting posture in kindergarten | a) Direct OT and/or PT intervention to improve postural control<br>b) Environmental adaptation of the chair (providing foot and arm rests) |

*The parent or caregiver.* As does any parent of a child with chronic illness, the parent or caregiver of a child with MD needs strong support structures and oftentimes direction. The parent witnesses continual skill regression over time and is constantly reminded of the continued care and assistance the child will need. Providing support and appropriate direction to parents, who in turn can empower their children, is a focus of occupational therapy intervention.

| Parent Characteristic | Seen as | Possible Strategy or Solution |
|---|---|---|
| 15-year-old with Duchenne's dystrophy | Parent sees the adolescent as depressed, unmotivated, and as withdrawing socially | a) Seek out participation in a MD support group for both the parent and child<br>b) Foster frequent family gatherings<br>c) Explore the need for professional counseling |

| Parent Characteristic | Seen as | Possible Strategy or Solution |
|---|---|---|
| 15-year-old with Duchenne's dystrophy | Parent sees the child as having a low self-esteem | a) Identify leisure tasks the child can participate in successfully<br>b) Have the child participate in noncompetitive leisure pursuits |

*The environment.* Environmental adaptation is a major role of occupational therapy in the intervention process of the child with MD. Adapting the environment is not only physical adaptation to objects or equipment, it also encompasses adaptation of routines, procedures, or methods. Often, these adaptations influence the way tasks are accomplished at school and in the home.

| Environmental Characteristic | Seen as | In | Possible Strategy or Solution |
|---|---|---|---|
| 12-year-old walks with the aid of braces and walker | Child has slower ambulation | Student does not have enough time to get to next class | a) Allow the child to leave classes a few minutes early to ambulate through less crowded hallways<br>b) Child may use a wheelchair to move from class to class |
| 18-year-old with progressing limb-girdle dystrophy | Child has less legible written work and a slower rate of writing | Student has difficulty with completion of written work | a) Allow more time for written work<br>b) Allow for a trial with keyboarding<br>c) De-emphasize written work and allow for more oral experiences<br>d) Allow the student to tape lectures rather than take written notes |
| 10-year-old with Duchenne's dystrophy | Child has decreased mobility | Child is denied physical education at school | a) Use lighter-weight equipment<br>b) Adapt tasks to incorporate the child<br>c) Allow the child to participate in the game by keeping score |

# CONGENITAL DISORDERS

## OSTEOGENESIS IMPERFECTA

Osteogenesis imperfecta (OI) is a generalized disorder of genetic origin that is characterized by the presence of brittle bones. The disorder involves not only the connective tissue of bone but also of the skin, ligaments, tendons, fascia, sclera, and middle and inner ear (Tsipouras, 1995). The most frequent manifestations of OI are brittle bones and deafness. Other complications include blue sclera (a graying of the whites of the eyes), thin skin, joint laxity, and bowing of the long bones in the upper and lower extremities (Fig. 6–2). Most forms of OI are caused by improperly formed bone collagen. In OI, children either have less collagen or a poorer collagen quality than normal. These collagen formation errors are the result of a genetic defect, with OI dominantly or recessively inherited. OI can also occur as a gene mutation. Although the actual number of persons with OI is not known, estimates range from a minimum of 20,000 to possibly 50,000 (Osteogenesis Imperfecta Foundation [OIF], 1996).

There are at least four distinct forms of OI, representing significant variability from person to person (OIF, 1996). Type 1 OI is the most common form. It is characterized by frequent bone fractures (most of which are prepubescent), blue sclera, and dental problems. Hearing loss begins in the early twenties and thirties. As adults, persons of this type have near-normal

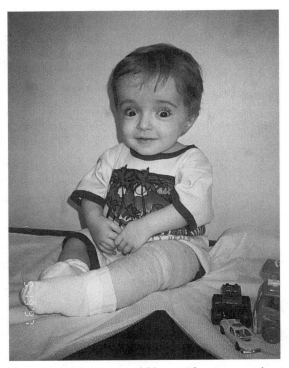

Figure 6–2 Three-year-old boy with osteogenesis imperfecta, type 3.

stature. In type 2 OI, newborns are severely affected (frequently fatally), with a very small stature, small chest, and underdeveloped lungs. In type 3 OI, fractures at birth are common, as is evidence of in utero fractures that are healing. In this type, stature is very small. Loose joints and poor muscle development in the arms and legs are noted, as is severe hearing loss. In type 4 OI, bones fracture easily (most are prepubescent). Loose joints and spinal curvatures are often present. Sclera is normal or near normal in color.

Presently, there is no cure for OI. Treatment is directed toward preventing and/or correcting the symptoms. Immobilization can lead to additional osteoporosis and muscle wasting, which in turn can lead to more fractures. Proper positioning and muscle strengthening should be fostered as soon as possible following a fracture. Exercise and weight bearing should be encouraged. Therefore, swimming and water play are activities that are frequently recommended to meet these goals. Braces are often used when the child is ready to stand to provide increased stability. Walkers and/or wheelchairs are used for mobility. Extensive dental work is usually required. "Rodding" is frequently considered to straighten and strengthen long bones and to prevent further deformity.

---

■ *THERAPEDS POINTER*

Rodding can be used to surgically manage deformities in OI. Rodding involves insertion of metal rods along the long bones. Rodding to the lower extremities (intramedullary rodding) is more common than of the upper extremities (humeral rodding). Rodding is performed to repair a nonunion fracture of a single bone, and/or to prevent deformity and recurrent fractures. Elongating rods have decreased the rod removal rate and increased the length of time between replacement operations. With rodding, improved motor skill development, functional independence, and social integration has been fostered. Refer to the following articles for more information and outcome research involving upper- and lower-extremity rodding:

- Gargan, M. F., Wisbeach, A., & Fixsen, J. A. (1996). Humeral rodding in osteogenesis imperfecta. *Journal of Pediatric Orthopedics, 16,* 719.
- Daly, K., Wisbeach, A., Sanpera, I., & Fixsen, J. A. (1996). The prognosis for walking in osteogenesis imperfecta. *Journal of Bone and Joint Surgery, 78,* 477.

---

Prognosis for OI is dependent on the number and severity of symptoms. Despite frequent fractures, activity restrictions, and short stature, many persons with OI lead productive and happy lives (OIF, 1996).

## ARTHROGRYPOSIS MULTIPLEX

Arthrogryposis multiplex describes a group of conditions characterized by the formation of multiple nonprogressive congenital contractures (Eilert & Georgopoulos, 1996; Hall, 1991; Hall, Reed & Driscoll, 1983). These contractures are present at birth; may be flexor or extensor in nature, asymmetrical or symmetrical; and may be noted in one, many, or all body joints (Fig. 6–3).

Upper-extremity deformities often consist of shoulder adduction and internal rotation, elbow extension, wrist flexion, and stiff extended fingers with poor thumb control. Lower-extremity deformities often consist of hip dislocations, extension or flexion contractures of the knees, and severe clubfoot. In most cases, muscle development is poor. Muscles may be represented only by fibrous bands, similar to muscle composition in MD.

The joint deformities appear to be secondary to a lack of movement by the child in utero. The most frequent cause of limitation of movement in utero relates to an underlying neurological abnormality, but it also has been associated with muscle and/or connective tissue abnormalities and in utero crowding in cases of a lack of amniotic fluid and twinning (Hall, 1991). Overall, 5 to 10 percent of cases of arthrogryposis have been considered to be myopathic, and 90 to 95 percent to be neuropathic (Banker, 1986).

Careful examination of the child with multiple joint contractures is important. Overall resting postures should be described. Contracture positions with measurements of active and passive ROM also require documentation, as do tendon positions. Given these findings, splinting needs should be eval-

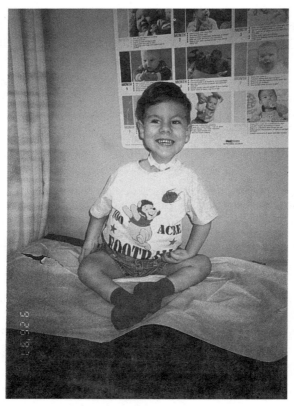

**Figure 6–3** Three-year-old boy with arthrogryposis multiplex.

uated and may be necessary even in neonates. Secondary to the movement limitations, performance of infant occupations may be impaired. For example, jaw limitations may interfere with the child's feeding status. Diaper changes may be difficult in cases of hip involvement. Play and manipulation skills are also often affected with upper-extremity involvement. Together, these findings provide the foundation for intervention planning.

Therapeutic intervention begins early in life. Because of poor muscle development and control, joint mobility cannot be maintained by spontaneous active motion. Therefore, activities relying on passive ROM are used and weight bearing is encouraged. Serial casting is contraindicated, because it often results in further joint stiffness and muscle atrophy (Eilert & Georgopoulos, 1996; Hall et al., 1983). Accordingly, the use of removable splints and aggressive therapy is the most effective conservative intervention for all joint deformities in arthrogryposis. Surgical release or correction of the affected joints is often necessary, as it is in cases of clubfoot and knee deformity. Tendon releases of the flexor carpi ulnaris can also be performed in the upper extremity to facilitate increased wrist extension. In young children, closed reduction of the dislocated hip is attempted, with open reduction completed if necessary before 18 months. Throughout the intervention process, the OT attempts to habilitate the child to age-appropriate occupations.

Long-term prognosis in arthrogryposis is extremely variable and is dependent on the level and number of joints involved. Most children will have average intelligence. Those with fewer joints involved and joints that respond well to intervention have a good prognosis for living independent, productive lives, but the prognosis is not as good for those with more joint involvement and severe handicaps. In these cases independent living and vocational barriers often persist.

## LIMB AMPUTATIONS AND DEFICIENCIES

Limb amputations can be of traumatic, pathological, or congenital etiology. Traumatic amputations are the result of accidental injury (e.g., automotive accident or power tool accident). Pathological amputations are completed in cases of a diseased condition of the part (e.g., tumor). Congenital amputations may be caused by teratogens (e.g., drugs or viruses), amniotic bands, or metabolic diseases (e.g., maternal diabetes) (Eilert & Georgopoulos, 1996). Congenital amputations are also often referred to as *limb deficiencies* (Table 6–2). Most of these amputations are spontaneous in nature and not genetically predetermined.

Amputations are further classified as terminal or longitudinal. In terminal amputation, all parts are missing distal to the level of involvement. For example, in a terminal elbow amputation, the forearm, wrist, and hand are absent. In longitudinal amputations, there is partial absence of structures in the extremity along one side or the other. For instance, in radial clubhand, the entire radius is absent, but the thumb may be incompletely developed or completely absent. Complex tissue defects are nearly always associated with longitudinal amputations in that the associated nerves and muscles are not usually completely represented when a bone is absent (Eilert & Georgopoulos, 1996).

Evaluation and intervention is dependent on the amputation type and in many cases is accomplished in a clinic exclusively for persons with amputa-

Table 6–2 **Limb Deficiency Classification**

| Type | Description |
| --- | --- |
| Amelia | Absence of an arm |
| Phocomelia | Limb that is missing the proximal part |
| Paraxial deficiency | Normal proximal portion of the limb with either the radial part of the arm and attached fingers underdeveloped or the ulnar part of the arm and attached fingers underdeveloped |
| Transverse hemimelia | Portion of a forearm or hand or part of all of the fingers are missing |

tions. Terminal amputations are first addressed by fitting the child with a prosthesis. Evaluation begins with determining joint involvement. Available ROM, strength, and skin integrity of the residual limb must then be established to provide a foundation for determining prosthetic needs. Lower-extremity prostheses are best fitted at the time the child is beginning to ambulate. By offering a prosthesis at this time, increased acceptance is fostered because the child needs the prosthesis for balancing and walking. Upper-extremity prostheses should be fitted as early as 6 months of age to foster bilateral hand activities. Children fitted with an upper-extremity prosthesis after 2 years of age are reported to have a higher rate of rejection (Eilert & Georgopoulos, 1996). Prosthetic options are many. Conventional prosthetics are more frequently used than myoelectric ones because they are often found to be more functional and cost effective given the frequent adjustments required with growth of the child. The terminal device can be changed to meet the demands of the occupation the child is engaged in. In any case, continual adjustments are needed as the child grows and skill levels change.

In longitudinal deficiencies, reconstructive surgery may be done to reduce deformity and stabilize the joints. In certain cases, surgical intervention entails removal of a portion of a limb so that a prosthesis can be fit at an earlier age. Postoperative intervention focuses on improving the neuromuscular status (ROM, muscle tone, strength, sensation, coordination) of the involved joints and/or prosthetic training in some cases. Application of these motor improvements to childhood occupations is the desired outcome.

With both limb amputations and deformities, occupational therapy intervention attempts to facilitate age-appropriate developmental and adaptive skill—whether habilitative, as in congenital amputations, or rehabilitative, as in traumatic and pathological amputations. In most cases, children learn to function with their prostheses or residual limb and lead full lives without activity limitations

# ▰▰▰ FROM THE BOOKSHELF

Further information regarding treatment of upper limb amputations can be found in Atkins, D. J., & Meier, R. H. (Eds.). (1988). *Comprehensive management of upper limb amputee.* New York: Springer-Verlag.

# THE OCCUPATIONAL THERAPY PERSPECTIVE

**Evaluation.** Evaluation of children with any of these congenital disorders often begins in infancy. As with most conditions, evaluation should begin with obtaining a thorough medical history. In doing so, information regarding childhood occupations is also gathered. History of past or current fractures in OI, past and/or scheduled surgeries in arthrogryposis and limb deficiencies, and movement restrictions all have significant implications for intervention. Additionally, the parents' or caregivers' overall understanding of the condition and acceptance of it should be explored to determine the need for further education and/or intervention. A comprehensive neuromuscular assessment often initiates the physical evaluation. Joint involvement is documented and joint-specific measurement of active and passive ROM are obtained. Proximal and distal muscle tone and skeletal obstructions are evaluated and may be found to be the cause of ROM limitations. Muscle strength is often assessed through observation of antigravity postures and movements during play, since the child is often too young to participate in manual muscle testing. Behavioral reactions are used to assess the sensory status of the child. Throughout all of these evaluation areas, the therapist must be aware of behavioral pain responses. Given neuromuscular status limitations, splinting and/or prosthesis needs are considered.

The child's overall developmental status also requires thorough evaluation. As previously discussed in this chapter, *The Vineland Adaptive Behavior Scales* (Sparrow et al., 1984), *BDI* (DLM, 1984), or *DPII* (Alpren et al., 1984) may be used. For assessment of motor skill the *PDMS* (Folio & Fewell, 1983), *Movement Assessment of Infants (MAI)* (Chandler, Andrews, & Swanson, 1980), or *Toddler and Infant Motor Evaluation (T.I.M.E.)* (Miller & Roid, 1994) may be used. The constructs represented in the aforementioned tests provide the building blocks from which adaptive living skills and occupations are built. Assessment of adaptive skills is often an ongoing process, and as the child continues to age and develop, acquisition of age-appropriate adaptive skill is monitored.

**Intervention.** Intervention goals focus on alleviating neuromuscular and developmental motor deficits so that age-appropriate occupations, including play and adaptive skill, can be fostered. Occupational therapy intervention is sometimes done in conjunction or piggy-backed with physical therapy intervention. On the treatment team, roles are often delineated to prevent duplication of services. For example, decisions will be made about who will coordinate the splinting and equipment needs of the child. With most of these congenital conditions, intervention is habilitative in nature. Short-term neuromuscular and motor improvements noted with intervention assist the child in working toward long-term goals of developmentally age-appropriate skills. Often, parent training and home programming are key components in the intervention process. Daily, ongoing intervention in the home usually elicits better treatment results than intervention that is given on a weekly basis.

As the child grows, environmental adaptation is often needed at home and at preschool. Adaptive equipment is used to promote independence during self-care and mobility. Adapting the environment allows for freer mobility and independence. Training with the equipment and daily application within the home and school assists the child in gaining control and independence, given significant neuromuscular limitations. Acceptance of the condition, its effects, and the overall intervention are important psychosocial factors to consider in the child.

*The child.* Child-based interventions attempt to facilitate normal developmental milestones and occupation by minimizing the effects of neuromuscular, skeletal, and motor deficits. Adaptive equipment (splints, prostheses, mobility aids, self-help aids, etc.) is integral in this habilitative process. Occupational therapy often works closely with and builds on other health-care professionals to attain team goals.

| Child Characteristic | Seen as | In | Possible Strategy or Solution |
|---|---|---|---|
| 24-month-old with arthrogryposis and with bilateral rigid elbow extensor contractures | Decreased hand to mouth activity | Self-feeding | a) Angled spoon<br>b) Use splints, maintaining maximal elbow flexion during meals |
| 5-year-old with a right transverse hemimelia who is not a candidate for a prosthesis | Lack of bilateral hand skill | Self-dressing skills | a) Teach the child hemi techniques for dressing<br>b) Use adaptive equipment (elastic shoe laces, button aid, etc.)<br>c) Adapt clothing |
| 12-year-old following a traumatic amputation of her dominant hand | Decreased fine and visual motor control with non-dominant hand | Writing tasks | a) Allow more time for written work<br>b) De-emphasize written work and allow for more oral experiences |

*The parent or caregiver.* Acceptance of any disabling condition in one's child is difficult. The fact that these conditions are congenital in nature often makes acceptance more difficult, as unwarranted guilt is experienced by the parent(s). Early education and support to the family is often needed. The aim of occupational therapy is to help the family solve problems and enable parents or caregivers to play, interact, and work freely with the child. Day-to-day difficulties with care for the child often are of initial concern to the parents, and therefore these difficulties are often where intervention begins.

| Characteristic | Seen as | Possible Strategy or Solution |
|---|---|---|
| 12-month-old with OI | Parents fear leaving the child (even for short periods) | a) Leave for short periods and gradually lengthen time away<br>b) Have trusted family members babysit |

| Characteristic | Seen as | Possible Strategy or Solution |
|---|---|---|
| | | c) Check local early intervention programs to see if respite services by trained professionals are available |
| 6-year-old with arthrogryposis (involving bilateral upper and lower extremity) who wants to participate in after-school activities with friends | Parents have anxiety about activities because the child may not be able to keep up with the others | a) Parents can encourage participation in noncompetitive activities<br>b) Have the child join recreational clubs (Boy or Girl Scouts, 4H, etc.) |
| 3-month-old child with Type 2 OI | Parents are afraid to move the child for fear of fractures | a) Teach the parent open-hand handling techniques<br>b) Put egg-crate padding in a pillow case and lay the child on it. Transfer the child and shift his or her weight by moving the padding. |

*The environment.* Adaptive equipment and environmental adaptation are widely used with most of these congenital conditions. They are key components of both medical and therapeutic intervention to promote increased self-help independence and overall developmental milestone attainment.

| Characteristic | Seen As | Possible Strategy or Solution |
|---|---|---|
| 4-year-old with type 3 OI | Nonambulatory, though increasing need for mobility | Assist the child in obtaining:<br>a) Cart<br>b) Electric wheelchair |
| 8-month-old with a congenital amputation prior to being fit with a prosthesis | Decreased ability to hold bottle and feed self with one arm or hand | a) Attempt using a ring bottle that can be held with one hand<br>b) Position the child so that the bottle can be stabilized against something (chest, furniture, pillow) |

■ *THERAPEDS POINTER*

For additional information on any of the above congenital conditions, contact their national association. These associations can provide educational materials, support and referral, and general information:

*Muscular Dystrophy Association*
3300 East Sunrise Drive
Tucson, AZ 85718-3208
1-800-572-1717

*Osteogenesis Imperfecta Foundation, Inc. (OIF)*
5005 West Laurel Street, Suite 210
Tampa, FL 33607
(301) 947-0083

*Avenues - National Support Group for Arthrogryposis*
P.O. Box 5192
Sonora, CA 95370
(209) 928-3688

---

## ▟▎▎ FROM THE BOOKSHELF

A good children's educational book to help teach genetic concepts and describe how genetic diseases occur is Balkwill, F., & Rolph, M. (1993). *Amazing schemes within your genes*. London: Harper-Collins.

---

# SCOLIOSIS

## THE CLINICAL PICTURE

Scoliosis refers to a lateral curvature of the spine, which is always associated with some vertebral rotation (Cassella & Hall, 1991; Eilert & Georgopoulos, 1991). It is classified by etiology, anatomical location, and direction. The most common type of scoliosis is so-called idiopathic scoliosis and constitutes 80 percent of all cases (Eilert & Georgopoulos, 1991). The other 20 percent of cases are caused by congenital vertebral anomalies or are secondary effects and relate to another condition or disease process. Diseases that may be associated with scoliosis include neurofibromatosis, Marfan's syndrome, cerebral palsy, MD, poliomyelitis, and myelodysplasia. The anatomical location of the scoliosis denotes the vertebral involvement, in either the thoracic or lumbar spine, with rare involvement of the cervical spine. The convexity of the curve is described as right or left and indicates the direction of the scoliosis. Therefore, a left thoracic scoliosis would refer to a thoracic curve in which the convexity is to the left.

This section will focus on idiopathic scoliosis. The term *idiopathic* means of unknown etiology. It is known that idiopathic scoliosis is genetic in origin; however, the mechanism of development remains unknown (Cassella & Hall, 1991). Current theories attribute neural mechanisms involving balance and coordination deficits as possible etiological factors (Yamada et al., 1984). Idiopathic scoliosis is subcategorized by age group: infantile (birth to 3 years), juvenile (3 to 10 years), and adolescent (>10 years). This categorization indicates the age at which the curve was discovered and diagnosed; however, this may not be the age at which the curve first started to develop.

Idiopathic scoliosis is four to five times more common in girls than boys (Eilert & Georgopoulos, 1991). The disorder is usually asymptomatic through the adolescent years and generally not associated with pain (Dell & Regan, 1987; Eilert & Georgopoulos, 1991). If scoliosis and pain are present, investigation to determine the source of pain is warranted.

Lateral curves are often first detected by parents. Lateral curves may also be discovered by pediatricians during routine visits. The majority of lateral curves, however, are discovered during school screenings. Often, a scoliometer is used in screenings to determine the angle of trunk rotation (ATR) to assist in making decisions regarding referral for formal diagnosis. An ATR of 5 degrees or more warrants an orthopedic referral (Dell & Regan, 1987). Imaging studies are required for diagnosis of scoliosis. The most valuable X rays are those taken of the entire spine in a standing position in both the anteroposterior and lateral planes (Eilert & Georgopoulos, 1991). If a curvature exists, the diagnosis is made and the curvature is measured using the Cobb method (Cobb, 1948).

Treatment decisions are based on the degree of curvature, skeletal maturity, and risk of progression. Curvatures of less than 20 degrees do not require treatment unless there is evidence of progression; therefore, these curvatures only require monitoring. Curvatures of 20 to 40 degrees require treatment, especially for the skeletally immature child and/or when progression is documented. Conventional treatment involves wearing a brace for prolonged periods. The goal of a bracing program is to prevent further progression of the curvature and to align the trunk over the sacrum. Permanent correction of the curvature is not expected (Dell & Regan, 1987; Eilert & Georgopoulos, 1991). This goal is reached in 80 percent of cases. The most effective method of curve control is to apply a direct force at the apex of the curve; however, since the spinal column is inaccessible, the force is applied indirectly on the ribs.

A newer modality being used in the treatment of scoliosis is transcutaneous muscle stimulation. Lateral electrical surface stimulation is applied to the paraspinal musculature on the convex side of the curve. It is a treatment modality that is very appealing, since the electrical stimulation is done at night and there is no bracing required during the day. Initial studies showed this modality to be as effective as bracing, but more recent studies have shown less favorable results (Dell & Regan, 1987). Therefore, bracing continues to be the recommended treatment for curves of 20 to 40 degrees. Curvatures of greater than 40 degrees resist bracing. Curvatures of greater than 60 degrees have been correlated with poor pulmonary function in adult life and therefore require surgical intervention. Curvatures of this severity are surgically corrected and maintained by posterior spinal fusion (Fig. 6–4). Postoperative correction is usually maintained by a subcutaneous rod. Curves of 40 to 60 degrees may also require surgical intervention if they are progressive, cosmetically unacceptable, or are causing decompensation of the spine.

The prognosis for scoliosis is dependent on the severity of the curve. Larger curves are predictive of a shorter life span and may progress through adulthood. Respiratory complications and disabling pain are often present during adulthood. On the other hand, small curves (less than 40 degrees) that have been compensated and do not progress may be well tolerated throughout life with little cosmetic concern. Therefore, early detection with appro-

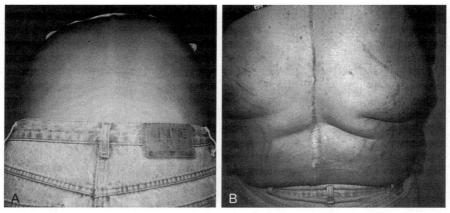

Figure 6–4 Presurgery (A) scoliosis and (B) postsurgical correction in an adolescent with Marfan's syndrome.

priate intervention is critical in preventing progression of the curve and the need for surgical correction. Consequently, school scoliosis screening programs can be instrumental in detecting and preventing deformity and disability.

## THE OCCUPATIONAL THERAPY PERSPECTIVE

**Evaluation.** Typically, OTs function as part of a team in the treatment of scoliosis. The focus and role of the OT on this team dependent on the overall severity of the curve and resulting intervention. For the child with a smaller curve that cannot be operated on, the overall intervention plan will likely include an exercise program coupled with a bracing protocol. These programs may be supervised by either OTs or physical therapists. The goal of these programs is to prevent further progression of the curve. Evaluation of these children should include analysis of posture, ROM, muscle strength, respiratory status, and functional levels. The child's overall developmental status should also be evaluated to anticipate difficulties with role function in play and school situations. Standardized evaluations for developmental and functional skill performance were previously noted in this chapter. Together, these findings serve as baseline data for comparison after the brace protocol has been initiated.

Proximal muscle strength and ROM, their impact on the child's overall posture, and the child's chest mobility may be compromised during initial stages of bracing. Therefore, decreased independence and/or tolerance during adaptive living, play, and school tasks may occur. The overall goals of the intervention team are to foster improved postural awareness to facilitate proper spinal alignment, maintain proper respiratory function and chest mobility, maintain muscle strength, and maintain ROM and spinal flexibility (Cassella & Hall, 1991). In doing so, a main goal for occupational therapy intervention is to resume adaptive living, play, and school performance to pre-bracing levels. The child should also be encouraged to resume normal pre-bracing activities.

For children with larger curves, surgical intervention is often required to straighten the curve and balance the trunk. Here, the goals of intervention are rehabilitative in nature, in that they attempt to restore function and child-hood occupation. Many times the child will be seen prior to surgery for eval-uation by an OT. Preoperative evaluation involves assessment of posture, ROM, muscle strength, respiratory status, and functional levels (adaptive liv-ing, play, school). At this time the child may be instructed in compensatory adaptive living tasks. The use of adaptive equipment to accomplish lower-body self-help tasks may be attempted at the preoperative visit(s). In doing so, the child may be more likely to participate postoperatively, given pain ex-pectations. Initial goals of intervention postoperatively are to encourage early mobility to prevent complications. As mobility improves, the rehabilitation process attempts to return the child to preoperative skill levels in all areas. Occupational therapy again will address daily living performance and will likely use adaptive equipment to improve function. Adaptation of play and school tasks, or positioning within them, may also be required.

---

### ■ THERAPEDS POINTER

Training for compensatory adaptive living tasks may be done pre-operatively by simulating the tasks within any prescribed move-ment limitations or suspected limitations (movement or pain). Ex-amples include:

- Donning socks with sock aid
- Donning pants with a dressing stick or reacher
- Donning shoes with a long-handled shoehorn
- Demonstrating use of elastic shoe laces

---

For all children with scoliosis, the psychosocial adjustment to the diag-nosis and intervention must also be considered throughout the therapeutic process. With brace application, the child may develop an inaccurate body image and self-concept. Stress may also be noted relating to social acceptance from peers and a change in activities. Anxiety and depression may be exhib-ited secondary to loss of control.

Psychological stress has been reported in one study on a group of ado-lescent children with scoliosis between the ages of 9 and 16 (Kahanovitz, Snow, & Pinter, 1984). Eight standardized tests were used to examine the psy-chological effects of treatment between children treated with transcutaneous muscle stimulation and those treated with a brace protocol. Brace patients re-ported more depression, helplessness, withdrawal, and hostility than trans-cutaneous muscle stimulation patients. They were also viewed by others as more hostile, uncooperative, and socially insecure. Not only is it important to take these factors into consideration at the initiation of intervention, but these are also important considerations when determining how the child is coping with the diagnosis throughout the therapeutic process.

**Intervention.** Intervention programs designed by OTs are based on evaluation findings and, as previously noted, the mode of medical intervention (i.e., bracing vs. surgical). In either case, the main focus of occupational therapy intervention is to promote continued independence—both physically and emotionally. Providing educational and environmental support is often a hallmark of this process.

*The child.* Following implementation of a bracing program or surgical correction of a curve, assisting the child to regain functional independence to resume his or her occupations is a goal of occupational therapy. Enhancing the psychosocial adjustment of the child is frequently an element that warrants attention and enhances with the improvement of these skills.

| Child Characteristic | Seen as | In | Possible Strategy or Solution |
|---|---|---|---|
| 14-year-old after surgical correction | Decreased trunk mobility | Lower-body daily living skills | a) Within restrictions, activity programs to improve mobility<br>b) Adaptive equipment can be used to compensate for decreased motion and promote independence |
| 8-year-old beginning a brace program | Anxiety | Play with toys or other children | a) Teach the child relaxation techniques<br>b) Use media (i.e., clay, leather, drawings) to work out feelings of aggression and/or anger<br>c) Role play anxiety-provoking situation with stuffed animals<br>d) Engage the child in play groups with other children |
| 10-year-old during a bracing program | Decreased socialization | School, home, and neighborhood | a) Facilitate peer interactions by taking children on outings and/or organizing activities<br>b) Enroll the child in a scoliosis support group |

*The parent or caregiver.* Grief and stress are often experienced by the parents of a child diagnosed with scoliosis. Parents feel grief for what is perceived as the loss of a normal child. OTs can assist the parents or caregivers in coping with the day-to-day difficulties they may encounter in raising the child and/or the difficulties directly experienced by their child. Often, this is accomplished through parent education.

| Parent Characteristic | Seen as | Possible Strategy or Solution |
|---|---|---|
| 9-year-old child beginning a bracing program | Parents feel stress and grief relating to the diagnosis and intervention | a) Encourage the parents to enroll in a support group<br>b) Consult with the child's teachers, guidance counselor, and orthotist to develop appropriate expectations |
| 11-year-old in a bracing program | Parent sees the child as having an impaired self-concept and decreasing autonomy | Give the child some control in the intervention process.<br>a) Based on physician time guidelines, allow the child to decide on the wearing schedule<br>b) Allow the child to choose the clothing he or she would like to wear while in the brace<br>c) Have the child clean the brace |

*The environment.* Adaptation of the environment is also often necessary as a result of either interventions. Adaptive equipment will often be used in the initial phases of bracing and postsurgery rehabilitation to promote daily living independence.

| Environmental Characteristic | Seen as | Possible Strategy or Solution |
|---|---|---|
| 5-year-old beginning a brace program | Child has difficulty getting up from the floor during circle time | a) Allow the child to sit on a stool or chair in circle time and allow the child to pick one other student to sit next to him or her also on a chair to prevent social stigma<br>b) Have the class all sit in chairs |
| 13-year-old with a brace, post surgery | Child is fidgety and has impaired attention in class because he or she cannot get comfortable in a chair | Allow the child to have a more comfortable chair to sit in within the classroom |

# JUVENILE RHEUMATOID ARTHRITIS

## THE CLINICAL PICTURE

Juvenile rheumatoid arthritis (JRA) is the most common pediatric rheumatic disease in North America (Cassidy & Petty, 1990). It has been estimated that 65,000 to 70,000 children in the United States are diagnosed with this disorder (Singsen, 1990). Girls are more often affected than boys, with onset occurring anytime during childhood.

JRA is characterized by chronic synovial inflammation of unknown cause. Definitive diagnosis of JRA requires at least 6 weeks of objective synovitis (Cassidy & Petty, 1990; Hollister, 1995; Rhodes, 1991). There are three patterns of presentation in JRA that provide a foundation for predicting possible sequelae and prognosis of the disease. They are systematic, pauciarticular, and polyarticular and are defined in Table 6–3. Assignment of one of these onset types occurs only after 6 months of active disease.

There is no one test available that can be used to diagnose JRA. There are laboratory findings, however, that are used to assist in diagnosing and classifying it (Hollister, 1995). Presence of rheumatoid factors and antinuclear antibodies may indicate the presence of active disease, with certain concentrations noted in different JRA subtypes. Therefore, these laboratory findings are often used in classifying JRA type. Imaging studies are also useful in diagnosing JRA. In early stages of the disease only soft tissue swelling and regional osteoporosis are seen. A more specific magnetic resonance imaging (MRI) of involved joints may indicate joint damage at earlier stages of the disease than with less-sensitive imaging studies. In the case of reported neck pain, cervical subluxation should be monitored.

Comprehensive intervention and early diagnosis are essential in minimizing deformity and promoting normal development. Following diagnosis, the intervention process begins with the child being seen by the treatment team for baseline evaluations. These baseline data will be used for comparison to determine treatment effectiveness and to document changes in the disease process. A comprehensive evaluation should include assessment of pain, edema, ROM, muscle strength, coordination, perception, and daily living independence. Splinting and adaptive equipment needs also must be determined. A thorough patient history should document the disease process to date, as well as identify interventions already in place (i.e., splinting, medication, exercise). Additionally, information about pain perception, difficulties with play or school performance, and task endurance should be gathered. Together, this information provides the foundation for goal setting and treatment planning and is used as a comparison to determine treatment efficacy.

Following the evaluation process, intervention often begins with education. The child, family, and friends are often frightened by the diagnosis. The school system may also have concerns about proper programming for the child given the diagnosis. To be effective, all need to be educated as to the course of the disease and related interventions. The immediate goals of physical medicine and therapeutic intervention are to relieve symptoms (i.e., ease

Table 6–3 **JRA by Onset Type**

| Type | Epidemiology | Presentation | Joint Involvement | Complications/ Side Effects | Prognosis |
|---|---|---|---|---|---|
| Systemic | 10% of cases<br>Equal male to female ratio<br>Onset at any age | Spiking fevers<br>Salmon-pink rash (often in the late afternoon or early evening<br>Pericarditis<br>Lymphadenopathy<br>Anemia<br>Increased white blood cell count | Often develops into polyarticular | Growth retardation<br>Delayed development of sexual characteristics | 50% develop severe chronic arthritis<br>Others have recurrent systemic manifestations |
| Polyarticular | 40% of cases<br>Onset at any age, peaking at age 1–3 years<br>Female-to-male ratio: 3:1 | Weight loss<br>Low-grade fevers<br>Adenopathy<br>Anemia<br>Positive RF (15–20%)<br>Positive ANA (40–60%) | 5 or more joints affected<br>Symmetrical in 75% of cases<br>Affects of wide variety of joints | Growth retardation<br>Delayed development of sexual characteristics<br>Subcutaneous nodules attached to tendon sheaths | Poor if rheumatoid factor (RF) positive; (increased possibility of disabling arthritis in up to 50% of cases)<br>Better if RF negative |
| Pauciarticular | 50% of cases<br>Onset under age 10, peaking at age 1–2 years<br>Male-to-female ratio: 5:1 | Positive ANA | 4 or fewer joints affected<br>Most commonly the knee, followed by ankle and elbow<br>Often asymmetrical | Iridocyclitis (chronic eye inflammation); 15–30% develop functional blindness | Good (few joints are affected, disability uncommon, increased percentage in early remission). |

pain and reduce joint inflammation), maintain joint ROM and muscle strength, and maintain or restore optimal function. Treatment modalities and techniques will be discussed within the occupational therapy perspective. In addition to therapeutic intervention, pharmacological treatment is vital in JRA medical management. Recently, nonsteroidal anti-inflammatory drugs (NSAIDs) have replaced aspirin in treatment of JRA. Although the anti-inflammatory potency is not different from that of aspirin, decreased frequency of dosing and diminished side effects appear to enhance compliance and justify their increased cost (Hollister, 1995). Adequate rest and good health habits are also important to JRA management.

Follow-up assessment of responses to treatment requires careful consideration. Assessment of self-help skill, play, neuromuscular status, ambulation, and pain are to be considered. Secondary to the lack of accurate and consistent reporting in some children, parent reports of subtle changes in play behavior and of the child's complaints are also often important in determining treatment effectiveness.

In the primarily articular forms, JRA steadily diminishes with age and ceases in about 95 percent of cases by puberty (Hollister, 1995). In few instances, symptoms persist into adult life. Difficulties after puberty often relate to residual joint damage from the active phase of the disease. Thus, presentation in the teen years is indicative of an adult rheumatic disease (Hollister, 1995).

## THE OCCUPATIONAL THERAPY PERSPECTIVE

**Evaluation.** Occupational therapy is typically one key component in JRA management. The evaluation process for occupational therapy often begins with assessment of pain and clarification of the child's perception of it. General pain should be assessed at rest, on weight bearing, and with motion. This is often done using a Likert scale. In assessing edema, joints are evaluated for presence of effusion, synovial thickening, heat, and redness (Rhodes, 1991). Overall edema is also often quantified by use of a Likert scale. Given pain and swelling limitations, ROM and muscle strength are next evaluated. Specific joint measures are recommended to document the disease process properly. ROM is determined by goniometer, whereas strength is measured by manual muscle test, and for grip and pinch strength by dynamometer and pinchmeter. If a child is too young to participate in manual muscle testing, using developmental postures to assess strength may be of benefit.

If neuromuscular limitations are present, aspects of gross and fine motor coordination are often impaired with effects on childhood occupations. The OT may be called on to evaluate both of these areas or may only perform fine motor testing if a physical therapist is also a member of the intervention team. For younger children, the *PDMS* (Folio & Fewell, 1983) may be used to assess gross and fine motor skills, whereas in the schoolaged child the *BOTMP* (Bruiniks, 1978) can be used to assess these same abilities. For JRA types complicated by iridocyclitis, perceptual testing must also be conducted. Visual perceptual abilities can be assessed using the *MVPT-R* (Colarusso & Hammill, 1996) or the *TVPS* (Gardner, 1982). Analysis of the results from fine motor and perceptual testing may also indicate a need to further evaluate visual-motor abilities. Given the impact visual-motor control difficulties can have on handwriting performance, visual-motor testing is often essential in determining academic programming. The *TVMS-R* (Gardner, 1995) or the *VMI* (Beery, 1967) may be used to assess visual-motor abilities.

---

■ *THERAPEDS POINTER*

Inflammation of the iris and ciliary body of the eye (iridocyclitis) develops in 10 to 50 percent of children with pauciarticular JRA (Singsen, 1993). Iridocyclitis usually develops concurrently with joint complaints, although it may develop 5 to 10 years later. It is often chronic and has great potential for ocular damage and vision loss or blindness. Children with iridocyclitis rarely have or complain of light sensitivity, red eyes, or visual change. Therefore, routine ophthalmological screening with slitlamp examination should be performed (Hollister, 1995; Singsen, 1993).

---

Splinting needs also must be assessed. Splinting can be used as both a rehabilitative and a preventive intervention. Contractures that do not improve with exercise warrant splinting to prevent further deformity and promote soft tissue lengthening. Splinting is also used to prevent deformity and maintain ROM. Children will often wear resting splints at night to minimize morning stiffness.

Neuromuscular or motor limitations or the presence of splints may result in adaptive-living skill deficits. In these circumstances, assessment of adaptive-living independence is essential to completing a thorough evaluation. Parent reports will often be used to obtain this information. When assessing self-help skill and levels of occupational independence, adaptive equipment needs must also be considered. The physical therapist on the team will often recommend mobility aids, but the OT is instrumental in recommending most other adaptive aids (raised toilet seat, shower chairs, jar and can openers, etc.). A major consideration during the evaluation is the impact of identified problem areas on play skill development. Adaptations to play activities may also be warranted. Social interaction difficulties may arise as the disease progresses and the child experiences more pain and loss of function. Given all of the above evaluation information, appropriate and effective treatment planning and intervention can be initiated.

**Intervention.** The intervention program should meet the physical, emotional, cultural, and developmental needs of the child based on evaluation findings and reflect his or her maturity level. Ideally, the program should be incorporated into the child's daily occupations, and therefore the program may encompass child, family, and/or school roles. Throughout the therapeutic process, child and family education are instrumental to clarify the current status of the disease and to provide predictive information of the possible future progression.

During acute phases, goals of intervention are preventive in nature.

Physically, therapy attempts to prevent ROM limitation, muscle weakness, and osteoporosis (Rhodes, 1991). Self-help independence and preservation of role performance should also be maintained. In this phase, proper rest and comfort are promoted. Therapeutic intervention should not advance the symptoms. Active, active-assistive, and passive ROM and isometric exercises are recommended. Conversely, during chronic phases of JRA goals are more rehabilitative in nature. Progressive-resistive exercise is incorporated as long as it does not increase the child's symptoms. Endurance also increases because of participation in general exercise programs. Whatever the phase, closely monitoring the child's symptoms to determine treatment effects (positive or negative) is important.

Pain, muscle weakness and atrophy, decreased endurance, and contractures are features of JRA (Singsen, 1993). Although pharamcological interventions can assist with pain, an exercise program is often used to manage neuromuscular effects. The goal of an exercise program depends on the phase of disease the child is in and thus may be used to prevent and/or maximize strength, ROM, and function. In doing so, the child can hopefully continue to participate in childhood occupations and role performance. Again, this program will likely be most effective and have maximal compliance if carried out within the child's daily routine. Therefore, these programs are typically given to the child and family as a home program and are monitored. In addition to exercise programs, positioning programs are often developed for contracture prevention. For trunk positioning, a good posture should be emphasized. Resting hand splints may be used to prevent wrist deformities, and elbow and knee bracing in extended postures may be used to maintain ROM of these joints. A soft cervical collar may be appropriate to maintain neck ROM and inhibit flexor deformities. Prolonged prone positioning can assist in the prevention of hip flexor contractures. If contractures do develop, serial casting, splinting, or soft tissue releases may be required to reduce them and the pain.

## ▟▐▌ FROM THE BOOKSHELF

Fess, E., & Philps, C. (1987). *Hand splints: Principles and methods* (2d ed.). St. Louis: C. V. Mosby.

---

Given particular state guidelines, other treatments can also be used within therapeutic intervention to alleviate joint stiffness and pain (Rhodes, 1991). Paraffin is often used to relieve symptoms in the feet and hands. Moist heat (whirlpool, hot packs, warm bath tub, or swimming pool) can also have positive effects. Maintaining body warmth to prevent stiffness is also recommended. Morning baths, warm pajamas, and electric blankets may be used in the home for optimal program carryover.

Issuing of and training with adaptive equipment is another focus of occupational therapy intervention. Everyday household adaptations (jar, can, and bottle openers; turning handles; door knob extensions; tub chair; and raised toilet seat) are used to prevent joint damage from repetitive motion.

Adaptive equipment is also used to maximize functional independence during self-feeding and dressing tasks, with equipment needs likely changing as the disease process and joint status also change. Children with JRA should be encouraged to be self-sufficient to an age-appropriate extent (Singsen, 1993). Often, adaptive equipment allows the child to maintain control over and independence during these activities.

*The child.* JRA often causes developmental motor changes that result in skill loss and increased dependence. Occupational therapy intervention attempts to promote developmental motor maintenance and/or improvements that maintain independence and function. Patient and family education is often vital in this process.

| Child Characteristic | Seen as | In | Possible Strategy or Solution |
|---|---|---|---|
| 10-year-old in acute phase of polyarticular JRA | Decreased fine motor dexterity | Dressing | a) Have child wear pullover shirts and elastic pants<br>b) Adapt shirts with Velcro<br>c) Teach the child to close snaps with his or her palms<br>d) Use zipper pulls |
| 8-year-old with polyarticular JRA beginning chronic phase | Slowly decreasing pain, stiffness, and edema, with the child becoming more active | Sports often continue to be restricted to prevent exacerbation | Child should be encouraged to participate in swimming and bicycling |
| 7-year-old with pauciarticular JRA | Overall joint stiffness (especially in the knees, elbows, and wrists) | The morning | a) Morning bath or whirlpool<br>b) Electric blanket on a timer to come on an hour before the child is to get up<br>c) Night splints to maintain ROM |

*The parent or caregiver.* Parents often initially have difficulty with accepting the diagnosis of JRA and the resultant changes the disease has on their child. Education about the disease process and interventions is often useful in helping the parent make the transition from this stage to one that is more helpful to their children. Assisting parents to solve problems arising from the day-to-day difficulties arising from a child with JRA within the home is often one role of occupational therapy. Educating them along with the child on use of adaptive equipment is essential for treatment carryover in the home.

| Parent Characteristic | Seen as | Possible Strategy or Solution |
|---|---|---|
| Child with pauciartic-ular JRA | Parents feel they have no control over the disease process | a) Attend an exercise group with the child<br>b) Attend classes with the child to learn energy conservation, joint protection, work simplification to apply within the home |

*The environment.* As skill-level changes occur, environmental adaptations are often necessary for the child to maintain and promote increased independence. Adaptations within the environment also are important in prevention of further joint stress and deformity.

| Environmental Characteristic | Seen as | Possible Strategy or Solution |
|---|---|---|
| Home interactions | Joint stress | To prevent joint stress, equip the home with knob and handle turns, door knob extensions, raised toilet seats, etc. |
| 12-year-old with increased joint pain (especially knee and ankle) | Increased difficulty with ambulation and a slower rate of ambulation | a) Have the child use a wheelchair for long distances<br>b) Allow the child more time to get from place to place |

# WRAPPING IT UP

Physical status changes characterize these neuromuscular disorders. These changes often lead to skill loss (MD, JRA) or delayed acquisition of developmental milestones (congenital conditions). In many cases pain is present and dysmorphic features are noticeable. The occupational therapy process can be preventive, habilitative, or rehabilitative in nature. Occupational therapy interventions attempt to minimize the effects of the neuromuscular and motor deficits on play, self-care, school, and leisure performance. Often, adaptive equipment and/or environmental adaptation is used within the intervention process. Family education and programming are essential given the impact these conditions have on daily living performance. Prognosis for these conditions is variable, although it does appear that improved prognosis is noted when the child receives the benefit of appropriate interventions.

## ▮▮▮ FROM THE BOOKSHELF

A good resource for parents and families is Miller, N. B. (1994). *Nobody's perfect: Living and growing with children who have special needs.* Baltimore: Brookes Publishing.

Case-Smith, J., Pratt, P. N., & Allen, A. S. (1996). *Occupational therapy for children.* (3d ed.). St. Louis: C. V. Mosby. For additional study, this text has a nice section on intervention organized by performance area.

---

## CASE STUDY

Sam is a 4-month-old African-American child diagnosed at birth with osteogenesis imperfecta, type 3. He was referred through his state's early intervention system for both occupational and physical therapy evaluations to determine intervention needs. During the evaluation, Sam's mother reported that he has had two previous fractures (left humerus and left femur) and that his right radius was currently fractured. His forearm was currently immobilized with a removable splint. Findings indicate that his overall muscle tone and antigravity strength were diminished. Bowing of bilateral femur and humerus was present. Active and passive ROM at bilateral shoulder was limited to approximately 100 degrees and Sam had difficulty with directional reach task above his shoulders when supine or in a supported sit. He demonstrated no bilateral hand play or manipulation. He did not attempt to hold his bottle. He required moderate assistance to maintain an upright sit. His mother reports that Sam is never positioned in a prone position for fear of fractures while weight bearing on his elbows. She typically positions Sam in a supine position on the top of two folded quilts. She positions him in his car seat on top of a towel with the straps loose because she feels one of his fractures was caused by a strap pulling too hard on his arm as the car bounced. While discussing evaluation findings, Sam's mother noted that she needs to return to work soon and does not know what she can do about intervention. If possible, she would like intervention to be coordinated through the local early intervention system and provided within Sam's day care setting. Currently, she does not know where she is going to take Sam for day care while she works. She wants to take him to their church's day care, but she has not checked out the program or any other day care centers to date. She expresses fear of leaving Sam with anyone for prolonged periods for fear of new fractures.

1. What can be done to ease Sam's mother's anxiety about leaving Sam in the care of others?
2. What considerations or recommendations should be made about the day care setting she chooses?

   Availability of trained aides to meet self-care needs
   Accessibility, positioning needs, mobility needs
   Daily programming within the program
   Transportation (from daycare for trips within the day)
   Necessary environmental adaptations or needed adaptive equipment

3. What types of interventions appear appropriate? How will they be best coordinated with the day care *and* the family for optimal benefit of Sam?

## Real-Life Lab

Sam is now 3 years old. He continues to be nonambulatory, although he does stand for brief periods. Sam is in need of a standing frame and a cart or wheelchair for mobility. Additionally, he is in need of adaptive equipment to improve his independence with both self-feeding and dressing. For feeding, he needs equipment that will compensate for ROM limitations at his wrists and forearms. In order to dress himself, he requires assistance primarily with lower-body care. The family has limited insurance coverage and does not qualify for Disabled Children's Program funds. The equipment loan closet at the local early intervention system is quite limited. The family would like to know how much all of the recommended equipment will cost so that they can budget and prioritize. Use the following form to compile the information.

| Item | Catalog or Company | Function of Item or Skill Addressed | Unit Cost |
|------|--------------------|-----------------------------------|-----------|
|      |                    |                                   |           |
|      |                    |                                   |           |
|      |                    |                                   |           |
|      |                    |                                   |           |
|      |                    |                                   |           |
|      |                    |                                   |           |
|      |                    |                                   |           |
|      |                    |                                   |           |
|      |                    |                                   |           |
|      |                    |                                   |           |
|      |                    |                                   |           |
|      |                    |                                   |           |
|      |                    |                                   |           |

# References

Alpren, G. D., Boll, T. J., & Shearer, M. S. (1984). Developmental profile II. Los Angeles: Western Psychological Services.

Atkins, D. J., & Meier, R. H. (Eds.). (1988). Comprehensive management of upper limb amputees. New York: Springer-Verlag.

Balkwill, F., & Ralph, M. (1993). Amazing schemes within your genes. London: Harper-Collins.

Banker, B. Q. (1986). Arthrogryposis multiplex congenita: Spectrum of pathologic changes. Human Pathology, 17, 656.

Beery, K. E. (1989). Developmental test of visual motor integration: Administration and scoring manual. Chicago: Follette.

Bruiniks, R. H. (1978). Bruiniks-Oseretsky test of motor proficiency examiner's manual.

Circle Pines, MN: American Guidance Service.

Cassella, M. C., & Hall, J. E. (1991). Current treatment approaches in the nonoperative and operative management of adolescent idiopathic scolosis. *Physical Therapy 71*, 897.

Cassidy, J. T., & Petty, R. E. (1990). Juvenile rheumatoid arthritis. In Schumacher, H. R. (Ed.). *Textbook of rheumatology* (2d ed.). New York: Churchill Livingstone.

Chandler, L., Andrews, M., & Swanson, M. (1980). The movement assessment of infants. Rolling Bay, WA: MAI.

Cobb, J. R. (1948). Outline for the study of scoliosis: Instructional course lectures. Ann Arbor, MI: The American Academy of Orthopaedic Surgeons.

Colarusso, R. P., & Hammill, D. D. (1996). *Motor-free visual perception test—revised manual.* Novato, CA: Academic Therapy Publications.

Daly, K., Wisbeach, A., Sanpera, I., & Fixsen, J. A. (1996). The prognosis for walking in osteogenesis imperfecta. *Journal of Bone and Joint Surgery, 78,* 477.

Dell, D. D., & Regan, R. (1987). Juvenile idiopathic scoliosis. *Orthopaedic Nursing, 6,* 23.

Eilert, R. E., & Georgopoulos, G. (1995) Orthopedics. In Hay, W. W., Groothuis, J. R., Hayward, A. R., & Levin, M. J. *Current pediatric diagnosis and treatment* (12th ed.). East Norwalk, CT: Appleton & Lange.

Emery, A. E. H. (1991). The muscular dystrophies. In Emery, A. E. H., & Rimoin, D. L. (Eds.). *Principles and practice of medical genetics* (2d ed., Vol. 1). Edinburgh: Churchill Livingstone.

Emery, A. E. H. (1987). *Duchenne muscular dystrophy.* London: Oxford University Press.

England, S. B., Nicholson, L. V. B., & Johnson, M. A. (1990). Very mild muscular dystrophy associated with the deletion of 46% of dystrophin. *Nature, 343,* 180.

Fisher, A., Bryze, K., & Magalhaes, L. (1998). School assessment of motor and process skill: Research edition. Fort Collins: Colorado State University.

Folio, M. R., & Fewell, R. R. (1983). *Peabody developmental motor scales and activity cards manual.* Chicago: Riverside.

Gardner, M. F. (1982). *Test of visual-perceptual skills (non-motor) manual.* Los Angeles: Western Psychological Services.

Gardner, M. F. (1995). *Test of visual-motor skills—revised manual.* Los Angeles: Western Psychological Services.

Gargan, M. F., Wisbeach, A., & Fixsen, J. A.

(1996). Humeral rodding in osteogenesis imperfecta. *Journal of Pediatric Orthopedics, 16,* 719.

Goertzen, M., Baltzer, A., & Voit, T. Clinical results of early orthopedic management in Duechenne muscular dystrophy. *Neuropediatrics, 26,* 257.

Hall, J. G. (1991). Arthrogryposis. In Emery, A. E. H., & Rimoin, D. L. (Eds.). *Principles and practice of medical genetics* (2d ed., Vol. 2). Edinburgh: Churchill Livingstone.

Hall, R. G., Reed, S. D., & Driscoll, E. P: Part 1: Amyoplasia: A common, sporadic condition with congenital contractures. *American Journal of Medical Genetics, 15,* 571.

Hollister, J. R. (1995). Rheumatic diseases. In Hay, W. W., Groothuis, J. R., Hayward, A. R., and Levin, M. J.: *Current pediatric diagnosis and treatment* (12th ed.). East Norwalk, CT: Appleton & Lange.

Kahanovitz, N., Snow, B., & Pinter, I. (1984). The comparative results of psychologic testing in scoliosis patients treated with electrical stimulation or bracing. *Spine, 9,* 442.

Miller, L. J. (1988). *Miller assessment for preschoolers—revised edition.* San Antonio: The Psychological Corporation.

Miller, L. J., & Roid, G. H. (1994). The T.I.M.E.: Toddler and infant motor evaluation. Tucson: Therapy Skill Builders.

Muscular Dystrophy Association. (1995). *Facts about muscular dystrophy.* Tucson: Muscular Dystrophy Association.

Newborg, J., Stock, J. R., & Wnek, L. (1984). *Battelle developmental inventory examiner's manual.* Allen, TX: DLM Teaching Resources.

Osteogenesis Imperfecta Foundation (OIF). (1996). Fast facts on osteogenesis imperfecta. Tampa, FL: Osteogenesis Imperfecta Foundation.

Rhodes, V. J. (1991). Physical therapy management of patients with juvenile rheumatoid arthritis. *Physical Therapy, 71,* 910.

Robinson, A., & Linden, M. G. (1993). Genetic neuromuscular disorders. In Robinson, A., & Linden, M. G. (Eds.). *Clinical genetics handbook* (2d ed.). Boston: Blackwell Scientific.

Schanzenbacher, K. E. (1989). Diagnostic problems in pediatrics. In Pratt, P. N., & Allen, A. S. (Eds.). *Occupational therapy for children* (2d ed.). St. Louis: C. V. Mosby.

Singsen, B. H. (1993). Juvenile rheumatoid arthritis. In Schumacher, H. R. (Ed.). *Primer on the rheumatic diseases* (10th ed.). Atlanta: Arthritis Foundation.

Smith, S. E., Green, N. E., Cole, R. J.,

Robison, J. D., & Fenichel, G. M. (1993). Prolongation of ambulation in children with Duchenne muscular dystrophy by subcutaneous lower limb tenotomy. *Journal of Pediatric Orthopedics, 13,* 336.

Sparrow, S. S., Balla, D. A., & Cicchetti, D. V. (1984). *Vineland adaptive behavior scales.* Circle Pines, MN: American Guidance Service.

Tsipouras, P. (1995). Osteogenesis imperfecta. In Beighton, P. (Ed.). *McKusick's heritable disorders of connective tissue* (5th ed.). St. Louis: C.V. Mosby.

Uniform Data Systems. (1993). *The Wee functional independence measure.* Buffalo: Uniform Data Systems.

Worton, R. G., & Brooke, M. H. (1995). The X-linked muscular dystrophies. In Scriver, C. R., Beaudet, A. L., Sly, W. S., & Valle, D. (Eds.). *The metabolic and molecular bases of inherited disease* (7th ed., Vol. 3). New York: McGraw-Hill.

Yamada, K., Yamamoto, H., Nakagawa, Y., et al. (1984). Etiology of idiopathic scoliosis. *Clinical Orthopedics, 184,* 50.

# 7

# The Visual and Auditory Systems

Susan Miller Porr, MEd, MS, OTR

*But the eyes are blind. One must look with the heart . . .*
—Antoine de Saint-Exupéry, *The Little Prince*

*Being blind cuts you off from things, but being deaf cuts you off from people.*

—Helen Keller

**KEY POINTS**

- Vision and hearing provide us with important information about the world in which we live.
- Children with impairments in sensory systems often have delays in other areas of development including motor skills, language, and socialization.
- Advances in medicine and technology have offered new opportunities to children with vision and hearing losses.

## BEGINNINGS

My daughter recently went to a local production of the Helen Keller story. For many of us, Helen Keller embodies the triumph of the human spirit over multiple sensory handicaps. We are fascinated, as my child is, with the beauty of sign language and the skill with which the visually impaired navigate in their world. But we stand outside of these worlds. We do not fathom the overwhelming implications of these sensory system deficits for the children who live without sound or light.

In this chapter the mechanisms of the eye and the ear are briefly reviewed. The causes of visual impairment and hearing impairment are explored. New advances in technology and medicine have impacted on both areas of disability. Children with hearing impairments (HI) and/or visual impairments (VI) provide new challenges for therapists, who team with others to provide interventions throughout life.

# VISUAL IMPAIRMENTS

## THE EYE: A REFRESHER COURSE

The eye, as everyone has been told since grade school, "works like a camera" (Figs. 7–1 and 7–2). The outside covering of the eye, the "camera case," is the *sclera*. The *extraocular muscles* of the eye act as both as the tripod and the swivel for the camera, allowing the eyeball to be moved in the eye socket. The colored portion of the eye, the *iris,* acts as the camera's shutter, controlling the light that enters the eye. The *pupil* is the hole in the center of the iris. The *cornea* covers the iris and is the first refractor that light encounters when entering the eye. The *lens,* which sits behind the body of fluid known as the *aqueous humor,* changes shape constantly to focus on objects near and far. Be-

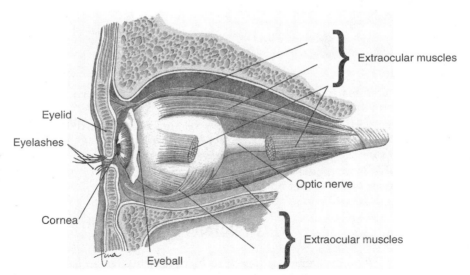

Figure 7–1 Lateral view of the left eye. Note the extraocular muscles. (Adapted from V. C. Scanlon & T. Sanders [1991]. Essentials of Anatomy and Physiology, ed 2 [p. 199.], Philadelphia, F. A. Davis.)

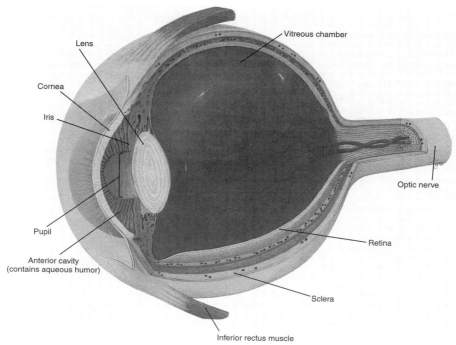

Figure 7–2  Internal anatomy of the eyeball. (Adapted from V. C. Scanlon & T. Sanders [1991]. Essentials of Anatomy and Physiology, ed 2 [p. 200.], Philadelphia, F. A. Davis.)

hind the lens is the *vitreous humor,* which is a jelly-like substance. The *retina,* at the back of the eye, which acts as film, imprints images in reverse (upside down and back to front). The optic nerve carries this information to the occipital lobe of the brain where perception and interpretation of the visual image are done.

From the time light hits the cornea and travels through the lens to the retina until the brain receives the image, processing problems can occur. These may result in visual impairments (Batshaw & Perret, 1986; Moore, 1980; Stiles & Knox, 1996).

## ∎∎∎ FROM THE BOOKSHELF

Stiles and Knox, just cited, comes from a wonderful resource, *Children with Visual Impairments: A Parents' Guide* edited by M. C. Holbrook (1996a). This book is part of the Special Needs Collection published by Woodbine House. It is comprehensive and jargon-free. It was a "must have" for my own professional library!

# THE CLINICAL PICTURE

There are numerous factors that may explain why vision in a child might be impaired. The workings of the extraocular muscles may be compromised by nerve or muscle damage, as in the child with cerebral palsy. Strabismus (improper alignment of the eyes) resulting from birth or trauma also compromises one's visual skills. Nystagmus, a rhythmic oscillation of one or usually both eyes, can impair a child's visual acuity, especially that used for distance vision (Stiles & Knox, 1996).

When the lens and cornea are "out of synch," vision problems known as refraction errors can occur. Refraction refers to "the process by which the cornea and lens of the eye bend light rays so that they are focused on the retina" (Stiles & Knox, 1996, p. 33). Nearsightedness (myopia) and farsightedness (hyperopia) are refraction errors known to many people who wear glasses or contact lenses. Astigmatism, which causes the eye to see blurry images, comes from unevenness in the cornea (a lumpy cornea).

Hyperopia and astigmatism are common in young children and infants (Batshaw & Perret, 1986). Researchers have noted that the human infant's vision develops quite rapidly over the first several months of life but does not reach the acuity level of adults until the ages of 6 to 9 months. This qualitative improvement in a baby's vision is attributed to the emerging visual cortex in the infant's brain (Adkinson & Braddick, 1990).

Although we normally associate glaucoma with adults about 5 percent of children who are blind are impaired by glaucoma. This disease is caused by an increase in internal pressure in the eye arising from a blocked flow of aqueous humor. This pressure increase causes damage to the optic nerve and subsequent visual impairment. In children glaucoma may arise from an infection, be the result of a malformation, or be caused by a chromosomal change (Batshaw & Perret, 1986; Rothenberg & Chapman 1994). Functionally, children with glaucoma have high degrees of astigmatism and nearsightedness (Stiles & Knox, 1996).

Children, like adults, may also have cataracts, which can cause visual loss. Vision is decreased when the lens of the eye becomes more opaque (cloudy) and light is not able to reach the retina. This results in a vision change for the child. Of the blindness seen in children, 15 percent can be attributed to cataracts. The cataracts may be congenital, such is in children with congenital rubella, or caused by trauma to the eye. Some children with certain syndromes (i.e., Turner's syndrome, Down syndrome) may be at risk for cataracts. By removing the lens of the eye, the cataract can be corrected. For children with congenital cataracts, this removal of the lens is done promptly (in the first 3 months of life) to promote normal development of vision. Children then wear special contact lenses or glasses that substitute for the eye's lens and allow for improved vision (Rothenberg & Chapman, 1994; Stiles & Knox, 1996).

There are a wide variety of causes for blindness, but the most common causes of blindness from birth are eye malformations or prenatal viral infections (e.g., rubella). One of the other causes of blindness in infants, retinopathy of prematurity (ROP), has been markedly decreased in recent years owing to changes in the medical interventions used with premature infants.

■ *THERAPEDS POINTER*

Cases of ROP arose almost exclusively when premature babies received high levels of oxygen ($O_2$) for treatment of respiratory distress syndrome (another complication of prematurity). This intense $O_2$ level destroyed the blood vessel network in the infant's retina. When the baby was returned to normal levels of oxygen, a disorganized network of blood vessels grew back. This caused excessive scar tissue and detachment of the retina, resulting in blindness. When medical professionals realized the association between ROP and high $O_2$ levels, changes in therapeutic levels of $O_2$ were made. Today, infants with respiratory distress syndrome get lower percentages of $O_2$ (30 to 45 percent) and are monitored by an ophthalmologist while receiving the treatment.

The risk of ROP is related to the infant's weight and level of prematurity. The more premature a baby is and the lower the birth weight, the greater the chances are of ROP occurring. The greatest risk is for infants born before 28 weeks' gestation who "weigh in" under 1500 g (about 3 lb, 5 oz.).

Children with ROP are usually candidates for long-term eye care because of refraction errors such as nearsightedness and astigmatism. Glaucoma may also develop later in these children (Batshaw & Perret, 1986; Stiles & Knox, 1996).

VI can also be caused by an inherited disease or by changes that affect vision in other ways than acuity (the clarity or sharpness of the image). For example, color blindness affects a child's ability to distinguish among certain colors. This trait, which impacts on vision, is more often seen in males and tends to be hereditary (Rothenberg & Chapman, 1994).

Amblyopia, commonly referred to as "lazy eye," results when the image from one eye is suppressed. When one eye functions better than the other (i.e., via better visual acuity), the brain may selectively ignore vision in one eye to prevent blurry or double vision. Over time this may cause permanent vision loss in the eye not being used. If detected before the visual system matures (about age 9), the amblyopia can be treated. Treatment is accomplished using a patch to cover the "good" eye, thus forcing the lazy eye to work (Stiles & Knox, 1996). Patching can be done anywhere from months to a year after detection of the condition.

Cortical blindness describes VI that is not related to the actual structure and processes in the eye itself (i.e., the cornea, lens, retina, eyeball). This term applies to VI that comes from the processing areas for vision—either in the neural path to the brain (optic nerve) or in the brain itself.

When all of the above causes for blindness are considered, the incidence of blindness in children is 0.4/1000. The majority of children who are blind are born with a VI or become so within the first year of life (46 percent are born blind; 38 percent become blind before a year old) (Batshaw & Perret, 1986). *Blindness* is defined as having less than 20/200 visual acuity in both eyes or a vision field of less than 20 degrees even when corrected. *Note:* A vision field is that area in front of the eye that can be seen without the eye moving (Rothenberg & Chapman, 1994).

Children with VI who do not meet the criteria for blindness are considered to have low vision. Although these children may have usable vision, they may be hampered by losses in visual acuity, color or depth perception, or visual field deficits. All of these low-vision impairments impact on the way developmental skills are acquired and functional tasks are completed (Beaver & Mann, 1995). Although children have similar needs to adults who acquire VI later in life, the issues in pediatric treatment of low vision are different. Children with VI do not have the same repertoire of skills or fund of visual knowledge that their adult counterparts have acquired over years of living (Faye et al., 1984).

## DIAGNOSIS AND INTERVENTION

Children with VI, as noted, may be blind or have a lesser degree of impairment. Because vision develops in children in a specific patterned manner, the child with total vision loss is easier to diagnosis (Batshaw & Perret, 1986). Children with lesser degrees of vision loss are more difficult to catch because they exhibit "normal vision behavior" (Faye et al., 1984, p. 429). Regardless of the level of the problem, VI has effects on the way a child adjusts to the world.

---

■ *THERAPEDS POINTER*

Just what is 20/20 vision anyway? This magic pair of numbers refers to a measurement of visual acuity taken using the Snellen eye chart. This chart consists of letters that are $^3/_8$ in high. The person who has 20/20 vision can read letters this size ($^3/_8$ in) from a distance of 20 feet from the chart. If one's vision is poorer than 20/20, the second number in the pair will be larger. For example, if Susie has 20/80 vision, then she sees from 20 feet what a person with "normal" vision sees from 80 feet. For children and others who can't identify letters, a similar chart has been designed that uses pictures (i.e., apples, houses) to obtain the same information (Holbrook, 1996b).

---

Diagnosis of a vision problem in an infant or young child is a challenging task. The most accurate assessment is generally parental report. However, tools are available that can objectify the process if this is desired. In infants optokinetic nystagmus can be used to determine the integrity of the visual pathway. Its absence is always a concern, but the presence of this reflex does not always reflect an intact visual pathway. This reflex generally appears at 29 to 30 weeks' postconceptual age and as such can be used with infants born prematurely (Hoon, 1996). Additional assessment may include testing for a blinking reflex and pupillary constriction when the child's eyes are exposed to light.

When infants are of at least term age, fixation and following, preferential looking, and visual evoked potential tests can be added to examine visual functions. However, it may be difficult to sort out nonattending behaviors and to account for differences arising from behavioral states at very young ages (Hoon, 1996). It is important to note that these early tests of visual function may not have adequate predictive validity; that is, they may not give the evaluator valid information about how the visual system will function later in life (Hoon, 1996).

In children of even toddler age, observation can be very useful. Offering visually interesting toys and noting the response can be a valuable way to begin. The STYCAR Test, Allen cards, and the Snellen chart can all be used to obtain some information about visual function. All require the active participation of the child.

---

■ *THERAPEDS POINTER*

Tests of Visual Acuity in Children (Adapted from Hoon, 1996)

STYCAR Test: Utilizes single-letter cards, charts, small toys, and graded white balls. Can be used to determine acuity with children who do not talk.

Allen cards: Designed for children able to identify line drawings. Children are shown line drawings and when the examiner is certain they can identify the drawings, the distance from card to eye is changed to obtain an acuity reading.

Snellen chart: Most common tool for determining acuity; requires the identification of letters. May underestimate visual acuity in children who do not have confidence in their ability to identify the letters.

---

Ophthalmologists have access to tools to help with diagnoses. Ophthalmoscopes are used to look at the back of the eye to check for problems. Slit lamps can be used to look for damage or malformations in the cornea or the lens of the eye. High-tech diagnosis may involve the use of an electroretinogram. This machine records the electrical activity of the retina in a graphic way (similar to the way an EEG (electroencephalogram) records brain activity. It is used to determine retina dysfunction or disease (Rothenberg & Chapman, 1994).

Determining the impact of a VI on development presents other challenges. Although some professionals suggest that even with typical intellect children with blindness or VI will experience significant delays (Menacker & Batshaw, 1997), others disagree. Part of the difficulty in identifying delays in development is related to the fact that overall development in children without sight progresses differently from development in children with sight. Children without sight deal with the environment in significantly different ways than their counterparts with sight, and a simple developmental comparison is therefore thought to be inappropriate. Davidson and Simmons (1992) suggest that "The uniqueness of development [in children without sight] must be matched by the uniqueness of approach to clinical assessment if proper account is to be taken of the specialized characteristics of a blind child" (p. 222).

A specialized assessment tool has been designed by Nesker-Simmons and Davidson, the Simmons-Davidson Developmental Profile (Nesker-Simmons & Davidson, 1992). This tool is designed to identify skills and needs in context of each role the child assumes. The evaluation has two components, one to obtain information on what the environment provides, and a second to determine how the child functions within the context of the environment. Areas to observe include orientation and mobility, language, exploration and play, social and emotional development, and academic performance. This assessment process also capitalizes on interviews with the parents and other significant adults in the world of the child. The need for specialized assessment tools and processes for children without sight is echoed by Brombring & Tröster (1994). These investigators suggest that no evaluation tool can fairly compare development in very young children with blindness with their sighted peers because no tools available are "blind neutral." Thus, if you choose to use specific assessment tools, it is best to be very sensitive to the fact that children with blindness are likely to follow a different developmental course from their sighted counterparts.

The professional team involved with the child with VI may include a variety of people. Parents, teachers of the visually impaired, ophthalmologists, social workers, educational psychologists, pediatricians, and therapists may all be involved in the care of these children. Within these multidisciplinary teams there is a need for a key person to coordinate services and needs for the child with VI (Youngson-Reilly, Tobin, & Fielder, 1994). This case manager concept is believed to provide better support and communication to the parents of the child.

The interventions used for a child with blindness or low vision are dependent on several factors, including: (1) the nature and severity of the problem, (2) the age when impairment occurred, (3) the family situation, and (4) the type of team involvement. As noted, medical personnel are involved with diagnosis and with the monitoring of the physical aspects of the disease or impairment. Other members of the team are involved with programming, education, and training for children with VI. Issues specific to children with VI include mobility, written communication, the development of functional independence in activities of daily living (ADL), and the use of technology both in the educational and vocational settings (*Resource Guide*, 1995).

Orientation and mobility (O&M) specialists may be unique to the team. These persons are specifically trained to assist those with VI to navigate in a sighted world. Teachers of the visually impaired are also trained in specific skills to help these children use their residual vision and make use of other sensory cues.

Many times a transdisciplinary approach is used to provide integrated comprehensive programming. OTs have both traditional roles and new models to demonstrate in serving children who have VI.

## INTERVENTION FROM THE
## OCCUPATIONAL THERAPY PERSPECTIVE

Numerous roles in a variety of settings have been played by OTs working with persons with VI. Therapists have traditionally been involved with persons with vision loss as "low vision specialists" in vision rehabilitation (Donovan, 1994). Others have addressed the needs of their young clients through early intervention programs or school settings. As OTs, the "adaption people," become involved with mandated assistive technology (AT) services, new interventions for this population become feasible (Brown, Castro, Lauck, & McSorley, 1996)

As Donovan (1994) indicated, the role of the OT is to help persons with VI achieve functional independence through activity. This concept can be very different for children depending on their age, level of disability, and the demands of the environment in which they function. Table 7–1 illustrates the assessment areas therapists might consider as they work with children with VI.

Occupational therapy interventions are driven by the results of assessment and evaluation. For the child with VI, foundation skills based on sensory input are often delayed. In the seeing population, 80 to 90 percent of learning takes place through the visual system (Johnson-Martin, Jens, Attermeier, & Hacker, 1991). To allow infants or toddlers with VI to progress, use exploration experiences based on sound and touch to give them alternatives.

As noted above, the development sequence for the child with VI may differ from that for children with sight. Because vision fosters the development of balance and stability (Johnson-Martin et al., 1991), and typical muscle tone has been associated with visual perception, deviations from typical gross motor development would be expected. Mobility skills may be particularly delayed compared to sighted infants. Sitting may appear at about 8 months of age, and the onset of walking may be delayed until well beyond the child's second birthday because of the lack of visual input (Menacker & Batshaw, 1997). There are some reports of delays in language acquisition (Menacker & Batshaw, 1997) or language syntax (Teplin, 1995). Early social interaction cues such as smiling may be late to develop, but generally children with VI are quite able to form emotional attachments to familiar and important people in their environment at about the same time as their sighted counterparts (Teplin, 1995).

Although written literature often recommends positioning a child with VI on the stomach to foster the development of neck and trunk strength, the therapist must be cautious about the use of this position. In the prone position typical infants lift their heads to look around and begin a visual exploration of the environment. This avenue of exploration is not available to a child with VI, and as such one must question the utility of this intervention. Certainly neck and trunk strength can be increased by working these muscles against gravity, but a better approach may be to engage the child in a game in which the parent tilts the child toward and away from gravity. If the parent is talking, laughing, and encouraging the child to maintain the head upright during this game, strength can be worked on, and the task is much more entertaining. The fact that the head is moving through space during such a

Table 7–1  **Assessment Components for the Child with VI**

| Age of child/ status | Toddler/VI since birth | 4th-grader/VI after traumatic brain injury (TBI) | High schooler in supported work program/VI since infancy from adverse drug reaction |
|---|---|---|---|
| Mobility | Address balance, reflexes, righting reactions<br>Observe methods of movement: walk, crawl, cruise, other | Consult with orientation and mobility specialist<br>Address barriers in school and play settings | Determine mobility on a variety of surfaces<br>Evaluate ability to use forms of transport such as bus and taxi<br>Assess workplace mobility issues |
| Play/leisure | Assess type of play done (solitary, group)<br>Observe how present play items are used<br>Determine child's use of other senses for play, i.e., touch, hearing | Do a play history to determine play skills/ activities prior to injury<br>Survey child as to present leisure interests | Determine present leisure activities<br>Determine student's balance of work, leisure, ADL<br>Generate ideas for new personal and social leisure outlets |
| ADL | Evaluate level of functional indepen- dence in feeding, dressing, toileting (if applicable) | Assess present functional inde- pendence in all areas of ADL (Are they age- appropriate?) | Assess for functional independence in ADL<br>Determine level of assistance needed for job site and job coach information |
| School/ vocational | Evaluate fine motor skills for preschool readiness (if applicable) | Determine need for adaptions in school-related areas, i.e., writing, personal organi- zation, and possible AT needs | Review present levels of function in school for gaps or needs<br>Assess AT use and future needs<br>Determine level of work skills, interests, and behaviors |

game also activates the vestibular system, which should further facilitate neck extensor contractions.

Other early areas of intervention include games to encourage reaching for sound cues, language development, and activities that encourage tactile exploration of a variety of materials with both hands (Teplin, 1995). It is important to note that children with VI will need to learn to use both hands to explore their environment; one hand acts as a reference point, and the other explores from this point. It is therefore appropriate to work on games and activities that capitalize on the use of both hands.

Play and social skills are at risk of not developing as would be expected of a child with sight. Play may be more repetitive and social skills more rudimentary because the child cannot use visual models to further their understanding of the situation. Thus, intervention that focuses on play and social interaction with both typical peers and adults is important for children with VI.

As children with VI acquire gross motor skills and foundation skills, the therapist may move to interventions in the area of ADL. Here consultation with teachers, low vision specialists, and vision consultants becomes very helpful. These persons regularly work with persons with VI and often are well versed in "the tricks of the trade." For example, tactile cues, such as Velcro sticky dots, help the child with VI to position clothing and know front from back for dressing. Consistent placement of eating utensils and teaching preschoolers to track around the plate by touch help them to be "clean plate clubbers" at meal time. Becoming familiar with AT that the child may use in preschool or childcare settings is also valuable for the therapist working with the visually impaired.

## ▰▰▰ FROM THE BOOKSHELF

> Several books on intervention for children with VI are available from the Blind Children's Center (4120 Marathon St., P.O. Box 29159, Los Angeles, CA 90020-0159; 213-664-2153). Many are available to parents at no cost. Some examples include:
> * *Talk to Me* and *Talk to Me II:* A language guide.
> * *Move with Me:* A guide for movement development.
> * *Learning to Play*
> * *Dancing Cheek to Cheek:* A guide for the development of social, play, and language skills.
> * *Reaching, Crawling, Walking . . . Orientation and Mobility for Preschool Children Who Are Visually Impaired.*

> ■ *THERAPEDS POINTER*
>
> Tactile cues may come in many different forms and are used by many persons with VI. Press-on earrings can be used as tactile dots for marking objects for toddlers and preschoolers. Adhesive dots in both standard and jumbo size are available commercially. These can be used by teachers, staff, and parents for marking a variety of things from maps to the TV remote control in the home. Exceptional Teaching Aids (1-800-549-6999) is one resource for these items.

As the child with VI becomes ready for entry into elementary school, the extent of the vision problem should be known (Batshaw & Perret, 1986). The OT working in the schools will be asked for adaptive strategies for many different situations. Incorporating tactile cues into organizational strategies may be useful (i.e., for identifying personal belongings). At this point in time the "reading, writing, and 'rithmetic" program will need team consideration. Will the student be able to use a print magnifier to augment the child's residual vision to see printed materials? Will braille be taught for language and reading? Will additional assistance in mobility training be needed for the student to navigate the school environment? These questions and more will all be raised by the new school setting and require OT input on the multidisciplinary team. In fact, the intervention strategies will vary for each child with VI that a therapist encounters.

---

**■ THERAPEDS POINTER**

Assistive technology (AT) changes so rapidly that this week's invention will be next week's old news. To help get a perspective on the AT that may be useful with children with VI, examples have been divided into three categories: high tech, low tech, and no tech. This array will change continuously, and therapists are advised to stay in touch or use AT resources that are easy to access.

*No-tech adaptions:* Use of a peer tutor to transcribe papers that the child with VI gives orally; large-print books; "white cane" assistance for school and community mobility; textured number shapes to assist learning of counting and math concepts; use of beaded keychains as tactile markers in personal clothing, i.e., coats, sweatshirts.
*Low-tech adaptions:* Use of a tape recorder for oral test answers or playing books on tape; hand magnifiers to enlarge print for those with low vision; use of inexpensive telescopes to see the board in class. (These items may require basic initial training for the child but are easily used with introductory information.)
*High-tech adaptions:* Computers can be used with children with VI in a variety of ways: software can be used that has enlarged fonts for easier reading. Other software has voice output that reads back word processing information to the writer. Optical scanners are now able to "read" printed materials from texts using synthesized speech. Closed-circuit TV offers enlargement capacities for print also. Braille is available via computer in several ways. Software is now available to actually print the raised dot type. Braille displays can augment keyboards and are a possibility for proficient braille readers. (These items are more sophisticated than low-tech adaptions and may require more comprehensive training and customized adaptions for each user.)

Information from Beaver & Mann, 1995; Donovan, 1994; Faye et al., 1984.

---

As students with VI move into adolescence, a therapist may need to pull out more psychosocial interventions. High school students with VI may be upset or angry over their difficulties in keeping pace academically with their peers. Students who have low vision or are blind must deal with the stresses of not fitting the norm. Teen rites of passage such as driver's licenses and independent dating may be unobtainable or challenging at best for this population (Faye et al., 1984).

The future may loom large as transition from school to the work environment becomes a reality. For individuals with VI there are resources that are not available to individuals with other disabilities. It is critical to contact these special organizations for information and assistance on making the transition to adult life. Organizations that may be of some help in this process are listed in the Therapeds Pointer below.

---

■ *THERAPEDS POINTER*

Resources helpful in planning for individuals with VI:

*American Foundation for the Blind*
11 Penn Plaza
Suite 300
New York, NY 10001
(800) 232-5463 or (212) 502-7600

*American Printing House for the Blind*
1839 Frankfurt Avenue
P.O. Box 6085
Frankfurt, KY 40206-0085
(800) 223-1839 or (502) 895-2405

*Hadley School for the Blind*
700 Elm Street
Winnetka, IL 60093
(800) 323-4238 or (708) 446-8153

*HEATH Resource Center*
One Dupont Circle, NW
Suite 800
Washington, DC 20036-1193
(800) 544-3284 or (202) 939-9320

*Helen Keller National Center for Deaf-Blind Youths and Adults*
111 Middle Neck Road
Sands Point, NY 11050
(800) 255-0411 or (516) 944-8900, (516) 944-8637 (TDD)

*Library of Congress National Library Service for the Blind and Physically Handicapped*
1291 Taylor Street, N.W.
Washington, DC 20542
(800) 424-8567

*Recording for the Blind & Dyslexic*
20 Roszel Road
Princeton, NJ 08540
(800) 221-4792 or (609) 452-0606

In addition, the American Foundation for the Blind can be found at the following Web site: http://www.afb.org/afb/index.html

---

OTs may help young people with VI to make the move from school to work more smoothly with consultations and direct interventions. Determining interests and skill levels in a particular vocational area may be a therapist's role in conjunction with other team members. Helping these teenagers to access community services (e.g., public transportation, job counseling) and to use them are valuable contributions an OT can make. Students with VI pursuing higher education may need a different adaption than was used in the high school setting. For example, the student with VI entering the community college setting may find a reader service that can also provide explanations, and tutoring may be more beneficial than textbooks on tape (Faye,

1984). Knowledgeable foresight and an integrated preplanned program help the student with VI move forward with life.

# HEARING IMPAIRMENTS

## THE EAR: THE BASICS

"If a tree fell in the forest and nobody was there to hear it, would it make a sound?" Most of us have been asked to ponder this question at sometime in our educational past. Although sound is a physics issue, our ears allow us to be aware of the world around us and to share in the excitement of speech and language. The ear is essentially a three-part structure (Fig. 7–3). The external ear, *the auricle,* catches sound waves and guides them into the skull through the ear canal. This internal tunnel leads to the *tympanic membrane,* known to most as the eardrum. This membrane divides the external ear from the middle ear. It also acts mechanically by vibrating and causing the move-

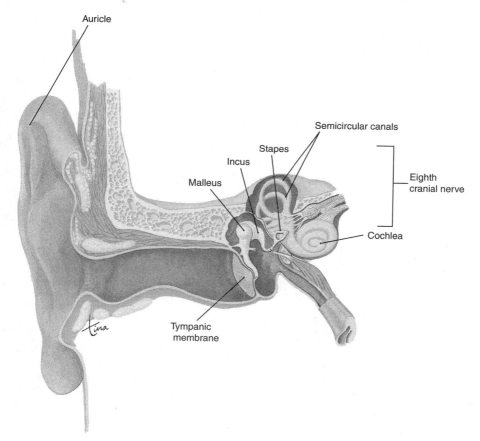

Figure 7–3  Outer, middle, and inner ear structures as shown in a frontal section through the right temporal bone. (Adapted from V. C. Scanlon & T. Sanders [1991]. Essentials of Anatomy and Physiology, ed 2 [p. 206], Philadelphia, F. A. Davis.)

ment of the three small bones (the malleus, incus, and stapes) in the middle ear cavity. The middle ear also houses one end of the *auditory tube* (a.k.a. the eustachian tube), which leads from the middle ear to the the nasopharynx area (back of the throat behind the nose). Although the main purpose of the auditory tube is to equalize ear pressure with atmospheric pressure, many parents feel there is another subversive purpose to this structure. It serves as a prime route for infection from the nasopharynx area to the ear and subsequent earaches and hearing problems may result (Moore, 1980).

The bones of the middle ear pass vibrations along to a second membrane known as the *oval window*. This window divides the middle ear from the inner ear. In the inner ear the mechanical energy that was once sound waves is converted to electrical energy. This is done via the *cochlea*, which encases fluid and hair cells connected to the auditory nerve. When fluid movement changes in the snail-shaped cochlea, the hair cells send sound information via the *auditory nerve* to the temporal lobe of the brain. This is the "hearing center," where sound is interpreted and given meaning (Batshaw & Perret, 1986).

The inner ear also houses the *vestibular apparatus*, which influences balance, stability, and movement. The vestibular system consists of semicircular canals and otolith organs, both innervated by the eighth cranial nerve. The semicircular canals are likely the portion of the vestibular system with which most of us are familiar. You may recall that the semicircular canals are paired, with three in each inner ear. They are oriented in three different planes, to give us information about movement in three-dimensional space. The receptor region in the canals is the cristae ampullaris. Within the cristae are hair cell receptors embedded in the cupula, a gelatin-like substance that surrounds the hair cell projections. The hair cells here respond to angular movement, both acceleration and deceleration. Sensory input from this region therefore gives the body information about rotary movements of the head (Moore, 1980; Fisher, 1991) and contributes to our dynamic equilibrium. When not appropriately modulated, the input from these sensory organs contributes to motion sickness in some people (Fisher, 1991).

Two otolith organs exist: the utricle and the saccule. Within the otolith organs is a specialized sensory receptor region known as macula. The macula also houses hair cell receptors. Otoliths, or calcium carbonate crystals, are embedded in a gelatinous substance that surrounds the hair cell projections. Within the utricle the hair cells are systematically oriented in different planes, which allows for detection of head movement in three-dimensional space again. Head tilt, gravity, or linear acceleration will activate these receptor cells. The utricle also responds to slower linear movement.

Functionally, if the goal of an intervention is to develop or facilitate postural support or postural reactions, linear activities that activate the utricle will be the best approach. Alternatively, if phasic or transitional postural reactions are the goal of therapy, activation of the semicircular canals will be more appropriate (Fisher, 1991).

## THE CLINICAL PICTURE

Hearing loss may be the result of a malfunction in the external ear, the middle ear, the inner ear, or a combination of these. Conductive hearing losses involve those hearing impairments that are in the external and/or middle ear that impact on how sound is moved through these areas. Sensorineural hearing losses are those hearing impairments that stem from problems in the cochlea or in the auditory nerve. A child with a sensorineural hearing loss is more likely to have vestibular problems than is a child with a conductive hearing loss, because of the origin of the problems. A mixed problem may arise when both conductive and sensorineural problems are present (Batshaw & Perret, 1986).

The definition of hearing impairment (HI) covers everything from mild loss to deafness. These losses may be bilateral (both ears) or only involve one ear (unilateral). The categories of HI based on types of sounds lost and the implications of that level of loss are found in Table 7–2.

For a young child, a hearing loss is a double problem because speech development is dependent on the cues one gets from hearing others speak. Adults who develop later-in-life hearing losses have an auditory repertoire to help fill in the blanks they may miss because of their HI. Many children with HI have never been exposed to or formed these auditory perceptions, so they are at a loss for using many of the speech cues hearing children depend on for speech acquisition (Northern & Downs, 1991).

The cause of hearing loss for about half of the children with HI is not known (Batshaw & Perret, 1986). When a hearing problem is identified, its source may be one of many possibilities. Structural problems in the external ear or ear canal may be the cause of hearing loss. Genetic conditions account for numerous cases of HI, including hereditary deafness. Infections both before and after birth may also cause hearing loss. For example, rubella and herpes in the mother during pregnancy are tied to cases of hearing loss in infants. After birth a bout with meningitis may be the cause of childhood hearing loss. In about 20 percent of meningitis cases the auditory nerve may be affected in some way (Batshaw & Perret, 1986). Other causes of deafness include drugs

---

Table 7–2 **Categories of Hearing Impairment**

| Category | Range (dB) | Functional Description of the dB Level | Implications |
|---|---|---|---|
| Mild loss | 15–30 | A whisper (about 20 dB) | May see inattention and/or mild speech and language delay |
| Moderate loss | 30–50 | Conversation levels of speech: soft, 45 dB; loud, 55 dB | Child misses speech in conversations; may help to have amplification; learning problems seen |
| Severe loss | 50–70 | Loud music from a radio (65 dB) | No spontaneous speech in children at this level; serious need for early intervention; can hear own voice sounds |
| Profound loss (deafness) | 70 or more | City traffic (75 dB) A factory with loud machinery (100 dB) | May react to very loud sounds; severe speech and language problems |

*Source:* Adapted from Northern & Downs, 1991; Rezen & Hausman, 1985.

that damage the auditory part of the inner ear (cochlea) and disease syndromes associated with hearing loss.

The most common cause of mild to moderate hearing loss in children is chronic infection of the middle ear, otitis media. In many cases of chronic middle ear infection, ventilation tubes (also known as PE [pressure-equalizing] tubes) are placed surgically to prevent infection by aiding drainage of the middle ear area. Children at particular risk for otitis media include those with head and neck malformations (e.g., Down syndrome or cleft palate). Middle ear infection affects the eardrum, causing a conductive hearing loss (Arnold, 1996).

Hearing loss is the most common disability in the United States (Kent & Izen, 1989). It occurs in 1 percent of all children. Of this group, 2 out of 1000 children have a profound level of deafness, with the majority of these having experienced deafness from birth (Batshaw & Perret, 1986). HI impacts both on the child and the family. Normal family communications may be lost because the child with HI has speech- and language-acquisition difficulties. School programming may also be affected by this lack of communication, producing the subsequent isolation of the student with HI (Northern & Downs, 1991). To prevent future problems and decrease the impact of this disability, early identification of and interventions for the HI are recommended (Drews, Yeargin-Allsopp, Murphy, & Decouflé, 1994).

## DIAGNOSIS AND INTERVENTION

Parents and those who provide daily care to infants and toddlers are often the first to notice a severe hearing loss. A baby who seems to sleep too well may have a hearing problem (Kent & Izen, 1989). In the 6- to 7-month range infants with profound hearing loss will stop cooing. They do not get the auditory feedback from the environment to progress with these early speech patterns. Children with HI frequently do not develop the baby talk associated with the normal development of infants in the 9- to 12-month range (Batshaw & Perret, 1986). When a severe hearing loss is suspected at this early age, new medical testing is available to diagnose the presence of the HI and the degree of the disability. This can be done as early as 8 to 10 months of age (Kent & Izen, 1989). Early detection of a hearing problem allows for optimal intervention and programming.

---

■ *THERAPEDS POINTER*

Infants are difficult to assess for the level of hearing loss that may be present. When typical audiometry tests are not successful, a brainstem auditory evoked response (BAER) test may be done. In this test the brain's response to sound is charted via an EEG (electroencephalogram). This reading is taken via electrodes that are attached to the outside of the skull. Information regarding neural activity related to sounds is then evaluated (Batshaw & Perret, 1986; Kent & Izen, 1989).

---

Although more severe loss of hearing such as that described above can be diagnosed early, identification of children with mild or moderate loss is not as quick or easy. These children are often picked up through general school screenings. In spite of the fact that overreferral from these screenings has been seen, it is important that children are identified through this process. Of children who fail their initial hearing screening, 10 percent are further diagnosed with persistent hearing problems (Batshaw & Perret, 1986).

Once a child is determined to need more specific auditory testing, several different evaluation methods and tools are used. The audiologist on an intervention team is specially trained in the diagnosis and treatment of hearing loss (Kent & Izen, 1989). He or she may gather information from observing the child's behavior. Additional audiometric testing includes the measuring of the threshold for hearing sounds as well as hearing specific speech sounds and processing sound (Rothenberg & Chapman, 1994). The physical structure of the ear is evaluated using an otoscope. More sophisticated evaluation may include the use of tympanometry to determine how the eardrum is functioning (Newby & Popelka, 1992).

Additional medical testing for hearing loss may include a brainstem evoked auditory response (BAER) noted in the preceding Therapeds Pointer (Batshaw & Perret, 1986; Kent & Izen, 1989). This test assesses whether auditory information is actually getting to the brain. This type of testing is done with infants and with children whose disabilities make regular audiometric testing difficult and inaccurate. The BAER does not determine how the information is processed once it gets to the brain.

Once the diagnosis and extent of the disability are known, other members of the professional team are also involved in programming for the child with HI. Along with physicians and audiologists, teachers of the hearing impaired, school psychologists, social workers, parents, and speech and language therapists may be members of the intervention team. OTs may be involved as school therapists, members of augmentive communication teams, or providers of assistive technology (AT) expertise. Interventions for children with HI integrate medical and education plans as well as family support and social services issues.

Medical interventions for children with HI often include amplification of sound via hearing aids. The style of hearing aid most often used by children (infants or teens) is the device that fits behind the ear (Bentler, 1993). The style of aid that fits in the ear is not often used in pediatrics, because children's ears grow rapidly, making frequent changes necessary. Other alternatives for direct amplification are FM radio systems, which provide the student with a direct link to the teacher's voice in a classroom. These systems (also known as auditory trainers) help to filter out background noise that may be distracting to the student with the hearing disability.

---

■ *THERAPEDS POINTER*

One of the latest advances in medical technology is the use of cochlear implants to improve the perceptions of speech in those children who have profound sensorineural hearing loss. These implants are actually electrodes that are surgically implanted into the child's inner ear. The electrodes directly stimulate the auditory nerve. The brain then interprets this stimulation as sound. The initial results of this technique have been very successful. There have been few physical complications from the surgery. Because of the newness of this technology, long-term side effects of direct neural stimulation are not known (Bentler, 1993; Newby & Popelka, 1992).

Children with HI come with their own personal needs and areas for intervention. The primary focus for each child depends on the severity of the hearing disability and the time the hearing loss occurred in the child's life (Batshaw & Perret, 1986). For young children, communication and speech are primary areas of concern. The child's inability to communicate may also create family problems, since parents have difficulty knowing how to interact with their nonhearing child (Northern & Downs, 1991). Barriers for the school-age child with HI include the forementioned communication issues as well as social isolation that comes with the inability to communicate with peers in the "hearing" world (Batshaw & Perret, 1986). For teenagers with HI, vocational choice becomes an important concern. Interventions in the educational arena from early intervention to school-to-work transition planning all need to be child-focused and outcome-oriented.

The goal of educational interventions for the child with HI is to assist the student in achieving his or her highest potential (Northern & Downs, 1991, p. 323). How that is accomplished will vary with each child. Children with HI usually have needs in the areas of receptive language, and they also have speech and language problems (Newby & Popelka, 1992). Goals of educational intervention are focused in four primary areas: (1) language, (2) positive mental health, (3) intelligible speech, and (4) communication with others (peers, family, community) (Northern & Downs, 1991). The entire team of professionals will be responsible for some piece of the educational pie when it comes to intervening with a child with HI.

---

### ■ THERAPEDS POINTER

Having a rudimentary level of skill in sign language is a valuable tool for a therapist to acquire. Finger spelling will allow basic communication for those persons with HI who are readers. For younger children learning the basic signs for daily living activities (i.e., eat, drink, play) and positive reinforcement (i.e., good work, please, and thank you) will be invaluable. Local bookstores have reference texts for learning signs. A course at the local community college or a learning center may be the easiest (and most fun) because instructors' real-life gestures are more readily imitated.

---

Although the areas of intervention may have been delineated for students with HI, the "best" method for achieving these goals is still controversial. Three basic styles of teaching and communication are in use, with each one having its own advocacy group. The "basics" for each are outlined in Table 7–3. It should be noted that although the majority of schools for children with deafness or HI have adopted the total communication method, research has yielded inconsistent results regarding the "best" mode for teaching and communication (Newby & Popelka, 1992; Northern & Downs, 1991).

## ▟▊▌ FROM THE BOOKSHELF

An excellent resource for therapists involved with children learning sign language is *Pre-Sign Language Motor Skills* (Dunn, 1982). This book looks at the physical aspects of learning sign language. It includes valuable information regarding "pre-sign" assessment, fine motor movement patterns, and sign language teaching techniques. It's one to put on the professional bookshelf.

Laura Rankin's *The Handmade Alphabet* (1991) contains beautifully artistic renditions of the manual alphabet. Each drawing is linked to a word that begins with that letter. The author-artist prepared this volume as a tribute to her stepson who is deaf. It is a visual delight!

Trends in working with children with sensory impairments in general have moved toward functional programming. Needs for children with HI go beyond the classroom. Life-skills models address issues such as communication, social skills, independent daily living skills, and problem solving (Sacks & Bullis, 1988). Interventions in these areas target the real-life components one needs to be successful beyond the front door of one's house or school.

**Table 7–3 Educational Styles Used with Students with HI**

| | |
|---|---|
| Auditory/oral | • Supports the idea that students with HI can use speech meaningfully and can communicate in a spoken manner.<br>• Uses spoken language alone in class and teaching.<br>• Students depend on speech or speech reading (known earlier as lip reading) for communication information. |
| Manual | • Advocates of this method feel auditory information is not useful for the person with severe hearing loss.<br>• Uses a visual system such as gestures or sign language for communication.<br>• American Sign Language (ASL) is the most commonly used sign language; it is not a translated oral language but an independent language system.<br>• Signing Exact English (SEE method) involves signs for oral English with word-by-word signing |
| Total communi-<br>cation | • Uses components of both manual and auditory oral methods.<br>• In "total" schools have seen students' preference for manual communication (sign language) as sign is easier to use. |

*Source:* Adapted from Newby & Popelka, 1992; Northern & Downs, 1991; Sacks & Bullis, 1988.

## INTERVENTION FROM THE
## OCCUPATIONAL THERAPY PERSPECTIVE

OTs are involved with children with HI throughout the childhood and adolescent years. Earlier identification of hearing losses helps these children to receive services as "at-risk" candidates in infant and toddler programs. School therapists may be involved with students who are hearing impaired in special programs (e.g., state schools for students with HI) or in inclusionary programs on school campuses. Vocational readiness and work-related skills may be the focus of a therapist's program with a teenager with HI.

The assessment process for each child with HI will be different depending on the setting, the individual's age and needs, and the level of the child's disability. Although the components of the assessment process (i.e., fine motor, play, ADL, foundation skills) may be familiar to the therapist, the communication aspect of the assessment may be unique for the professional. Challenges during both assessment and intervention may be communication-based. It may be difficult to explain test directions to these children without interpreter assistance. It is also difficult to know what a child is thinking if communication skills are limited (Northern & Downs, 1991). Observations, interviews, and actual task performance may provide more information for the therapist than attempts to use standardized testing tools. Integration of knowledge from a variety of professional sources will provide the most complete assessment picture of the child with HI.

---

■ *THERAPEDS POINTER*

The Leiter International Performance Scale (LIPS) is one of the few standardized tests available for testing the intelligence of individuals with language and speech problems. This includes persons with HI, those who do not speak English, and others who may have difficulty with reading or speaking.

The test uses a wooden frame and stimulus cards; directions are given in pantomime. Tasks range in ability from preschool matching of colors and shapes to higher level classification and pattern completion items.

LIPS can be given to individuals from 2 to 18 years old. Raw scores are converted to mental ages. The developmental format of the test helps with program planning following the testing. Test reviewers have noted problems with reliability and validity; standardization has also been faulted. Despite these concerns, the LIPS is a useful diagnostic tool for atypical assessments (Reynolds & Mann, 1987).

---

Once assessment has been completed and strengths and needs of the child with HI have been determined, intervention strategies and plans may be put into place. The table accompanying gives examples of three different scenarios of youth with HI who are seen by OTs to address their different and varied needs.

| The Scenario— | | |
|---|---|---|
| | **Fourth-grade** | |
| **Preschool child** | **student with HI** | **A group of adolescents** |
| **with HI (hereditary)** | **is also learning** | **with HI and severe** |
| **being taught sign** | **disabled in written** | **language delays in state** |
| **language** | **language area** | **school** |
| Assessment Information re needs | Fine motor skills for isolating fingers and using hands for sign are weak | Student's written performance is poorer because of illegibility, poverty of content, and grammar errors | Staff has determined that social skills for group are lacking in areas of social "niceties"—turn taking, peer interactions, etc. |
| OT Interventions | Consult with preschool teacher re presign activities for motor skills: finger puppets, clothespin games, rubber band exercises (Dunn, 1982)<br><br>Also OT does colleague consultation with speech language therapist to determine which functional signs have easiest motor components | Collaborative meeting re student's writing program: OT to explore software for keyboarding (alternative to handwriting) and writing software with topic cues (for generating story ideas) for trial with student<br><br>OT also asks for sentences on specific topics during cursive handwriting practice sessions | The middle school team develops social skills training program involving role playing, positive reinforcement, and correction process.<br><br>OT and speech and language therapist do role playing in social skills group; OT also checks for generalization of skills on community outing to local fast-food restaurant (scenario adapted from Rasing & Duker, 1993) |

These are only examples of the variety of challenges and opportunities OTs have when working with children with HI. As with the population of students with visual impairments, AT has provided assistance to many children and adults with hearing losses. OTs have both evaluation and training roles in the AT realm (Compton, 1993; Kent & Izen, 1989).

■ *THERAPEDS POINTER*

As was noted earlier in this chapter, AT changes at a rapid pace. What's here today may be new and improved tomorrow. Technology provides a way for persons with HI to access the speaking world and to communicate with others.

Alternatives to human speech are provided through augmentative and alternative communication (AAC) devices. These electronic tools may have voice output that can be programmed, in many cases specifically for the user. These machines have become smaller, more sophisticated, and more user friendly. OTs can help a communication team determine a child's motor skills that are best-suited for accessing an AAC.

Youth with HI also need a means for accessing spoken language on a daily basis. Use of the telephone may be challenging for the teen with HI who wants access to the school social circle. Amplification handsets are available for regular telephones for those with milder degrees of hearing loss. A telecommunication device for the deaf (TDD) provides transcription of a telephone conversation as it takes place. Therapists can provide opportunities for students to access, use, and generalize their skills in this area of AT (Compton, 1993).

---

New technology, improved medical techniques, and integrated programming for children with HI have improved the prognosis for their success. When there are no other disabling conditions, the severity of the hearing loss and the age when it occurred often impact on rate of progress and achievement of highest potential (Batshaw & Perret, 1986). When other conditions compound the issue of hearing (or visual impairment), then the life plan becomes more complex and challenging.

# A WORD ON MULTIPLE IMPAIRMENTS

Children with impairments of more than one sensory system offer multiple challenges. In fact, there are several conditions (e.g., rubella) where vision and hearing deficits occur together (Faye et al., 1984). This knowledge helps professionals to double check on other sensory involvement in at-risk children, but the findings may be devastating for families. The outcomes for children with sensory impairment as part of a dual- or multiple-disability diagnosis are much poorer than for those with single-system involvement. When other issues such as cognitive deficits are involved, the pace of progress will be much slower. It is imperative that teams working with children with multiple conditions cooperate, communicate, and coordinate in their efforts (Talbott, 1992).

As one can imagine, the assessment process for children with dual sensory impairments or multiple conditions is not the typical "use a standardized test" situation. Assessment and programming for those youths with dual or multiple sensory impairments should use a "top-down" approach (Marchant, 1992). Instead of taking a developmental approach (which builds on a foundation of sequential skills), look at what the child needs to succeed in life tasks. With slowed rates of skill acquisition, a developmental model might never allow a successful endpoint to be reached.

The intervention plan for a child with dual sensory impairments needs to capitalize on all the child's senses and skills. This is truly a place to plan and address all the issues (child, family, community, safety) as a team, demonstrating ongoing flexibility as new challenges arise. OTs, with their task analysis skills and training in facilitating acquisition of skill in the activities of daily living (ADL) can be valuable to a child's professional team. As Marchant (1992) notes, "Skills that are taught to students with dual sensory handicaps should be those that the student needs to function in all the different environments in his or her daily life" (p. 114). Therapists have the opportunity to capitalize on their skills while intervening with this population to provide what's best for these children.

## WRAPPING IT UP

Children with sensory impairments often demonstrate needs that benefit from occupational therapy intervention. As professional team members, therapists can add their life skills knowledge to the professional team's data base on a child. When vision, hearing, or both senses are impaired, one's life experiences are vastly altered from the norm. With new technologies, both assistive and medical, the prognosis for independence for those with VI or HI has improved. When combined with functional programming, technology and teamwork can provide both light and sound at the end of the tunnel.

---

### CASE STORY

Todd is an 8-year-old student who is legally blind, has mild cerebral palsy (CP) (left hemiplegia), and is within normal limits for cognitive skills. He has recently completed first grade at a state school for the blind and is moving back home to attend his local school district elementary school. Information from the state school team indicated that Todd has needs in dressing, organizational skills, and academics in the written language area.

1. As the OT who will be working with Todd, what additional assessment information would you want to know beyond the fact that he is not able to tie his shoes, do fasteners, or hang his coat up? Where or how might you get this information?
2. How might you go about teaching Todd to tie his shoes? (Don't forget he has CP and blindness.) What factors would help you determine if and when this was an appropriate goal for Todd in the ADL area?
3. Who might you contact for additional resources about Todd's case: people? agencies? references?
4. What team members might be involved at the school level with Todd's written language needs?

---

## Real-Life Lab

You are the OT who is helping a high school student who is deaf make a transition to a local office job. This is your first experience with a youth who is totally deaf. The office manager wants to know if he needs to change the telephone system in his office to accommodate the student's needs.

1. Familiarize yourself with a telecommunication device for the deaf (TDD). See how this works and report back to your colleagues.

2. Call the local telephone company to find out what resources they have for persons with hearing impairments. Pick up any resource pamphlets they have for your future reference file.

3. What additional communication strategies might your team devise to help this student (and office staff) with this transition?

4. Explore the legal obligations of businesses in regard to accommodations for workers with disabilities on the job. Information regarding the Americans with Disabilities Act (ADA) is a starting point.

---

# References

Adkinson, J., & Braddick, O. J. (1990). The developmental course of cortical processing streams in the human infant. In Blakesmore, C. (Ed.). *Vision: Coding and efficiency.* New York: Cambridge University Press, pp. 247–253.

Arnold, J. E. (1996). Otitis media. In Rakel, R. E. (Ed.). *Conn's current therapy 1996.* Philadelphia: Saunders, pp. 200–202.

Batshaw, M. L., & Perret, Y. M. (1986). *Children with handicaps: A medical primer* (2d ed.). Baltimore: Brookes.

Beaver, K. A., & Mann, W. C. (1995). Overview of technology for low vision. *The American Journal of Occupational Therapy, 49,* 913–921.

Bentler, R. A. (1993). Amplification for the hearing impaired child. In Alpiner, J. G., & McCarthy, P. A. (Eds.). *Rehabilitative audiology for children and adults* (2d ed.). Baltimore: Williams & Wilkins, pp. 72–105.

Brombring, M., & Tröster, H. (1994). The assessment of cognitive development in blind infants and preschoolers. *Journal of Visual Impairment & Blindness, 88,* 1, 9–18.

Brown, M., Castro, I., Lauck, V., & McSorley, J. (1996). *The use of technology to encourage language development in blind and multiply impaired children.* Presentation materials from Washington State School

for the Blind Assistive Technology Conference (February 29–March 1, 1996), Vancouver, WA.

Compton, C. L. (1993). Assistive technology for deaf and hard of hearing people. In Alpiner, J. G., & McCarthy, P. A. (Eds.). *Rehabilitative audiology for children and adults* (2d ed.). Baltimore: Williams & Wilkins, pp. 441–469.

Davidson, I. F. W. K., & Nesker-Simmons, J. (1992). Young blind children: Towards assessment for rehabilitation. *International Journal of Rehabilitation Research, 15,* 219–226

Donovan, N. J. (1994). The role of occupational therapy in vision rehabilitation. In Albert, D. M., & Jakobiec, F. A. (Eds.). *Principles and practice of ophthalmology* (Vol. 5—Clinical Practice). Philadelphia: Saunders, pp. 3683–3696.

Drews, C. D., Yeargin-Allsopp, M., C. C., & Decouflé, P. (1994). Hearing impairment among 10-year-old children: Metropolitan Atlanta, 1985 through 1987. *American Journal of Public Health, 84,* 1164–1166.

Dunn, M. L. (1982). *Pre-sign language motor skills.* Tucson: Communication Skill Builders.

Faye, E. E., Padula, W. V., Padula, J. B., Gurland, J. E., Greenberg, M. L., & Hood,

C. M. (1984). The low vision child. In Faye, E. E. (Ed.). *Clinical low vision* (2d ed.). Boston: Little, Brown, pp. 437–475.

Fisher, A. G. (1991). Vestibular-proprioceptive processing and bilateral integration and sequencing deficits. In Bundy, A. C., Fisher, A. G., & Murray, E. A. (Eds.) *Sensory integration: Theory and practice.* Philadelphia: F. A. Davis, pp. 71–107.

Holbrook, M. C. (1996). *Children with visual impairments: A parent's guide.* Bethesda, MD: Woodbine House.

Holbrook, M. C. (1996). What is visual impairment? In Holbrook, M. C. (Ed.). *Children with visual impairments: A parent's guide.* Bethesda, MD: Woodbine House, pp. 1–20.

Hoon, A. H., Jr. (1995). Visual impairments in children. In Capule, A. J., & Accardo, P. J. (Eds.). *Developmental disabilities in infancy and childhood* (Vol. 2, 2d ed). Baltimore: Brookes, pp. 461–477.

Johnson-Martin, N. M., Jens, K. G., Attermeier, S. M., & Hacker, B. J. (1991). *The Carolina curriculum for infants and toddlers with special needs* (2d ed.). Baltimore: Brookes.

Kent, D. D., & Izen, J. M. (1989). Communication disorders. In Logigian, M. K., & Ward, J. D. (Eds.). *A team approach for therapists: Pediatric rehabilitation.* Boston: Little, Brown, pp. 171–183.

Marchant, J. M. (1992). Deaf-blind handicapping conditions. In McLaughlin, P. J., & Wehman, P. (Eds.). *Developmental disabilities: A handbook for best practices.* Boston: Andover, pp. 113–123.

Menacker, S. J. & Batshaw, M. L. (1997). Vision: Our window to the world. In Batshaw, M. L. (Ed.). *Children with disabilities* (4th ed.). Baltimore: Brookes, pp. 211–240.

Moore, K. L., (1980). *Clinically oriented anatomy.* Baltimore: Williams & Wilkins.

Nesker-Simmons, J., & Davidson, I. F. W. K. (1992). *The Simmons-Davidson Developmental Profile: A guide to its use.* Toronto: Heron.

Newby, H. A., & Popelka, G. R. *Audiology* (6th ed.). Englewood Cliffs, NJ: Prentice Hall.

Northern, J. L., & Downs, M. P. (1991). *Hearing in children* (4th ed.). Baltimore: Williams & Wilkins.

Rankin, L. (1991). *The handmade alphabet.* New York: Dial.

Rasing, E. J., & Duker, P. C. (1993). Effects of a multifaceted training procedure on the social behaviors of hearing-impaired children with severe language disabilities: A replication. *Journal of Applied Behavior Analysis, 25,* 723–734.

*Resource Guide.* (1995). Portland, OR: Oregon Commission for the Blind.

Reynolds, C. R., & Mann, L. (Eds.). (1987). *Encyclopedia of special education* (Vol. 2). New York: Wiley and Sons.

Rezen, S. V., & Hausman, C. (1985). *Coping with hearing loss: A guide for adults and their families.* New York: Dembner.

Rothenberg, M. A., & Chapman, C. F. (1994). *Dictionary of medical terms for the nonmedical person* (3d ed.). Hauppauge, NY: Barron's.

Sacks, S. Z., & Bullis, M. (1988). Vocational education of persons with sensory handicaps. In Gaylord-Ross, R. (Ed.). *Vocational education for persons with handicaps.* Mountain View, CA: Mayfield, pp. 417–444.

Saint-Exupéry, A., de [translated by Woods, K.]. (1971). *The little prince.* New York: Harcourt, Brace.

Siegel, J. C., Marchetti, M., & Tecklin, J. S. (1991). Age-related balance changes in hearing-impaired children. *Physical Therapy, 71, 3,* 183–189.

Stiles, S., & Knox, R. (1996). Medical issues, treatments, and professionals. In Holbrook, M. C. (Ed.). *Children with visual impairments: A parent's guide.* Bethesda, MD: Woodbine House, pp. 21–48.

Talbott, R. E. (1992). Communication disorders. In McLaughlin, P. J., & Wehman, P. (Eds.). *Developmental disabilities: A handbook for best practices.* Boston: Andover, pp. 96–112.

Teplin, S. W. (1995). Visual impairment in infants and young children. *Infants and Young Children, 8, 1,* 18–51.

Youngson-Reilly, S., Tobin, M. J., & Fielder, A. R. (1994). Patterns of professional involvement with parents of visually impaired children. *Developmental Medicine and Child Neurology, 36,* 449–458.

# 8

# *The Cognitive System*

Susan Miller Porr, MEd, MS, OTR

*Examinations, checkups, and impressions are important, but actual performance under everyday living conditions is what counts—How does it work? What can it do? How far can it be pushed? What are the load limits?*
*And so it is with the brain. The structure is vitally important, the function even more so—and the two inexorably intertwined.*
—Ray Wunderlich, MD (from Wunderlich, 1970, p. 4)

## KEY POINTS

- Mental retardation and learning disorders involve exceptionality in cognitive functioning. The impact of the symptoms for both these disabilities goes far beyond "thoughts and thinking."

*Regarding mental retardation*

- Mental retardation is a symptom. The causative factors can be singular or multiple in nature.

- Mental retardation definitions look at both cognitive function and the adaptive nature of the individual with retardation.

- The movement encompassing deinstitutionalization, normalization, and now inclusion reflects a major environmental intervention that has had far-reaching effects for persons with mental retardation.

- OTs may provide services for persons with mental retardation throughout the life spans of these individuals in multiple settings in the community.

*Regarding learning disorders*

- The group of children with learning disorders is a heterogeneous one, with the severity of the situation varying widely from child to child.

- The scatter of strengths and needs seen in individuals with learning disorders is often reflected as very different behaviors and skill outcomes across settings.
- Learning disorders are seldom "outgrown": remedial steps, compensation, and adaptation allow for increasing success in functioning over a lifetime.
- Intervention techniques for both the learning disorder and the mentally retarded populations involve multiple disciplines; long-term commitments; and consistency across home, school, and community settings.

## BEGINNINGS

In this chapter the topics of mental retardation (MR) and learning disorders (LD) will be discussed. Both of these involve the area of cognition, and their impact is far-reaching. As with many of the pediatric situations discussed in this book, the lifelong nature of these entities goes beyond a "variation in thinking." The complex clinical pictures for both MR and LD will be addressed.

Evaluation processes and intervention strategies for working with these two groups are discussed. Often professionals from multiple disciplines are involved with children having either diagnosis. A system perspective to intervention services involves many people on many fronts for successful outcomes to be achieved (Crnic & Reid, 1989).

Occupational therapy services may be provided throughout the childhood and the adolescent years for both the LD and MR populations. Assessment is ongoing throughout the childhood years, because new functional challenges must be met by these children. OTs also find themselves and their services "growing up" in new roles as these youth grow, too. Group homes, supported work, and advanced technology may require innovative therapy strategies as therapists work in both traditional and nontraditional roles.

## MENTAL RETARDATION

### THE CLINICAL PICTURE

Mental retardation is defined by the *Diagnostic and Statistical Manual of Mental Disorders*, 1994 [*DSM-IV*] as "significantly subaverage intellectual functioning." According to the *DSM-IV*, the onset of this cognitive impairment appears before the age of 18. This definition also looks at the adaptive functioning of the individual with cognitive deficits. Adaptive functioning refers to that set of skills children need to achieve age-appropriate independence. Issues of self-care, play skills, and social skills may be included in this area.

The actual definition of MR has become more complex over the years (Szymanski & Kaplan, 1991). Originally MR was reflected by one's deficits in the area of personal independence. In the early 1900s, as psychometric testing came into being, the intelligence quotient (IQ) became an additional parameter. The *DSM-IV* (1994, p. 40) provides the following scale for categorizing the population with MR according to IQ scores:

IQ 50–55 to about 70: Mild MR
IQ 35–40 to 50–55: Moderate MR
IQ 20–25 to 35–40: Severe MR
IQ below 20–25: Profound MR

MR is a symptom that reflects central nervous system (CNS) dysfunction (Rubin, 1989). The causes of MR may be one or many. Origins of MR might include problems in the development of the CNS prior to birth (e.g., spina bifida), errors in metabolism or chromosomal abnormalities (e.g., Down syndrome), outside events (e.g., head injury or meningitis), and/or environmental conditions or problems such as lead poisoning or poor maternal nutrition during pregnancy.

---

### ■*THERAPEDS POINTER*

A *syndrome* is a collection of signs and symptoms that together present a picture of a particular disease or disorder (Rothenberg & Chapman, 1994). Two of the more common syndromes that are characterized by mental retardation are Down syndrome and fragile X syndrome.

Down syndrome is the most common of the chromosomal abnormalities. Children with this syndrome are usually short in stature, have obliquely placed eyes, and are usually mentally retarded. Health concerns that may impact on these children's activity levels include heart complications and bowel defects that are often associated with this syndrome.

Fragile X syndrome is the most commonly inherited form of MR (Runyon, 1993). It, like Down, is a syndrome caused by a chromosomal abnormality. More knowledge about fragile X has become available as increasingly sophisticated laboratory procedures make chromosome study more feasible.

The level of impairment among individuals with fragile X syndrome is highly variable. Males with this syndrome tend to be lower functioning than females. The clinical picture of the male with fragile X syndrome is one of a child with a more prominent chin and ears; increased testes size after puberty; and a long, narrow face (Menkes, 1995). Females with this syndrome usually have fewer prominent physical characteristics. MR, hyperactivity, and learning problems have been seen in both males and females with fragile X. There has also been documentation of increased autistic-like behaviors in males with this syndrome (Menkes, 1995; Runyon, 1993).

---

Information on the prevalence of MR depends on how and what category system (such as that found in the *DSM-IV* noted above) is used. Resources (Crocker & Nelson, 1992; Szymanski & Kaplan, 1991) indicate that between 1 and 3 percent of the general population has significant deficits in intelligence. Although test scores and definitions may quantify and clarify MR, the ensuing issues are complex. Often the key to successful community integration is the level of one's adaptive skills. There is a wide variation in functioning among individuals who may, for programming purposes, be "classified" at the same level or category. Descriptive information regarding the skills of children with a particular level of MR is only the springboard for personalizing and tailoring evaluation and interventions for each individual.

Identifying MR in a child may come soon after birth or later in childhood. Children may be regarded as at risk for MR at birth as a result of premature birth, trauma at birth, or an established risk (e.g., signs and symptoms of a specific syndrome such as Down). Mothers have been found to be both accurate and specific estimators of MR in their youngsters (Pulsifer, Hoon, Palmer, Gopalan, & Capute, 1994), possibly prompting earlier identification. Other children may be brought to their family physician because of slow development in areas such as mobility or communication. The enactment of Public Law 99-457 has increased the availability of "child find" services that emphasize the early identification and intervention with developmental disabilities, including cognitive impairments.

## PARAMETERS AND POSSIBILITIES

General characteristics of children with MR include: slower learning of skills, memory difficulties, and decreased "generalizing" of a skill across different settings (Ward, 1989). These children and adolescents seem to like to work for external rewards. In plain English this means learning is doable, although it may take a longer time, and offering a prize may help. Newly acquired skills need to be practiced often and everywhere they are needed!

Individuals with mild MR frequently acquire basic reading and math skills. They may receive vocational training in semiskilled jobs (e.g., restaurant help staff or grocery shelf stocker). They often have demonstrated needs in the areas of social competence ("fitting in") and in the use of leisure time. Many children with mild retardation become competent in their adult life roles with little or no supervision.

Individuals with moderate retardation may be notably slower in acquiring those basic self-care skills such as toilet training or dressing as toddlers and preschoolers. Social skills needed for success in the school setting are often a "need" area for these children. Ward (1989) suggests that parents' and professionals' greatest assistance to these children may be in fostering appropriate social skills development.

For children with moderate MR, survival skills in the areas of money use, reading at a level adequate for determining safety and community needs, and writing (i.e., legal signature) may be enhanced through interventions. Students exhibiting a moderate degree of MR may not be academically successful beyond the second-grade level, but may work in the community with training (*DSM-IV*, 1994). These people usually need some support or supervision. Adolescents with moderate levels of MR may be seen working in a school cafeteria or bagging groceries with supervision at a local market. "Job coaching," a form of graded work supervision, has become more prevalent with this population in work settings.

Three to four percent of the population exhibiting MR is considered severely retarded. Children in this category often need programs focusing on basic self-care and structured work skills and behaviors. Independence in these areas is often a key determinant of the later placement of these individuals outside the home. Group homes that offer supervised living conditions are a placement goal for many students after leaving the home and school settings.

Children diagnosed with profound MR have global developmental deficits and delays in many functional areas. These individuals are essentially dependent on caregivers for all areas of self-care, including feeding, dressing, and toileting. Issues of concern for this population include medical problems arising directly or indirectly from severe CNS impairment. These may include seizures, skin breakdown from immobility, and nutritional issues from poor feeding skills (Crocker & Nelson, 1992). Although this group of children makes up 1 percent of the population with MR, the challenges of providing for these individuals are numerous. Parents and caregivers for this population need respite from the physical care demands, support groups for social and emotional assistance, and concrete information regarding resources and services (Syzmanski & Kaplan, 1991).

## EVALUATION: ASSESSING NEEDS AND DETERMINING STRENGTHS

The evaluation process may be initiated via a screening tool used at a local developmental center or at a public health setting in the local community. Screening tools are used to identify initial "red flag" areas that warrant additional testing. The *Denver-II* (Frankenburg, Dodds, Archer et al., 1990) is a restandardized version of the *Denver Developmental Screening Test (DDST)* (Frankenburg et al., 1975), one of the oldest and best known of developmental screenings (Glascoe, Byrne, Ashford, Johnson, Chang, & Strickland, 1992). This screening tool is used by pediatricians, public health nurses, preschool staff, and other developmental specialists to identify young children (birth to 6 years) whose development is "not on the norm" with peers. The *DDST* may have a tendency to underrefer children with needs; the *Denver-II* has been found to do just the opposite, tending to overrefer from the normal population (Glascoe et al., 1992; Greer, Bauchner, & Zuckerman, 1989). The *Miller Assessment for Preschoolers* (MAP) (Miller, 1982) was designed by Dr. Lucy Miller (an OT) to identify children who may have mild to moderate developmental delays. It can be used with children from 2 years, 9 months to 5 years, 8 months. It is also classified as a screening test, but does provide a format that gives an evaluator more information (Stowers & Huber, 1987).

Assessment tools frequently used include measures of intelligence (IQ tests) such as the *Wechsler Intelligence Scales for Children, Revised (WISC-R)* (Wechsler, 1974) and the *Kaufman Assessment Battery for Children (KABC)* (Kaufman & Kaufman, 1983). These tests are usually administered by licensed psychologists on the assessment team. They yield information regarding intelligence. (The *KABC* also provides achievement information [Shea, Towle, & Gordon, 1987]). As a therapist, one can often glean pertinent information from cognitive testing by talking with the team psychologists regarding a child's performance on these tests.

## ▮▮▮ FROM THE BOOKSHELF

*A Therapist's Guide to Pediatric Assessment* (King-Thomas & Hacker, 1987) is an excellent resource for one's professional library. It provides pediatric test information, discusses the testing process, and includes valuable reviews of materials used across pediatric disciplines.

Measures of adaptive behaviors are frequently used in assessing children suspected of having cognitive delays. These measures help to provide a picture of the child's patterns of functioning on a daily basis. The *Vineland Adaptive Behavior Scales* (Sparrow, Balla, & Cicchetti, 1984) are widely used in determining independence levels for youth in the domains of communication, daily living skills, socialization, and motor skills. These scales are useful across a wide age range (birth through 18 years) and use a semistructured interview format for eliciting information. OTs as well as social workers, psychologists, and other professionals may use this tool for evaluation purposes with appropriate training and a background in developmental disabilities.

The variety of professionals using the assessment tools noted above suggests that the evaluation process for MR spans multiple disciplines. A team or collaborative approach to this task is beneficial to the child involved in the process. This teaming allows for a sharing of information, helps to avoid redundancy in testing, and presents a more global picture of the child for those involved in interventions. As the complexity of a child's situation increases (e.g., the child with MR is also deaf), assessment challenges increase and workable plans take many professionals' integrated input.

Like the evaluation process, the intervention process is likely to be interdisciplinary. Because MR has lifetime implications, children with this diagnosis have chronic long-term needs to be met. Community-based early intervention programs frequently see these children first. Transitioning to a school program may be the first of many life-span issues to be dealt with by parents, children, and the professional team helping them. Later intervention needs may concern social skills as teenagers, job and work behaviors for leaving school, and appropriate skills for independent or group home living. MR is a complex issue and varies greatly from person to person (Szymanski & Kaplan, 1991). Interventions from all disciplines that are holistic, family- and child-centered, and well-integrated will be most likely to have the greatest positive impact.

## INTERVENTION FROM AN OCCUPATIONAL THERAPY PERSPECTIVE

OTs may be involved with issues related to MR for numerous years of a child's life. Assessment needs and procedures change as the child and family deal with new life transitions. Early assessment and follow-up interventions may focus on gross motor and hand skills. For example, a child with Down syndrome may have delayed acquisition of the pincer grasp and low muscle tone, resulting in poor sitting skills and hand function for finger feeding.

As the child enters "formal school" academics, school-related daily living tasks and social demands change. An OT in this setting might assist a child with skills needed for successful "survival" in the classroom. For example, the new first-grader with Down syndrome may lack the finger strength to unzip his or her backpack. The therapist provides fine motor interventions for the child to enhance "backpack management" and also looks at other components of this task, such as organization of the pack, skills needed for other fasteners on the pack, and the body scheme demands for donning and doffing this ever important school day accessory!

A classroom teacher for children with moderate MR may request an OT consultation to help develop new "workshop" activities focused on job skills with fine motor components. Community outings often benefit from OT input: barrier assessments for local restaurants, education of others in the community, and research of local activities may all come under the OT intervention umbrella.

As adolescents with MR look toward leaving the school system, realistic future planning needs to be accomplished. Here OT input regarding an individual's self-care skills, work behaviors, and socialization helps to determine appropriate living and working placement following exit from the school setting.

---

■ *THERAPEDS POINTER*

Each child with MR will come with varied strengths and needs to be assessed. In devising an assessment plan it will be necessary to look at the child's day and collect information regarding those areas in which a child must function throughout the 24 hours. Age, disability, and the environment may factor into the assessment process. The tasks to consider below may help one to make a mental or actual checklist of areas to be considered:

| | |
|---|---|
| ___ Wake and sleep patterns | ___ Dressing skills |
| ___ Play/leisure skills | ___ School-related skills |
| ___ Social skills | ___ Personal care/toileting skills |
| ___ Mobility skills | ___ Feeding/eating skills |
| ___ Work/vocational readiness | ___ Foundation areas: reflexes, balance, strength, ROM, sensory/perceptual status |

Programming for children with MR is based on the information received from evaluation. A therapist plans intervention to teach a skill, remediate for a need area, or compensate for a deficit. OTs and their strategies may be as varied as the children and adolescents with whom they work. The suggestions below look at the child, the parent or caregiver, and the environment (setting and/or system).

---

## The Child

In working with the child with MR, independence in self-care and competency in social skills are important for the "normalization" process. It is also important to factor in the amount of time it may take one to learn a new skill with deficits in cognition. The process many times is doable, but the pace is slow.

| Situation/Issue | Seen as | In | Possible Solution |
|---|---|---|---|
| Child with Down syndrome has poor trunk stability because of low muscle tone | Poor sitting in preschool chairs; he "melts" into the table | Classroom | 1. Trial of direct treatment for increasing proprioceptive input<br>2. Adapt chair to provide more outside support (i.e., footrest, arm supports) |
| Student with moderate MR is nonverbal but has good hand skills | Possible candidate for sign language | School and social settings | 1. Consult with speech therapist regarding hand skills for sign language<br>2. Demonstrate sign language patterns to student and assess her skill<br>3. Share assessment results with speech therapist to integrate into sign language program in class |
| 12-year-old child with profound MR has multiple sensory and motor deficits | "Problem feeder" because of length of time needed to feed snack | After-school respite program | 1. Observe feeding process for positioning, feeder skills, feeding process<br>2. Consider nutrition consultation<br>3. Share results with respite staff<br>4. Do a feeding demonstration |

## The Parent

Parents of children with MR come with a variety of skills, needs, and coping strategies. As with many chronic-care situations, the severity of the situation, internal and external supports, and the availability of community resources impact on a parent or caregiver's role. Transitions may be crises or challenges depending on the resources for parents dealing with these changes with their children.

| Situation/Challenge | Parent Need/Concern | Possible Solution |
|---|---|---|
| 9-year-old with mild MR seeks afterschool activity and friends | Parent anxiety re child's ability to keep pace with peers and "have friends" | 1. Consult with parent re local activities such as scouts, recreation programs<br>2. Ask for child's input on interests<br>3. Encourage "play dates" at house with school peer |
| 11-year-old girl with moderate MR is reaching puberty | Parent concern regarding sexuality issue and menstrual period | 1. Research available printed materials on topic<br>2. Offer, in conjunction with |

| Situation/Challenge | Parent Need/Concern | Possible Solution |
| --- | --- | --- |
| | | nurse, informal "brainstorming" session for parents<br>3. Assist parent, staff, and student with these self-care needs |

## ▉▉ FROM THE BOOKSHELF

Josh Greenfeld in *A Child Called Noah* (1972) captures the essence of one family's life growing up together with a child who is severely brain damaged. His use of a diary format allows one to see a father's reflections on the search for answers for his child in the late 1960s and early 1970s. Great insights!

## *The Environment*

Children with MR have been moved through various systems, for example, the schools, mental health systems, and community programs, in many ways in the past. Changing the system from the self-contained classrooms to the inclusion models seen today has taken planning, vision, and flexibility from many of those involved with the environment. Several examples of OT input for "systems change" follow.

| Situation/ Characteristic | Environmental/ System Impact | Possible Solution |
| --- | --- | --- |
| Students who are nonverbal with MR ride rural bus route each day | Transportation manager is concerned for safety of children regarding their needs if an accident occurs or a child doesn't get off bus at correct stop | OT with special education staff consider systems for accessing information on each child including 1) an information file box on bus; 2) "rider license": ID-type card for each child to wear; 3) mobile phone access for bus driver to get assistance |
| A child with profound MR and multiple disabilities is at serious risk for "coding" (cardiac arrest) in school | Systems that are not medically based, e.g., schools, have a great need for education re medically fragile children, many of whom are profoundly retarded (therapists and school nurses are frequently the only people with *any* medical background in this setting) | 1. Develop good professional relations with local doctors working with these children.<br>2. Help the system to access the needed medical information to reduce the anxiety level of the staff (this needs to have parent consent).<br>3. Encourage the system to develop procedures for dealing with specific medical emergencies. |

## MENTAL RETARDATION: WRAPPING IT UP

OTs intervene with the mentally retarded over a period of many of their childhood years and within numerous settings. As working members of interdisciplinary teams, OTs have the knowledge of life skills to offer. They also may straddle the medical and community border to provide valuable transition information. OTs also become "advocates through activity" so that persons with MR are viewed for their contributions rather than their differences.

# LEARNING DISORDERS

## THE CLINICAL PICTURE

The term "learning disorders" (LD) has recently been defined in the *DSM-IV* (1994) as a diagnosis where a child's skills as measured by standard achievement tests are "substantially below" ability (as measured by an IQ test). In lay language this means a child is not demonstrating in school tasks what her or his ability suggests she or he is capable of doing. This definition of LD indicates that the difference between skills and ability is the crux of the problem. It is important to note that the difference is intrinsic to the child (Kirk & Kirk, 1983) and not attributed to an external source (e.g., environmental deprivation). These learning difficulties are attributed to CNS dysfunction (Gottsman & Cerullo, 1989; Kirk & Kirk, 1983; Levine, 1990).

The entire issue of LD has been somewhat evolutionary in the literature. "Labels" for the group of children with learning difficulties have changed on a regular basis. The terms "learning disabled," "learning impaired," and "minimally brain dysfunctioned" have all been applied to these children at various times. Although the jargon of the professionals continues to change and be re-examined, the children remain as a heterogeneous group with learning difficulties. These learning disorders impact on children's school successes, their self-esteem, and their social relations with peers and adults. Silver (1991) noted that each child with an LD will have a personal profile of strengths and needs.

Because the definition of "learning disordered" has changed over the past 10 to 15 years, the estimates of children presenting with LDs have also fluctuated. Tucker and colleagues (1983) reported that experts have estimated between 0 and 3 percent of the pediatric population may exhibit LD. Later research (Silver, 1991) suggested that no true numbers regarding prevalence could be given because of the forementioned differences in who belongs to the group at any one time. Diagnosis is frequently made at the age of 6 to 7, which coincides with most children's entrance into the school realm.

Assessments and interventions for children with LD may involve many different professionals' skills. From the medical standpoint, an accurate history, including birth and pregnancy background, a developmental summary, and family information, is needed (Kandt, 1984). During the neurological examination the practitioner may see "soft signs" of CNS disorder. These minor abnormalities may include clumsy gait, poorer finger control than peers, and difficulties in accuracy and speed with fine motor skills.

Educators see many children with LD on a regular basis. It is often these professionals who are the first to informally assess at-risk children and recommend further evaluations. Educational characteristics of children with LD may include: (1) difficulties in specific academic areas; (2) attention problems, including difficulties "tuning in" (selective attention) and "staying tuned in" (seen as distractibility); (3) poor memory for visual and/or auditory input; (4) deficits in the language skills areas; and (5) limited or inflexible problem-solving strategies. In the social skills areas these children often don't "read" the subtle cues in groups and may be impulsive. Peer relations may be hampered by these traits (Levine, 1990; Warren & Taylor, 1984). Problematic friendships may subsequently affect self-esteem. This "vicious circle" may contribute to the high dropout rate among LD students. It has been noted (*DSM-IV*, 1994) that about 40 percent of these students drop out of school.

As noted earlier, teachers are often the persons to refer a child for suspected learning problems. Educators see children whose performance is considered "within normal limits" on a regular basis. They have a good understanding of the wide range of normal skills in children and are often on target with informal assessments of students' needs. Formal assessments for children with LD include ability tests (IQ) as well as achievement tests. The *Wechsler Intelligence Test for Children, Revised* (Wechsler, 1974) (see section on assessment for MR for more information) is often used by a licensed psychologist to test a child's abilities in the verbal and performance areas designated by the test. The results of this testing are compared with achievement testing information. These latter tests may be administered to the child by psychologists, special education staff, or other designated trainer-examiners.

Two of the more commonly used achievement tests are the *Wide Range Achievement Test, Revised* (WRAT) (Jastak & Wilkinson, 1984) and the *Woodcock-Johnson Psycho-Educational Battery* (WJ) (Woodcock, 1977). Both testing tools evaluate a student's skills in the areas of reading, math, and spelling. The WJ provides more complex tasks in the areas of reading comprehension and math skills (Feinstein & Aldershof, 1991). (For the OT, reviewing the writing samples in these tests provides one more piece of information regarding a student's fine motor abilities.)

Information from multiple sources, including parents, school professionals, and the assessment team, provides a profile of strengths and needs from which interventions may be planned for children with LD. Interventions with these children may be complex and multidimensional. Levine (1990) noted the need to identify and use the specific "skill patterns" of children with LD. Others (Carbo & Hodges, 1988) have noted that learning styles for children at risk (which includes LD youth) when accommodated result in improved academic performance and fewer discipline problems.

---

■ *THERAPEDS POINTER*

Learning styles information is based on the idea that not all people learn the same way. Because OTs spend time with children in a "teaching-learning" mode, some knowledge regarding learning styles may be beneficial for one's future practice. Tips from learning styles–based instruction include: (1) learning styles and instruction styles should be matched, (2) checklists for determining learning style can be used for identifying a child's particular learning style (see Carbo & Hodges [1988] for more information), and many at-risk students benefit from tactile and kinesthetic modalities when learning new things. (Now doesn't that sound like an OT talking?)

P.S. Do you know what your learning style is?

---

Educators who work with learning-disordered children often use a remediation-compensation approach to academic instruction. Remedial strategies in the areas of math and writing are often the focus of educators' programs. Compensations for handwriting and memory-strengthening activities may be adjuncts to assistance provided by computer technology. Counselors may also be involved with social skills programs. Wanat (1983) notes that social skills training programs have provided, in some cases, significant improvement in self-concept of children with LD. All of these strategies are focused at creating successes for children in the settings in which they are asked to participate—school, play, and peer groups. OTs, as collaborators with educators, provide adaptations, task analysis, and alternative strategies in these activities to foster student success.

Professionals are frequently well attuned to "finding out what's wrong," but it is also important to look at "what's right" with these children and use their strengths. Finding a hobby that a child with a learning disorder may excel at may be an answer. A structured social activity with peers such as scouting or a "low-key" community gymnastics class may be more rewarding for a child with LD than a sandlot softball game. OTs, with their holistic perspectives on person and function, may provide this important link.

## INTERVENTION FROM AN OCCUPATIONAL THERAPY PERSPECTIVE

### *Assessment*

OTs have training in both the physical and psychological realms of human functioning. Children with LD frequently demonstrate needs in both these areas, which can be assessed by a therapist. Assessment tools such as the *Bruininks-Oseretsky Tests of Motor Proficiency* (*BOTMP*) (Bruininks, 1978); *Quick Neurological Screening Test* (*QNST*) (Mutti, Sterling, & Spalding, 1978); *The Perceptual Motor Assessment for Children* (*P-MAC*) (Dial, McCarron, & Amann, 1988); and the *Sensory Integration and Praxis Tests* (*SIPT*) (Ayres, 1986) provide additional information to team evaluations. These instruments test areas of sensorimotor processing that are the foundations for many school skills. Play histories and observations in a variety of places (i.e., classroom, cafeteria, art class, playground) also provide therapists with information on the daily functioning of these children in the school setting (Dunn & DeGangi, 1992). The American Occupational Therapy Association's *Classroom Applications for School-Based Practice* (Royeen, 1992) provides excellent information for therapists assessing children with LD in the school setting. It provides a wealth of information on both standardized and more informal tools OTs can use to gather information on students with LD.

---

■ *THERAPEDS POINTER*

Sensory integration (SI) refers to a theory developed in the 1960s by Dr. Jean Ayres, an OT and researcher. It is based on the theory that our CNS takes information from the outside world, organizes it, and uses it to produce useful responses directed toward specific goals. How incoming sensory information (i.e., touch, vestibular, proprioceptive ["joint sense"]) is perceived and used determines the "quality" of those specific responses.

At the present time direct interventions with SI procedures may best be used for the clinical setting, where equipment and time factors can be easily adapted. Therapists in school and community settings may find the tenets of SI valuable as they consult with parents and others regarding the behaviors and responses of certain children with LD.

For further information on SI check out "Sensory integration and neurodevelopmental treatment for educational programming" by Winnie Dunn and Georgia DeGangi, in *Classroom Applications for School-Based Practice* from AOTA Self Study Series. This work gives practical suggestions for using SI theory in functional outcome-based settings. Both assessment information and theory explanation are offered.

---

Reviewing the tests of other disciplines provides evaluation information and may also prevent redundant testing. For example, the visual-perceptual tests are often used by psychologists and educators in their work. A therapist's test choice in this area may complement information already obtained by other professionals. Interviewing the child regarding likes and dislikes in school and play activities is often enlightening (and candid!) and adds an additional piece to the "assessment puzzle."

---

■ *THERAPEDS POINTER*

Many professionals use paper-and-pencil tests of visual motor integration. Psychologists, educators, and OTs are all users of these tests, such as the *Test of Visual Motor Integration* (*VMI*) (Beery & Buktenica, 1967) and *The Test of Visual Motor Skills* (*TVMS*) (Gardner, 1986). Removing the motor component of the testing by using a motor-free test such as the *Motor Free Visual Perception Test* (*MVPT*) (Colarusso & Hammill, 1972) is often helpful. This assists in sorting the fine motor from the visual-perceptual components of a problem area such as handwriting.

---

Once this assessment puzzle has been put together, the picture of the child with LD should become clearer. Strategies for assisting the child include collaborative (team) approaches, practical adaptations, and direct interventions when needed. The child, the parents, and the setting may all be changed or become "change agents" in this process. The examples below are only the springboard for problem solving with LD students.

## *Interventions*

**The child.** School is the work of childhood and when work is hard or boring or stressful, life is tough! Children with LD need strategies to help them feel more competent about their work. The following interventions can be applied in a variety of settings.

| Student Characteristic | Seen as | In This Setting | Possible Solution or Strategy |
|---|---|---|---|
| 9-year-old boy with LD doesn't "work" in art class | Lazy student by the art teacher | Art class | Since the child does not have "flexible strategies," creative efforts are difficult. The OT:<br>1. Tries direct services focused on shape drawing and illustration.<br>2. Meets with art teacher to brainstorm possible projects using child's present skills level.<br>3. Provides child with copy of *The Anti-Coloring Book* (see From the Bookshelf following) for home practice. |
| Fifth-grade student has not demonstrated needed handwriting quality or skills in either print or cursive writing | Unable to complete schoolwork | Social studies class | 1. Determine with child which format (print or cursive) works best for speed for classwork.<br>2. Use only chosen format for guided practice for 4–6 weeks.<br>3. Consider word processing alternatives. |

## FROM THE BOOKSHELF

*The Anti-Coloring Book* (Striker & Kimmel, 1984) series holds lot of therapeutic potential. These paperback coloring-type books provide a framework for a child's illustration with some cues as to what to draw. They have more illustration demands than a printed coloring book but are less intimidating than a blank page of paper for the "reluctant artist."

**The parent or caregiver.** Adults who love, work with, and care for youth with LD are at times frustrated, perplexed, and amazed with these children. (Sometimes all of these feelings happen at the same time!) Concrete, practical strategies for succeeding in daily life often are the most well received by these adults.

| Child Characteristic | Adult or Parent Issue | Possible Strategy or Solution |
|---|---|---|
| 7-year-old dawdles with morning routine | "Mornings are crazy— we're all late because of . . . " | 1. Suggest prompts be given verbally and with visual cues (call the child's name *and* stand in the doorway of the bedroom). 2. Lay out clothes the child can manage the night before (dressing skills may be problematic). 3. Consider use of checklist with reward for timely completion of tasks. |
| 11-year-old "gifted" LD student never turns in work— it's "lost" | Teacher gives student failing grade because of lack of completed assignments | 1. Talk with teacher about additional organizational strategies to use with the child. For example, a separate "in" box for child's papers. 2. Present organizational strategies for all students in a workshop format; include "how to's" for assignment book use, calendars, and binder organization. |
| Group of fourth-grade students with LD need additional practice in fine motor skills | Teachers request ideas for combining fine motor skills and academics. | 1. Hold a "make it–take it" session for teachers to design or fabricate folder games using both areas. 2. Provide additional ideas from OT perspective during the informal session. |

■ *THERAPEDS POINTER*

Teachers are great "hands-on" people and enjoy new ideas for their classes. Set up a "make it–take it" session after school or during an in-service day. Provide the materials to make several games that combine OT goals with classroom goals. For example, second-grade teachers may need ideas to increase spelling practice, and you as the OT would like to see alternatives to written lists offered for spelling practice. Combination strategies might include: (1) packets with Wikki Stiks (Omnicor, Inc., Phoenix, AZ [602–870–9937]) and paper squares; the Wikki Stiks can be used in forming letters of words, then (2) use the paper and a crayon to do "rubbings" of the words for individual spelling sheets. (*Note:* Wikki Stiks are colored, wax-covered strings that resemble pipecleaners. They can be cut, folded, braided, and twisted into letters, shapes, and numerals. Check a good local toy story for your supply.)

The opportunities here are endless. With the coffeepot going and some good colleague collaboration everyone will go home happy!

---

**The environment.** Children with LD are frequently challenged by their environment. Because many have problems with focused attention and distractibility, sensory overload may be an issue in one setting. In another, more structured place with fewer distractors, work may be completed with no problems at all. Adapting the environment both via setting changes and materials alterations may prove to be beneficial.

| Environmental Issue | Outcome or Result | Possible Strategies |
|---|---|---|
| "Arty" fourth-grade teacher has classroom that is a visual collage. | Distractible 10-year-old with LD is on "visual overload." | 1. Educate teacher re sensory overload for LD child; suggest visually "quiet" area for child's desk. 2. Provide a "carrel" type desk for child to reduce visual distractors and help with focusing. |
| Reading workbooks issued to third-grader with LD do not accommodate child's large printing. | Child's work is difficult to read because of crowding and answers are incomplete because the child runs out of room on the lines provided. | 1. Have child write answers on a separate sheet of paper. 2. Use enlarger on photocopy machine to enlarge entire workbook pages (check with publisher to get permission for doing this!) |

## LEARNING DISORDERS: WRAPPING IT UP

Children with LD are an interesting blend of "strengths and needs." The "soft signs" of neurological dysfunction often make for "hard times" in the school of life for these children. Subtle fine motor problems, difficulties with attention to task, and deficits in social competence make successful progress in childhood tasks challenging for these students. OTs with their diversified training can make valuable contributions to the often complex interventions process. Using one's knowledge of the sensory system, focusing on task analysis of skills for children with LD, and collaborating with others for a "systems" approach to problem solving may be key in intervening with this population.

**A step beyond.** Poll your colleagues as to their estimates of the time it takes to feed a severely disabled child a lunch-type meal (drink, meat, vegetable). All feeding is done by staff personnel. Then interview the staff at a program servicing these children (or parents) to check your estimates.

---

### CASE STORY

Chris is an 8-year-old student with profound mental retardation and multiple sensory and motor deficits. He is nonambulatory and dependent on others for all of his self-care needs. He is enrolled in self-contained classroom and receives several therapy services. As his OT you have been working with the staff on oral feeding skills. Concerns have been raised regarding Chris's need to gain weight. Despite the introduction of additional snacks and more calorie-dense meals, Chris has a documented weight loss over the past 5 months. The length of time it takes to feed him at meals in the classroom and at home has also reportedly increased. Parents and caregivers attribute this to frequent gagging episodes and the apparent increased effort Chris must expend to eat orally.

At Chris's annual checkup at the medical center developmental clinic, the need for a gastrostomy tube (a type of feeding tube) has been brought up. A gastrostomy tube is placed into the abdominal wall during a surgical procedure. It allows for artificial feeding. The tube feeding will allow Chris to grow and develop better, according to his medical team.

This is a new situation for you as an OT and you need more information. You generate a list of questions and set out to get some answers. The questions are:

1. What does a gastrostomy tube do and how does it work?
2. Does a child get both oral and tube feedings? Who decides this?
3. What exactly goes into the tube to feed the child?
4. Who will educate the staff at the school when Chris returns from surgery and how will this procedure be taught to the school staff?

The following is a "search and find out" activity from real life. Team up with your peers to interview an OT who works with children who are tube fed. A dietitian with pediatric experience may be a valuable resource for this question, too.

An excellent resource to get you started is *Feeding and Nutrition for the Child with Special Needs* by Marcia Dunn Klein and Tracey Delaney (published by Therapy Skill Builders, 1994). This complete notebook has a wealth of information on feeding for professionals and parents alike.

---

## Real-Life Lab

**1.** As a school therapist you have evaluated a fourth-grade student with a learning disorder. Because of his labored handwriting efforts and the illegible quality of his written work, you recommend a word processing program for the classroom computer. *Note:* The student you have assessed has some visual tracking problems and may benefit from large type, too.

To assist his regular classroom teacher you have offered to preview and research three different programs for the school to consider for purchase. The program should be usable for regular education students in the class also.

**a.** Locate catalogs for software vendors for children. (A local computer store may help you or the librarian at a school fieldwork site may have some information. Most vendors also have toll-free numbers so you can call for information.)

**b.** In the section on word processing software in the catalog, check to see (1) what type of computer the software is made for, (2) whether the type (font) size can be changed, and (3) whether the software is "kid friendly" (i.e., picture directions or easy reading directions).

**c.** After you have located several choices you think would work, complete the accompanying chart. The first line has been filled in with a fictitious choice to clarify this task. (Your answers should be *real*, not fiction!)

| Software Name | Source | Cost | Pros (+) | Cons(−) |
|---|---|---|---|---|
| 1. Kids' Writing Company | Adventures in Computing | $24.99 | + Low cost<br>+ Picture cues with directions<br>+ 3 styles of letters in type | − Only for Macs<br>− No spell checker in program<br>− Requires laser printer |
| 2. | | | | |
| 3. | | | | |

**2.** A local sheltered workshop has contracted your services (25 hours) to help them design a class for their new employees on social behaviors on the job. (New employees are high school age, 17–19.] The majority of the employees have moderate degrees of mental retardation, are ambulatory, and are essentially independent in all self-care areas. In the past this sheltered workshop has placed employees in a local greenhouse caring for plants, in a fast-food restaurant on the cleanup team, and in a local video store. The levels of interaction with the public are varied and newly placed employees are initially in supported work positions. (Supported work indicates the new employees will have "coaches" and other adaptations to help them in the workplace initially; this assistance is reduced as employees become proficient at their jobs.) List three or four tasks you would need to accomplish to start your plan of action. Some of the spaces have been filled in to help you get started. (*Hint:* You have not been to the workshop site yet.)

| Action Plan | | | |
|---|---|---|---|
| **To Do** | **To Ask** | **To See** | **To Check Out** |
| *Visit past job sites and observe workers (what info will this give you?) | *Is there a need for practice in travel etiquette on bus, or is other transportation used? | * | * |
| | | * | |
| | | | * |
| * | | * | * |
| * | * | | |

# REFERENCES

Ayres, A. J. (1986). *Sensory integration and praxis tests.* Los Angeles: Western Psychological Services.

Beery, K., & Buktenica, N. A. (1967). *The Beery-Buktenica test of visual motor-integration.* Cleveland: Modern Curriculum Press.

Bruininks, R. H. (1978). *The Bruininks-Oseretsky test of motor proficiency.* Circle Pines, MN: American Guidance Service.

Carbo, M., & Hodges, H. (1988). Learning styles strategies can help students at risk. *Teaching Exceptional Children.* Summer 55–58.

Colarusso, R. P., & Hammill, D. D. (1972). *Motor free visual perception test.* Novato, CA: Academic Therapy Publications.

Crnic, K. A., & Reid, M. (1989). Mental retardation. In E. J. Marsh & R. A. Barkley (Eds.). *Treatment of childhood disorders.* (pp. 247–285). New York: The Guilford Press.

Crocker, A., & Nelson, R. P. (1992). Mental retardation. In M. D. Levine, W. B. Carey, & A. C. Crocker (Eds.). *Developmental-behavioral pediatrics* (2d ed.) (pp. 500–509). Philadelphia: W. B. Saunders.

*Diagnostic and statistical manual of mental disorders (DSM-IV).* (1994). Washington, DC: American Psychiatric Association.

Dial, J. G., McCarron, L., & Amann, G. (1988). *The perceptual-motor assessment for children.* Dallas: McCarron-Dial Systems.

Dunn, W., & DeGangi, G. (1992). Sensory integration and neurodevelopmental treatment for educational programming. In C. B. Royeen (Ed.), *AOTA self study series: Classroom applications for school-based practice* (pp. 1–72). Rockville, MD: American Occupational Therapy Association.

Feinstein, C., & Aldershof, A. (1991). Developmental disorders of language and learning. In J. M. Wiener (Ed.). *Textbook of child and adolescent psychiatry* (pp. 206–220). Washington, DC: American Psychiatric Press.

Frankenburg, W. K., Dodds, J., Archer, P., et al. (1990). *The Denver II: Technical manual.* Denver: Denver Developmental Materials.

Frankenburg, W. K., Dodds, J. B., Fandal, A. W., Kazuk, E., & Cohrs, M. (1975). *The Denver developmental screening test.* Denver: Denver Developmental Materials Inc.

Gardner, M. F. (1986). *TVMS: Test of visual motor skills.* San Francisco: Children's Hospital of San Francisco.

Glascoe, F. P., Byrne, K. E., Ashford, L. G., Johnson, K. L., Chang, B., & Strickland, B.

(1992). Accuracy of the Denver-II in developmental screening. *Pediatrics, 89,* 1221–1225.

Gottsman, R. L., & Cerullo, F. M. (1989). The development and preliminary evaluation of a screening test to detect school learning problems. *Journal of Developmental and Behavioral Pediatrics, 10* (2), 68–74.

Greenfeld, J. (1972). *A child called Noah: A family journey.* New York: Harcourt Brace Jovanovich.

Greer, S., Bauchner, H., & Zuckerman, B. (1989). The Denver developmental screening test: How good is its predictive validity? *Developmental Medicine and Child Neurology, 31,* 774–781.

Jastak, S., & Wilkinson, G. S. (1984). *Wide range achievement test—Revised.* Wilmington, DE: Jastak Associates.

Kandt, R. S. (1984). Neurological examination of children with learning disorders. *Pediatric Clinics of North America, 31* (2), 297–315.

Kaufman, A. S., & Kaufman, N. L. (1983). *Kaufman assessment battery for children.* Circle Pines, MN: American Guidance Service.

King-Thomas, L., & Hacker, B. (Eds.) (1987). *A therapist's guide to pediatric assessment* Boston: Little, Brown.

Kirk, S. A., & Kirk, W. D. (1983). On defining learning disabilities. *Journal of Learning Disabilities, 6* (1), 20–21.

Klein, M. D., & Delaney, T. A. (1994). *Feeding and nutrition for the child with special needs.* Tucson, AZ: Therapy Skill Builders.

Levine, M. (1990). Learning disorders. In J. A. Stockman (Ed.). *Difficult diagnosis in pediatrics* (pp. 41–48). Philadelphia: W. B. Saunders.

Menkes, J. (1995). *Textbook of child neurology* (5th ed.). Baltimore: Williams & Wilkins.

Miller, L. (1982). *Miller assessment for preschoolers.* Englewood, CO: The Foundation for Knowledge in Development.

Mutti, M., Sterling, H. M., & Spalding, N. V. (1978). *Quick neurological screening test* (rev. ed.). Los Angeles: Western Psychological Services.

*New illustrated Webster's dictionary of the English language* (1992). New York: PMC Publishing.

Pulsifer, M. B., Hoon, A. H., Palmer, F. B., Gopalan, R., & Capute, A. J. (1994). Maternal estimates of developmental age in preschool children. *Journal of Pediatrics, 125* (1), 18–24.

Rothenberg, M. A., & Chapman, C. F. (1994). *Dictionary of medical terms for the nonmedical person* (3rd ed.). Hauppauge, NY: Barron's Educational Series.

Royeen, C. B. (Ed.). (1992). *AOTA self study series: Classroom applications for school based practice.* Rockville, MD: American Occupational Therapy Association.

Rubin, I. L. (1989). Management of children and adults with severe and profound central nervous system dysfunction. In I. L. Rubin & A. C. Crocker (Eds.). *Developmental disabilities: Delivery of medical care for children and adults* (pp. 390–397). Philadelphia: Lea & Febiger.

Runyon, D. (1993). Fragile X syndrome. In S. W. Ekvall (Ed.). *Pediatric nutrition in chronic diseases and developmental disorders: Prevention, assessment, and treatment.* New York: Oxford University Press.

Shea, V., Towle, P. O., & Gordon, B. N. (1987). Psychological and cognitive tests. In L. King-Thomas & B. J. Hacker (Eds.). *A therapist's guide to pediatric assessment* (pp. 287–332). Boston: Little, Brown.

Silver, L.B. (1991). Developmental learning disorders. In M. Lewis (Ed.). *Child and adolescent psychiatry: A comprehensive textbook* (pp. 522–528). Baltimore: Williams & Wilkins.

Sparrow, S. S., Balla, D. A., & Cicchetti, D. V. (1984). *Vineland adaptive behavior scales.* Circle Pines, MN: American Guidance Service.

Stowers, S., & Huber, C. J. (1987). Developmental and screening tests. In L. King-Thomas & B. J. Hacker (Eds.). *A therapist's guide to pediatric assessment* (pp. 43–142). Boston: Little, Brown.

Striker, S. G., & Kimmel, E. (1984). *The anti-coloring book.* New York: Henry Holt.

Szymanski, L. S., & Kaplan, L. C. (1991). Mental retardation. In J. M. Wiener (Ed.). *Textbook of child and adolescent psychiatry* (pp. 143–168). Washington, DC: American Psychiatric Press.

Tucker, J., Stevens, L., & Ysseldyke, J. E. (1983). Learning disabilities: The experts speak out. *Journal of Learning Disabilities, 16,* 6–14.

Wanat, P. E. (1983) Social skills: An awareness program with learning disabled adolescents. *Journal of Learning Disabilities, 16,* 35–38.

Ward, J. D. (1989). Mental retardation. In M. K. Logigian & J. D. Ward (Eds.). *A* team approach for therapists: *Pediatric rehabilitation* (pp. 63–81). Boston: Little, Brown.

Warren, S. A., & Taylor, R. L. (1984). Education of children with learning problems. *Pediatric Clinics of North America, 31* (2), 331–343.

Wechsler, D. (1974). *The Wechsler Intelligence Scale for Children—Revised.* San Antonio: The Psychological Corporation.

Woodcock, R. W. (1977). *Woodcock Johnson psycho-educational battery: Technical report.* Allen, TX: DLM Teaching Resources.

Wunderlich, R. C. (1970). *Kids, brains, and learning.* St. Petersburg, FL: Johnny Reads.

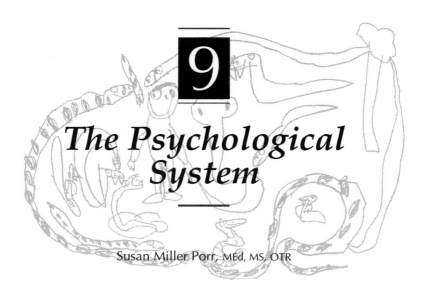

# 9

# The Psychological System

Susan Miller Porr, MEd, MS, OTR

*If the human mind was simple enough to understand, we'd be too simple to understand it.*

—Emerson Pugh

**KEY POINTS**

- Deficits in the psychological system, while invisible to the viewer, often impact globally on the child and his or her world.
- There are frequently overlapping diagnoses within this area with children having more than one psychosocial diagnosis.
- Having a diagnosis in one area of the psychosocial realm may predispose a child toward another diagnosis, e.g., children with ADHD may be more likely than their peers to become depressed.
- OTs have historically been involved with patients who exhibit psychosocial dysfunction. Action and activity-oriented treatments have long been used for remediation with this population.

# BEGINNINGS

This chapter will overview selected key diagnoses in the psychosocial area seen by pediatric OTs. Included will be information regarding children with attention deficit disorder; pervasive development disorder in its various forms, and emotional handicaps, highlighting depression, conduct disorder, and defiant behavior.

Occupational therapy intervention with children who have psychosocial needs is multifaceted. After understanding the clinical aspects of the disorder, disease, or syndrome, the therapist is involved with the assessment of the child and the numerous situations composing that child's world. Intervention often includes the family, the play and school settings, and input from multiple professionals involved with a particular child's case. To function at one's personal optimal level within the demands of the setting is a continual challenge for children with psychosocial dysfunction.

# ATTENTION DEFICIT DISORDER

## THE CLINICAL PICTURE

Attentional disorders (ADs) have become some of the most commonly encountered biopsychological diagnoses in the pediatric population today (Reiff, Banez, & Culbert, 1993; Leung, Robson, Fagan, & Lim, 1994). Children who present with AD are most often described as inattentive and impulsive. Although "being hyper" in a motoric sense is frequently associated with AD, it has been recognized that not all children demonstrate this characteristic. The *Diagnostic and Statistical Manual of Mental Disorders,* 4th edition (*DSM-IV*) (1994) formally names this set of characteristics attention deficit hyperactivity disorder (ADHD), but differentiates between the subset of children who have excess motor activity and those who mainly demonstrate inattentiveness and impulsivity.

Children with AD come in all shapes and sizes and from all kinds of backgrounds. Although males tend to populate the ranks of AD—the ratio is 6:1—characteristic behaviors tend not to be sex-biased. Parents of children with AD often report "he was a fussy infant who cried all the time" or "she only ate her baby food lukewarm." Being highly sensitive to changes in sensory input is often associated with children who demonstrate AD later in life (Kaplan, Sadlock, & Grebb, 1994). In contrast, some children with AD may be very competent in a structured setting such as school but may have more difficulty with free play or more open situations involving new situations and transitions (e.g., the neighbor's birthday party at the local pizza parlor).

As these children move into the preschool years, they may be notably more active than their peers and have difficulty staying seated for short circle time activities. Teachers may note that the child never completes an activity center in the classroom, and there's often an empty work folder to prove it.

In the elementary grades one may see a more observable difference between the children exhibiting AD without hyperactivity and those who are more motorically active. Those children exhibiting the hyperactive component of AD may be noisier, more aggressive, and less mature than their counterparts (Reiff et al., 1993). Conversely, children with AD but without hyperactivity may be seen as unmotivated and slower to process academic materials than their class mates. These children, because they do not cause classroom disruptions, are often diagnosed later in their school career. This may put them at greater risk for low self-esteem and poor peer interactions, both recognized problems that may accompany an ADHD diagnosis (Leung et al., 1994).

It was thought at one time that children "outgrew" their attention deficits and the accompanying hyperactivity. It is now recognized that ADHD may be chronic and lifelong. Varying sources report percentages of cases ranging from 15 to 20 percent to 50 to 70 percent persisting into adulthood (Kaplan et al., 1994). These adults appear to be at higher risk for divorce and substance abuse than their peers.

The diagnosis of AD in the pediatric population has been widely recognized. *Why* it exists is still a medical mystery. Although the exact etiology (cause) is not known, genetic factors, prenatal trauma, exposure to toxins, and neurotransmitter abnormalities have all been cited as possible contributing factors (Kaplan et al., 1994; Leung et al., 1994; Reiff et al., 1993).

Both the diagnosis and treatment of children with AD are multidisciplinary in nature. Diagnosis includes a developmental history and medical evaluation to rule out other health problems (i.e., visual, metabolic, or neurologically related). Psychological or psychiatric evaluation may be done to determine the mental health status of the child. Social evaluations help to assess the strengths and needs of the family unit. Interviews and observations of the child across settings also become valuable diagnostic tools, as the behavior of children with AD frequently fluctuates from place to place. One tool that can be used across disciplines is a behavior checklist. These checklists are often a good starting point for assessing a child's capabilities with age-expected or age-appropriate behaviors (Rudel, 1988). The Achenbach and Conners rating scales are two of the checklists more commonly used with the ADHD population (Achenbach & Edelbrock, 1983; Conners, 1969).

---

■ *THERAPEDS POINTER*

The Achenbach and Conners rating scales are paper-and-pencil scales administered by a person observing a child. Both have separate formats for use with a parent and with a teacher. Rating scales are reported to be less biased than self-reports. They can also be used with children who are unable to report themselves (because of a language or cognitive deficit). Evaluators have noted that the major drawback of rating scales is a possibly subjective viewpoint from the rater (i.e., Johnny's parent or the third-grade teacher). It should be noted, though, that raters such as teachers see normal behavior on a daily basis and frequently accurately perceive what's within normal limits and what is not (Martin, Hooper, & Snow, 1986). Table 9–1 compares the two rating scales.

---

Table 9–1 **Comparison of Achenbach and Conners Rating Scales**

| The Basics | Achenbach Child Behavior Checklist | Conners Parent Rating Scale |
|---|---|---|
| Age | 4–16 | 3–17 |
| Rater | Parent or teacher | Parent or teacher forms available |
| Highlights | Quick to give (about 15 min)<br>Looks at bands of behavior<br>118 responses<br>Looks at leisure skills (usable OT evaluation information) | Has list of "problem" behaviors<br>Has 48 items |

Interventions used with children with AD are also multidimensional and should be integrated to provide the standard of care needed for the most successful outcomes. Medical professionals may recommend the use of stimulant drugs, which affect the way specific neurotransmitters interact with the frontal lobe of the brain, which modulates attention and impulsivity (Hancock, 1996). The most commonly used stimulant drugs for treating AD are Ritalin (methylphenidate hydrochloride), Dexedrine (dextroamphetamine sulfate), and Cylert (pemoline).

Educational interventions are used in conjunction with the drug therapy. Many children with AD do better with small, structured classrooms. Assisting children with organization skills and adjusting workloads to attention spans foster school success. Helping these students to become "experts" at something helps to raise their self-esteem and provides them with "positive strokes" they may not receive in other venues.

## INTERVENTIONS FROM THE OCCUPATIONAL THERAPY PERSPECTIVE

OTs often become the liaison members of a team, because they see children with AD across numerous settings. In the assessment stages therapists frequently make a home visit to obtain information from parents or daycare providers. Testing provides information regarding the child's attention span, activity level, and "work" style in a structured one-to-one setting, as well as fine motor skill data. Clinical observations may provide a strength and needs profile of the child in the areas of play, school skills, and activities of daily living (ADL) as he or she functions throughout the typical day.

An OT intervention checklist may include some or all of the following:

1. Interview with the parent and/or childcare person (via telephone or as a home visit).
2. Observations of the child in several settings, preferably one structured (i.e., classroom or daycare activity) and one nonstructured (i.e., recess or outdoor play).
3. Standardized or formal testing in the fine motor area using age-appropriate materials (i.e., *Peabody Developmental Motor Scales* [Folio & Fewell, 1983] or *Bruininks-Oseretsky Tests of Motor Proficiency* [Bruininks, 1978]).
4. Specialized testing in a specific area, such as visual perception or sensory integration (often-used tests of visual perception and visual motor skill include the *Developmental Test of Visual Motor Integration* [Beery & Buktenica, 1967], the *Test of Visual Motor Skills* [Gardner, 1986], and the *Motor Free Visual Perception Test* [Colarusso & Hammill, 1972]; Jean Ayre's *Sensory Integration and Praxis Tests* [1986]) is used for determining deficits in sensory integrative functioning.
5. Task observations of ADLs needed for successful completion of the day. These may include dressing and feeding skills as well as school-related skills (packing a backpack) and/or play-related activities (riding a tricycle, dressing a Barbie doll) depending on the age of child. In these areas, the "how-it-is-done" qualities are as important as the "what-is-done" factors. For children with AD, the

functional skills may be present, but the performance of these skills is erratic, impulsive, or incomplete.

6. Review of pertinent records and materials provided by other disciplines. This activity helps to prevent redundancy in testing, may give insight into why a child performs "your tasks" in a certain way, and encourages integration of information.

7. Other—there will always be an "other" category to allow the therapist to customize assessment procedures for a specific child. Local policy or institutions may also direct the content of this category for the therapist.

After assessment is completed and information has been shared with parents and other appropriate professionals, the intervention planning takes place. Ideally, this is done in an integrated manner with other members. Below are some possible ways OTs may intervene with children who have AD. Techniques and strategies may include direct services to the child, program planning with other professionals, and/or "brainstorming" and consultation with parents and other invested adults. Suggestions below look at the child, the parent, and the environment or the system.

**The child.** In working with children with AD consider how the characteristics of the disorder (impulsivity, inattention, hyperactivity) may affect daily functioning in school, play, and ADL.

| Characteristics | Seen as | In | Possible Solution |
|---|---|---|---|
| Impulsivity | Multiple clothing choices in dressing for school but never complete dressing | Home | Set out clothes prior to event with child's input into choice (this puts parameters on the dressing task) Use a timer to complete dressing routine (to encourage focused activity within a time limit) |
| Hyperactivity | Out-of-seat behavior in preschool circle | School | Provide set boundaries via carpet squares, tape, or "hula hoops" on floor |
| Inattention | Failure to get classroom assignments down for homework | School | Child copies all assignments from the board at beginning of day Copy checked by peer "buddy" prior to end of day |

**The parent.** Parents and care providers for children with AD are frequently asked to carry out large portions of intervention, because they see the child on the most regular basis. It is important to determine what parents feel is the cause of behaviors and how they work with their child. It is not uncommon for parents of children with AD to have negative thoughts regarding their skills and their child's situation (Reiff et al., 1993). Again, the characteristics of the disorder provide a springboard for planning interventions with the parents.

| Characteristics | Seen by Parents as | Possible Solution |
|---|---|---|
| Inattentiveness | "Not paying attention to what I say." | Provide multiple cues when giving directions, i.e., put hand on shoulder and look at child as you say directive. Ask the child to repeat direction that has just been given. |
| Low self-esteem | Lack of enthusiasm about family activities. | Find a new hobby or activity to explore with child where everyone's a novice. Consider child's strengths in choice. |
| Hyperactivity | "He never sleeps and I'm exhausted." | Teach parent sensory "calming" activities to use at bedtime. Address the sleep issue with other medical professionals. |

**The system or environment.** Adapting the environment or changing the system may be one of the least restrictive and most expedient ways a therapist can intervene with a child who demonstrates AD. Many times an adaptation in the system allows for a workable temporary solution, while a more permanent remediation may come with time. For example, a child may be learning "self-talk" strategies to slow down his or her impulsiveness in test-taking settings. Meanwhile the system may provide for one-to-one instruction for tests with coaching of self-talk skills also provided. (Self-talk, or private speech, is the way a child thinks "out loud" as a self-directing mechanism [Berk & Landau, 1995].)

| Characteristics | System or Environmental Impact | Possible Solution (ST = short term, LT = long term) |
|---|---|---|
| Impulsiveness | Unsafe conditions for child on preschool nature walks | ST: Make "hand-holding contract" with child for outside activities LT: Teach child "danger" concepts and "Stop, Look, and Listen" skills |
| Motor coordination problems plus inattention | Handwritten school work is not completed on time | ST: System allows for oral presentations by student LT: Investigate use of computer and motor control program to improve handwriting skills |
| Fine motor problems plus inattention, plus impulsivity | Taking of schoolwide standardized tests is challenging for child | ST: Provide adapted environment for test situation, i.e., small group, separate room as per regulations |

| Characteristics | System or Environmental Impact | Possible Solution (ST = short term, LT = long term) |
|---|---|---|
| | | LT: Work on test-taking skills, i.e., self-talk for pacing, "bubble-dot" test form accuracy to move back to less restricted environment |

## WRAPPING IT UP

OTs have training in both the psychosocial and the physical skills intervention realms. The merging of these areas to promote optimal functioning for children with AD is critical. The biopsychological nature of AD requires intervention in the many areas that make up a child's daily world.

# PERVASIVE DEVELOPMENTAL DISORDERS

The grouping of disorders known as pervasive developmental disorders (PDDs) encompasses the better-known diagnosis of autism as well as the more recently defined entities of Rett syndrome and Asperger syndrome. These early developmental disorders are marked by the global deficits and/or delays seen in the acquisition of appropriate social, communication, and cognitive skills (Tsai & Ghaziuddin, 1991). Although there are overlapping signs and symptoms within the PDD group, the clinical pictures are somewhat different. Autism will be looked at first from the clinical standpoint. Additional clinical information regarding the differing diagnoses of Asperger and Rett syndromes will also be presented. Intervention will focus on the entire group of PDD. (*Note:* The terms *Asperger's syndrome* and *Asperger's disorder* will be found in the literature as well as Asperger syndrome; the same is true for Rett syndrome, where *Rett's syndrome* or *Rett's disorder* is used to mean the same as the above in other texts and articles.)

## AUTISM: THE CLINICAL PICTURE

Autism as a diagnosis was first described by Leo Kanner in 1943. Kanner, a psychiatrist at Johns Hopkins, identified a group of 11 children with a set of similar characteristics. These children seemed to prefer being alone, demonstrated aloofness, and seemed to be obsessed with keeping routines. Early causes for this "morbid self-absorption" were attributed to cold, unfeeling mothers (Minshew & Payton, 1988). The "refrigerator mothers" were purported to have poorly nurtured their infants, causing the autism.

It is recognized now that the etiology of autism is neurobiological in nature. Although no specific cause has been consistently identified in research, genetic factors may be involved and the pathology appears to be at the cellular level in the nervous system (Minshew & Payton, 1988; Tsai & Ghaziuddin, 1991). Seizures often are seen in the population with PDD, a sign of nervous system involvement (Nelson, 1984). The prevalence of autism has been reported to be 2 to 5/10,000 (Elliott, 1996). The male-female ratio of occurrence of autism is reported to be 3 to 4:1.

The child diagnosed with autism will have had an onset of characteristic behaviors prior to the age of 30 months (Tsai & Ghaziuddin, 1991). Often, social issues initially trigger concerns for parents of autistic children. Failing to bond with a mother may occur. The infant with autism gives a parent little "baby" socialization in the form of eye contact, smiles, or other social awareness.

Social deficits and/or deviations may continue to emerge as the child moves into toddlerhood. Unusual attachments to specific toys or objects may occur. These children may not have a people preference, demonstrating an unnatural lack of separation anxiety when left by parents (Kaplan et al., 1994).

As children with autism move into the school years, the social skills deficits continue to set them apart from their peers. These children have problems making friends and maintaining social relationships. They may not demonstrate the accepted level of empathy when a classmate falls or a peer becomes upset. Teenagers with autism may acknowledge the desire for friendships but are socially inept in pursuing goals to that end. Being unable to display the appropriate emotions in the correct social setting is a dilemma that follows these adolescents into adulthood.

In the area of intellectual functioning, the majority of children with autism are mentally retarded. (Seventy percent have an IQ of less than 70. [Kaplan et al., 1994].) Some of these children have "super skills" in specific cognitive areas. Evidence of this "Rainman" talent may be seen as superior musical abilities, spatial skills (e.g., doing difficult puzzles easily), or memorization skills for volumes of minute details.

Communication dysfunction is one of the defining characteristics of autism. This problem encompasses both the verbal and nonverbal areas of communication (Tsai & Ghaziuddin, 1991). Children with autism often do not attend to, much less read, body language, which is critical in many social situations. Their speech may be marked by echolalia, the repetition of particular words or phrases in a stereotypical pattern. The use of language to communicate seems to be meaningless for many children with autism. A child may recite from memory a lengthy poem but have no understanding of the content of his or her recitation. This limited communication repertoire has serious implications for the child in our social verbal world.

Behavioral issues surrounding autism may be manifestations of the clinical picture. Children with autism are often very resistive to change. Alterations in schedules, breakfast foods, or caregivers may cause moodiness or outbursts. Some professionals feel that the response to sensory input is different for children with autism (Kaplan et al., 1994). This may be reflected behaviorally in some cases. For example, a low tolerance for certain sensory information, a loud noise may trigger an emotional outburst beyond what one would expect for the situation. High threshholds for pain may also be manifested as self-injurious behavior like scab picking or head banging.

Children with autism may have scattered strengths in the motor skills area. They may excel at fine motor activities that require spatial skills, i.e., puzzle completion or building blocks. Activities that involve imitation, such as a game of Simon Says, can be the ultimate challenge for an autistic student in a social play setting.

## ▟▌▌ FROM THE BOOKSHELF

Josh Greenfeld's books on his son Noah look at the impact of having a child with a severe disability from a father's perspective. Greenfeld addresses his son's early years with an autistic-type disorder in *A Child Called Noah* (1972) (see Chapter 8). Additional titles include *A Place for Noah* (1989) and *A Client Called Noah* (1989). *Nobody Nowhere* (1992) by Donna Williams is the autobiography of an autistic woman. *Emergence: Labeled Autistic* (1986) by Temple Grandin and M. M. Scariano is a classic in the field of autism. It is a true account of one woman's life with autism. It is a hopeful book, well worth reading.

Autism is a chronic condition with lifelong ramifications. The majority of children with autism will require a supported living situation as adults. New practices such as job coaching in employment and residing in group homes as adults have made functional living a more "normalized" process for this population.

## Rett's Syndrome: The Clinical Picture

Rett's syndrome is the "new kid on the block" of the PDD group. It was initially described by an Austrian doctor, Andreas Rett, in 1966. It received more recognition in the 1980s as a larger pool of patient information was made available. Before then children with Rett's syndrome were classified as autistic.

Rett's syndrome is a progressive degenerative neurological disorder with several signs and symptoms that set it apart from autism. The disease appears to occur exclusively in girls (Holm, 1985). Females with this disease have reportedly normal development through the first 7 to 12 months, whereas in autism the disorder frequently is noted in infancy and prior to 30 months of age. In Rett's syndrome a rapid degeneration of both physical and cognitive skills is seen between the age of onset and about 3 years of age. Classic symptoms include periods of breathholding and hyperventilation, "handwringing" or other stereotypical hand movements, delayed walking, and ataxia.

---

■ *THERAPEDS POINTER*

OTs have been using splints of various types to improve hand function in girls with Rett's syndrome. Elbow splints have been used during feeding to break up stereotypical hand patterns (Sharpe & Ottenbacher, 1990). In another case, dorsal wrist splints helped a young woman with Rett's syndrome to develop more refined hand skills (i.e., active grasp and emerging release, also a pinch pattern) (Kubas, 1992). Although the gains have been variable, they have been in the positive direction. OTs add this splinting contribution to the team as they foster functional hand use in children.

---

Later in childhood a plateau may be reached where fewer degenerative changes are seen. Girls may become more autistic-like in their behavior, and seizures may occur. Adolescence may bring increases in spasticity and the onset of a scoliosis. Walking skills may decrease and girls may become wheelchair-bound. Little information is presently available on adult patients with Rett's syndrome. The majority of females with Rett's syndrome who have been followed have survived into their 40s (Tsai & Ghaziuddin, 1991).

At the present time there is no known cause for Rett's syndrome. Some speculation has been offered regarding genetic mutations or metabolic dysfunction. Because the syndrome is so newly defined, information and research regarding etiology are still sparse. With the identification of new cases and the study of present cases, more background information will become available for medical research.

## ASPERGER SYNDROME: THE CLINICAL PICTURE

Asperger syndrome is a form of PDD that has just recently received its own diagnostic category in the *DSM-IV* (1994). In comparison to other children with PDD, those with Asperger syndrome seem to have fewer language deficits but exhibit qualitative social skills impairments (Elliot, 1996).

The child with Asperger syndrome may have grossly normal language skills on first observation. On closer study one finds deficits in social communication skills, both in the verbal and nonverbal areas. Like other forms of PDD, there is a great interest in stereotypical patterns of behavior in children with Asperger syndrome. Cognitive skills for these children tend to be within normal limits (Elliot, 1996; Nelson, 1984).

Although Asperger syndrome seems to be a milder form of PDD, the social language area is the most dysfunctional. Children with this syndrome have stilted conversational style. Conversational gesturing is minimal or awkward. They do not read social situations well and hence act or react inappropriately. It may appear on the surface that skills are intact, but this is often an inflexible repertoire that is not easily altered by the child if the situation changes. In older children and adults with Asperger syndrome, one may see difficulties with social-emotional relationships and unusual preoccupations (Elliot, 1996).

The specific cause of this syndrome is not yet known. Boys outnumber girls in this diagnostic category, but more cases are needed for research and study. The reported prognosis for children with Asperger syndrome is mixed (Tsai, 1991). Unresolved questions regarding this new category will require more research and larger patient pools for answers.

## INTERVENTIONS FOR PDD

A diagnosis of PDD has a global impact on a child and his or her environment. The intervention approach for each child is individualized. Programming should reflect the assessment information gathered by the professionals working with the child. Interventions include behavioral methods, parent support and counseling, structured educational programming, and in some cases drug therapy (especially for seizure control).

Assessment for children with PDD is an interdisciplinary process. Physicians often serve as a referral source and as the monitors of health status of these children (Schanzenbacher, 1985). Speech and language clinicians focus on the communication needs of this population. Educators, along with therapists, help to determine the strengths and needs in the functional world for children with PDD. The status of social, self-care, and job-related skills for these individuals often determines the focus of future programming (Tsai & Ghaziuddin, 1991). Developmental tests (i.e., the *Peabody Developmental Motor Scales* [Folio & Fewell, 1983]), parent interviews, and structured observations often yield valuable assessment information. There are also several evaluations that have specifically been designed for children with autism that may provide useful information.

---

■ *THERAPEDS POINTER*

*The Psychoeducational Profile* (*PEP*) (Schopler & Reichler, 1979) has been designed for specific use with children with autism. It takes a developmental approach and looks at skills and behaviors in seven different areas, including imitation; perception; fine motor, gross motor, and eye-hand coordination; cognition; and verbal skills. It has been reported (Nelson, 1984) that this assessment provides a profile of the child's regular strengths and weaknesses. Limitations of the *PEP* include a lack of reliable statistics, a decreased reliability when given to children over 6 years of age, and a small normative sample.

---

Strategies used for changing behaviors are frequently in the realm of the psychologist or psychiatrist on an intervention team. Implementation of a behavior management program may be done by all team members working with the child. In some settings there may be an intervention specialist who provides information and training to other team members working with a child with PDD.

The need for support and respite for parents and caregivers of children with PDD cannot be underestimated. Because social deficits and gross communication dysfunctions are traits of PDD, parents get little positive reinforcement for their efforts from their children. The use of a support system or parent group may be a lifeline for a frazzled parent at the end of a long week with a child with PDD. As Nelson (1984) notes, "The fact remains that parents [of children with PDD] must still bear a burden that very few would assume voluntarily" (p. 260).

Table 9–2 **Behavior Common to PDD and Medication as Intervention**

| Behavior | Medication |
| --- | --- |
| Uncontrollable motor activity, continued self-injurious behavior (SIB), persistent assaultive behavior | Antipsychotics, i.e., haloperidol or thioridazine<br>Anticonvulsants (i.e., valproic acid)<br>Lithium |
| Mental age inappropriate hyperactivity and inattention | Stimulants (i.e., methylphenidate)<br>Clonidine |
| Marked sleep disturbances, i.e., refusal to go to sleep, frequent wakenings, waking early | Tricyclic antidepressants |
| Marked anxiety | Tricyclic antidepressants |
| Repetitive, obsessive, or compulsive behaviors | Selective serotonin uptake inhibitors (these drugs change the way the chemical serotonin is used in the body) |
| Seizure disorders | Anticonvulsants |

*Source:* Adapted from Elliot, 1996.

Educational programming provides academic skills, work skills, and self-care skills for many children with PDD. Classrooms tend to be structured to provide predictability for children who often resist transitions. Self-care, basic academics, and fundamental social skills lessons make up many early-learning programs for children with PDD. Community-living skills may be the focus in older grades as students prepare to move into vocational settings beyond the school realm. These community outings also help to determine the social skills needs of children with PDD. Educational programming should be "intensive and sustained" (Tsai & Ghaziuddin, 1991, p. 185).

Medical professionals may often be involved with children with PDD as specific symptoms warrant. Pharmacological treatment for seizures or hyperactivity may be beneficial. The intent of this therapy is to treat the symptom, not "cure" the disorder (Tsai & Ghaziuddin, 1991). Table 9–2 reviews some of the more common behaviors associated with PDD and the medications used to ameliorate them.

Medical follow-up of children with Rett's syndrome is somewhat different from that involved with other cases in the area of PDD. The progressive, degenerative nature of this syndrome makes goal-setting challenging. For example, toilet training for a child with Rett's syndrome may look like a viable goal early on. However, as ambulation and balance deteriorate, the progress toward goal success may be limited because of physical and neurological changes.

## INTERVENTIONS FROM AN OCCUPATIONAL THERAPY PERSPECTIVE

OTs working with children with PDD may use formal assessments such as those mentioned earlier. This formal information is often used in conjunction with structured observations of the child performing daily living activities such as feeding, dressing, and playing. Specialized assessments for visual-perceptual skills, sensory integration, and reflexes may also provide additional information for the assessment profile. Results of the assessment provide the foundation for the child's individualized intervention planning.

The OT, as the activity specialist on the intervention team, has an important role. Being able to analyze a specific task and adapt it for the child with PDD is a critical skill. Knowing about the stereotypical patterns of many children with PDD, the possible aberrations in their sensory processing during tasks, and their lack of social skills for group tasks, all shape the therapist's intervention planning. The following are examples of strategies and techniques that may be used by OTs intervening with children with PDD and their environment.

**The child.** The child with PDD has many obstacles to overcome to fit well into the world. The characteristics of poor communication, ineffective social skills, and poorer use of imitation for learning all provide areas of intervention for OT expertise. The following examples are a potential springboard for problem solving regarding these children.

| Characteristic | Seen as | In | Possible Strategy or Solution |
|---|---|---|---|
| Ineffective social skills | Failure to keep "personal space" | Social conversation | Cue child with signal during talks in class. Use community outings, e.g., McDonald's or post office, to check skills in real world. Practice social greeting (i.e., handshake) upon arrival to class each day. |
| Poor imitation skills | Difficulty in learning new game in class | Physical education (PE) class | Get advance info on class tasks from PE teacher. Practice components in therapy sessions giving manual cues to child. Participate with child in class. |
| Repetitive behavior | Need for child to be verbally cued to take each bite off a fork | Preschool class at snack | Consult with behavior specialist to plan program to "extinguish" behavior |

**The parent.** As has been noted already, parenting a child with PDD is a monumental task because of the lack of positive feedback a parent gets from his or her child. This lack of interaction goes far beyond the isolation of a moody teenager or the tantrums of a "terrible two." Parents of children with PDD may rely on others informally or formally for support. They also become very creative with solutions to practical problems, making them at times a great resource for therapists.

| Characteristic | Seen by Parents as | Possible Strategy |
|---|---|---|
| Lack of creative play or self-initiation in play tasks | Child "self-stimulates" during leisure or downtime at home | Incorporate a leisure skills "training" program into class curriculum. |
| Rigid behavior and sensory issues in dressing | Child will wear only one set or type clothing —"he wears the *same* thing every day!" | Help to determine if the sensory character (i.e., texture) is pleasing factor in garment. Introduce small changes in clothing style or texture. Decide the uniform look is OK. |
| Inappropriate social skills | "We can't take her anywhere—she just doesn't know how to act." | Target where parent would like to take child. Help parents to analyze these places in terms of sensory overload for child with PDD. Incorporate class trips to these places when possible. |

**The environment or system.** The environment impacts on all people daily and they impact on their surroundings. For children with PDD, negotiating this environment is a major life task every day. Their capacity to deal with environmental changes is often behaviorally an extremely stressful task. Sensory input may be interpreted by their systems in entirely different ways. For children and adolescents who inherently are alone in their own world, the environment presents a challenge.

| Characteristic | System or Environmental Impact | Possible Strategy |
|---|---|---|
| Child has heightened auditory awareness. | All noises in surroundings are stressful, especially loud noises. | Provide a "quiet" room for stressful times, possibly with headphones or quiet music. |
| Child does not transition well. | Room is not functionally organized to foster transition. | Organize room into non-cluttered work areas. Provide "map" of work areas in room. Adopt "work check-in" procedure at each area to structure routine. |

## WRAPPING IT UP

Children with PDD require comprehensive programming that demands the combined skills of many team members. OTs, with their functional approaches to life skills and their activity analysis strategies, have much to offer these children. The "best" programs for these children combine parental insights and skills and professional expertise with ongoing questioning regarding "what's the next step? . . . ."

# CHILDREN WITH EMOTIONAL HANDICAPS: SELECTED CASES

Children with emotional handicaps have been seen by occupational therapy professionals over the years. The settings in which these children are seen today have changed. With moves toward deinstitutionalization of mental health patients, these children are in classroom settings, preschool programs, and group home and/or day programs.

The emotional handicaps to be discussed are depression and conduct disorder and defiant behavior. These are only highlighted examples of what might be seen by a pediatric therapist. These conditions have diagnostic criteria presented in the *DSM-IV* (1994). (This manual provides definitions, criteria for diagnosis, and a multiaxial assessment strategy; it is an excellent resource.)

## DEPRESSION: THE CLINICAL PICTURE

The key diagnosis of a major depressive disorder often entails using the *DSM-IV* criteria. The manual indicates a "depressive mood" will be present for 2 weeks to be considered a major depressive disorder. It is challenging to diagnose depression in children because of their limited verbal abilities. Although the signs and symptoms are similar to those seen in depressed adults, these may be described in "kid terms." For example, children may be "down in the dumps" or "unhappy" (depressed mood). They may state that they are "mad at everyone" (increased irritability) or that "nobody likes me" (hopelessness and poor self-esteem).

Children who are depressed may also act out their feelings when they are not able to describe them. The preschooler who has "lost his zip," the weepy 7-year-old, and the kindergartener who has a "sick tummy" may all be trying to demonstrate their feelings through ways other than language (Brent, Puig-Antich, & Rabinovitch, 1992). Additional red flags suggesting depression include sleep and/or appetite changes, drug or alcohol abuse, and excessive risk taking in behavior. Suicidal ideation and/or behavior is a major concern with depressed children and adolescents.

---

■ *THERAPEDS POINTER*

- There has been a major increase in suicidal behavior in the past 15 to 20 years
- Suicidal ideation means one has thoughts about suicide; this is especially high risk if the person verbalizes or acknowledges a "plan" for suicide.
- Trigger factors for children and adolescents regarding suicide include a major loss, an interpersonal conflict, or a disciplinary situation.

---

*Source:* Brent et al., 1992.

Within the realm of depressive disorders there are several "variations on a theme" that may be differently diagnosed by a medical professional. A child may exhibit a reactive depression. This is a depressed mood most often attributed to a change in one's life or a major life adjustment (Levine, Brooks, & Honkoff, 1980). The death of a loved one, a move to a new home, or a divorce may trigger this type of depression. A child may also be diagnosed as dysthymic. This type of depression tends to be a milder, chronic depressive pattern. These children appear to be apathetic, have crying spells, and be irritable or cranky on a daily basis. The pattern may wax and wane, but seldom are children symptom-free for periods of 2 months or more.

The occurrence of depression in children is reported to be about 2 percent of the pediatric population (Brent et al., 1992). Prior to adolescence, depression occurs about equally in boys and girls. After the age of 15, females are about two times as likely to be depressed as males.

One specific cause for depression is not presently known. Biochemical factors, genetics, and environmental stress have been indicated. It should also be noted that depression may be present along with other psychosocial problems such as learning disabilities, attentional disorders, or substance abuse.

**Children with depression; interventions and management.** Although the diagnosis of depression is a medical one, many other people may be involved with the intervention and management of depression in children. Often the parents, teachers, or caregivers note the change in a child's behavior that sends up the "red flat" for depression.

Approaches to managing depression may be multiple. Physicians are involved in the initial diagnosis. They conduct medical examinations to rule out a medical problem as the possible cause of the depression. They may also be involved with prescribing medicines to help with the symptoms of depression.

Pharmacological treatments may include the use of antidepressants, tranquilizers, and other medications. These are often included as part of a team treatment approach, which also provides individual therapy for the child as well as family therapy. Child psychologists may help a child to develop competence and internal resources for dealing with stressors. Social workers and family therapists may also help to investigate external resources and supports that may add to a child's feelings of competency. This may also increase the stability of the environment within which the depressed child functions.

**Interventions from an occupational therapy perspective.** OTs are often integral members of professional teams working with children who are depressed. This has been considered a highly specialized intervention area for pediatric therapists over the past several decades (Burnell, 1985). Being able to relate well to other team members and share treatment goals becomes important, because structuring and consistency are often critical need areas for children with depression and other emotional problems.

*The child.* The child with depression may be challenging to work with for activity-based OTs. The lack of motivation to do, a common sign of depression, makes initial starts in intervention difficult. Some examples of possible intervention strategies are presented in the following chart.

| Characteristic | Seen as | Possible Strategy or Solution |
|---|---|---|
| Poor self-esteem | Constant negative comments about self | Contract with child during treatment session to diminish negative comments and/or find 2–3 positive aspects of self and task |
| Lethargy, lack of motivation | Sitting, doing "nothing" all day | Introduce a physical activity in treatment program, i.e., walking or aerobics (with medical OK) |
| Irritability | Cranky behavior | Assess for sensory integration deficits |

*The parent.* Parents of depressed children may have a twofold impact on their children. They may be contributing to a depressive situation and they also have to deal with the child in the depressed state. Teaming with other professionals (i.e., social work or psychology) may be vital regarding parents and their depressed child.

| Characteristic | Parent Role | Possible Strategy or Intervention |
|---|---|---|
| Poor self-esteem in the child | Attempts to bolster child but lacks the skills | Refer to community resources for "positive parenting" classes |
| Depressed affect because of home problems | Parent is an abused spouse in poor situation | Refer to social worker on team; help parent to seek help |

*The environment or system.* The environment cannot be separated from the child when considering depression. The impact of life stressors, discord in the home situation, and possible abuse can be overwhelming to the depressed child. Although the OT can assist with changing the environment, most likely total team effort will be needed to make a positive impact.

| Characteristic | System or Environmental Impact | Possible Strategy |
|---|---|---|
| Child has frequent mood swings | Child lacks friends because of unpredictable affect | Consider student education about depression for peers in class (with parents' prior consent) |
| Child has suicidal ideation | Teachers and other adults are concerned about child's presence in school | Refer to psychology or psychiatry, and educate staff on warning signs of suicide |

## OPPOSITIONAL DEFIANT DISORDER
## AND CONDUCT DISORDER:
## THE CLINICAL PICTURES

Oppositional defiant disorder (ODD) and conduct disorder (CD) are two of the disruptive behavior diagnoses described and categorized in *DSM-IV* (1994). These two disorders are similar in that children and adolescents with these diagnoses are noted to be "more troubling than troubled" (Egan, 1991, p. 276).

In contrasting the two disorders, one finds children with ODD to be the "undercover" defiants, whereas their cohorts with CD are more aggressive and tend to break age-acceptable societal norms blatantly. Children with ODD frequently ignore parental and adult requests, seem to have greater problems with peer relationships than normal, and may be underachievers in school. Their disruptive behavior may be more often seen at home and in school because they are covert in their actions.

Children and adolescents with CD are often labeled as "antisocial." Their behaviors frequently violate the rights of others. These violations may include fighting with peers and destroying property. Extreme examples include torturing animals and setting fires (Malmquist, 1991). Disobedience and an uncooperative attitude are regularly seen within this population. Both ODD and CD have symptoms that must be present for at least 6 months for a diagnosis to be made.

These problems must also be severe enough to impact on the daily lives of these juveniles. The prevalence of both diagnoses is difficult to determine because in the past criteria for diagnosis varied and overlapping diagnoses commonly occurred (i.e., AD and ODD). The common range for antisocial behavior is reported to be from 5 to 20 percent, depending on the population surveyed. Males are five times more often labeled as having antisocial behavior. Confusion in studies measuring conduct disorder, as to *what* is being measured, makes obtaining numbers challenging (Malmquist, 1991).

Determining the cause for disruptive behavior such as ODD and CD becomes more difficult when the actual diagnoses may be elusive. Behavioral problems are often viewed by professionals from their own "territorial niche." The child with ODD is acting out for the school psychologist, an "underachiever" for the teacher, and "a bad boy" for the neighbor whose house was egged. Factors contributing to the cause of both diagnoses may include personality traits, unstable home situations, and other environmental influences. The complexity of these behavioral problems precludes one from solving the problem by eliminating the risk factors—it's not that easy!

### ▮▮▮ FROM THE BOOKSHELF

*There Are No Children Here* (Kotlowitz, 1992) is a journalist's story of growing up in inner-city Chicago, with many of the environmental hazards of being "on location" there as a child. It gives one insight into where behaviors may come from and what triggers certain actions. Food for thought!

Treatment approaches for ODD and CD vary widely depending on the treatment setting. Various approaches by other professionals have included group therapies, family therapies, and various individual treatments. The use of behavior modification, that is, token economies, has been tried, as have trials with varying drugs. Some of the more successful approaches have been programs that teach problem-solving skills to these children. The subjects are taught to look at behavioral issues, decide where the problem is, and consider appropriate solutions to the dilemmas (Lewis, 1991). Lewis also noted that community-based programs using adult "buddies" as positive social models for students with CD have been used.

In summary, interventions for CD and ODD have been varied in type and success rate. It has been noted that this behaviorally disordered population appears to have chronic long-term needs for multiple services. There appears to be no one right answer. Ongoing research into interventions and longitudinal outcomes are both needed and being pursued.

**Interventions from an occupational therapy perspective.** The intervention approach used by an OT in working with behaviorally disordered children may depend both on the needs of the child and the setting in which he or she is being seen. In residential settings, therapists may have more opportunities for cohesive team interactions than in school or day programs. Below are some examples of need areas demonstrated by a hypothetical 12-year-old boy with ODD and some different interventions in certain settings. (*Note:* The severity of a child's symptoms may determine the location of treatment, and as this changes, so does the environment for intervention.)

| Characteristic | Setting | Intervention Strategy |
|---|---|---|
| Poor self-esteem | Residential program | Work with child to choose new craft skill to master; complete project in individual treatment sessions on child's unit |
| Poor self-esteem | Self-contained school classroom | Student works with group plan and prepares lunch using cooperative skills; upon completion each participant lists positive skills of others in the group |
| Poor self-esteem | Integrated classroom | Observe child in social setting, i.e., lunch or playground. Role play through difficult social situations and assign "homework" of trying new problem-solving strategies; consider "cotreating" with school counselor |
| Noncompliance with rules | Residential setting | As part of intervention team OT contributes list of rules to be followed by child to "earn" special activity pass (token economy or award system for positive behaviors) |

| Characteristic | Setting | Intervention Strategy |
|---|---|---|
| Noncompliance with rules | Self-contained classroom | May use similar approach to above box with "team approach" to earning points or rewards to foster "positive peer pressure" to comply with rules |
| Poor cooperative skills | Middle school integrated classroom | Provided "wilderness" training experience for group to learn team building/cooperative skills |

## WRAPPING IT UP

Children with emotional handicaps often endure the "invisible illness" stigma. Because they do not have visible signs of a problem (i.e., crutches or glasses), their illnesses may lack credibility with others around them. Just "snapping out" of the blues or "acting right for a change" is no more feasible for them than walking without crutches or seeing the chalkboard without glasses for their peers with physical impairments. Research into the whys of these disorders as well as a comprehensive review of the components of effective interventions may yield much needed information for future intervention programs.

## CASE STORY

Karen is an 8-year-old girl in a cross-categorical (mixed-diagnoses) classroom in a rural school district. She was diagnosed 2 years ago with Rett syndrome after an initial diagnosis of autism at the age of 34 months. She demonstrates the characteristic "handwringing" pattern and the breath holding typical of Rett's syndrome. She has become more unstable in her gait over the past 6 months and mobility in the classroom requires assistance. Her OT goals over the past year have focused on feeding skills (with silverware) and on toileting skills in conjunction with physical therapy goals. Karen is nonverbal and her cognitive skills are estimated to be in the range of 26 months developmentally.

At a back-to-school team meeting in September, Karen's summer program was explained by her mother. Team members present included the physician following Karen, the classroom staff, the OT, the PT, and the school social worker. The mother indicated her frustration with Karen's lack of progress in the area of toilet training and her concern that Karen no longer "finger-fed" herself and that spoon feeding required constant physical assistance from a parent or adult.

1. What adaptations might you make to the feeding program in hopes of increasing independent feeding skills in Karen?
2. With the physical therapist you assess Karen's present toileting status in the home and school bathrooms. Sitting balance appears to be "precarious" on the commode.

a) What recommendations or adaptions might you make in light of this assessment? Consider health-and-safety issues in your recommendations.

b) How might the fact that Rett's syndrome is progressive and degenerative in nature influence your recommendations?

## Real-Life Lab

**1.** You are the staff OT for a private residential school for autistic children. You have been working with the recreation therapist to enhance the weekend leisure program for your residents. The staff has requested ideas for games or activities that individuals may do alone or with another resident where feasible. A local service organization has just donated $200 for this project.

**a)** What items or activities might be part of your wish list? Why?

**b)** Check out a local toy store for new ideas. List one or two activities that you have found (include brand and cost). Consider ways the items could be adapted for children with autism of various intellectual levels.

**2.** You are a therapist in private practice who has just evaluated an 11-year-old boy with an attentional disorder. During the feedback session, the parents request recommendations for summer camp programs for their child. What resources might provide them with further information regarding this request? (Be specific, names and titles of resources are needed. "At the library" is not the answer to this question!)

**3.** Head to the library and find the July 1996 issue of *OT Practice* (see References for full citation). The article "Autism: Defining the OT's Role in Treating This Confusing Disorder" is an excellent review of the various roles of the OT in working with autism and PDD. After reading this article by Bethany Stancliff, ponder with your colleagues the following:

**a)** What does the federal law say about children with autism receiving OT services?

**b)** What are some of the emotions parents experience when dealing with their child's disability and its impacts on the family?

**c)** What skills or knowledge do OTs have to offer parents in this situation, and likewise, what skills or knowledge do parents have to share with therapists?

## References

Achenbach, T. M., & Edelbrock, C. (1983). *Manual for the child behavior checklist and revised child behavior profile*. Burlington: University of Vermont, Department of Psychology.

Ayres, A. J. (1986). *Sensory integration and*

*praxis tests*. Los Angeles, CA: Western Psychological Services.

Beery, K., & Buktenica, N. A. (1967). *The Beery-Buktenica test of visual motor integration*. Cleveland: Modern Curriculum Press.

Berk, L., & Landau, S. (1995). Private speech of learning disabled and normally achieving children in classroom academic and laboratory contexts. In M. E. Hertzig & E. A. Farber (Eds.). *Annual progress in child psychiatry and child development 1994* (pp. 394–417). New York: Bruner/Mazel.

Brent, D. A., Puig-Antich, J., & Rabinovitch, H. (1992). Major psychiatric disorders in childhood and adolescence. In M. D. Levine, W. B. Carey, & A. C. Crocker (Eds.). *Developmental-behavioral pediatrics* (2nd ed.) (pp. 569–588). Philadelphia: W. B. Saunders.

Bruininks, R. H. (1978). *The Bruininks-Oserestsky test of motor proficiency examiner's manual*. Circle Pines, MN: American Guidance Service.

Burnell, D. P. (1985). Children with severe emotional or behavioral disorders. In P. N. Clark & A. S. Allen (Eds.). *Occupational therapy for children* (pp. 456–470). St. Louis: C. V. Mosby.

Colarusso, R. P., & Hammill, D. D. (1972). *Motor free visual perception test*. Novato, CA: Academic Therapy Publications.

Conners, C. K. (1969). A teacher rating scale for use in drug studies with children. *American Journal of Psychiatry, 126* (6), 152–156.

*Diagnostic and statistical manual of mental disorders* (1994). Washington, D.C.: American Psychiatric Association.

Egan, J. (1991). Oppositional defiant disorder. In J. M. Wiener (Ed.). *Textbook of child and adolescent psychiatry.* (pp. 276–278). Washington, D.C.: American Psychiatric Press.

Elliott, G. R. (1996). Autistic disorder and other pervasive developmental disorders. In A. M. Rudolph, J. Hoffman, & C. D. Rudolph (Eds.). *Rudolph's pediatrics* (20th ed.) (pp. 168–170). Stamford, CT: Appleton & Lange.

Folio, M. R., & Fewell, R. R. (1983). Peabody *developmental motor scales and activity cards* (manual). Allen, TX: DLM Teaching Resources.

Gardner, M. F. (1986). *TVMS: Test of visual motor skills*. San Francisco: Children's Hospital of San Francisco.

Grandin, T., & Scariano, M. M. (1986). *Emergence: Labeled autistic*. New York: Warner Books.

Greenfeld, J. (1972). *A child called Noah: A family journey*. New York: Harcourt Brace Jovanovich.

Greenfeld, J. (1989). *A place for Noah*. New York: Harcourt Brace Jovanovich.

Greenfeld, J. (1989). *A client called Noah*. New York: Harcourt Brace Jovanovich.

Hancock, L. (1996, March 18). Mother's little helper. *Newsweek*, pp. 51–59.

Holm, V. (1985). Rett syndrome: A progressive developmental disability in girls. *Developmental and Behavioral Pediatrics, 6* (1), 32–35.

Kaplan, H. I., Sadlock, B. J., & Grebb, K. A. (1994). *Kaplan and Sadlock's synopsis of psychiatry, behavioral sciences, clinical psychiatry* (7th ed.). Baltimore: Williams & Wilkins.

Kotlowitz, A. (1992). *There are no children here*. New York: Anchor Books.

Kubas, E. S. (1992). Use of splints to develop hand skills in a woman with Rett syndrome. *American Journal of Occupational Therapy, 46* (4), 364–368.

Leung, A. K., Robson, W. L., Fagan, J. E., & Lim, S. H. (1994). Attention deficit hyperactivity disorder: Getting control of impulsive behavior. *Postgraduate Medicine, 95* (2), 153–160.

Levine, M. D., Brooks, R., & Shonkoff, J. (1980). *A pediatric approach to learning disorders*. New York: John Wiley & Sons.

Lewis, D. (1991). Conduct disorder. In M. Lewis (Ed.). *Child and adolescent psychiatry: A comprehensive textbook* (pp. 561–573). Baltimore: Williams & Wilkins.

Malmquist, C. (1991). Conduct disorder: Conceptual and diagnostic issues. In J. M. Wiener (Ed.). *Textbook of child and adolescent psychiatry* (pp. 279–287). Washington, D.C.: American Psychiatric Press.

Martin, R. P., Hooper, S., & Snow, J. (1986): Behavior rating scale approaches to personality assessment in children and adolescents. In H. M. Knoff (Ed.). *The assessment of child and adolescent personality* (pp. 309–352). New York: The Guilford Press.

Minshew, N. J., & Payton, J. B. (1988). New perspectives in autism, part I: The clinical spectrum of autism. *Current Problems in Pediatrics, 18* (10), 561–610.

Nelson, D. (1984). *Children with autism and other pervasive disorders of development and behavior: Therapy through activities*. Thorofare, NJ: Slack.

Reiff, M. I., Banez, G. A., & Culbert, T. P. (1993): Children who have attentional disorders: Diagnosis and evaluation. *Pediatrics in Review, 14* (12), 455–465.

Rudel, R. G. (1988). *Assessment of developmental learning disorders.* New York: Basic Books.

Schanzenbacher, K. (1985). Diagnostic problems in pediatrics. In P. N. Clark & A. T. Allen (Eds.). *Occupational therapy for children* (pp. 78–113). St. Louis: C. V. Mosby.

Schopler, E., & Reichler, R. J. (1979). *Individualized assessment and treatment for autistic and developmentally disabled children.* (Vol. I). *Psychoeducational profile.* Baltimore: University Park Press.

Sharpe, P. A., & Ottenbacher, K. J. (1990). Use of an elbow restraint to improve finger feeding skills in a child with Rett syndrome. *American Journal of Occupational Therapy, 44,* 328–332.

Stancliff, B. (1996). Autism: Defining the OT's role in treating this confusing disorder. *OT Practice,* July, 18–21, 23–29.

Tsai, L. Y. (1991). Other pervasive developmental disorders. In J. M. Wiener (Ed.). *Textbook of child and adolescent psychiatry* (pp. 192–205). Washington, D.C.: American Psychiatric Press.

Tsai, L. Y. & Ghaziuddin, M. (1991). Autistic disorder. In J. M. Wiener (Ed.). *Textbook of child and adolescent psychiatry* (pp. 169–191). Washington, D. C.: American Psychiatric Press.

Weller, E., & Weller, R. (1991). Mood disorders in children. In J. M. Wiener (Ed.). *Textbook of child and adolescent psychiatry* (pp. 240–247). Washington, D.C.: American Psychiatric Press.

Williams, D. (1992). *Nobody nowhere: The extraordinary autobiography of an autistic.* New York: Avon Books.

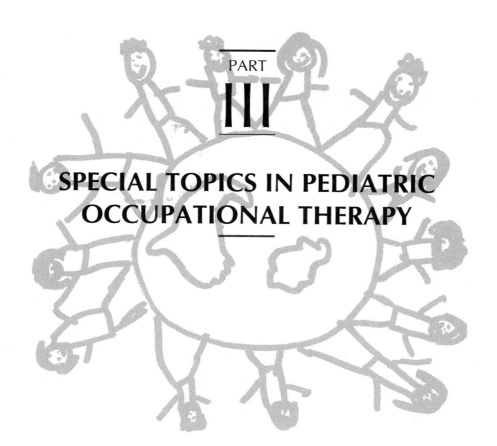

# SPECIAL TOPICS IN PEDIATRIC
# OCCUPATIONAL THERAPY

# 10

# *Working in the Neonatal Intensive Care Unit*

Jayne T. Shepherd, MS, OTR
Judith Kytle Hanshaw, BS, OTR
Shelly J. Lane, PHD, OTR, ATP, FAOTA

## KEY POINTS

- Therapists working in newborn intensive care units (NICUs) require extensive knowledge and training *before* entering neonatal practice.
- Postconceptual age and a variety of medical terms are used to define the medical status and capabilities of babies who are premature or critically ill.
- Babies who are premature or critically ill require specialized medical treatment and equipment and the help of a variety of team members.
- The sound, light, and caregiving practices of the NICU environment may negatively impact the growth and development of the baby.
- Parents and all professionals working with babies need to learn the engagement and disengagement signals of each individual baby to modify their own behaviors and to adapt the environment.
- It is essential for therapists to acknowledge parental feelings and teach parents how to read their baby's cues so that they can care for and play with their baby.
- Assessment and intervention practices in NICU are tailored to each individual baby as the physiological cost of interaction can be life-threatening if not administered appropriately.
- Therapists and all NICU staff train parents to learn about their baby's

uniqueness, condition, and care so that they become progressively more confident in their caregiving and parenting abilities.

As medical care for neonates has advanced, more babies are surviving premature birth or a critical illness. Often they find themselves in the highly technical environment of the newborn intensive care units (NICUs). OTs have worked NICUs for more than 20 years, and as such find increasingly fragile babies on their caseloads (Dewire, White, Kanny, and Glass, 1996; Rappaport, 1992). This is a highly specialized field for therapists that requires extensive knowledge and training of medical, environmental, and social variables that affect the fragility of babies. It is estimated that less than 1 percent of OTs work primarily in the NICU setting (AOTA, 1996) and The American Occupational Therapy Association (AOTA) now recognizes work in NICU as an advanced practice area (AOTA, 1993).

The purpose of this chapter is to expose the therapist to the complexity of the NICU environment and basic assessment and treatment techniques for the baby and the family in the NICU. It does not purport to teach a therapist to work in the NICU. Sweeney (1993) suggests that therapists need to earn their trust and acceptance in NICU by first being a professional guest and later becoming an integrated NICU team member when they understand the complexity of the environment.

This chapter first defines the terminology, diagnoses, abbreviations, and equipment that may be used when a neonate enters NICU. It will then identify the impact of the NICU experience on the family and baby. Basic evaluation and treatment concepts will be discussed, and the therapist will be given resources for parents and for further training in NICU practice.

# DEFINITIONS

## Newborn Classifications

There are a variety of terms used to describe babies, and the NICU environment has more terminology and abbreviations to learn than most other environments. Medically, newborns are classified according to their gestational age, birth weight, the relationship between age and weight, and developmental risk. As a baby is born, physicians attempt to determine their gestational age (GA) or the number of weeks the baby has been in utero since conception. They examine the baby and give him or her a postconceptional age (PCA). Based on the PCA, they classify the baby as premature, full term, or post term. The survival rates for babies born prematurely and who receive care in the NICU vary according to the PCA. Babies born at 23 weeks PCA have a survival rate of 5 to 25 percent, with an increase in the survival rate of 3 to 4 percent per day of life (Brazy, 1997). The older the baby's PCA, the more likely the baby will survive. By 27 weeks, it is estimated that there is a greater than 90 percent survival rate (Brazy, 1997). The birth weight of the neonate is measured in grams and is classified as low or average (see Table 10–1 for a pound-gram conversion chart and Table 10–2 for inch-centimeter conversion chart).

Birth weights that are low are subclassified as low (LBW), very low

Table 10–1    **Weight Conversion Chart from Pounds and Ounces to Grams**

|  | | **POUNDS** | | | | | | | | |
|---|---|---|---|---|---|---|---|---|---|---|
|  | **0** | **1** | **2** | **3** | **4** | **5** | **6** | **7** | **8** | **9** |
| **0** | 0 | 454 | 907 | 1361 | 1814 | 2268 | 2722 | 3175 | 3629 | 4082 |
| **1** | 28 | 482 | 936 | 1389 | 1843 | 2296 | 2750 | 3203 | 3657 | 4111 |
| **2** | 57 | 510 | 964 | 1417 | 1871 | 2325 | 2778 | 3232 | 3685 | 4139 |
| **3** | 85 | 539 | 992 | 1446 | 1899 | 2353 | 2807 | 3260 | 3714 | 4167 |
| **4** | 113 | 567 | 1021 | 1474 | 1928 | 2381 | 2835 | 3289 | 3742 | 4196 |
| **5** | 142 | 595 | 1049 | 1503 | 1956 | 2410 | 2863 | 3317 | 3770 | 4224 |
| **6** | 170 | 624 | 1077 | 1531 | 1984 | 2438 | 2892 | 3345 | 3799 | 4252 |
| **7** | 198 | 652 | 1106 | 1559 | 2013 | 2466 | 2920 | 3374 | 3827 | 4281 |
| **8** | 227 | 680 | 1134 | 1588 | 2041 | 2495 | 2948 | 3402 | 3856 | 4309 |
| **9** | 255 | 709 | 1162 | 1616 | 2070 | 2523 | 2977 | 3430 | 3884 | 4337 |
| **10** | 283 | 737 | 1191 | 1644 | 2098 | 2551 | 3005 | 3459 | 3912 | 4366 |
| **11** | 312 | 765 | 1219 | 1673 | 2126 | 2580 | 3033 | 3487 | 3941 | 4394 |
| **12** | 340 | 794 | 1247 | 1701 | 2155 | 2608 | 3062 | 3515 | 3969 | 4423 |
| **13** | 369 | 822 | 1276 | 1729 | 2183 | 2637 | 3090 | 3544 | 3997 | 4451 |
| **14** | 397 | 859 | 1304 | 1758 | 2211 | 2665 | 3118 | 3572 | 4026 | 4479 |
| **15** | 425 | 879 | 1332 | 1786 | 2240 | 2693 | 3147 | 3600 | 4054 | 4508 |

*(OUNCES label is along the left vertical axis)*

Table 10–2    **Conversion of Centimeters to Inches (2.5 cm = approximately 1 inch)**

| Centimeters | Inches | Centimeters | Inches | Centimeters | Inches |
|---|---|---|---|---|---|
| 25.4 | 10 | 43.2 | 17 | 61.0 | 24 |
| 26.7 | $10^1/_2$ | 44.4 | $17^1/_2$ | 62.2 | $24^1/_2$ |
| 27.9 | 11 | 45.7 | 18 | 63.5 | 25 |
| 29.2 | $11^1/_2$ | 47.0 | $18^1/_2$ | 64.8 | $25^1/_2$ |
| 30.5 | 12 | 48.3 | 19 | 66.1 | 26 |
| 31.8 | $12^1/_2$ | 49.5 | $19^1/_2$ | 67.4 | $26^1/_2$ |
| 33.0 | 13 | 50.8 | 20 | 68.7 | 27 |
| 34.3 | $13^1/_2$ | 52.1 | $20^1/_2$ | 69.9 | $27^1/_2$ |
| 35.6 | 14 | 53.3 | 21 | 71.2 | 28 |
| 36.8 | $14^1/_2$ | 54.6 | $21^1/_2$ | 72.5 | $28^1/_2$ |
| 38.1 | 15 | 55.9 | 22 | 73.8 | 29 |
| 39.4 | $15^1/_2$ | 57.2 | $22^1/_2$ | 75.1 | $29^1/_2$ |
| 40.6 | 16 | 58.4 | 23 | 76.4 | 30 |
| 41.9 | $16^1/_2$ | 59.7 | $23^1/_2$ | 77.6 | $30^1/_2$ |

(VLBW), or extremely low birth weight (ELBW). As with gestational age, survival decreases with decreasing birth weight. After the neonate is given a PCA and a weight, the relationship between these two classifications is determined by plotting them on a weight to gestational age relationship graph. The adequacy of weight for PCA is classified such that babies fall into appropriate (AGA), small (SGA), or large for gestational age (LGA).

■ *THERAPEDS POINTER*

Medical Classifications for Gestational Age and Weight

| GESTATIONAL AGE CATEGORIES | | |
|---|---|---|

A full-term baby has an average gestation of 40 weeks, ± 2 weeks. Thus, full term is considered 38 to 42 weeks' gestational age. Other gestational age categories are as follows:

| | | |
|---|---|---|
| Preterm (PT) | | 28–37 weeks PCA |
| Extremely preterm | | <28 weeks PCA |
| Posterm | | >42 weeks PCA |

| BIRTH WEIGHT CATEGORIES | | |
|---|---|---|
| | **Grams** | **Pounds/Ounces** |
| Average newborn birth weight | >2500 | >5 lb, 8 oz |
| Low birth weight (LBW) | 1500–2500 | 3 lb, 5 oz–5 lb, 8 oz |
| Very low birth weight (VLBW) | 1000–1499 | 2 lb, 3oz–3 lb, 4 oz |
| Extremely low birth weight (ELBW) | <1000 | <2 lb, 3 oz |

| WEIGHT-TO-GESTATIONAL-AGE RELATIONSHIPS | |
|---|---|
| Appropriate for gestational age (AGA) | Between 10th and 90th percentile |
| Small for gestational age (SGA) | <10th percentile |
| Large for gestational age (LGA) | >90th percentile |

Babies who are premature, full term, or postterm may be classified as AGA, SGA, or LGA. For example, a baby may be full term but may have intrauterine growth retardation (IUGR), which classifies him as SGA. Or a premature baby may have an estimated PCA of 30 weeks, but he is LGA because he weighs more than most babies born at 30 weeks' PCA. Similarly, a postterm baby may be SGA if his weight is in the 9th percentile for babies born at 43 weeks.

Yet another classification for babies in the NICU is their future risk status, which will determine their eligibility for intervention post hospitalization. Vergara (1993a) suggested that babies with prenatal, perinatal, or postnatal complications, or a family history of risk be labeled "at-risk," whereas neonates who have been in a NICU environment be classified as at "high risk" for developmental delays. Unfortunately, these definitions are not universally applied. Each state has had the opportunity to develop independent definitions of these terms and as such, classification by risk varies among states. Further, IDEA (Individuals with Disabilities Education Act) allows each state to determine eligibility for services, and in some states being placed in a risk category is sufficient to qualify a baby for early intervention, whereas in other states this is not the case. Therapists should consult their state regulations to determine how risk is classified for babies, and how this impacts eligibility for early intervention services when the baby leaves the NICU.

## NICU ABBREVIATIONS AND TERMINOLOGY

Specific medical terminology or abbreviations are used to discuss the needs and care of high-risk neonates. Appendix A at the end of this chapter gives a sample listing of these abbreviations and terms. When first entering the NICU, therapists may keep a list of frequently used terms in their pocket to help decipher medical charts and conversations with other professionals. It is suggested that therapists add to this list as they encounter new abbreviations or terms.

## THE NICU ENVIRONMENT

While supporting the life of the baby, NICU environments are overloaded with a wide variety of sounds, bright lights, strong odors, and varying temperatures. This is quite a change from the intrauterine environment. Here the baby experiences rhythmic swooshes, bubbles, and gurgles with a steady maternal heartbeat. The mother's voice and some environmental sounds are audible as the baby floats in dark, warm fluid (Weibley, 1989). When the baby arrives in the world and subsequently NICU, he or she is surrounded by the noise of technology enabling their survival. Noise level is often comparable to that of auto traffic (Gottfried et al., 1981). In many NICU environments, there are continuous bright lights and cold air, and the baby is generally placed on a firm nonmoving bed surface. It has been reported that the baby in the NICU is disturbed 132 times per day and has brief undisturbed rest on an average of only 4 to 10 minutes (Korones, 1985). This environment may constitute a sensory overload for the immature nervous system of the neonate. Sensory development is altered by the sudden drastic change from intrauterine to extrauterine survival. Babies born prematurely may be highly reactive and overwhelmed by all the inappropriate sensory overload present (Hunter, 1996b), and may have difficulty adapting or habituating to overwhelming stimuli. Their responses may tend to be disorganized, overreactive, and physiologically draining. Furthermore, their reactions may cause hypoxic events and/or create maladaptive behavior that may affect later developmental outcomes (Hunter, 1996b). NICU staff and consultants can modify the baby's environment to eliminate unnecessary stimulation, assist the baby to respond in a more organized manner, and provide the opportunity for the baby to calm herself. The success of modifying the environment depends on administrative support and on the nursing staff who are present for 24 hours and can identify which events appear most stressful, painful, or disruptive to the baby who is suffering from sleep deprivation. Table 10–3 compares the intrauterine and extrauterine environments and gives approaches to adapt the NICU (Hunter, 1996b; Weibley, 1989). Some of these low-tech adaptations are easy to do, whereas others require administrative support to change the physical environment.

**Table 10–3   Characteristics of the Neonatal Environment and Gentle Adaptations**

| Intrauterine | Extrauterine | Gentle NICU |
|---|---|---|
| **Tactile:** | | |
| Constant maternal proprioceptive input; soothing, moist and warm support | Invasive/painful touch from medical procedures; dry air; lack of tactile support | Nesting; comfort the infant to offset harsh input; gentle touch during rounds and at bedside when awake or when upset; stuffed animals support limbs, chest, back; parent strokes or massages |
| **Vestibular:** | | |
| Maternal rocking movements with active and inactive periods; gentle rocking and fluid support while baby is in a flexed position | Reduced movements; equipment restraints; flat position maintained | Position in flexion; use gel pads or water mats; hammock; give frequent position changes |
| **Auditory:** | | |
| Audible maternal body sounds; distorted maternal speech and environmental sounds | Equipment sounds; painful loudness; constant noise; variety of sounds and voices | Speaking to infant; use whole name and gender; soft music or tapes of family voices; quiet time where staff monitor voice volume; acoustic ceilings; carpet on floors; NICU rounds away from beds; low voice page system; partitions; phones and alarms with flashing lights; move noisy equipment to another room; insulate equipment so not as noisy |
| **Visual:** | | |
| Enclosed darkness with occasional red light dimness | Constant overhead lights (usually fluorescent) | Sunscreens on windows or shades; bedside lights with rheostat dimmers; lights out for quiet time; covers for isolettes and cribs; cyclic lights; cool lights; mobiles or family photos; use of flashlights when "quiet time" |
| **Thermal:** | | |
| Constant warmth; consistent temperature | Extreme heat variations; high risk for heat loss when incubator portholes are opened or baby is fed, changed, or medical procedure performed; dry and cool surroundings | Heat probe monitoring; extra blankets; sensitive thermostats; hats; reduced handling; clustered caregiving |

**Parent/Caretaker:**

| | | |
|---|---|---|
| Chooses where she will be and how she cares for herself and unborn baby | Lacks privacy; holding difficult; inconsistent nursing care; social chatter among staff; lack of family togetherness; feelings of depersonalization | Screens; love and gentle care is top priority; parents are center of care; parents are welcomed & informed of infant's day; acknowledge the "whole" baby by touch and voice; family visiting rooms; parent overnight rooms; sibling visits; personalize the baby's bed site; primary nursing model; clustered caregiving to enhance longer sleep cycles |

*Source:* Compiled from Frank, Maurer, & Shepherd (1991); Hunter (1992); Weibley (1989).

## TEAM MEMBERS IN NICU

There are many professional staffs that provide special care to the baby in NICU and his or her family. As an OT you need to be aware of all available NICU services. These services help support your program, enhance the care of the baby, eliminate duplication of services, promote teamwork, increase communication, and focus on achieving therapeutic interdisciplinary health care for the baby. Listed below are some of the staff who have a unique impact on occupational therapy (Semmler & Butcher, 1990).

The *neonatologist* is a pediatrician with advanced training in the care and management of babies (term and preterm) who are sick. He or she is usually the one who refers the baby to occupational therapy for an evaluation and treatment.

The *nursing staff* is responsible for coordinating the daily care for the baby. They administer medications and procedures, alert the physician to any medical changes, and are often the main people who communicate daily with the baby's family. When appropriate, nurses and OTs collaborate with each other to determine the best techniques to feed and position the baby, and to discuss the baby's ability to interact and learn from the environment with or without modifications. The success of the occupational therapy program in the NICU is dependent on nursing staff support and implementation of therapeutic suggestions.

The *pastoral care chaplain* provides the family and staff with spiritual comfort and may perform baptisms in the NICU. They assist in grief counseling and may receive a referral from the OT.

The *nutritionist* or *dietitian* plans the caloric diet needed to improve the baby's weight gain and assists the family in learning how to monitor the baby's nutritional needs. The nutritionist or dietitian collaborates with OT and nursing to determine when it is developmentally appropriate to introduce oral feedings.

The *speech therapist* may also be involved in determining the feeding needs of the baby by assessing swallowing through the use of a barium swallow test. They also assess early oral-motor movements to manipulate food and develop early language skills.

The *physical therapist* assesses and treats neonates with congenital, structural, and motor disabilities. He or she uses active and passive movement patterns to help the baby progress in gross-motor skills and consults with the OT about positioning, equipment, and lower-extremity splinting or casting needs.

The *respiratory therapist (RT)* monitors breathing problems and provides specialized equipment to support the respiratory efforts of the baby. OTs consult with RTs in ways to adapt the breathing equipment so the baby can move and explore his environment, use items at midline, and maintain skin integrity.

Discharge planning begins the day the baby enters NICU. OTs work with parents, social workers, and community health nurses to help the baby make the transition smoothly to home. They also work together and give the family a referral to an early intervention program.

*Social workers* help families who may need financial assistance or information about medical insurance, housing, equipment location (e.g., car seats, strollers, bath chairs), or accessing other services or agencies (e.g., substance abuse program or temporary housing). They may provide counseling to the family, provide parent role models, and coordinate discharge planning.

The *community health nurse* visits the home prior to and after discharge. This nurse facilitates the role of the local health department, identifies home health agencies or early intervention agencies in the area, and assists in compiling and disbursing the OT's report and recommendations for follow-up.

## THE EFFECT OF NICU ON FAMILIES

As most parents are waiting for their baby to be born, they are developing an image of their baby and of themselves as parents (Galinsky, 1987). When a baby is born early or is born with medical complications, these parental images are shattered and many medical decisions need to be made. Instead of holding and nurturing their bundle of joy, these parents are unexpectedly thrown into the NICU with professionals controlling the care of their baby (Olson & Baltman, 1994). This environment and the baby can be very frightening to parents, as can the numerous professionals who are using unfamiliar abbreviations and terminology. This foreign language and environment often make parents feel uncomfortable, and they may avoid coming to the NICU or feel inhibited to actively participate in their baby's care.

During this period in the NICU, parents may be in shock and may deny that their baby has any problems or they may feel a wide range of emotions such as loss, anxiety, or anger (Olson & Baltman, 1994). Some parents may grieve for the "perfect baby" or the parenting experience they had expected. Other parents may blame themselves for a genetic problem or for the early birth of the baby (e.g., "I shouldn't have had that aspirin" or "I should have slowed down more"). Mothers and fathers may feel incompetent that they could not produce a healthy baby, or they may blame each other for the baby's problems. Feelings of guilt and grief along with the hormonal changes in a mother after birth may lead to depression. Detachment and emotional distancing from the baby may occur because of all the tubes and machines, the parents' fear that their baby is going to die, or the parent's anger. Acknowledging feelings and teaching parents how to care for their baby is essential (Holloway, 1994). Parents need to discuss their concerns and vent their frustrations. It may also help parents to seek counseling or a join a support group if needed.

---

### ■ *THERAPEDS POINTER*

In addition to acknowledging parental needs and stresses, therapists can be instrumental in involving families in treatment. This involvement may serve to lessen the fears and increase the investment of the family in the processes and procedures of the NICU. Here are some ideas:

- Have families bring in pictures of family members from home
- Bring in toys (give suggestions of types of toys if they ask)
- Dress the baby in clothes from home instead of the hospital clothes
- Provide adaptive positioning devices
- Talk about the uniqueness of the baby
- Post bedside pictures of the baby with an explanation of what they can do
- Have family members watch and be part of the treatment process

---

All members of the family are affected when the baby remains in NICU for an extended period of time. Families are often separated from each other. Siblings may stay with other people while Mom and Dad are running to the hospital. Depending on the siblings' ages, they may not understand why they are being left or why their parents are so concerned about their new brother or sister. Family functions change and need flexibility at this time. Daily living activities, recreation, socialization, education, affection, and work routines and activities are impacted. If available, families may need to rely on others to do some of these daily living tasks. Financial concerns are usually great, because NICU environments are extremely expensive. Parents need to make decisions about returning to work or school and if they need to apply for assistance for medical bills. Families without insurance or with limited insurance often seem extremely stressed by the financial implications of having a child in NICU and providing for this child when he or she comes home. Financial concerns may impact how often the parent can be at the hospital (e.g., money for transportation or babysitters for siblings) and the type of medical treatment the parents seek for their baby. Typical emotional supports or ways to relieve stress (e.g., friends, family members, exercise, recreational activities) are unavailable or may change because of the time spent with the baby. Some parents feel they cannot talk to their friends who haven't "lived the NICU experience," and they may benefit from talking to other parents of NICU graduates. In retrospect, other parents just may wish that NICU staff would ask about their well-being as well as the babies.

■ *THERAPEDS POINTER*

Therapists must be alert to the needs of the parents as well as to the needs of the baby. Some simple questions can be asked of the parents to let them know you care about them as well as their baby:

- How are *you*?
- How is your family?
- What have you done to take care of yourself?
- What did your baby do today?
- What can I do to help?

The medical stability of babies in NICU is often turbulent. Parents are asked to make medical decisions that may affect the baby's ability to survive. Ethically, it is very important that parents are given all of the facts needed to make informed decisions about medical procedures. Parents have the right to choose supportive care versus aggressive treatment when great suffering or a high probability of mortality is evident (Harrison, 1993). These decisions can be controversial and heart wrenching to families and may be impacted by their own personal beliefs and values. Healing practices and customs may surface that are different from typical NICU procedures. When discrepancies between family decisions and NICU staff recommendations exist, Baker (1995) suggests that the goal of the family be compared to the goal of the NICU staff, and if the baby will not be harmed, the family's decision or request should be supported.

## ▟▎▎ FROM THE BOOKSHELF

BOOKS FOR SIBLINGS
Hawkins-Walsh, E. (1985). *Katie's premature brother.* Omaha: Centering Corporation. (Box 3367, Omaha, NE 68103).
Lafferty, L. (1995). *Born early: A premature baby's story for children.* Grand Junction, CO: Songbird Publication Company. (P.O. Box 4260, Grand Junction, CO 81502).
Murphy-Melas, E. (1996). *Watching Bradley grow.* Georgia: Longstreet Press.
Walden, M., & Congdon, B. (1992). *A special gift for Mike: For brothers and sisters of premature or ill babies.* Houston: Texas Children's Hospital, Office of Educational Resources.

### *Families with Special Needs*

In NICU, therapists are often introduced to families with special needs. These mothers and fathers may be teenagers or may have mental illness, mental retardation, AIDS, physical disabilities, drug or alcohol dependency, or may be abused by others within their environment. The therapist places his or her own values aside and supports these families in becoming competent caregivers for their baby while at the same time being vigilant to protect the baby from harm. When working with these parents, the therapist thinks about the mother's developmental or medical needs and evaluates who is available in the family or community to support this family. Social workers, early intervention programs, and family members themselves are instrumental in identifying and utilizing these supports. Many NICUs will not release babies from the hospital until an identified support person is trained in the baby's care and passes cardiopulmonary resuscitation techniques.

Case-Smith (1993) has identified five roles for the OT working with families in NICU. They are:

1. Facilitate positive interactions between the baby and family members.
2. Collaborate with parents on the care of their baby.
3. Share information in a supportive manner.
4. Encourage informal support systems for parents.
5. Recognize and honor the individuality of families and be flexible and responsive to their unique needs.

## NEONATAL EQUIPMENT

Equipment typically used in the NICU environment is listed in Table 10–4. Therapists need to understand the purpose of the equipment and be prepared to use it, or respond to it, at times. For example, alarms often sound when working with a baby because of a pulled or twisted wire; it saves noise and nursing time if the therapist knows how to turn off the alarm or reset it. On-the-job training as well as in-service training is necessary before using any of this equipment.

Other equipment may be used in the NICU environment besides those listed on Table 10–4. Therapists always need to ask about the equipment's purpose, precautions when using it with a baby, and when and how to use the equipment if it is appropriate. As medical technology in the NICU increases, some equipment becomes obsolete while new equipment is introduced. Open and honest communication with other NICU professionals about your comfort level and knowledge about the equipment is essential. It is recommended that a skilled therapist or nurse review your competency in operating the equipment in NICU. Many hospitals have competency checklists that are completed for all new staff working in the NICU environment.

## INFECTION CONTROL

All NICU employees have the responsibility to prevent the spread of infection. Any infection can seriously compromise or become fatal to a baby who is medically fragile. Iatrogenic infection is a result of surgical procedures or physician treatment. A nosocomial infection is a result of contact during a hospital stay. Infections are transmitted by direct touch, airborne particles, and physical objects like toys or equipment or clothing. A thorough 3-minute handwashing scrub with a germicide solution upon entry to the unit is the

Table 10–4  **Typical Equipment Used in the NICU**

| | |
|---|---|
| Bag and mask ventilation | A quick way to give oxygen to a baby by squeezing a bag attached to a face mask. |
| Cardiorespiratory monitor | Provides a visual and a numerical tracing that correlates with the heart and breathing rate of the neonate. Audible alarms are elicited if rates are not within the present ranges. |
| Chest tubes | A plastic tube placed into the chest to remove air or fluid from a lung(s). |
| CPAP (continuous positive airway pressure) | Low-pressure air is given to the baby to support breathing (e.g., via a nasopharyngeal tube or an endotracheal tube). |
| Enteral nutrition | Feedings to the digestive system via oral, nasogastric, or gastrostomy tubes. |
| Parenteral nutrition | Feedings are given intravenously to the digestive system. |
| Incubator | An enclosed clear plastic bed that maintains body temperature. It often has a temperature sensor attached to the infant's skin. Portholes are used to care for the baby. |
| Infusion pumps | Controls parenteral fluids into the peripheral veins, arterial lines or central venous catheters (C-line). Allows for slow advanced feeding volumes. |
| Mechanical ventilation | A variety of machines that control breathing by keeping the airway open and inflating the lungs. Oxygen is delivered from 100% to 0% via nasal or oral intubation. |
| Nasal cannula | Flexible plastic tubing that carries moist oxygen into the infant's nares. |
| Oxygen hood | A plastic hood attached to a moist oxygen source is placed over the baby's head. |
| Pulse oximeter | Noninvasive method that continuously assesses arterial oxygen saturation with a sensor wrapped around the infant's hand or foot. Pulse rate must approximate heart rate on the cardiorespiratory monitor. |
| Radiant warmer | An open bed with an overhead heater used during critical care (for easy access). |
| Transcutaneous oxygen monitoring | An electrode placed on the infant to measure oxygen and carbon dioxide levels in the blood. |

*Source:* Compiled from Hunter, 1996b; Semmler & Butcher, 1990; Vergara, 1993a.

best defense in controlling infection. Fifteen-second scrubs between babies, and 1-minute scrubs when departing NICU are also recommended. Most NICUs require all staff who are in physical contact with the baby to wear gowns and gloves. Equipment used by the OT is cleaned between treatment sessions with a 1:10 bleach solution to water to destroy infectious organisms.

OTs need to know the NICU infection control, guidelines for isolation, visitation procedures for students and families, and staff policies and procedures for the NICU in which they work (Semmler, 1990). Guidelines for personal illnesses, open cuts, symptoms, and personal hygiene (e.g., jewelry, nail length, hair containment) are usually delineated. Therapists follow all procedures carefully if they wish to become welcome members of the NICU team.

## TYPICAL MEDICAL CONDITIONS SEEN IN THE NICU

Numerous diseases and difficulties may lead a baby to enter the NICU after birth. Some babies may enter because of prematurity, low birth weight, or complications during delivery. Other babies may have a medical emergency or a congenital disability that needs immediate treatment or monitoring by a NICU team. Table 10–5 lists a variety of medical conditions and definitions seen in NICU and the possible role of the occupational therapist in working with these babies. This table divides diagnoses into orthopedic, gastrointestinal, respiratory, sensory, neurological, and genetic disorders. Infectious complications and cardiac problems are also discussed. The reader is encouraged to read additional and more detailed information about the medical needs of babies in NICU.

## ▮▮▮ FROM THE BOOKSHELF

FOR THERAPISTS TO LEARN ABOUT MEDICAL CONDITIONS IN NICU
Hunter, J., Mullen, J., & Vergara, D. (1994). Medical considerations and practice guidelines for the neonatal occupational therapist. *American Journal of Occupational Therapy, 48*(6), 546–559.
Semmler, C. (Ed.) (1989). *A guide to care & management of very low birth weight infants.* Tucson, Arizona: Therapy Skill Builders.
Semmler, C., & Hunter, J. (1990). *Early occupational therapy intervention: Neonates to three years.* Gaithersburg, MD: Aspen.
Vergara, E. (1993a, b). *Foundations for practice in the neonatal intensive care unit and early intervention: A self-guided practice manual, vol. 1, 2.* Rockville, MD: American Occupational Therapy Association.

## ASSESSMENT AND INTERVENTION IN THE NICU

Perhaps even more than with other areas of occupational therapy, assessment of a baby in the NICU must be closely tied to intervention. Ideally the process is seamless, and the therapist works with the family and other team members to identify strengths and needs of the baby as they together develop a plan for intervention during subsequent interactions with the baby. Thus, in this section we will address assessment and intervention together.

Table 10–5 **Definitions of Health Complications in Neonates and Occupational Therapy Intervention**

| Diagnosis | Definition | Occupational Therapy Intervention |
|---|---|---|
| | **ORTHOPEDIC** | |
| Brachial plexus injuries | Temporary or permanent upper-extremity paralysis resulting from damage to brachial plexus during difficult birth. Nerve roots, trunks of plexus may be bruised, stretched, or torn | Prevention of more damage to the nerve structure, prevent contractures |
| Erb's palsy | Damage to nerve roots of C-5 and C-6. Best prognosis and most common; involvement of small hand muscles | Teach positioning and handling to protect limb, PROM, dressing, bathing, carrying, soft splint |
| Erb-Duchenne-Klumpke palsy | Damage to C-5 to T-1; breech extraction | " |
| Klumpke's palsy | Damage to C-8 to T-1 | " |
| Congenital dislocated hips | Genetic, mechanical, or hormonal factors to produce displaced or subluxed femoral heads | Consult with orthopedist about splinting and positioning harness; positioning equipment |
| Arthrogryposis multiplex congenita | Congenital curved joints with persistent flexor contractures; most common in all four limbs; muscle insertions may be displaced | Early and intensive casting, splinting, PROM to all joints; 4 times a day for 30 minutes |
| | **GASTROINTESTINAL** | |
| Gastroschisis | A protrusion of the large and/or small intestines outside of the body with no membrane covering. Often associated with intestinal malrotation. | Surgery is immediate; high risk for infection. Post-op positioning; sensory enrichment; nonnutrient stimulation; slow feeders due to GI absorption or motility problems. |
| Jejunal, dudodenal, or ileal stenosis or atresia | Specific portions of the intestine are narrowed, absent, or closed; 30% of duodenal cases have other major anomaly or chromosomal abnormality. | Nonnutrient oral stimulation prior to repair; sensory enrichment; self-calming techniques as these babies tend to be irritable. |
| Necrotizing enterocolitis (NEC) | In premature births, major cause of death when not | Gentle handling; positional options; sensory stimulation. |

|  | | |
|---|---|---|
|  | discovered in early stage. Intestinal immaturity; gastrointestinal tract mucosal injury; bacteria invades and causes ruptures and gangrenous intestines, which require surgery. | Environment changes; self-calming positions; nonnutrient stimulation. |
| Omphalocele | Ventral wall defect in the abdomen; viscera herniates into the base of umbilical cord; membrane covered | Gentle handling post surgery; enrichment; positional options to include weight bearing but not prone; oral stimulation. |
| Gastroseophageal reflux (GER) | Absent or delayed swallowing or choking; gargling noises shortly after feeding; frequent spit-ups; vomiting; cause unclear | Positioning with sling or seat to support baby at top of crib at a 60 degree angle; slow or smaller feedings held at 90 degrees; some thickened formula; encourage use of pacifier |

### RESPIRATORY

|  | | |
|---|---|---|
| Bronchopulmonary dysplasia (BPD) | Radiographic progression of lung changes with acute lung disease; prolonged assistive ventilation; injury from positive-pressure and prolonged high oxygen concentration that damages lung tissue; and scarring that obstructs exchange of oxygen and carbon dioxide. | State control; self-calming; early oral stimulation; positioning; sensory enrichment; developmental follow-up. |
| Extracorporeal membrane oxygenation (ECMO) | Sophisticated life support using modified cardiopulmonary bypass to rest the lungs; minimizes complications of barotrauma for respiratory failure. | Positioning gel pad for skin integrity; nonnutrient stimulation; tactile stroking; PROM to all limbs; follow-up. |
| Meconimum aspiration syndrome (MAS) | Aspiration of meconium into the tracheobronchial tree; intrauterine stress causes early passage of meconium. | Nonnutrient stimulation; slow-paced feeding. |
| Apnea | Respiratory pause for more than 15–20 seconds; cause is CNS immaturity; damage is obstructive and there is often infection or illness. | Positioning, feeding safety, graded sensory stimulation, State control, low endurance, sensitive to environmental overload. |

*continued on following page*

Table 10–5—*continued*

| Diagnosis | Definition | Occupational Therapy Intervention |
|---|---|---|
| | **SENSORY** | |
| Hearing loss | Reported in 2–10% of infants weighing less than 1500 grams; infections; asphyxia; malformations; specific medications | Hearing screening; sensory stimulation; environmental control; parent teaching |
| Retinopathy of prematurity (ROP) | Increase or injury to the blood vessels of the retina; abnormal vascular formation | Low light; stimulation; contrasting colors and flashing lights (if no seizure history) |
| | **NEUROLOGICAL** | |
| Hypoxic-ischemic encephalopathy (HIE) | Perinatal asphyxia; hypotonia; seizures; lethargy; incomplete reflexes; fetal distress; prognosis depends on duration of asphyxia. | Minimal stimulation protocol; PROM; tactile stimulation; positional support; oral stimulation. |
| Hydrocephalus | Abnormal collection of cerebral spinal fluids (CSF); obstruction or stenosis in ventricles occluding CSF flow; causes dilation and abnormal head growth; usually a shunt is placed in the ventricle to drain CSF. | Gel pad for head if shunted; low lights; feeding precautions; sensory processing delays; positioning. |
| Periventricular leukomalacia (PVL) | Scarring; necrosis of white matter around the ventricles; cystic formation seen on ultrasound; may result in cerebral palsy or developmental delay. | Positioning; oral stimulation; graded sensory stimulation; guarded feeding prognosis; working on self-calming techniques. |
| Intraventricular hemorrhage (IVH) | Bleeding into the cerebral ventricles and surrounding brain tissue; occurs within first 24 hours after birth of babies born prematurely. | Special seating; car seat or car bed adaptations; cautious oral stimulation; feeding and aspiration precautions; low sensory diet; adapt environment; splinting, infant massage; close follow-up. |
| | Grade I—germinal matrix bleed. Grade II—intraventricular bleed without dilation. | |

Grade III—intraventricular bleed with ventricle dilation or hydrocephalus; 80% have developmental delays.
Grade IV—intraventricular and intraparenchymal bleeding; shunt placement is typical; 90% have severe delays; hydrocephalus typical.

### INFECTIOUS COMPLICATIONS

| | | |
|---|---|---|
| Sepsis | Early onset; first 5 days; generalized infection in the blood; it can localize and produce osteomyelitis or meningitis. | Be cautious of handling; universal precautions; temperature instability; maintain optimal thermal environment so there is no heat loss. |
| Bacterial sepsis | Spreads. | " |
| Group B/Streptococci | Difficult to treat; serious; 10–20% mortality. | " |
| CMV (cytomegalovirus) | Herpes virus passed from the mother; 90% subclinical signs; liver enlargement; jaundice; intrauterine growth retardation (IUGR); microcephaly. | " |
| Herpes | Acquired in utero; birth; after birth can spread or localize. | " |
| Rubella | Viral infection to fetus if Mom acquired before 12–16 weeks of pregnancy; cataracts; deafness; heart defects; seizures; mental retardation. | " |
| Acquired Immune Deficiency Syndrome (AIDS) | Virus attacks body's immune system via contact with maternal blood; breast milk; 50% symptomatic 1st yr.; 4–6 months; 75–80% die by 2 yrs if AIDS (not HIV+). Thrush; failure to thrive; sepsis; renal disease; CNS dysfunction; developmental delay or losses. | " |

*continued on following page*

Table 10–5—*continued*

| Diagnosis | Definition | Occupational Therapy Intervention |
|---|---|---|
| Anemia | Low hemoglobin count with reduced red blood cells; pale; bruising; inactive and lethargic; tachypnea and tachycardia; congestive heart failure (CHF) | " |

### CARDIAC COMPLICATIONS

| Diagnosis | Definition | Occupational Therapy Intervention |
|---|---|---|
| Patent ductus arteriosus (PDA) | Failure of the duct to close at birth in babies born prematurely; confirmed by murmur, ECG; fluid overflow and hypoxic episodes | Monitor; duct usually closes with medication or surgery. |
| Coarctation of aorta | Narrowing or malformation of the aorta; causing blood pressure problems and cyanosis | Feeding adaptations; positioning needs; nonnutrient stimulation; cluster care; environmental control. |
| Tetrology of Fallot | A group of defects; large ventricular septal defect (VSD) and pulmonary stenosis; right ventricular hypertrophy; hypoxic episodes of increasing cyanosis; crying; failure to thrive (FTT) | Nonnutrient vs. nutrient feeding; low stimulation; positioning; cluster care to perform procedures |

### GENETIC DISORDERS

| Diagnosis | Definition | Occupational Therapy Intervention |
|---|---|---|
| Trisomy 21 (Down syndrome) | Congenital heart; hypotonia; flat face; simian crease; slanted eye folds; unstable atlanto-odontoid joint; frequent ear infections; mental retardation | Positioning; sensory enrichment; oral stimulation; feeding adaptions; parent teaching and intervention; follow-up; splinting; PROM; positioning; car-bed fitting; cluster care |
| Trisomy 18 | Hands fisted and feet deformed; small jaws, all tube-fed, FTT, micro-cephaly; mental retardation; 10% survive 1st year | " |
| Cornelia De Lange syndrome | Facial abnormalities; severe prenatal growth; micromelia; high arched palates; projective vomiting; failure to thrive, IQ less than 50 | Reflux positioning; oral stimulation; sensory diet modified; intervention follow-up |

| | | |
|---|---|---|
| Pierre Robin sequence | Tongue obstructs airway; micrognathia; cleft palate; respiratory and feeding problems; severe hypotonia; retracted tongue; glossoptosis | Prone bed adaption; positioning; special bottles; sensory stimulation; infant intervention |
| Cleft lip or palate | Occurs by 8th week of gestation; failure of upper lip and/or central closure of palate. Cleft palate varying degree of surgery and speech difficulties; recurrent otitis media | Feeding abilities needing special bottles, techniques, parent teaching, coordination of other medical follow-ups; plastics; genetics; breastfeeding potential |

*Source:* Compiled from: Hunter (1996b); Hunter, Mullen, & Vergara (1994); Semmler (1989); Semmler & Hunter (1990); and Vergara (1993a, b)

## ASSESSMENT PROCESS

There is no set procedure for assessing babies in the NICU. Many factors influence what assessments are appropriate and possible for the baby. Medical stability may be the most critical factor to consider when beginning an assessment, as it will determine the amount of handling and extent of disturbance the baby will be able to tolerate during an assessment. For example, an unstable baby cannot tolerate much handling without compromising physiological stability, whereas stable babies can tolerate a more thorough assessment with handling. When the baby is unstable, the OT may begin the assessment process by evaluating equipment needs and availability, as well as the environmental strengths and needs. These are critical factors for the high-risk baby, and an appropriate place to begin the process. In this way intervention can be begun without needing to disturb the baby for direct assessment.

When a hands-on assessment can be accomplished, the therapist must remember the PCA and chronological age of the baby. In addition, the therapist must know what can be reasonably expected of a baby at the different ages. Table 10–6 describes the typical behavior of a stable baby who is born prematurely, between PCA 26 and 38 weeks.

Before beginning an assessment or intervention, the therapist should use these general "developmental milestones" to determine what systems and skills need to be assessed or treated. For example, a baby born at 26 weeks PCA is not physiologically ready to respond to a light source, but at 32 weeks PCA, one would expect some response from the baby when stimulated with light. Additionally, a baby at 26 weeks PCA will have little or no ability to obtain an active alert state, but by 30 weeks, the baby may alternate between active and drowsy states.

Other factors, such as the time available for intervention, the reason for referral, the family needs, and the delineation of roles and expertise of team members (Vergara, 1993a), influence what areas are assessed. The following guidelines are suggested for assessing babies in NICU (Hunter, 1996b; Semmler & Hunter, 1990; Vergara, 1993a):

Table 10–6   **Typical Behaviors of Infants Born Prematurely**

| Behavior | 26 weeks | 28 weeks | 30 weeks | 32 weeks | 34 weeks | 36 weeks | 38 weeks |
|---|---|---|---|---|---|---|---|
| Movement patterns | Patterns Global hypotonia UE more active Occasional flexion/ extension of legs Isolated lateral head motion | Generalized hypotonia at rest No flexor recoil in UE No grasp with toes Tremors common No attempt to align head or body | Flexion in thighs Arms recoil Active movement more controlled No weight bearing on feet | Thighs and hips are flexed Some weight on feet Active motions more controlled Head-righting smoother Improved head control Increase in flexor motor tone | Hip flexion, frog leg posture UE grasp and traction maintained Resists PROM in knees Extends hips and knees in supported standing Movements are smoother | Wide variety of resting postures Flexion in all limbs and trunk Brisk leg recoil Resists knee extension Active wide movements | UEs recoil in 2–3 seconds Smooth, purposeful movements Extension dominates flexion Resists full extension of knee, hip, & shoulder |
| State control | Rapid eye movement Sleep in a restless mode Fleeting alert and drowsy times No energy for interaction | Brief wake periods More stupor, sleep Continuous tongue or mouth motions | Alert and drowsy states Easily stressed by environment Cries are prolonged and maintained | Active sleep decreases, quiet sleep increases Increased alert time Less irritable | Periods of quiet and active sleep Crying more frequent to pain or hunger Awakes to stimulation | Less random movements Slow and regular respirations | Quiet sleep increases Equal times for activity and sleep Longer periods of alertness All states are present |
| Feeding | | Gavage feeding | Hands to mouth beginning Suck and swallow coordination beginning | Begins breast and/or bottle feeding Hand to face orientation | Latches more on breast Hand-to-mouth movements Cries when hungry | Vigorous cry before feeding Established feeding routine | Lips tightly sealed; no spillage of liquid Sucking vigorously |

|  | 1 | 2 | 3 | 4 | 5 | 6 | 7 | 8 |
|---|---|---|---|---|---|---|---|---|
| *(feeding)* | | Unable to coordinate with breathing | | | Begins to coordinate suck, swallow, and breathing | | | Feeds every 3–4 hours Coordinates suck, swallow, and breathing |
| Sensory | Eyes open but no processing Ears flat and shapeless | Minimal response to light Poor visual acuity If vision too intense (focus), baby may have an apnea spell Touch and pain well differentiated Immediate response to touch Hearing; prefers Mom's voice; increased respirations Reflexive smile | Hearing well developed Not attentive to light source | May respond to light stimuli Some alerting responses Facial expressions to auditory stimuli May briefly focus | May orient to stimuli Visual fixates for 10 seconds Widens eyes to auditory input Horizontal tracking begins Less averse to touch | | Better ability to orient to sound Visually tracks in all directions Turns head to sound | Displays visual preferences Fixates 15 seconds Turns head to auditory stimulus |
| Reflexes | *Moro*—slight extension in UE; hands react *Rooting*— | *Moro*—UE no extension or abduction *Rooting*— | *Moro*—easily elicited and vigorous *Rooting*— | *Moro*—complete UE abduction and extension *Rooting*— | Same as 32 weeks | | *Moro*—complete and brisk *Rooting*— | *Moro*—perfect *Rooting*—perfect *Sucking*—like |

*continued on following page*

Table 10–6—continued

| Behavior | 26 weeks | 28 weeks | 30 weeks | 32 weeks | 34 weeks | 36 weeks | 38 weeks |
|---|---|---|---|---|---|---|---|
| | *Rooting*—slight yawn to side/upper lip | yawns not the lower lip | incomplete | complete and intense | | perfect, weak head turn | full-term baby |
| | *Sucking*—brief pattern | *Sucking*—chewing motion | *Sucking*—better synchrony | *Sucking*—active and good | | | |
| | *Gag*—absent | *Gag*—tongue protrusion | | *Gag*—fair quality and active | | *Gag*—better | |
| | *Palmar*—improved response | *Palmar*—localized | *Palmar*—in fingers and wrist | *Palmar*—stronger than traction | | *Palmar*—firm | |
| | *Doll's eyes*—absent | *Doll's eyes*—absent | *Doll's eyes*—absent | *Doll's eyes*—beginning | | *Doll's eyes*—present; head does not follow | *Doll's eyes*—present |
| | *Automatic walking*—trace | *Automatic walking*—improves | *Automatic walking*—improves | *Automatic walking*—tip-toes | | *Automatic walking*—present, but not sustained | *Automatic walking*—automatic, full weight support |

*Source:* Adapted from Creger (1989), Hunter (1992; 1996b); Semmler (1989).

- Assess as much as possible without disturbing the baby. Thus, it is essential to perform a thorough chart review (demographics, past and current medical status) and gather as much information from the nurses, other professionals, and family before beginning an assessment.
- Avoid duplicating assessments of other professionals and use teamwork to assess the baby; assess the environment during the assessment. This can be done without disturbing the baby and may be done at various times of the day, since the routine of the NICU changes with each hour.
- Assess what is necessary, not every aspect of neonatal development.
- Assess at an optimum time according to the baby's schedule (e.g., feeding, sleeping, routine medical care).
- Avoid handling the neonate as much as possible. Observation of the baby can be used to gather an abundance of information, and the baby need not be disturbed at all.
- Allow time for the baby to respond, because responses are often delayed.
- Know and monitor vital signs to pace the assessment (e.g., What is the baby's normal range for heart rate, oxygenation levels, breathing rate?)
- Recognize baby engagement and stress or disengagement cues. Keep in mind that although there are general cues to look for (e.g., gaze aversion, hiccups, gagging), each baby is unique and a behavioral sign of stress in one baby may not be a sign of stress in another baby. If possible, look for relationships between behavioral signs and vital sign changes during the assessment process.
- Involve parents in the process when possible and appropriate.
- Report results in terminology that other professionals and parents can understand.
- Find something positive to say about every baby you assess.

## INTERVENTION CONCEPTS

"The main goal of neonatal intervention is to optimize the baby's potential for development" (Vergara, 1996a, p. 121). This can best be done by the primary caregivers for the baby, generally the family. In addition, it is dependent upon the development of good caregiver-baby interaction, something that can prove to be a challenge for babies born prematurely or at risk because of other health concerns. Thus, intervention must be geared toward assisting caregivers where needed as they try to establish sound interaction skills with their baby. This process can be a tricky one because of the medical needs and fragility of the baby. Primary caregivers (parents) may in fact need information and need to learn the skills that will enable them to read and respond to their baby's cues. However, even parents who once believed themselves to be competent in their parenting skills may feel at a loss with a small, medically fragile baby. They may look to the therapist as the "expert." As tempting as this role may be to play, the therapist must give it back to the parent, helping them where needed, but often just supporting them as they adapt their own parenting skills to a new situation (Holloway, 1997). As we explore evaluation and intervention below, consider how you would give this information to a parent or primary caregiver.

As noted earlier, babies who are premature may be more sensitive to stimulation, depending on their age, illness, and individual personality. The immature brain and unstable homeostasis systems interfere with the baby's ability to respond to sensory input. The neonatal therapist needs to protect the immature baby from inappropriate stimulation that could compromise physiological stability. The baby's behavioral cues and his physiological reactions (e.g., heart and respiration rates, oxygenation levels) determine appropriate intervention. All input strives to minimize stimulation and is developmentally appropriate for the baby's age. Input is varied in many ways, such as the type, quantity, timing, patterning, amount, and quality of stimulation. The intervention is organized as part of a developmental plan and is coordinated with other caregivers in the NICU. It is ideal to plan your intervention for times when the neonate is

- Stable, not deprived of deep sleep
- Not fatigued by medical procedures
- More organized in states of alertness
- In a supportive, calm, and nurturing environment (Lester & Tronick, 1990).

Hunter (1996b) suggests the following key points for the new neonatal therapist to remember when working with a neonate in NICU: (1) consider the environmental factors and the baby's response to them; (2) let the baby's needs determine the timing and sequencing of input; (3) observe the baby's ongoing cues; (4) modify the pace and techniques of stimulation to facilitate stability; and (5) reassess movement and handling when signs of stress, avoidance, and withdrawal appear. Therapists constantly monitor the baby's state, physiological reactions, and the needs of the parents when planning treatment.

## EVALUATION AND INTERVENTION AREAS

There are many potential areas for assessment and intervention with the neonate who is in NICU. The environment, the baby's physiological state regulation, and interactive behavior with staff and parents are first and foremost. A large portion of the evaluation here can be done observationally, and as such it is an ideal place to begin. Given sufficient physiological stability, sensory, neuromuscular, motor, and feeding skills should be considered, as should positioning and handling. Finally, discharge planning and equipment needs for both the NICU and the home are assessed. We will look at each of these in turn.

### Environment

Assessing the NICU environment prior to even touching the baby helps the therapist understand what sensory stimulation is occurring for the baby. Hunter (1996b) advocates assessing the macro and the micro environment. In the macro environment, the entire physical layout of the NICU is considered:

noise level (e.g., talking, phones, alarms), lighting capabilities (e.g., all or none or individual lighting), crowdedness, and the amount of activity occurring within the room. For example, if the NICU is at full capacity and there are two or three critically ill babies who require numerous procedures or resuscitations, the room's activity is increased and the stress level of nursing may be high (Hunter, 1996b). These conditions are noted on an assessment as they may affect the baby's ability to interact with the therapist or family.

In the micro environment, note specifically where the baby is placed in the isolette or crib. Is the isolette near the nurses' station, the door, the window, the telephones, or other babies who have many medical procedures or self-regulatory problems? Can the baby be shielded from the light and sound intrusions? Within the isolette, are there positioning aids available, and what is the visual environment like for the baby inside? Are there pictures or items from home and are there too many or too little of them? By assessing and modifying the NICU environment first, a more accurate assessment of other aspects of baby skill can be performed.

Intervention for environmental issues will require a team effort. Although the therapist may be able to assess the environment and make suggestions, the primary care staff will be responsible for carrying out any suggested modifications. As such, it is critical to have an interactive team work together on environmental issues. Refer back to Table 10–3 for examples of how to modify the sensory environment.

## Infant State and Interactive Behaviors

Als, Lester, Tronick, and Brazelton (1982) developed a conceptual framework to assess the behavior of babies who are premature. Their framework is divided into five developmental subsystems: physiological or autonomic responses, motor responses, state control, attention and interactional behavior, and self-regulation. Tables 10–7 and Table 10–8 use the subsystems defined by Als and colleagues to describe baby engagement and disengagement behaviors.

Table 10–7    **Infant Signs of Attention and Self-Regulation That Allow Engagement**

| Attentional or Interaction Signs | Self-Regulatory Behaviors |
|---|---|
| Smiling | Visual looking |
| Mouthing | Sucking |
| Cooing | Hand to face or mouth |
| Relaxed face | Grasping |
| "OOh face" | Fisting |
| Relaxed limbs | Hand clasp |
| Minimal motor movement | Foot clasp |
| Smooth movements | Leg bracing |
| Alertness | Postural change |
| | Pushing or bracing against the crib |
| | Flexing all extremities and trunk |
| | Shifting to lower states (light sleep or drowsy) |

*Source:* Adapted from Gardner et al. (1993); Vergara (1993a).

Table 10–8  **Infant Signs of Stress That May Cause Disengagement**

| Autonomic Signs | Motor Signs | State Signs |
|---|---|---|
| Color changes (mottling, flushing, blueness, paleness) | Hypotonia | Gaze aversion |
| | Flailing movements | Glassy eyes |
| | Trunk arching | Staring |
| | Hyperextension of extremities | Irritability |
| | Frantic, disorganized movements | Panicked look |
| Changes in vital signs (heart rate, respiratory rate, blood pressure, oxygen saturation) | Squirming movements | Twitching |
| | Posturing (salute, sitting in air, airplane) | Grimacing |
| | | Deep sleep |
| | Finger splaying | Diffuse sleep states |
| | Tongue thrusting | Lack of alertness |
| Vomiting | | |
| Gagging | | |
| Hiccups | | |
| Flatus | | |
| Diarrhea | | |
| Sneezing | | |
| Yawning | | |
| Burping | | |

*Source:* Adapted from Als (1982); Als et al. (1982); Brazelton (1984); Gardner et al. (1993); and Vergara (1993a).

When parents and professionals are aware of these behaviors, they are able to adjust how they respond to their baby, and they can learn how to develop reciprocity in the interaction cycle.

## ▄▌▐ FROM THE BOOKSHELF

The following books have excellent pictures of engagement and disengagement signals to educate parents and staff:

Creger, P. J. (Ed). (1989.) *Developmental interventions for preterm and high-risk infants. Self study modules for professionals.* Tucson: Therapy Skill Builders.

Harrison, H. & Kositsky, A. (1983). *The premature baby book: A parents' guide to coping and caring in the first years.* Tucson: Therapy Skill Builders.

Hussey, B. (1988). *Understanding my signals.* Palo Alto: VORT.

Semmler, C. (Ed.) (1989). *A guide to care & management of very low birth weight infants.* Tucson: Therapy Skill Builders.

Unlike the full-term baby, the baby who is premature may not develop these subsystems simultaneously, and she may demonstrate disorganized or stress behaviors. Responses to input may be inconsistent and require systematic observations of the baby over a period of time. Parents and all professionals working with these babies need to learn the engagement and disengagement signals of the individual baby in order to modify their own behaviors or the environment. These modifications help the baby become more self-regulated and willing to engage in interaction. Self-regulatory behaviors help a baby maintain or develop equilibrium. This can be challenging, since some reported behaviors of stress may not indicate disorganization and/or stress in all babies.

Interventions are focused on avoiding stress-related events and facilitating self-regulation and engagement in the baby. How self-regulation and engagement are facilitated will depend on the baby, but some guidelines can be garnered from available literature. Generally you will want to contain the baby to reduce extraneous motor activity. This may involve swaddling, or perhaps containment props within a crib or isolette. This will be discussed more below when we address positioning of the baby. The therapist will also want to determine what sensory channels lead to stress reactions in the baby, and what leads to attention and orientation (Brazelton, 1984). Typically, fragile babies cannot address multiple input channels simultaneously and self-regulate, so often the therapist will be using just touch, or just a calm voice, or just slow movement to aid a baby in organizing his or her behavior. Specifics on these issues will be addressed below as well. Numerous studies have shown an increased weight gain, a lower incidence of medical complications, improved developmental outcomes, and shorter hospital stays for babies who have learned self-regulatory behaviors (Als et al., 1994).

Neonatal arousal or consciousness is generally classified into six major behavioral states (Als, 1982; Brazelton, 1984; Gardner et al., 1993). The baby's state can affect his responses to the environment or stimuli, his feeding abilities, and his motor skills. The definitions of these states are outlined in Table 10–9.

When assessing the baby's state, it is important to document what events occurred prior to, during, and after the observation. Observations take place while the baby is lying in the incubator or during medical procedures, feeding, or during times the parent or professional is interacting or playing with the baby. The baby's ability to move between states (e.g., range, quality, and frequency) is noted, as well as the baby's sleep-wake cycle (Brazelton, 1984). the baby's overall irritability and the physiological cost to the baby when moving between states also is noted (Vergara, 1993a). Smooth transitions between states usually demonstrate neurological maturation and integrity (Hunter, 1996b), but this is usually not expected until a baby's PCA is more than 36 weeks. Aside from PCA, state control may be affected by the baby's medical condition or the environment. For example, babies exposed to alcohol and other toxic substances in utero may have disorganized state control or have greater difficulty attaining a state that permits environmental investigation and interaction.

---

### ■ *THERAPEDS POINTER*

**Physiological Cost**
Stress behaviors are often reflected physiologically by increased heart rate, increased respiration rate, lowered blood oxygen saturation, and higher caloric expenditure. These physiologic mechanisms "cost" the baby energy. The end result of higher physiological costs is slower weight gain, potentially more medical complications, and consequently more hospital time for the baby.

---

Table 10–9 **Newborn States and Behaviors**

| Newborn States | State Level | Behaviors |
|---|---|---|
| Sleep states | State 1: Deep sleep | • Sleeping with regular breathing<br>• Facial expressions are relaxed<br>• Closed eyelids without movement underneath<br>• Activity is not present<br>• Arousal is difficult<br>• Slow changes between states |
| | State 2: Light sleep | • Closed eyelids, movement underneath<br>• Irregular breathing<br>• Low activity level<br>• Startles, moves randomly<br>• Sucks intermittently |
| Transitional state | State 3: Drowsy, semidozing | • Eyelids opened or closed<br>• Fluttering eyelids or heavy lids<br>• Rapid and shallow respirations<br>• Startles intermittently<br>• Fussing possible<br>• Response to sensory stimuli delayed<br>• Changes states smoothly to sleep or alert |
| Awake states | State 4: Quiet alert (Best time for interaction) | • Bright eyes, opened intermittently<br>• Focus on stimuli source<br>• Motor activity minimal<br>• Appears to process information |
| | State 5: Alert | • Eyes opened or not opened<br>• Awake and aroused<br>• Motor activity increased<br>• Increased tonus<br>• Signs of discomfort (e.g., grimace, facial expressions, postures)<br>• Diffuse fussing but not crying |
| | State 6: Crying | • Intense crying<br>• Rhythmic, strong crying *or*<br>• Sounds of crying are absent, weak, or strained<br>• Grimace or cry face<br>• Respirations shallow, irregular<br>• Difficult to distract infant and disrupt crying |

*Source:* Compiled from Als et al. (1994); Brazelton (1984); and Gardner et al. (1993).

## *Sensory*

When a baby is physiologically stable, the baby's response to sensory stimuli is recorded during assessment and intervention. As stated earlier, there is no set protocol on how to proceed with assessment and intervention of the sensory systems. Each individual baby needs to be observed to determine her responses to and need for sensory activities. Vergara (1993a) states that sensory systems are assessed separately in the following developmental sequence: tactile, proprioceptive, and vestibular (underlying senses); then auditory and visual. Brazelton's assessment of neonates evaluates the baby's orientation, reactivity, and habituation to the stimuli (Brazelton, 1984). Orientation is the baby's ability to locate the source of the stimuli by turning his head, gazing toward, or moving toward the source. Reactivity refers to how the baby responds to the various types of stimuli presented by the therapist. Does the baby react and how? Does she cry, grimace, blink, or ignore the stimuli? Optimally, reactivity is assessed when the baby is in a transitional or awake state. Habituation occurs when the response to a stimulus diminishes over time until the stimulus has no significance to the baby. During this time, we see an initial orientation to the stimulus, and a gradual inhibition of the orienting response, or a blocking out of irrelevant stimuli (Brazelton, 1984).

When assessing and treating babies, sensory stimuli are presented one at a time and enough time is given to allow the baby to respond. The therapist also watches for signs of stress that may occur within 5 or 10 minutes after the activity (Hunter, 1996b). Later, multiple sensory stimuli, usually tactile or vestibular paired with visual or auditory, may be given while noting the baby's response to this procedure. If possible, this is done immediately prior to nursing or medical procedure when the baby is going to awakened anyhow.

---

■ *THERAPEDS POINTER*

**The NICU Assessment Kit**
Essential elements in your testing kit for NICU: tactile gloves, bell, variety of rattles with different sounds and handles, brightly colored disks, flashlight, red ball, and a soft powder puff.

---

Orientation to *tactile* input may be determined using light stroking, deep touch or massage, or cuddling the baby against the body. Light stroking may lead to increased arousal, but in typical babies it does not cause alarm. Deep touch, massage, and cuddling are viewed as calming inputs, used to help the baby to relax or become more organized. The therapist assesses the baby's responses as positive (e.g., self-calms, alerts, or increased physiological stability) or negative (e.g., avoids touch, cries, appears to not feel the touch, or has physiological alterations). In addition, the therapist can offer input on different body parts (e.g., the back, the tummy, the arms or legs) and determine where on the body and which type of touch appears to be more calming for a particular baby. In general, as the CNS matures, the baby has more positive responses, especially to tactile stimuli generally viewed as calming, and fewer avoidance reactions (Vergara, 1993a). Babies who are born prematurely search for boundaries and tactile confinement, which is lost at birth. The baby is unable to explore her body because of decreased active postural tone and reduced spontaneous movement. Medications and limb restraints may prevent movement exploration of the body as well as the macro and micro NICU environment. Intervention then may include the following:

- *Swaddling and nesting* to provide physical and tactile body containment
- *Stroking* done gently but firmly to prevent hypersensitive responses
- *Relaxing touch* applied slowly, firmly, and rhythmically

Touch can become adverse if applied too softly and too long or if fast touch is applied rapidly and intermittently. The caregiver tries to avoid tickling and stroking over the mouth, feet, palms, and genital areas.

---

### ■ *THERAPEDS POINTER*

**Tactile Treatment Ideas**
Nesting with soft fabrics, bendy bumpers, snuggles up, and blanket rolls to keep the baby in a more flexed posture which helps him feel more secure. Machine-washable sheepskin, powder puffs, soft stuffed animals, baby massage, and skin-to-skin/kangaroo care also offer the baby tactile input which is generally viewed as calming and leading to better behavioral organization (Vergara, 1993a).

---

During the intrauterine experience, the baby is used to vestibular stimulation from movement in the amniotic fluid. *Vestibular* experiences can be powerful tools to change a baby's state so she is able to focus on the environment (Vergara, 1993a). To assess the baby's reactivity to the vestibular system, note responses to movement when changing positions in the incubator or when being held, changed, or carried.

- Do positional changes increase the baby's level of arousal?
- Does he cry or widen his eyes with changes from a horizontal to a vertical position?
- Does slow rocking, walking, or holding the baby over the shoulder help her become more self-regulated?
- What position and type of vestibular stimulation is most favorable to the baby?

Generally, positional changes increase the baby's level of arousal, and most babies do not find them disturbing. Rocking and walking are also typically calming. Sometimes hammocks in the crib, oscillating waterbeds, or gel mats provide the vestibular stimulation needed to help calm an irritable baby and help him become more self-regulated. These devices need to be chosen cautiously as they may increase or decrease physiological stress for the baby.

*Proprioceptive* stimulation occurs when the baby is handled by a caregiver. *Handling* occurs when a caregiver moves or touches the baby while providing routine case. Slow-motion and gentle touch when diapering, carrying, lifting, bathing, feeding, and dressing are often recommended. The therapist and caregiver must avoid sudden and abrupt motions that would startle the neonate and may cause physiological stress in the heart rate, respiration rate, oxygenation, and color (Semmler, 1990). The basic principles for handling are:

1. Minimize the contact or reposition to help comfort the baby and maintain his calm level of energy.

2. Observe the baby's reaction to being handled and note any physiological changes
3. Hold the baby's limbs close to the body and in flexion to help calm her.
4. Provide slow, gentle motions to help the baby maintain his state of control and stability.
5. Apply normal sensory motor experiences during routine care by supporting the baby and giving distal control (Creger, 1989).

When handling a baby who is medically fragile, it is important to remember some basic principles. The baby's head is to be fully supported and close to midline with the neck in a neutral or slightly flexed position. This allows the baby to be able to see what is going on in the environment and discourages neck or whole body extension. If the trunk and hips are kept slightly flexed and the shoulders in protraction and forward, the hands will be in midline where the baby can see them and perhaps use them. When lifting a baby from supine, keep the shoulders forward, head in midline, hips in flexion, and then lift slowly. In prone, keep the baby's hands on her stomach, head supported and trunk resting on your forearm and her legs flexed. Handling and holding a baby who is critically ill or premature takes practice. It is recommended that everyone first practice on a well baby before working with the baby in NICU.

Carrying a baby may be done with the baby on your shoulder. In this position your hand is under the baby's buttocks, his back and shoulders are rounded, and his legs tucked as he curls in toward your body (Fig. 10–1). Carrying can also be done with the baby facing away from you. In this position the baby's lower back is rounded, her arms are folded on her chest, and your hands are supporting her buttocks and legs in flexion (Fig. 10–2). When carrying the baby in your arms, the baby's shoulders should be rounded forward, his head in midline, and his legs bent. In this position the baby looks as though he is in a nest (Fig. 10–3).

To diaper the baby, gently roll the baby to the side and place the diaper under her. Alternatively, you can flex one leg at the hip, leaving the other leg extended while placing the diaper under him. While dressing the baby, use your hand to go inside the arms or leg sleeves and gently guide the baby's foot or hand through the sleeve. Creger (1989) has beautiful clear baby photos demonstrating these techniques in his book. The baby is more content and stable when she is handled in the same manner for all her care and not stressed by rapid and abrupt movements.

Once a baby is mature enough to handle tactile, proprioceptive, and vestibular stimulation, auditory and visual sensory systems can be assessed. In a noisy NICU environment, auditory awareness may be diminished. *Auditory* stimulation such as heartbeats and other soothing sounds similar to the intrauterine environment can be calming to a baby. Vergara (1993a) suggests that auditory sounds paired with tactile containment may be the best way to calm an irritable baby. Orientation to auditory stimuli is tested when a baby is presented with a shaking rattle or other noise on the right or left side of his head. The therapist sees if the baby is aware of the sound. Can he locate the source of the sound (orientation), and what is his reaction to the sound? The following questions may be asked:

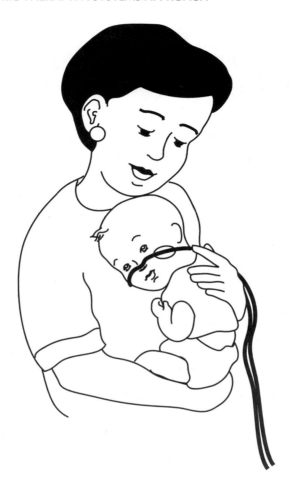

Figure 10–1 Carrying the premature infant nestled on your chest. (Adapted from the Therapy Skill Builders neonatal pictures series.)

- Does she turn toward a rattle, or, if Mom is talking to the baby, does she look up at her?
- Do sounds startle the baby?
- What type of noise is calming to him and what is alerting (e.g., voices, singing, music, phones, alarms)?

For the baby with possible auditory losses (e.g., weighing less than 1500 grams, intraventricular hemmorhage, rubella exposure, or cytomegalovirus infection), this evaluation may need to be modified. It is helpful if the therapist has a variety of sound toys to try to elicit a response. Various sizes of bells, rattles, squeak toys, and musical toys produce an array of sounds that may be heard by the baby with a hearing loss. Therapists also observe the baby's responses to noises within the environment.

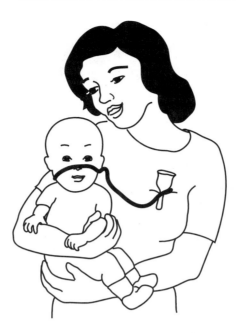

Figure 10–2 Carrying the baby facing away from you. (Adapted from the Therapy Skill Builders neonatal pictures series.)

When the baby is physiologically stable and term age, habituation to sounds may be tested. The therapist may ring a bell or rattle by the baby's ears and note the baby's response after ten trials of bell ringing (e.g., startle, eye movement, squirming, facial expressions). After the first few trials, a typical response is orientation, followed by the inhibition of this response. In the NICU, the therapist observes if the baby can block or tune out the stimuli, and notes the number of trials it takes to accomplish the habituation. Did the motor activity or heart rate or respirations decrease or increase? The baby who is premature may have a decrease in motor activity but an increased heart rate that does not diminish over trials. Therefore, therapists should be cautious about sensory input with such babies. Elevated heart rates use energy and calories, and they are physiologically costly (Vergara, 1993a). If a baby is unable to habituate and responds to all stimuli at the same or increased level of intensity, environmental modifications and parental teaching are indicated. If parents can learn about their baby's sensory preferences, they can modify home environments to be more comfortable for the baby. For example, if a baby is extremely sensitive to sound, the bedroom of choice for this baby may be far away from the kitchen or family room where noise is usually high.

At 32 to 33 weeks PCA, babies can *visually* focus but this may not be beneficial. Focusing may increase stress or may become obligatory because the baby cannot stop focusing (Glass, 1993; Hunter, 1996b). At about 36 weeks, you may assess the baby's ability to focus on the caregiver's face. How long does she focus and is there a physiological cost for focusing? When intro-

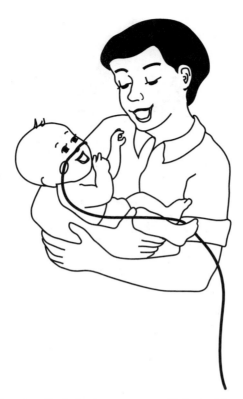

Figure 10–3 Carrying the baby in your arms. (Adapted from the Therapy Skill Builders neonatal pictures series.)

ducing inanimate objects, place them 6 to 9 inches from the baby's face and have the caregiver's face out of the baby's visual field (Vergara, 1993a). Glass (1993) suggests using three-dimensional objects with simple forms and not high-contrast colors. When placing visually stimulating objects (e.g., mirror, mobiles, toys, pictures) in the isolette or crib, be sure the baby can escape from the stimulus. Glass further recommends covering isolettes with plain fabrics facing the baby to avoid overstimulation.

Parents and caregiving staff need to be made aware of the baby's visual preferences. By knowing how visual stimuli affect the baby, caregivers can adapt their behaviors to get the best response from the baby. For example, if a baby has a difficult time breaking a gaze from an object, placement of the object in the isolette in relation to the baby's position and ability to move must be considered. Babies who have been exposed to rubella, who have Down syndrome, or retinopathy of prematurity may need some environmental adaptations to help them use their residual vision. For example, the therapist may do one or all of the following: lower the light level of the room, use flashlights with colored cellophane, provide toys and mobiles with bright contrasting colors or black-and-white images. If the baby is physiologically ready, pairing the visual stimuli with vestibular or tactile inputs may also be helpful.

Some babies may habituate to the visually stimulating NICU, and they may need assistance in learning how to focus on one object or face. Once the baby is able to focus, he may visually be able to track people or objects (approximately 36 to 38 weeks PCA). Vergara (1993a) cautions therapists to avoid stimulating sensory processing abilities in an immature baby, because this may be detrimental to the baby's cognitive and perceptual development.

## *Neuromuscular*

While observing and handling the baby, the therapist determines the baby's reflex development, muscle tone, range of motion, postural control, and soft-tissue integrity. Therapists test for the presence or absence of reflexes according to the baby's PCA. An assessment describes the response to the stimulus (e.g., quality; timing, quick/delayed; symmetrical/asymmetrical) and determines if the reflexes interfere with function (Borland, 1989). Most reflexes are elicited by PCA of 36 weeks. While the baby is resting or moving, the tone in his head, trunk, arms, and legs is noted. Is the tone high or low and are there asymmetries? Babies born prematurely often have not developed physiological flexion, which develops the last trimester of pregnancy. Since premature muscle tone develops in caudocephalic direction (feet to head), flexor tone gradually develops in the lower extremities and progresses to the upper extremities. Even at term age, the baby born prematurely does not have the same flexor tone quality as the full-term newborn (Hunter, 1996b).

Hypotonia is common in neonates born before 32 weeks and interferes with the development of physiological flexion. Babies in the NICU are often placed supine for extended periods of time because of ventilators, oxyhoods, or their critical medical status (e.g., those with respiratory distress syndrome or bronchopulmonary dysplasia or those on extracorporeal membrane oxygenation [ECMO]). When in supine, flexion must be accomplished against the resistance of gravity, which is extremely difficult for the baby born prematurely. Since the baby cannot move against gravity, he lies in an extended posture pressing against the supportive surface in search of containment. The frog leg posture or "M" position of the legs and the "W" posture of the arms develops from the prolonged extension, lack of neck and trunk coactivation, and the difficulty these babies experience in attempting to flex against gravity (Vergara, 1993a).

Passive and active ROM in the neck and extremities, and especially the hands or feet are assessed. Again, the PCA of the baby or the baby's diagnosis (e.g., intraventricular hemorrhage [IVH], brachial plexus injuries, hip dislocations, Down syndrome, arthrogryposis) may determine how much or how little flexibility is available. For example, a typical baby born at 27 to 28 weeks PCA will have full if not hyperextensive passive ROM without resistance. But a baby born with arthrogryposis may have flexor contractures that are almost fixed. Therefore, therapists need to be aware of the baby's condition before performing ROM.

Postures are noted when the baby is asleep or awake. Does she have any fixed postures? What type of head and trunk control does the baby have and does he have enough stability to be able to interact with the environment when he is awake? For most babies seen in NICU, postural control is limited and external positioning devices are needed.

The baby in the NICU may have many attachments to her body (e.g., intravenous fluids, leads from monitors, splints, dressings, and positioning aids) and may move more or less than typically developing babies. The skin of the baby who is premature or LBW may be very translucent and thin, and thus susceptible to break down. Therefore, it is important to evaluate the baby's soft tissue integrity. Are there red spots or any places where the skin is being sheared? Are there any potential areas that may need to be protected or ROM is contraindicated (e.g., babies with Erb's palsy, brachial plexus injuries, hip dislocations, chemical rickets, or those who are taking the drug Lasix [furosemide]).

The baby's movement with gravity eliminated and against gravity is evaluated. Is the movement smooth or jerky and is there a balance of flexion and extension? Can the baby get his hands to his face? Can she reach out and use a primitive grasp? Again, the PCA will help one to know when the baby is capable of doing these tasks. In general, movements develop in the following sequence: random, uncoordinated movements; reflexive movements; reciprocal movements; and then a wide variety of purposeful movements that are executed smoothly (Creger, 1989).

## *Positioning*

The position of the baby is assessed in the incubator or crib, or in the baby seat, tub seat, high chair, stroller, or car seat if they are being used in the NICU environment. When the baby is at rest, the therapist assesses his position to determine if the baby can interact with his environment visually as well as motorically. The therapist questions if the baby is in any position that could lead to deformities (e.g., subluxations, head flattening, or contractures) after a period of time or a position that may be dangerous for the baby (e.g., cannot clear an airway while in prone, or interference of equipment).

The baby in NICU may be extended with little flexion in her body, and she may have minimal voluntary movement to change her position. The baby's attachment to life-saving machines (e.g., ventilators, ECMO machines) may also limit the baby's movement or the variety of positions available. After carefully assessing the baby's favorite position as well as his ability to assume a variety of positions, equipment may be ordered with collaboration with parents and nursing. Positioning a newborn baby properly is essential to prevent postural abnormalities, to stimulate positive sensory motor input during hours spent without physical contact, and to enhance the baby's behavioral response to his environment. The most common postural deformities seen in babies spending time in the NICU are progressive flattening of the head into a narrow and elongated "preemie shape" head (doliocephaly); external rotation deformities of the limbs (e.g., the "W" posture of the upper extremities, and the "M" posture or frog-leg posture of the lower extremities); external torsion or rotation of the tibia; and decreased depth of the rib cage (Hunter, 1992).

Intervention will vary depending upon the medical equipment, medical restrictions, and neonate's physiological stability. Therapeutic positioning goals are far-reaching, and include the following (Creger, 1989):

- Promote newborn flexion.
- Facilitate midline orientation.
- Facilitate symmetrical positioning.

- Enhance self quieting and behavioral organization.
- Prevent bony deformities.
- Minimize muscle imbalance.
- Maintain skin integrity.
- Provide vestibular input.
- Enhance proprioceptive input to the body.
- Provide security and containment.
- Facilitate relaxation.
- Improve digestion.
- Assist in temperature regulation.
- Provide a variety of well supported positions.

A variety of positions are assessed and how each affects the baby is noted. Success is measured by watching the monitors, observing the baby reactions in the position for at least 30 minutes, and providing the least-restrictive space for comfort and control (Case, 1985). As an OT, positioning strategies are used to enhance behavioral and developmental learning. For example, while in prone, a diaper roll placed under the hips encourages flexion and reduces abduction of the hips (Fig. 10–4), while a blanket roll around the body helps swaddle the baby to help him feel more secure and contained (Fig. 10–5). A diaper roll lengthwise under the baby's body from chest to hips helps with security as well. In sidelying, a blanket roll behind the baby from shoulder to hips and another roll between her arms and legs help to keep the baby in the sidelying position to help her see and get her hands to midline (Fig. 10–6). In supine, nest the baby using three diaper rolls. Place two rolls under the shoulders and along each side to push the arms forward, and place one roll under the knees to break up the extension pattern. In supportive sitting, try to keep the body symmetrical with hips and knees flexed, shoulders forward, and the head in midline with slight flexion. To facilitate sitting, use a soft blanket roll under the knee and side rolls for lateral support (Creger, 1989). Table 10–10 gives the medical and developmental factors to consider when choosing positioning options.

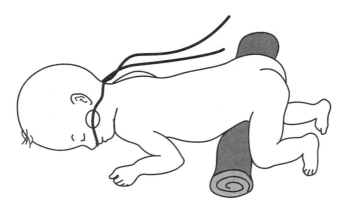

Figure 10–4 The diaper roll under the hips encourages flexion and reduces the hip abduction. (From the Denver Children's Hospital. Creger, P. J. [Ed]. [1989]. *Developmental interventions for preterm and high-risk infants: Self-study modules for professionals* [p. 109]. Tucson, AZ: Therapy Skill Builders.)

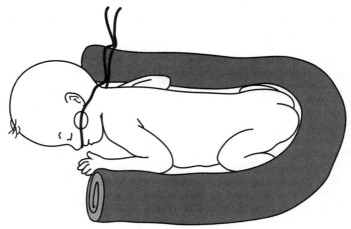

Figure 10–5 The blanket roll swaddles the baby to make him feel more secure. (From the Denver Children's Hospital. Creger, P. J. [Ed]. [1989]. *Developmental interventions for preterm and high-risk infants: Self-study modules for professionals* [p. 110]. Tucson, AZ: Therapy Skill Builders.)

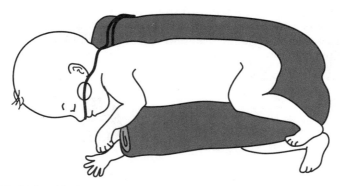

Figure 10–6 The side-lying position helps the baby to see his environment and to get his hands to midline. (From the Denver Children's Hospital. Creger, P. J. [Ed]. [1989]. *Developmental interventions for preterm and high-risk infants: Self-study modules for professionals* [p. 112]. Tucson, AZ: Therapy Skill Builders.)

Table 10–10 **Medical and Developmental Factors to Consider for Positioning Options**

| Medical Factors | Developmental Factors |
|---|---|
| | ***PRONE*** |

**Advantages**

Improved oxygenation and ventilation (despite increased total "work" of breathing) in infants with and without ventilatory support.[1,8,16,18,23]

Better gastric emptying than in supine or on left side (unless feeds pool regardless)[25]

Less reflux—especially if head of bed is elevated 30 degrees[3,19,20]

Decreased risk of aspiration[11]

Term and preterm infants sleep more and cry less when prone rather than supine[4,6]

Less energy expenditure when prone rather than supine[17]

Less sleep apnea in prone than in supine in term infants[12]

Best position to expose diaper rash to air or heat lamp

Facilitates development of flexor tone

Facilitates hand-to-mouth pattern for self-calming

Facilitates active neck extension and head raising

Improved coping with extrauterine environment (i.e., if sleep more, cry less)[4]

May decrease persistent head turning to the right and skull asymmetry

**Disadvantages**

Access for medical care is more difficult

Agitated or active infant may self-extubate

Visual exploration more difficult for baby

Face-to-face social contact more difficult

***SUPINE***

**Advantages**

Easier access to infant for medical care

Supine (in hammock) increases sleep time for preterm infants (vs. "flat" supine)[5]

Easier visual exploration by infant

Supine (in hammock) may facilitate midline position

Easier to position head in midline (than in prone)

**Disadvantages**

Decreased arterial oxygen tension, lung compliance, and tidal volume than in prone[1,16,23]

More reflux than in prone at any time, or than in upright sitting if infant is awake[19,20]

Greater risk of aspiration than in prone or right sidelying[11]

Term and preterm infants sleep less and cry more in supine than prone[4,6]

Supine hammock may decrease respiration if infant had decreased lung compliance (i.e., respiratory distress syndrome)[5]

Greater energy expenditure in supine than prone[17]

Encourages extension rather than flexion (increased muscle tone with hyperextension of head, neck, and shoulders)[2]

Encourages external rotation positional deformities of arms and legs (with later delayed hands-to-midline or out-toeing gait)

*continued on the following page*

Table 10–10—*continued*

| Medical Factors | Developmental Factors |
|---|---|
| | **SIDE-LYING** |

**Advantages**

Right side: better gastric emptying than in supine or left side-lying (about same as prone)[25]

Infant with unilateral lung disease has better oxygenation with good lung positioned uppermost[10]

Encourages midline orientation of head and extremities

Counteracts external rotation of limbs; promotes flexion and extremity adduction

Facilitates hand-to-mouth pattern for self-calming

Facilitates hand-to-hand activity

**Disadvantages**

Left side: decreased gastric emptying than in prone or right side-lying[25]

May be difficult to maintain flexed position with irritable or hypertonic extended infant

**SITTING**

**Advantages**

Alternative position (for variety and skin integrity)

Upright is an alerting posture

Encourages infant visual exploration

Encourages social interaction

May allow use of swing for older neonatal intensive care unit infants

May help temporarily "break up" (relax) high tone

**Disadvantages**

Infant seat or car seat elevated 60 degrees increased frequency and duration of reflux[20]

More upright (90 degrees) position increases heart rate and mean[22] arterial pressure in preterm infants

Semireclined position may decrease oxygen saturation in some preterm infants[24]

May be difficult to properly position baby without slumping or slouching of head and trunk[22]

**HEAD POSITION AND MIDLINE POSITION**

**Advantages**

Head in midline seems to decrease intracranial pressure/intraventricular hemorrhage[9]

Elevation of head of bed 30 degrees may reduce intracranial pressure[9]

Head in midline may improve head shape

Midline positioning reduces asymmetry and encourages development of flexion

Waterbeds (and water pillows) may reduce head flattening[7,13,15,21]

**Disadvantages**

May create pressure sore if too long on firm surface

Head midline positioning is difficult in prone

---

1. Alastair, A. H., Ross, K. R., & Russell, G. (1979). The effect of posture on ventilation and lung mechanics in preterm and light-for-date infants. *Pediatrics, 64*, 429–432.
2. Anderson, J., & Auster-Liebhaber, J. (1984). Developmental therapy in the neonatal intensive care unit. *Physical and Occupational Therapy in Pediatrics, 4*, 89–106.

3. Blumenthal, I., & Lealman, G. T. (1982). Effect of posture on gastroesophageal reflux in the newborn. *Archives of Diseases of Childhood, 57*(7), 555–556.

4. Bottos, M., & Stafani, D. (1982). Letter. Postural and motor care of the premature baby. *Developmental Medicine and Child Neurology, 24,* 706–707.

5. Bottos, M., Pettenazzo, A., Giancola, G., Stefani, D., Pettena, G., Viscolani, B., & Rubaltelli, F. F. (1985). The effect of a containing position in a hammock versus the supine position on the cutaneous oxygen level in premature and term babies. *Early Human Development, 11,* 265–273.

6. Brackbill, Y., Douthitt, T., & West, H. (1973). Psychophysiologic effects in the neonate of prone versus supine placement. *Journal of Pediatrics, 82,* 82–83.

7. Fay, M. J. (1988). The positive effects of positioning. *Neonatal Network, 8,* 23–28.

8. Fox, M., & Molesky, M. (1990). The effects of prone and supine positioning on arterial oxygen pressure. *Neonatal Network, 8,* 25–29.

9. Goldberg, R. N., Joshi, A., Moscoso, P., & Castillo, T. (1983). The effect of head position on intracranial pressure in the neonate. *Critical Care Medicine, 11*(6), 428–430.

10. Heaf, D. et al. (1983). Postural effects of gas exchange in infants. *New England Journal of Medicine, 308,* 1505–1508.

11. Hewitt, V. (1976). Effect of posture on the presence of fat in tracheal aspirate in neonates. *Australian Paediatric Journal, 12,* 267.

12. Hoshimoto, T. et al. (1983). Postural effects on behavioral states of newborn infants: A sleep polygraph study. *Brain Development, 5,* 286–291.

13. Kramer, L. I., & Pierpont, M. E. (1976). Rocking waterbeds and auditory stimuli to enhance growth of preterm infants. *Journal of Pediatrics, 88*(2), 297–299.

14. Mansell, A., Bryan, C., & Levison, H. (1972). Airway closure in children. *Journal of Applied Physiology, 33,* 711–714.

15. Marsden, D. J. (1980). Reduction of head flattening in preterm infants. *Developmental Medicine and Child Neurology, 22,* 507–509.

16. Martin, R. J., Herrell, N., Rubin, D., & Fanaroff, A. (1979). Effect of supine and prone positions on arterial oxygen tension in the preterm infant. *Pediatrics, 63*(4), 528–531.

17. Masterson, J., Zucker, C., & Schulze, K. (1987). Prone and supine positioning effects on energy expenditure and behavior of low birth weight neonates. *Pediatrics, 80*(5), 689–692.

18. Mendoza, J., Roberts, J., & Cook, L. (1991). Postural effects on pulmonary function and heart rate of preterm infants with lung disease. *Journal of Pediatrics, 118,* 445–448.

19. Meyers, W. F., & Herbst, J. J. (1982). Effectiveness of position therapy for gastroesophageal reflux. *Pediatrics, 69*(6), 768–772.

20. Orenstein, S., Whitington, P., & Orenstein, D. (1983). The infant seat as treatment for gastroesophageal reflux. *New England Journal of Medicine, 309,* 760–763.

21. Schwirian, P., Eesley, T., & Cuellar, L. (1986). Use of water pillows in reducing head shape distortion in preterm infants. *Research in Nursing and Health, 9,* 203–207.

22. Smith, P., & Turner, B. (1990). The physiologic effects of positioning premature infants in car seats. *Neonatal Network, 9,* 11–15.

23. Wagaman, M. J., Shutack, J. G., Moomjian, A. S., Schwartz, J. G., Shaffer, T. H., & Fox, W. W. (1979). Improved oxygenation and lung compliance with prone positioning of neonates. *Journal of Pediatrics, 94*(5), 787–791.

24. Willett, L, et al. (1986). Risk of hypoventilation in premature infants in car seats. *Journal of Pediatrics, 109,* 245–248.

25. Yu, V. Y. H. (1975). Effect of body position on gastric emptying in the neonate. *Archives of Diseases in Childhood, 50,* 500–504.

*Reprinted by permission:* Hunter, J. (1996). The neonatal intensive care unit, Table 22–7: Medical and developmental considerations of positioning options. In Case-Smith, J., Allen, A., & Pratt, P. *Occupational therapy for children,* (3d ed.) (pp. 600–601). St. Louis: Mosby.

---

### ■ *THERAPEDS POINTER*

Questions to ask after a baby has been positioned:

- Does visual alertness increase or decrease?
- Is general arousal increased or decreased?
- Have respiration patterns changed?

- Are movements in flexion facilitated?
- Is hand to mouth movement facilitated?
- Is the baby more or less active?
- Is body temperature compromised?
- Is pressure on the skin well distributed?
- Is this the best position after feeding?
- Does the skin have red marks?

There are commercially available positioners as well as handmade items. Positioners are effective if they decrease the therapy time, prevent deformities, decrease overstimulation, and conserve the baby's energy so he can gain weight (Case, 1985). While developing or purchasing a positioner, think about the following criteria for positioning devices found in Table 10–11.

OTs make positioning devices out of numerous materials such as foam, rubber tubing, baby blankets, diapers, stockinet, soft fabric, triwall, sheets, and egg-crate mattress pads. Other items may be available to purchase such as gel pillows, gel mattresses and wedges, reflux pants or slings, reflux wedges, inflatable inner tubes, soft sacks, snuggle buntings, bendy bumpers, snuggle ups, boppy cushions, water pads/mattress, artificial sheepskin, and stuffed animals. When deciding on the appropriate equipment, therapists, parents, and team members should discuss what has worked best in the past and what is acceptable to the family.

■ *THERAPEDS POINTER*

A great source for equipment designed for the baby who is premature. This company sells slings, isocovers, wedges, gel mattresses, snuggleups, bendy bumpers, diapers, tee shirts, etc.:

Developmental Care Products
Children Medical Ventures, Inc.
542 Main Street
S. Weymouth, MA 02190
Phone: 1-800-377-3449

Table 10–11 **Checklist for Positioning Devices**

| | |
|---|---|
| • Corrects the position | • Has minimal loose parts |
| • Secures body safely | • Comforts the baby |
| • Has access for diaper change | • Fits in bed size |
| • Allows for gavage feeding | • Does not disrupt nursing care |
| • Allows for intravenous lines | • Is cleanable or disposable |
| • Uses with little instruction | • Requires little storage space |
| • Is cosmetically appealing | • Is inexpensive |

*Source:* Adapted from Semmler (1989).

## Splinting

A neonatal OT may be the only person on the team to recognize a deformity that would profit from splinting. It is recommended that you receive a prescription from the physician and consult with an orthopedist if it is a mechanical or structural deformity (e.g., brachial plexus injury; arthrogryposis, IV burn, hip dislocation). Splinting on a small baby is difficult because of reduced skin surfaces and shaping of a very small splint. It is best to use two people: one to hold the correct position and the other to mold the shape of the splint. The purposes of a splint are to prevent contractures, immobilize, and support and to maintain or increase ROM (Vergara, 1993a). Splinting restricts active or passive movement and it is essential to supplement the splint wearing with a stretching exercise program.

Precautions for splinting are observed to prevent additional injuries. The baby's skin is thin and can result in burns and/or breakdowns. Remove the splints often to check the skin areas and be sure there are no reddened, creased, or pressure areas. Check the skin for edema, which happens when the straps are too tight and restrict the blood flow. Apply stockinet, or a sock to cover the splint to protect the baby's face or body from injuries when the baby moves rapidly in a disorganized manner.

Baby splints need more frequent modification because of rapid growth and/or changes in the soft tissue. Since babies do not express discomfort, it is crucial to check the newly made splint once per hour for 4 hours and then once every 4 hours. Post a clear instruction sheet including a picture or photo to help the nurses and family apply the splint correctly. Most common referrals for splinting are club feet, cortical thumbs, tight hand web spaces, foot drop, IV burns over a joint, wrist drop, bone agenesis, joint deformities, joint contractures, and postsurgery immobilization.

## Feeding

Feeding is typically a major focus for caregivers in the NICU. The course of development for feeding skills, and even the potential for oral feeding, is highly dependent upon infant characteristics including the degree of prematurity and medical complications. Both assessment and intervention for feeding skills will depend on these factors. Because feeding of the infant in the NICU requires some special skills and knowledge, it will be dealt with here. Further information on feeding can be found in Chapter 5.

A full-term infant comes complete with oral anatomical features that support safe and skilled feeding. As described briefly in Chapter 10, the full-term infant has a relatively large tongue, small oral cavity, and sucking "fat pads" in the cheeks. As a result of the large tongue and small oral cavity, the tongue, soft palate, and epiglottis are in close proximity, leaving little room for tongue mobility. The fat pads provide a means of compressing the nipple for milk expression. Together these anatomical features promote efficient suck and allow the infant to breath through the nose (Hunter, 1990; Morris & Klein, 1987). The infant born prematurely is not graced with these anatomical features, and as such will not be an efficient oral feeder, even in the absence of medical complications, until such features mature. Generally adequate feeding skills may emerge between 34 and 35 weeks' gestational age in healthy infants born prematurely (Wolf & Glass, 1992). Prior to this time the infant will likely exhibit poorly coordinated oral-motor skills and poorly developed oral reflexes. Coupled with the likelihood of muscle tone alterations, inadequate postural stability, and limited energy resources, the introduction of oral feeding prior to this age must be carefully considered; it is generally inadvisable.

Neonates who are at high risk may be unable to tolerate oral feedings and may have difficulty making the transition from alternative tube feedings to bottle and or breast feedings. The feeding experience is vital not only for physical growth and brain development, but also for the psychological bonding between mother and infant (Creger, 1989).

The very small and immature neonate receives his nutrients by IV feedings. The premature digestive system is unable to digest formula and the food is accessed through the veins. Infants who are sick, unstable, and premature may use gavage tube feedings. A plastic tube is inserted into the mouth or nose and passed directly down into the stomach. By a variety of different-size syringes, the formula is passed down the tube for the infant with no oral feeding experience. Neonates who are unsafe or incapable of sucking may receive a gastrostomy tube that is surgically placed directly into the stomach (Hunter, 1990). Nonoral feeding experiences may produce some side effects: irritation of the mucosa in the digestive system, stimulation of the vagal response and aspiration, and the reduction of sensory oral responses such as taste and touch (Glass & Wolf, 1994).

Infants born prematurely have a high likelihood of developing medical complications that will potentially interfere with the infant's ability to become a successful oral feeder. Many of these complications are defined in Table 10–8, so only the impact they may have on feeding will be addressed here. Respiratory distress syndrome (RDS) can lead to a cascade of events with cardiac and pulmonary sequella. Such complications make breathing effortful for the infant and come at a high physiological cost. Infants working hard to breathe cannot be expected to be efficient with oral feedings; that is, they cannot take in sufficient calories orally to support their physiological needs. RDS can give way to other pulmonary problems, such as bronchopulmonary dysplasia (BPD). This is a chronic pulmonary difficulty and can interfere long term with an infant's oral feeding ability due both to the pulmonary compromise seen with this disease, and to the behavioral, motor, and sensory issues that develop as a result of BPD (Wolf & Glass, 1992).

Necrotizing enterocolitis (NEC) can interrupt the development of oral feeding skills as well. NEC may mandate that oral feedings be discontinued, and surgery may be needed to resect portions of the bowel. Reintroducing oral feedings must proceed slowly when the infant is again medically stable and is often characterized by setbacks (Wolf & Glass, 1992). Gastroesophageal reflux (GER), while not precluding oral feedings, can certainly complicate the picture. Infants with GER may or may not vomit, but either way run a risk of aspiration of food and consequent pulmonary problems, as well as esophagitis.

Other complications that may mitigate against oral feedings include those related to the specific child. Children born with cleft palate, some of the trisomy syndromes (i.e., trisomy 18, trisomy 13), syndromes that cause skeletal deficits (Cornelia De Lange's syndrome), facial anomalies (Opitz syndrome, Pierre Robin syndrome), and other congenital disabilities (i.e., Prader-Willi syndrome) may all have difficulty becoming adequate oral feeders.

This is far from an exhaustive list of complications that have the potential to interfere with the development of oral feeding skills in the infant born prematurely. The caregiver and therapist may need to provide substantial support, great patience, and skilled intervention for the baby to become an adequate oral feeder. Assessment of oral feeding potential must be carried out carefully, keeping in mind the medical status of the infant.

The feeding assessment process involved here must be comprehensive. Therapists must be prepared to gather information from the medical chart (e.g., congenital anomalies, pertinent medical interventions, or perinatal history), from the caregivers (parents and nursing staff) and from observation of the infant *prior to* beginning a hands-on evaluation. Observations should include

- Presence of feeding tubes and other life-support systems
- Body symmetry at rest
- Muscle tone during various behavioral states
- Activity of the infant
- Behavioral state and state variations
- Reactivity to environmental inputs
- Calming and self-organizing skills
  (Adapted from Harris, 1986; Hunter, 1990.)

Following this initial information-gathering process, a "hands-on" evaluation can begin. Harris (1986) recommends use of a gloved finger in and around the infant's mouth to determine the structure of the oral cavity (i.e., structure of the palate and mandible) as well as to evaluate the tongue for tone, position, and mobility. At this time the therapist will also be able to determine if the infant has a typical gag reflex, and check the rooting reflex. Presence or absence of a tonic bite reflex and nonnutritive sucking can be assessed at this time as well. In addition to this information about the oral mechanisms, the therapist will want to examine reflexes that will impact feeding, including the Moro reflex and the neck and labyrinthine reflexes.

Oral-motor skills, both nutritive and nonnutritive, can be assessed if the infant is medically stable. It is important to note that these two oral functions are discrete; success in one does not mean success in the other (Wolf & Glass, 1992). During the evaluation of both patterns the therapist should determine if the suck is coordinated with swallow and breathing, is rhythmic, and is efficient. Breathing should continue throughout nonnutritive sucking, and through most stages of nutritive sucking (Hunter, 1990).

Nonnutritive sucking emerges by about 32 weeks' gestation age, and should also be rhythmic and characterized by bursts of sucking with intervals of rest. Typically nonnutritive sucking rates are faster, but rests are longer than seen with nutritive sucking. Nonnutritive sucking can be seen spontaneously during sleep and can be elicited in all states with the exception of deep sleep and crying (Hunter, 1990). Evaluation involves use of the therapist's gloved finger or a pacifier and observation of the sucking pattern. During evaluation of the physical skills involved in sucking, the therapist will also want to note how effective nonnutritive sucking is as a self-calming tool for the infant. Nonnutritive sucking is seen as different from nutritive sucking, but it is also seen to support the development of this later skill (Schwartz, Moody, Yarandi, & Anderson, 1987; Vergara, 1993a). As such, it is generally considered important development step in preparing an infant for oral feeding. It may also be useful during the feeding process, because it has been suggested to facilitate digestion (Vergara, 1993a). Since use of nonnutritive sucking for infants not ready for oral feedings can be critical in circumventing the potential development of oral tactile hypersensitivity, it is a crucial skill to evaluate even when the infant is not ready for oral feeding.

An efficient nutritive sucking pattern can be seen as early as 34 weeks' gestation and is characterized by an initial continuous burst of rhythmic sucking (30 to 70 seconds in duration) followed by intermittent bursts and pauses (Wolf & Glass, 1992). In typical infants the majority of intake occurs within the first 4 minutes of a feeding; within 15 to 20 minutes nutritional intake is complete if the infant is an efficient feeder (Hunter, 1990). When evaluating nutritive sucking, the oral structures of the jaw, cheek, palate, chin, lips, and tongue must be considered, as should the ability to lick, compress, and develop suction on the nipple, the ability to push food to the back of the mouth, and the ability to close the pharynx during feeding. According to Vergara (1993a), selecting an appropriate nipple is a critical aspect of the feeding assessment. The concept that breathing is interrupted briefly during the normal swallow process is now generally accepted (Hunter, 1990). In fact some incidences of apnea and oxygen desaturation can be expected during continuous sucking episodes, even in full-term infants (Mathew, 1988). The physiological cost of this process, and the ability of the infant to recover from these brief episodes, will be the deciding factors in determining if oral feedings are to be used functionally.

---

■ *THERAPEDS POINTER*

**Nipple Selection**
This will be a "nonscientific" procedure, one of trial and error. You may need to work with the nipple a bit before giving up on it, turn it in the mouth, put it in part way, pull it out a bit to promote sucking again when a long rest period has occurred. There is no perfect answer!

Standard: Amber in color, what most of us are familiar with; can be inserted part way into the mouth if the infant has a strong gag reflex
Red: Softer, narrower at the base than the amber; may be useful for a weak suck
Blue: Smaller than red and somewhat softer; offers a more steady flow of liquid, may be useful for a weak suck; may be useful for infants with small mouths or strong gag
NUK: Contour nipple, made to resemble the mother's nipple; shape may enhance ability to compress the nipple and express formula, may promote better suction; inverted may be useful for infants with cleft plate

---

Unfortunately, with the need for NICU intervention, there are many procedures that are not ideal for the development of normal oral-motor sensitivity. Feedings via oral gastric tubing or the placement of endotracheal tubes can lead to hypersensitivity within the oral cavity that will potentially interfere with oral feeding. Hypersensitivity is noted as an exaggerated gag reflex that is elicited in the anterior portion of the mouth or even on the lips. Vergara (1993a) points out that the gag reflex will be more easily elicited with unfamiliar stimuli (i.e., a new nipple or pacifier, the therapist's finger). Hypersensitivity must be examined as a component of the overall assessment process in order to obtain a full picture of the infant's skills and needs.

Combining the information from this assessment process the therapist will know how the infant deals with environmental input of the NICU; how well the infant regulates behavioral state; how well the infant coordinates sucking, swallowing, and breathing; and how well the infant processes sensory input in the mouth. This information will need to be viewed in light of other evaluation information pertaining to muscle tone, reflex integration, symmetry, positioning, etc., to determine how to proceed. Refer to the above sections for further discussion of these areas.

Consensus exists that non-nutritive sucking should be initiated early in the feeding intervention process with infants in the NICU (Harris, 1986; Glass & Wolf, 1994; Wolf & Glass, 1992; Vergara, 1993a). Before beginning an oral-feeding intervention plan, the therapist must consult with the nurse regarding feeding times, success or failure with feedings, and the infant's unique personality. According to Hunter (1996b) and Creger (1989), the success of oral feeding a neonate is multifaceted and dependent upon the following characteristics of the infant:

1. Gestational age and weight
2. Medical stability
3. Physiological stability
4. Readiness and interest
5. Muscle tone
6. Energy level and endurance
7. Caregiver experience and attitude
8. Surrounding environment
9. Behavioral organization and interaction
10. Previous oral experiences
11. Daily care not physically draining
12. Level of arousal and endurance

Before each feeding, consider the surrounding environment: dim the lights, place the monitor on silent mode, alert the nurses and others of needing a quiet space around the infant's bed, divert noxious odors, and provide very little stimulation. Assemble your nipple and bottle supplies, get extra diapers and blankets, review the daily nursing record reporting attempts at feeding by mouth, and, if needed, change her diaper slowly. Before lifting the infant, be sure to check the oxygen gauge, the length of all the lines attached to the baby, and place all necessary feeding items within your reach. Approach the baby gently, speak softly, and stroke or massage his limbs and make visual contact. Contain her limbs near her body as you slowly lift her up into your arms, encouraging flexion and shoulder and hip stability. Sit facing the monitors, position his head in midline with slight neck extension to open the airway, and swaddle his arms and legs. Keep your eyes on a clock to measure specific behaviors and length of feeding. Remember at any time the neonate's medical and physiological readiness and stability must be maintained and you must discontinue the feeding when the infant is unstable (Vergara, 1993a).

A variety of nipples are available, and a neonatal therapist must consider the size, shape, firmness and size of the hole for the high-risk infant. You want to select the nipple that facilitates the feeding abilities and supports the neonate's behavioral and physiological stability. It has been recommended to try one nipple for 2 days before switching to allow the infant time to adapt to suck changes and textures. The warmer the formula, the faster the flow through the nipple and the thickness of the formula affects the strength of suck and control over the flow into the baby's mouth (Creger, 1989). Oral feeding is successful when the intake of calorically appropriate formula is within a 30-minute time period, when the infant is safe with no risk of aspiration, and when the feeding is pleasurable and interactive.

Oral hypersensitivity may be diminished by offering the infant positive oral experiences during intubation procedures, and by using nonnutritive sucking during oral gastric feedings, and at times not associated with feeding. Remember that familiar pacifiers must be used at first, because hypersensitive responses will be less with familiar objects. The therapist or parent can gradually introduce other pacifiers or toys for nonnutritive sucking as they are tolerated.

Clinicians often precede a feeding session with firm tactile input on trunk and extremities before working in the infant's mouth at all. This procedure will increase proprioceptive input to the body, and may decrease defensive or hypersensitive responses to touch. Firm pressure can be applied around the mouth, as tolerated by the infant. Helping the infant move her own hand to the face and oral area may also diminish the hypersensitive response to touch as well. The process of decreasing hypersensitivity should be carried out with careful attention paid to the infant's responses to touch. It is often best to initiate a feeding session with some form of tactile input in an attempt to diminish oral hypersensitivity before offering the infant food via nipple.

Determining the appropriate feeding intervention techniques for neonates is a skill that a neonatal therapist must develop with practice, self-study, seminars, and mentorship. Some general recommendations are

1. Place the whole nipple inside the mouth to suck and swallow.
2. Remove the nipple more often when the baby is in respiratory distress.
3. Apply jaw closure when baby cannot maintain lip close on nipple.
4. Gentle pulling of the nipple in and out of the mouth may renew the sucking pattern.
5. Place middle finger under the chin and apply gently pressure to help reduce large, excessive jaw motions.
6. Apply external support to the cheeks by pressing in a downward and forward direction to improve lip seal and intraoral pressure.
7. Apply perioral and then intraoral tactile stimulation to the facial area to help with hypersensitivity, hand-to-mouth exploration, firm tactile pressure on gums, tactile toothbrushes, etc.

8. Stroke the infant's tongue downward and forward to facilitate more rhythmical suck.
9. To facilitate swallowing, gently stroke along the side of the throat, keep the bottle in a horizontal level to reduce the flow of the nipple, use a slow-flow nipple, or use the Haberman feeder.
10. Infants with reflux must be fed upright; have smaller, more frequent feedings; and be placed prone with bed at 30 degrees.
11. Wrap an irritable infant in tight swaddle position and avoid direct eye contact.
12. Burp infants often by placing them across your lap, sitting up with your hands on the baby's upper chest, and pat the back.
13. Parents need to learn the most efficient and safe technique to feed their baby.
14. Provide adequate postural support in flexion and inhibit extension (Hunter, 1990; Creger, 1989; Semmler, 1989)

## *Parent-Infant Interaction and Play*

As stated earlier, feeding is a great time to promote attachment of the baby and the parent. This attachment may be delayed when the baby is placed in NICU. Separation from the parents, a variety of staff members caring for the baby, the multiple machines and procedures, and life-threatening episodes may hamper the attachment process (Holloway, 1994). It often takes weeks before the baby who is sick or premature becomes neurologically stable with some consistency in sleep-awake cycles. As the neonate's neurological system matures and self-regulation is more evident, he is ready to interact with the people and objects in his environment.

Our role is to demonstrate to parents the uniqueness of their baby. By teaching parents to read their baby's cues, they can understand what the baby likes and dislikes. If parents learn to read these cues, they can respond to their baby's cues with activities that are pleasurable to the baby. This response helps the baby to see that she can influence people in the environment and can have her needs met. As the parents respond to the baby's cues, it is possible that the parents and baby will begin their own interaction pattern. Hopefully, this pattern is positive to both the parents and the baby and it encourages more give-and-take interaction. By reading and responding to the baby's cues, caregiving may become more pleasurable to the parents and the baby. This is particularly helpful to first-time parents and parents who are dealing with fussy babies 24 hours a day. Mom and Dad may now feed Johnny as they can read his cues to help pace the flow of the milk. Or they know that slow rocking or deep stroking helps Johnny to become calm so that he can eat or play.

---

■ *THERAPEDS POINTER*

Remember that it takes a period of time for parents and babies to adjust to each other. Listed are a few ways to promote parent-baby interaction (Holloway, 1997):

- Encourage parents to play with the baby, not just doing medical procedures.

- Imitate the baby and be playful as you do it! (e.g., alter voices, raise eyebrows, make funny faces, play with toys yourself)
- Demonstrate how the baby responds and interacts to stimuli.
- Give a playful activity with each "skill" you are trying to teach.
- Know and use the parent's coping style.
- Give developmental information that includes play.
- Refer parents to follow-up services after discharge (they may feel more playful!).
- Refer parents and siblings to counseling, support groups, or play groups if appropriate.
- Respect the parent's attitude toward play and select culturally appropriate activities.
- Recommend or provide toys that provide the "right" stimulation for the baby according to her sensory preferences and cognitive and motor capabilities.

It is critical that therapists and other NICU personnel help parents to embed these times for interaction and play within typical routines (Holloway, 1997). For example, the parent and baby may play a little game of give and take during diapering or when the baby is in a quiet alert state. Singing in the car, playing peek-a-boo with a washcloth during bath time, and placing the baby down in a spot that has the "just right" level of arousal, may give the baby numerous opportunities to play and interact with his parents and siblings. Incorporating siblings into activities also can be helpful to make the sibling feel important and to increase the opportunities for the baby to play.

# TRANSITION AND DISCHARGE PLANNING

Discharge planning should begin as soon as the baby is medically stable. When discharge from the NICU is actually possible, parents may meet this transition with both excitement and fear. When they go home, they must fulfill all caregiving responsibilities and must feel competent about their abilities. If an infant continues to require specialized procedures or equipment (e.g., suctioning, monitors, oxygen), parents may need support as they systematically begin to learn how to perform these procedures (Vergara, 1993a). Therapists and all NICU staff are responsible for training parents to learn about their child's condition and care and to become progressively more confident in their caregiving abilities. Appendix B at the end of this chapter gives a list of resources for parents.

## EQUIPMENT FOR DISCHARGE

Therapists often assess what equipment the baby needs when he goes home. Once the baby is medically stable, parents are questioned about the baby equipment they have at home. Parents need to be ready with a crib, a car seat, a baby seat, head and body positioners, tub equipment, and any other medical or emergency equipment they may need. Because babies leaving the NICU environment are often very small, much of the typical seating and transportation equipment does not fit. Having a car seat that fits the baby is critical, but adaptations must be done in a manner that does not violate the manufacturer's warranty and makes the car seat safe for transportation. Restraining small babies in car seats is a law in 50 states, but fitting a tiny baby to a standard-size car seat is not recommended. Using blanket rolls for each side and between the crotch strap prevents sliding. Car seats with lap or chest shields are not approved. Nothing firm is to go behind the head, back, or under the hips to try to adapt the car seat. Your state transportation safety office can give you a list of approved car seats and loan programs for the baby who is medically fragile or who may need an approved car bed. Strollers, feeding seats, and tub seats may also require assessment and adaptations.

OTs often ask parents about their housing, the arrangement of rooms, the equipment that is being brought into the home, and emergency backup plans. For example, the OT may ask the following questions related to the baby's sleeping arrangements:

- Do you have a crib? What does it look like?
- Can it be adapted to be smaller?
- Does it meet safety standards as far as the width of the bars and the ability to raise and lower the rail?
- Can the baby's equipment be attached to it?
- Can the head of the mattress be raised if the baby has reflux after eating?
- Where is the crib located? (e.g., room placement and the distance from the parent's or sibling's rooms)
- Do you have a baby monitor to listen to the baby when the baby is sleeping and you are in other parts of the house?
- Where is the placement of the crib in relation to the ventilator or other equipment?
- Is emergency power backup available?
- What type of linens do you have for the crib and how many?
- What are your concerns about the crib?

Therapists ask questions about equipment to prepare the parents for the homecoming of the baby. There are many commercially made adaptation devices that can be used with a crib, or with baby seats and strollers, that will make the baby more comfortable and potentially assist the baby in self-regulation. The therapists will need to consider the options and discuss them with the parents to determine what they would like to include in their home environment.

## FAMILY LIFE ROUTINES

Systematic planning often helps the discharge to home go more smoothly. OTs help families integrate their baby into their family life by discussing the baby's and family's strengths and needs (Vergara, 1993a). By discussing ways to interact, calm, play, and prevent stress signals, parents can learn how to develop healthy and satisfying parent-child interactions. Therapists may work with parents on how to manage the daily routine of child care and how to access support systems and therapy services if needed. These discussions are essential for helping parents enhance their baby's potential and feel attached to their new baby.

## FOLLOW-UP CLINICS AND PRACTICES

Not all graduates of NICU will require early intervention services at the time of discharge. Some of these babies will require good developmental follow-up through a post-NICU follow-up clinic (e.g., BPD, spina bifida, cleft palate) or a pediatrician. Parents need to be given information on how to contact an OT or an early-intervention program if they feel their baby is not progressing developmentally or if they have other concerns. Parents need to be informed about our roles and how we can help them if they need services.

---

■ *THERAPEDS POINTER*

Discharge planning begins when the baby enters NICU. These are questions that need to be asked by the NICU team.

- Where will this baby live and with whom? Geographic location, physical, social and cultural environments all need to be considered.
- Who will be the primary caregivers?
- Do the primary caregivers understand the baby's medical needs and can they perform medical procedures and cardiopulmonary resuscitation (CPR)?
- Who is the backup person for this family if the main caregiver cannot be there? Can they perform medical procedures and CPR?
- What baby equipment does the baby have? (e.g., crib, car seat, baby seat)
- Have you alerted the power company, rescue squad, police and fire departments about your child's medical status? (Extremely important if the baby is on a ventilator and there is a power outage.)
- What early-intervention program services or medical services are in this family's geographic area?
- What formal and informal supports are available to you?

---

# FURTHER TRAINING FOR OTs IN NICU

## PRACTICE GUIDELINES

When entering NICU practice, therapists need guided clinical experience and supervision, and, if possible, an established mentor-protégé relationship

(Hunter, 1996a). A knowledge and skills position paper has been written by the American Occupational Therapy Association (1993) for OTs working in the NICU. These practice guidelines should make administrators consider if they can ethically and legally place untrained therapists in a specialty practice such as the NICU (Hunter, 1996a). Unfortunately, a study by Dewire, White, Kanny and Glass (1996) suggests that therapists have a lack of education or on-the-job training to obtain the knowledge and skills necessary to work in the NICU. In this study, 174 therapists who worked in the NICU responded to questions about their current practices, training, and opinions about the amount of education needed to work in the NICU. Respondents were asked to rate the knowledge and skills needed to work in the NICU on a Likert scale from essential to not important. Many of these "essential items" as delineated by AOTA (1993) were rated from 32 to 97 percent. This was particularly worrisome when ratings of agreement were between 81 and 84 percent for knowledge about common precautions and health complications of the neonate and safety and infection control guidelines, and facilitating feeding, oral-motor, motor, and postural control skills (Hunter, 1996a). Most disheartening was only a 77 percent agreement that therapists need skills in fostering the attachment of babies to their parents.

## EDUCATIONAL EXPERIENCES

Hunter (1996a) and Dewire et al. (1996) have suggested numerous ways to help therapists become better trained to work in a highly specialized field such as NICU. They have suggested that AOTA needs to continue to develop self-study guides, advanced workshops, and research and practice articles related to NICU. Some training suggestions for neonatal specialists to work in NICU are:

1. Work in pediatrics prior to entering the NICU environment.
2. Use AOTA's neonatal self study series (Vergara, 1993a, b) or other series (Creger, 1989).
3. Enroll in some graduate courses or continuing education courses in NICU practice to enhance knowledge and develop clinical reasoning skills.
4. Participate in on-the-job training with written and visual teaching materials and guidelines for when competencies are achieved to ease the new therapist into various areas of NICU.
5. Develop a mentorship experience with an experienced clinician.
6. Attend a 3- or 4-day workshop focusing on evaluation and treatment with time allowed for networking with other therapists.
7. Read and participate in outcome-based research in the NICU.
8. Surf the Internet for information and resources.
9. Provide inservices to OT students of other NICU staff to help keep your knowledge base current.

Because of all the technological advances, this field changes constantly and therapists need to keep abreast of the literature and to participate in preservice and inservice education. The courses, conferences, books, and videos listed in Appendix C at the end of this chapter are just the beginning in learning how to work with babies in the NICU. This is a highly specialized field that requires your personal willingness to devote the time to learn and to relearn as research tells us more about babies born with complex illness or prematurity. Review the case story of Billy, a baby who had an extremely rocky NICU experience. Using the information in this chapter, try to answer the questions at the end of the case study.

## PITFALLS FOR THERAPISTS WORKING IN THE NICU

Hunter (1993) suggests that the following six behaviors can lead to ineffective therapy in NICU:

1. *Assuming all NICUs and the roles of all neonatal therapists are alike.* Each NICU has its own culture and expectations for members of the team. Therapists must learn the rules and procedures for the environment in which they are working and their expected roles.
2. *Lacking an adequate NICU medical foundation.* NICU is an extremely complex environment with babies who are often fighting for their lives. Therapists who are uninformed about medical conditions, procedures, precautions, and best practices for assessment and intervention in NICU may be putting their patients and professional license at risk. Knowing the "typical development" of babies who are premature is essential.
3. *Transplanting traditional pediatric practice in NICU.* Typical assessment and intervention strategies for healthy babies or toddlers are often contraindicated in the NICU environment. Providing babies in the NICU with feeding or sensory experiences that do not consider their immature neurological systems may be detrimental to their growth and development. For example, the baby with spina bifida in NICU has very different medical needs when seen in early intervention. In NICU, the baby is often undergoing numerous surgeries to correct the congenital deformities, and it may be contraindicated to place the baby on his back or on one side if back or shunt surgery has occurred.
4. *Inaccurate evaluations or misleading interpretation of results.* Therapists need to be informed about the typical development of babies for their EGA. If uninformed, they may evaluate babies inaccurately and alert parents and staff to problems that will resolve within a few weeks of growth and development.
5. *Comfortable apathy.* As therapists become more familiar with the NICU environment, sometimes they "accept" environmental conditions, medical procedures, or occupational therapy practices as standard treatment. Therapists constantly need to update their skills and assess alternatives to provide babies with the best practice possible.
6. *Neglect of family.* Therapists in NICU are sometimes so overwhelmed by the complexity of the baby and NICU environment that they forget to involve the family in therapy. Or if families are unable to

stay with their baby, families may only come to see their baby at night or during the weekend. If at all possible, therapists and administrators need to be flexible with scheduling therapist time so that the family's needs can be met.

To avoid ineffective therapy or incompetency in the NICU environment, therapists are encouraged to understand the essential knowledge and skills necessary to practice in NICU and to obtain appropriate training and mentorship. Therapists in NICU must keep abreast of the literature and be willing to learn from parents and their children as well as other NICU team members. They need to be aware of community resources so that families and their children can receive appropriate follow-up care through their pediatrician and early-intervention services. Working in the NICU is challenging and requires a commitment to life-long learning.

# SUMMARY

Working in the NICU as an OT requires experience and specialized knowledge to develop appropriate programs for babies who are premature or critically ill. This chapter gave an overview of the typical areas for assessment and intervention in NICU but does not purport to train therapists to work in NICU. Therapists need to be aware of medical conditions and precautions, NICU terminology and equipment, and the effect of the NICU environment on the baby and her family. Roles for therapists may vary according to team membership, and therapists need to work with other team members to coordinate appropriate assessment, intervention, and discharge planning with these babies and their families. Through self-study, mentorship, and guided experiences, OTs can work in the NICU environment. This chapter lists numerous books, videos, and Web sites to help therapists and family members to obtain additional information about the happenings in NICU.

## CASE STORY

| NAME: | Billy | BIRTHDATE: | February 15, 1997 |
|---|---|---|---|
| PCA: | 26 weeks | APGARS: | 8(1)/8(5) |
| GENDER: | Male | RACE: | Black |
| BIRTH WT: | 590 grams | WEIGHT: | 1 lb, 4.5 oz |
| HOME: | Yarlmoro, Virginia | INSURANCE: | Medicaid |

**Social:** Mom is 23 years old and works as a cook for a local  military base. She is single and had limited prenatal visits. Billy is her first baby.

**Birth History:** Because of Mom's severe pregnancy-induced hypertension and a decreased fetal heart rate, Billy was born at 26 weeks PCA by cesarean section at a large metropolitan hospital. Delivery was complicated by the nuchal cord being wrapped twice around Billy's neck.

**Medical History:** Billy had respiratory distress and was given surfactant ×2 and was intubated. An unresolved PDA was corrected by surgery March 7 and a septic-abdominal distention and suspected NEC resolved itself. Cardiac arrest ×4, 3/20–3/27 all requiring chest compressions. 5/97 urinary tract infection and the ultrasound revealed a small right kidney. On 7/12 Billy was hypothermic and hypotensive and by 7/19 he had septic shock and global seizures. On 7/30, total body rash occurred because of an allergic reaction to phenobarbital. On 8/1, Billy went into renal failure and was placed on dialysis. Several attempts were made to wean Billy from the ventilator but they were unsuccessful because he maintained high levels of $CO_2$. He was sedated from 8/15 to 10/10 after a tracheotomy was performed. Hearing test: 10/25—severe loss in his right ear and a moderate loss in his left ear. Eye exam: stage III regression in both eyes but stable. Head ultrasound: normal with no IVH bleeds.

**Occupational Therapy:** Referral for positioning 3/29/97. Patient continues to self-extubate and is very irritable. OT followed three times a week to monitor positioning needs and to adapt his bed to reduce stimuli and agitation. First assessment on 6/15: eyes followed black-and-white objects when placed close to eyes (3 inches); sucked on pacifier when intubated; and presented with a weak palmar grasp in the left and right hands. On 6/22, Billy was more agitated and a sidelyer was made to prevent extreme arching of head and extubation. On 8/4, his right wrist hyperextended because of the skin rash and a Neoprene splint was made to support the wrist in neutral. The left thumb was tight in abduction, so a left thumb splint was made and worn at all times except for bath. OT was canceled from 8/15 to 10/17 because of Billy's sedation and $CO_2$ retention. Occupational therapy continued to consult with nursing on positioning, ROM, and splint applications. Billy was reassessed 10/18 when moved over to the intermediate nursery and on CPAP (continuous positive airway pressure). Results of this assessment were:

*States:* Active alert to crying, no self-quieting behaviors.

*Stress cues:* Arching eyebrows, drop in heart rate, arching, finger splaying, eye aversion, stooling, decrease in oxygenation.

*Environment:* Large crib, covered quilts, back row next to a window.

*Equipment:* Nasal gastric tube, HR/RR monitor, tracheotomy, pulse oximeter/ventilator with three feeds of plastic flexible tubing.

*Sensory responses:* Tactile: very defensive to input on face, hands, feet, and inside mouth; he is able to tolerate deep pressure. Billy responds negatively to any position change on the left side (vestibular). He appears to enjoy a static change of position in a seat or stroller. Billy visually follows 20 degrees in dim area but mostly avers human input. He prefers his black-and-white mobile in bed. Billy demonstrated no observable response to a variety of auditory inputs.

*Neuromotor:* Billy has a strong head preference to the right but can hold his head briefly in midline. He resists turning to the left. Billy's right UE is more active in shoulder mobility, and when in supported sitting, he can put his right fist to his lips. Billy's right wrist flexors are tight but there is no ROM limitation. Billy can sustain a grasp for 1 minute, but he has no eye-hand focus. Movements are sluggish, but his tone is normal. There is no active reach or batting, and the left UE is held more in retraction and he only grasps for 30 seconds. He has no purposeful actions. Billy's legs kick infrequently and he has low tone with no ROM limitations. He is not weight bearing.

*Positioning:* He has a low tolerance for prone position but he can clear his head for an airway. Sidelying allows his right hand to go to his mouth. Supine: distal motions but there is no purpose.

*Feeding:* Billy is orally defensive to nipples, pacifiers, or fingers. He no longer sucks and his tongue is flat and bunches up to force objects out of mouth. Unable to assess swallowing because he does not suck food in, but he is able to handle his own secretions. Billy is tube-fed all meals and nursing reports do not show evidence of Billy being hungry.

*Discharge plans:* Mom desires to take Billy home but needs to work and cannot identify two other support people to help her. Currently, we are seeking alternate placement in an infant nursing home until he can be weaned from the ventilator. OT has met Mom once and she is caring and willing to learn how to take care of Billy. After an extremely complicated medical history, the staff and Mom are still amazed at Billy's will to live.

1. List what all the abbreviations mean.
2. What precautions would you consider when working with Billy?
3. What are Billy's strengths, needs, and supports?
4. What are some strategies you can introduce to Mom to help Billy be more self-regulated?
5. What positions would you suggest for Billy?
6. Do you have any concerns about Billy's feeding capabilities for the future? What should you do?
7. What do you suspect are Mom's strengths, concerns, and needs for discharge?
8. If you were going to see Billy in follow-up clinic after being discharged to a nursing home or home, what would you assess and how?

# References

Als, H. (1982). Toward a synactive theory of development: Premise for the assessment and support of infant individuality. *Infant Mental Health Journal, 3,* 229–243.

Als, H. (1986). A synactive model of neonatal behavioral organization: Framework for the assessment of neurobehavioral development in the premature infant and for the support of infants and parents in the neonatal intensive care environment. *Physical and Occupational Therapy in Pediatrics, 6* (3/4), 3–53.

Als, H., Lawhorn, G., Duffy, F., McAulty, G. B., Gibes-Grossman, R., & Bickman, J. (1994). Individualized developmental care for the very low-birth-weight preterm infant. *Journal of the American Medical Association, 272*(11), 853–858.

Als, H., Lester, B. H., Tronick, E. Z., & Brazelton, T. B. (1982). Toward a research instrument for the assessment of preterm infant's behavior (APIB). In H. Fitzgerald (Ed.), *Theory and research in behavioral pediatrics, Vol. 1.* New York: Plenum.

American Occupational Therapy Association (AOTA) (1996). Member data survey, 1996. Bethesda, MD: Author.

American Occupational Therapy Association (AOTA) (1993). Knowledge and skills for occupational therapy practice in the neonatal intensive care unit. *American Journal of Occupational Therapy, 47,* 1100–1105.

Baker, J. G. (1995). Commentary: Parents as partners in the NICU. *Neonatal Network, 14,* 9–10.

Backes, L. E., Dietz, J., Price, R., Glass, R., & Hays, R. (1993). The effect of oral support on sucking efficiency in preterm infants. *American Journal of Occupational Therapy, 48*(6), 490–497.

Borland, M. (1989). Neuromotor development. In C. Semmler (Ed.), *A guide to care & management of very low birth weight infants.* Tucson: Therapy Skill Builders.

Brazelton, T. B. (1984). *Neonatal behavioral assessment scale* (2d ed.). Philadelphia: Lippincott.

Brazy, J. E. (1997). Chances for survival (on line). Available on the Worldwide Web: www.medsch@wisc.edu/childrenshosp/ parents_of_preemies/survival.html.

Case, J. (1985). Positioning guidelines for the premature infant. *Developmental Disabilities Special Interest Section Newsletter 8*(3). Rockville, MD: American Occupational Therapy Association.

Case-Smith, J. (1993). Family-centered care in the neonatal intensive care unit. In Vergara, E. (Ed.), *Foundations for practice in the neonatal intensive care unit and early intervention: A self-guided practice manual, Vol 2.* (pp. 241–246). Rockville, MD: American Occupational Therapy Association.

Creger, P. J. (Ed.). (1989). *Developmental*

interventions for preterm and high-risk infants: Self study modules for professionals. Tucson: Therapy Skill Builders.

Dewire, A., White, D., Kanny, E. & Glass, R. (1996). Education and training of occupational therapists for neonatal intensive care units. *American Journal of Occupational Therapy, 50*(7), 486–494.

Frank, A., Maurer, P., and Shepherd, J. (1991). Survey results on the light and sound in newborn intensive care units. *Physical and Occupational Therapy in Pediatrics, 11*(2), 27–45.

Galinsky, E. (1987). *The six stages of parenthood.* North Reading, MA: Addison-Wesley.

Gardner, S. L., Garland, K. R., Merenstein, S. L., & Lubehenco, L. O. (1993). The neonate and the environment: Impact on development. In G. B., Gardner & S. L. Merenstein (Eds). *Handbook of neonatal intensive care* (3rd ed.). (pp. 564–608). St. Louis: Mosby.

Glass, R. P. (1993). Development of visual function in preterm infants: Implications for early intervention. *Infants and Young Children, 6,* 11–20.

Glass, R. P., & Wolf, L. S. (1994). A global perspective on feeding assessment in the neonatal intensive care unit. *American Journal of Occupational Therapy, 48*(6), 514–526.

Gottfried, A. W., Wallace-Lande, P., Sherman-Brown, S., King, K., Coen, C., & Hodgman, J. (1981). Physical and social environment of newborn infants in special care nurseries. *Science, 214*(6), 673–675.

Harris, M. B. (1986). Oral-motor management of the high-risk neonate. *Physical and Occupational Therapy in Pediatrics, 6,* 231–250.

Harrison, H. (1993). The principles for family centered neonatal care. *Pediatrics, 92,* 643–650.

Harrison, H., & Kositsky, A. (1983). *The premature baby book: A parents' guide to coping and caring in the first years.* Tucson: Therapy Skill Builders.

Holloway, E. (1997). Fostering parent-infant playfulness in the neonatal intensive care unit. In Parham, D., & Fazio, L. (Eds.), *Play in occupational therapy for children* (pp. 171–183), St. Louis: Mosby– Yearbook.

Holloway, E. (1994). Parent and occupational therapist collaboration in the  neonatal intensive care unit. *American Journal of Occupational Therapy, 48*(6), 535–538.

Hunter, J. (1996a). Clinical interpretation of "Education and training of occupational therapists for neonatal intensive care units." *American Journal of Occupational Therapy, 50*(7), 495–503.

Hunter, J. (1996b). The neonatal intensive care unit. In Case-Smith, J., Allen, A., & Pratt, P. (Eds.), *Occupational therapy for children,* (3rd ed.) (pp. 583–647). St. Louis: Mosby.

Hunter, J. (1993). Therapist acceptance and credibility in the NICU. In Vergara, E. (Ed.), *Foundations for practice in the neonatal intensive care unit and early intervention: A self-guided practice manual,* Vol. 2. (pp. 255–258). Rockville, MD: American Occupational Therapy Association.

Hunter, J. (1992). *A NICU overview: The population and practice.* Presentation AOTA Annual Conference, Houston, Texas.

Hunter, J. (1990). Pediatric feeding dysfunction. In Semmler, C., & Hunter, J. (1990). *Early occupational therapy intervention: Neonates to three years.* Gaithersburg, MD: Aspen.

Hunter, J., Mullen, J., & Dallas, D. (1994). Medical considerations and practice guidelines for the neonatal occupational therapist. *American Journal of Occupational Therapy, 48,* 546–560.

Hunter, J., Mullen, J., & Vergara, E. (1994). Medical considerations and practice guidelines for the neonatal occupational therapist. *American Journal of Occupational Therapy, 48*(6), 546–559.

Hussey, B. (1988). *Understanding my signals.* Palo Alto: VORT.

Hyde, A. S., & Jonkey, B. W. (1994). Developing competency in the neonatal intensive care unit: A hospital training program. *American Journal of Occupational Therapy, 48*(6), 539–545.

Korones, S. (1985). Physical structure and function organization of neonatal intensive care units. In Gottfried, A. W., & Gaiter, J. L. (Eds.), *Infant stress under intensive care,* (pp. 7–22). Baltimore: University Park Press.

Lester, B. M., & Tronick, E. Z. (1990). Guidelines for stimulation with preterm infants. *Clinical Perinatology, 17*(1), xv–xvii.

Mathew, O. P. (1988). Regulation of breathing pattern during feeding: Role of suck, swallow, and nutrients. In Mather, O. P., & Sant'Ambrogio, G. (Eds.), *Respiratory function of the upper airway.* (pp. 535–560). New York: Marcel Dekker.

Morris, S., & Klein, M. D. (1987). *Pre-feeding skills.* Tucson: Therapy Skill Buliders.

Olson, J. A., & Baltman, K. (1994). Infant mental health in occupational therapy practice in the neonatal intensive care unit. *American Journal of Occupational Therapy, 48*(6), 499–505.

Rappaport, M. J. K. (1992). A descriptive analysis of the role of physical and occupational therapists in the newborn intensive care unit. *Pediatric Physical Therapy, 4*(4), 172–178.

Schwartz, R., Moody, L., Yarandi, H., & Anderson, G. C. (1987). A meta-analysis of critical outcome variables in non-sutritive sucking in preterm infants. *Nursing Research, 36,* 292–295.

Semmler, C. J. (1990). *Early occupational therapy intervention.* Gaithersburg, MD: Aspen.

Semmler, C. (Ed.). (1989). *A guide to care & management of very low birth weight infants.* Tucson: Therapy Skill Builders.

Semmler, C., & Butcher, S. (1990). *Handle with care: Articles about the at-risk neonate.* Tucson: Therapy Skill Builders.

Semmler, C. & Hunter, J. (1990). *Early occupational therapy intervention: Neonates to three years.* Gaithersburg, MD: Aspen.

Sweeney , J. (1993). Assessment of the special care nursery environment: Effects on the high risk infant. In Wilhelm, I. J. (Ed.), *Physical therapy assessment in early infancy* (pp. 13–34). New York: Churchill Livingstone.

Vergara, E. (1993a). *Foundations for practice in the neonatal intensive care unit and early intervention: A self-guided practice manual, vol. 1.* Rockville, MD: American Occupational Therapy Association, Inc.

Vergara, E. (1993b). *Foundations for practice in the neonatal intensive care unit and early intervention: A self-guided practice manual, vol. 2.* Rockville, MD: American Occupational Therapy Association.

Weibley, T. T. (1989). Inside the incubator. *Maternal and child nursing, 989*(14), 96–100.

Wolf, L. S., & Glass, R. P. (1992). *Feeding and swallowing disorders in infancy: Assessment and management.* Tucson: Therapy Skill Builders.

# Appendix A: Typical Terminology and Abbreviations Found in the NICU

A+B—apnea and bradycardia
ABG—arterial blood gas
AGA—appropriate for gestational age
Apgar—A system for scoring physical observations of newborn immediately after delivery.
APIB—assessment of preterm infant behavior
Apnea—cessation of breathing of 20 seconds or more
ASD—atrial septal defect
Asphyxia—deficient delivery of oxygen to the brain
Atelectasis—incomplete expansion of lungs
BAER—brainstem auditory evoke responses
Blood gas—test that measures amount of oxygen, carbon dioxide, and acid in baby's blood
BPD—bronchopulmonary dysplasia—chronic lung disease
Bradycardia—slow heart rate
BW—birth weight
CAT scan—computerized tomography of the brain
CBC—complete blood count
CHF—congestive heart failure
Cleft lip—an anomaly related to the failure of the maxillary process merging with the medial nasal elevation at six weeks in utero
Clubfoot—talipes equinovarus: the foot is turned medially and in plantar flexion. Talipes calcaneovalgus: the foot deviates laterally and is dorsiflexed.
CMV—cytomegalovirus
CPAP—continuous positive airway pressure
CPS—Child Protective Services
CPT—chest physiotherapy
CRF—chronic respiratory failure
CSF—cerebrospinal fluid
Deep sleep state—state in which infant is difficult to arouse
Doll's eye movement—when the newborn's head is turned the eyes remain in their original position. Characteristic of the first 10 days of life.
Dyspnea—difficult breathing
ECMO—extracorporeal membrane oxygenation
ELBW—extremely low birth weight
FAS—fetal alcohol syndrome—pattern of congenital craniofacial, limb, and cardiovascular defects associated with prenatal maternal alcoholism.
F.T.—full term
GA—gestational age
Gavage feeding—feedings via a tube passed through nose or mouth into stomach
GER—gastroesophageal reflux
Gravida—pregnancies
HAL—hyperalimentation
HFJV—high-frequency jet ventilation
HFOV—high-frequency oscillating ventilation
HFV—high-frequency ventilation
HIE—hypoxic ischemic encephalopathy

Hip dysplasia—may be congenital subluxation or dislocation of hip
HMD—hyaline membrane disease
HSV—herpes simplex virus
HTN—hypertension
Hypotonia—lack of muscle tone
ICH—intracranial hemorrhage
IDM—infant of diabetic mother
Intubation—insertion of tube into larynx for airflow exchange
IUGR—intrauterine growth retardation
IV—intravenous
IVDA—intravenous drug abuse
IVH—intraventricular hemorrhage
Lanugo—fine downy hair covers the infant
LBW—low birth weight
LGA—large for gestational age
MAS—meconium aspiration syndrome
MCA—multiple congenital anomalies
Meconium—initial feces of newborn
NC—nasal cannula
NEC—necrotizing enterocolitis—necrosis of small intestine/colon
Neonatal—1st month of life
NG—nasogastric gavage
NICU—neonatal intensive care unit
NJ—nasojejunal tube
NNS—nonnutritive suck
NPO—nothing by mouth
NS—nutritive sucking
$O_2$ sets—oxygen saturation
OD—right eye
OG—oral gastric tube
OS—left eye
$PaCO_2$—concentration of $CO_2$ in peripheral arteries
PDA—patent ductus arteriosus
PEEP—positive end expiratory pressure
PFC—persistent fetal circulation
Phototherapy—treatment of jaundice using ultraviolent light to convert bilirubin
Pneumogram—records respiratory movements
PO—by mouth
Premature—less than 37 weeks
PROM—premature rupture of membranes; passive range of motion
PTL—preterm labor
PVL—periventricular leukomalacia
RDS—respiratory distress syndrome
REM—rapid eye movements in light sleep state
Rentrolental fibroplasia—damage to retinal vessels causing blindness. Can be
    caused by high doses of oxygen therapy.
ROM—rupture of membranes
ROP—retinopathy of prematurity
SATs—oxygen saturation levels
SGA—small for gestational age
SIDS—sudden infant death syndrome
SROM—spontaneous rupture of membranes
Tachypnea—abnormal rapid breathing
TPN—total parenteral nutrition

*continued on following page*

TTN—transient tachypnea of the newborn
URI—upper respiratory infection
USG—ultrasound
VEP—vision evoke potential
VLBW—very low birth weight <1500 grams

*Source:* Adapted from Hunter (1996b); Semmler & Butcher (1990); Vergara (1993a).

# Appendix B: References for Parents

Tiny Treasures
3618 Crossroads Court
Eagan, MN 55123
Phone: 612/681-7818
E-mail: higginss@chem.wise.edu

Alexis Foundation
PO Box 1126
Birmingham, MI 48012
Phone: 810/543-1639
E-mail: WBUL63@Prodigy.com

Association for the Care of Children's Health (formerly Parent Care)
7910 Woodmont Avenue
Suite 300
Bethesda, MD 20814
Phone: 1-800-808-2224

Parents Helping Parents of Intensive Care Newborns
(for Western Pennsylvania, West Virginia and Eastern Ohio)
PO Box 268
Hilliards, PA 16040
Phone: 1-800-PHP-NICU (747-6428)

## ONLINE/INTERNET RESOURCES

**WWW Links:**
http://www.medsch@wisc.edu/childrenhosp;
http://weber@u.washington.edu/-neonatal/NICU-WEB;
http://galen@med.virginia.edu
http://neonatology@wbinet.nl

**Support Groups:**
After the NICU
Alliance of Genetic Support Groups
Preemie-L Discussion Group Home Page
Parenting the Premature Baby (discussion group)

**Preemie Links:**
Baby Web
The Congenital Heart Disease Resource Page
The Future of Children: Low Birth Weight
Kangaroo Care
KidSource OnLine
Lactation and related resources
National Information Center for Children with Disabilities
Neonatology on the Net

*continued on following page*

New Visions—for feeding, swallowing, oral-motor, and prespeech problems
Retinopathy of Prematurity, with pictures

**Vendors:**
Preemie Clothes
Preemie Resources
The Preemie Store
More Preemie Clothes
Go to Sleep Tapes
Bedtime Baby Beat—Heartbeat tapes

## BOOKS

**Caring for your baby:**

Gotsch, G. (1990). *Breastfeeding your premature baby.* LaLeche League.

Harrison, H. (1983). *The premature baby book: A parents' guide to coping and caring in the first years.* New York: St. Martin's.

Hyman, M. (1987). *The pain of premature parents: A psychological guide for coping.* Maryland: University Press of America.

Jason, J., & Van der Meet, A. (1989). *Parenting your premature baby.* New York: Henry Holt.

Ludington-Hoe, S., & Golant, S. K. (1993). *Kangaroo care: The best you can do to help your preterm infant.* New York: Bantam.

Manginello, F., & Digeronimo, T. F. (1992). *Your premature baby.* New York: Wiley.

Sears, W. (1996). *Keys to calming the fussy baby.* New York: NAL-Dalton.

Sledden, E. (1989). *When will life be normal? The healthy beginnings program for parents of premature infants.* Austin, TX: Hogg Foundation for Mental Health, The University of Texas.

Zaichkin, J. (1996). *Newborn intensive care: What every parent needs to know.* Petaluma, CA: NICU Ink.

**Autobiographies of parents who had babies in the NICU:**

Barsuhn, R. (1996). *Growing Sophia: The story of a premature birth.* St. Paul, MI: Nelson Publications.

DePree, M. (1996). *Dear Zoe.* San Francisco: Harper Collins.

Kennedy, N. (1995). *Baby hand and baby feet: Poems and sketches from the NICU.* Petaluma, CA: NICU Ink.

Mehren, E. (1993). *Born too soon: The extraordinary true story of one infant's fight to survive.* New York: Windsor.

# Appendix C: Educational References for OTs Working in the NICU

## ARTICLES

American Occupational Therapy Association (AOTA). (1993). Knowledge and skills for occupational therapy practice in the neonatal intensive care unit. *American Journal of Occupational Therapy, 47,* 1100–1105.

Dewire, A., White, D., Kanny, E., & Glass, R. (1996). Education and training of occupational therapists for neonatal intensive care units. *American Journal of Occupational Therapy, 50*(7), 486–494.

Hunter, J., Mullen, J., & Vergara, E. (1994). Medical considerations and practice guidelines for the neonatal occupational therapist. *American Journal of Occupational Therapy, 48*(6), 546–559.

Neonatal Intensive Care Unit (Special Issue). (1994). *American Journal of Occupational Therapy, 48*(6).

## BOOKS

Creger, P. J. (Ed.) (1989). *Developmental interventions for preterm and high-risk infants: Self study modules for professionals.* Tucson: Therapy Skill Builders.

Semmler, C. (Ed.) (1989). *A guide to care & management of very low birth weight infants.* Tucson: Therapy Skill Builders.

Semmler, C., & Butcher, S. (1990). *Handle with care: Articles about the at-risk neonate.* Tucson: Therapy Skill Builders.

Semmler, C., & Hunter, J. (1990). *Early occupational therapy intervention: Neonates to three years.* Gaithersburg, MD: Aspen.

Vergara, E. (1993a, b). *Foundations for practice in the neonatal intensive care unit and early intervention: A self-guided practice manual* (Vols. 1, 2). Rockville, MD: American Occupational Therapy Association.

## CONFERENCES, WORKSHOPS, SEMINARS

Developmental Interventions in Neonatal Care
Contemporary Forums
1900 Silvergate Drive
Dublin, CA 94506-2257
1-510-828-7100

Neonatal Individualized Developmental Care and Assessment Program (NIDCAP). This training program teaches and certifies the professional in observing infant behaviors and developing individualized intervention. It is offered in a variety of institutions across the United States.

Heidelise Als, PhD
Director of Neurobehavioral Infant and Child Studies
Harvard University Medical School
Children's Hospital
Boston, MA 02115

*continued on following page*

- *Feeding your Premature Baby*
  Media Services
  Sacred Heart Medical Center
  PO Box 2555
  Spokane, WA 99220-2555
- *The Neonatal Experience*
  Georgetown University
  Georgetown, D.C.
- *NICU Training Series* (for parents and staff)
  Polymorph Films
  118 South St.
  Boston, MA 02111
- *Your Baby and You*
  Therapy Skill Builders
  555 Academic Court
  San Antonio, TX 78204-2498

# 11

# *Children with Feeding and Nutritional Problems*

Dianne Koontz Lowman, EdD
Shelly J. Lane, PHD, OTR, ATP, FAOTA

*Because eating is an important daily living skill, essential to health and well-being, and critical throughout a person's life span, it falls within the occupational therapy domain of concern."*

—Avery-Smith, 1996, p. 846

## KEY POINTS

- Feeding and eating skills and proper nutrition are essential to survival and form a critical foundation for optimal development.

- Children with a variety of pediatric disorders and deficits are at risk for feeding, swallowing, nutritional, and growth difficulties.

- Difficulties in feeding skills may affect all aspects of the child's life, including growth, learning, communication, and interactions with others (Case-Smith & Humphry, 1996). Feeding skills have a long-term effect on the quality of life and on the degree of independence a child is able to achieve (Caretto, Francois, & McKinney, 1997).

- The feeding process is a critical time for family members to form relationships and impart culture, traditions, and values (Case-Smith & Humphry, 1996). It is critical for therapists working with families to remember that family members are constant in a child's life, whereas professionals and services will vary over the life span (Shelton & Stepanek, 1994). The elements of family-centered care presented in Figure 11–1 are critical for therapists working with children with feeding and nutritional problems.

■ Recognizing that the family is the constant in the child's life while the service systems and personnel within those systems fluctuate

■ Facilitation of parent/professional collaboration at all levels of care:

- care on an individual child

- program development, implementation, and evaluation;

- policy formation

■ Honoring the racial, ethnic, cultural, and socioeconomic diversity of families

■ Recognizing family strengths and individuality and respecting different methods of coping

■ Sharing with parents on a continuing basis and in a supportive manner, complete and unbiased information

■ Encouraging and facilitating family-to-family support and networking

■ Understanding and incorporating the developmental needs of infants, children, and adolescents and their families into service delivery systems

■ Implementing comprehensive policies and programs that provide emotional support to meet the needs of families

■ Designing accessible service delivery systems that are flexible, culturally competent, and responsive to family-identified needs

Figure 11–1  The elements of family-centered care.

- Feeding specialists represent a variety of disciplines, including but not limited to occupational, physical, or speech therapists; nurses; special educators; and family members. Difficulties in the feeding process may be complex and require a team of individuals from various disciplines (Hall, Yohn, & Reed, 1992).

# BEGINNINGS

In this chapter, the topics of feeding and nutrition are discussed. Because there are considerable differences in terminology, the following definitions are used:

- *Eating* refers to actively bringing food to the mouth by oneself (Avery-Smith, 1996).

- *Feeding* refers to being assisted in the activity of eating (Avery-Smith, 1996).
- *Oral-motor control* relates to use of the lips, cheeks, jaw, tongue, and palate (Wolf & Glass, 1992).
- *Oral-motor development* refers to feeding, sound play, and oral exploration (Morris & Klein, 1987). Feeding is a part of oral-motor skills, but there are oral-motor skills that may not involve food at all, such as oral-motor awareness, oral-motor exploration, and speech development (Clark, 1993).

This chapter will focus on oral-motor skills as they relate to feeding. The normal development of oral-motor problems will be outlined, including special conditions such as supplemental tube (or nonoral) feedings. Evaluation through the use of a holistic feeding observation are suggested. Intervention strategies, equipment, and resources for the clinician are discussed.

OTs may be involved in all aspects of planning for and development of a holistic feeding plan, working as a member of an interdisciplinary team (Avery-Smith, 1996). OTs can provide direct evaluation and intervention of the eating and feeding performance areas and performance components as delineated in *Uniform Terminology for Occupational Therapy—Third Edition* (AOTA, 1994).

# NORMAL DEVELOPMENT OF ORAL-MOTOR SKILLS AND FEEDING SKILLS

The normal development of oral-motor skills related to feeding involves the development of sucking from a nipple, drinking from a cup, munching and chewing solid foods, and coordinating the suck-swallow-breathe sequence (Case-Smith & Humphry, 1996). Maturation of these skills is closely tied to the physical maturation of the infant. Anatomically the infant's oral mechanisms differ considerably from those of the adult, a fact that plays a major role in oral-motor skill and efficiency in infancy. As can be seen in Figure 11–2, the infants' oral cavity appears to be filled by the tongue. This is a result of a small oral space and a different oral space–tongue size ratio than is seen in an adult. This, coupled with sucking fat pads to give the cheeks stability, offers a typical infant an enhanced ability to compress and suck on a nipple placed in the mouth. Early suckling patterns are the result of the limited mobility of the tongue in the mouth. As the infant grows and the size ratios in the mouth change, more mature oral-motor patterns emerge (Morris & Klein, 1987).

Oral skills develop concurrently and are closely related to the overall development of sensorimotor and cognitive skills. As a review and point of reference, a brief overview of normal sensorimotor, oral-motor, feeding, and cognitive development during the 3 years of life is presented in Appendix A at the end of this chapter. The importance of a basic knowledge of normal development is illustrated in the following description. Initially, feeding requires that the adult provide head support and head-trunk alignment to allow the infant to coordinate the suck-swallow-breathe sequence. Suckling occurs naturally in typically developing infants, and gives way to sucking as head and jaw stability appears. By 6 months of age, the typical infant has com-

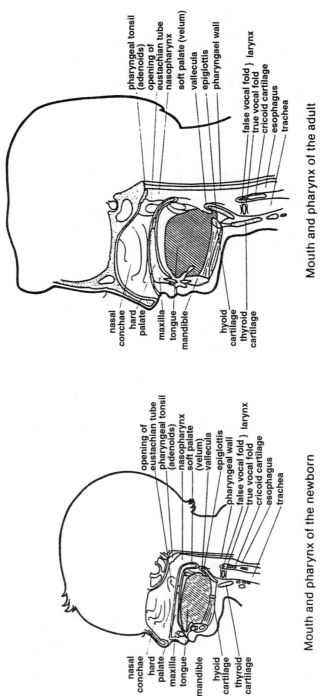

Mouth and pharynx of the newborn

Mouth and pharynx of the adult

Figure 11–2 Anatomical differences between the newborn and the adult mouth and pharynx.

plete head control and more jaw stability, allowing for better control of tongue movements. This stability allows him or her to suck from a bottle effectively, remove soft foods from a spoon, and begin to finger feed. The development of stability of the head and trunk are critical factors in the unfolding of oral-motor and feeding skills. As we will see later, the absence of this stability is linked to a variety of feeding difficulties.

The popularity of breastfeeding waxes and wanes in our society and is strongly influenced by cultural expectations and values. For some caregiver-infant dyads, breastfeeding may be the only choice for adequate nutrition. Often viewed as beneficial for both the mother and the infant, breast milk is easier to digest than formula, contains antibodies that increase the infant's immunity to infection, contains hormones and enzymes, and may lower the infant's risk of chronic disease (Danner, 1992a; Danner, 1992b; Klein & Delaney, 1994). Breastfeeding provides a quiet time for the interaction between the infant and mother, which promotes maternal-child bonding (Wolf & Glass, 1992).

Breastfeeding is undertaken when the infant has sufficiently coordinated sucking, swallowing, and breathing at full term. The physiology required for breastfeeding is slightly different from that used for bottle feeding. In breastfeeding, the infant's tongue is thrust up and forward to grasp the nipple. The gums and lips work together to create suction pressure. In bottle feeding, the infant's tongue thrusts forward to control milk overflow from the nipple; the gums and lips do not create compression (Wolf & Glass, 1992).

Infants born prematurely, and infants with other disabilities, may not be able to breast-feed initially; they can, however, still benefit from their mother's milk. The composition of preterm breast milk differs from the milk of full-term mothers; preterm milk contains more protein, fat, sodium, and chloride (Walker, 1992). Because bottle feeding can interfere with breastfeeding, some hospitals follow a *no-bottle protocol*. Oral stimulation is encouraged instead by finger feeding, suckling on a drained breast, or cup feeding. Premature infants who receive tube feedings should be transitioned to breastfeeding as soon as possible (Walker, 1992). Supplementary nutrition may be necessary when the infant first starts breastfeeding; previously pumped milk may be given through bottles or through the child's tube (Wolf & Glass, 1992).

As can be seen from Appendix A, eating skills are relatively mature by age 3. Further refinement of feeding and oral-motor skills continues between the ages of 3 and 5 years, as evidenced in the development of advanced skills such as drinking from a straw, blowing bubbles, or chewing gum. More in-depth information about normal development of eating is available from a variety of sources.

## ◢▮▮ FROM THE BOOKSHELF

The following books include detailed descriptions of normal sensorimotor, oral-motor, and/or feeding development:

- *Normal Development of Functional Motor Skills* (Alexander, Boehme, & Cupps, 1993)
- "Feeding and oral-motor skills" (Glass & Wolf, 1993), Chapter 8 in Case-Smith's *Pediatric Occupational Therapy and Early Intervention*.

# CHILDREN WITH FEEDING AND NUTRITIONAL PROBLEMS

## DIAGNOSIS AND IMPACT ON FEEDING AND NUTRITION

There is a general awareness that poor nutrition and consequent poor health can interfere with brain functions and learning. In fact, it has been stated that "The existing body of research shows a clear threat to the intellectual development of children who do not receive adequate nutrition" (Center on Hunger, Poverty, and Nutrition Policy at Tufts University School of Nutrition, 1995, p. 4). Severe malnutrition diminishes brain growth, whereas other nutritional deficiencies may lead to more subtle deficits in brain growth and function (Levy, 1996; Center on Hunger, Poverty, and Nutrition Policy at Tufts University School of Nutrition, 1995). Unfortunately, children with feeding difficulties are more vulnerable to such deficits. There are many clinical conditions that have the potential to affect feeding and nutrition adversely. As can be seen in Table 11–1, feeding, nutritional, and growth problems may be caused by neurological problems, congenital anomalies, endocrine disorders, gastrointestinal disorders, metabolic disorders, storage disorders, intrauterine growth retardation, chronic illness, cognitive or behavioral limitations, and psychosocial influences (Singer, 1990; Starrett 1991; Walter, 1994). In fact, most all childhood diseases and disabilities have the potential to affect feeding or nutrition negatively (Bazyk, 1990).

In addition to a direct impact of developmental disabilities on the child's ability to obtain sufficient nutrition to support growth, in some cases medications needed in the treatment of disability or disease can interfere with nutrition. For instance, a primary nutritional issue when children are on seizure medication relates to the interaction of anticonvulsant medication with foods. According to Horsley, Allen, and White (1996) anticonvulsant medications can change appetite, lower folic acid levels in the blood, and interfere with the activity of vitamin D. Anticonvulsants and other medication can also make the oral cavity sore or change sensitivity to taste, and these physical changes in the oral system will interfere with nutrient intake (Horsley et al., 1996; Powers & Moore, 1986). The therapist must be prepared to look at all aspects of the feeding difficulties in children with developmental disabilities. Of course, a team approach to feeding is preferable.

In-depth information is available about many of the clinical conditions listed in Table 11–1. For example, children with cerebral palsy have a high likelihood of displaying feeding or nutritional problems because of muscle tone abnormalities and delayed head and trunk control development. Considerable literature is available about this condition (Klein & Delaney, 1994; Morris & Klein, 1987). In this chapter, we highlight those conditions, such as Down syndrome, failure to thrive, fetal alcohol syndrome, prenatal substance exposure, and HIV/AIDS, for which information related to eating and feeding difficulties is less prevalent in the literature, and which are likely to appear in an OT's caseload. We will also briefly address behavioral issues that may surround feeding difficulties, because these cut across all categories of disability.

Table 11–1 **Pediatric Population at Risk for Feeding, Swallowing, Nutritional, and Growth Difficulties**

| Pediatric Disorders, Deficits, and Influences | Things to Look for Related to Feeding | Effects on Feeding and Nutrition |
|---|---|---|
| Neurological problems | | |
| Cerebral palsy | Poor sucking, swallowing, lack of head and trunk control, reflux, aspiration | Poor nutritional intake, failure to thrive, increased rate of infections |
| Traumatic brain injury | Depends on severity of brain injury and motor deficits but spasticity, ataxia, or tremor | Weight loss from reduced food intake, reflux, difficulties swallowing |
| Congenital anomaly syndromes | | |
| Down syndrome (Trisomy 21) | Hypotonia, inadequate lip closure, poor sucking, tongue protrusion | Overall developmental delay, persistent catarrh, and recurrent illness |
| Spina bifida | Problems with sucking, swallowing, gagging, oral sensitivity, gastrointestinal problems | May lose food out of mouth, discomfort sitting during feeding, poor nutrition |
| Cleft lip and/ or cleft palate | Poor oral suction, poor intake, nasal regurgitation, choking and gagging, excessive air intake | Slow weight gain, psychological or emotional problems that may impact eating |
| Prader-Willi syndrome | Low muscle tone during infancy; later voracious appetite and constant search or food | Obesity, microdontia, enamel defects, and dental caries |
| Pierre Robin anomaly | Airway obstruction, tracheostomy may be necessary | May require supplemental tube feedings |
| Endocrine disorders | | |
| Hypothyroidism (childhood or juvenile) | Hoarse voice, poor feeding, mental retardation | Growth retardation, delayed bone and dental maturation |
| Hyperthyroidism (neonatal— Graves' disease) | Infants born to mothers who have Graves' disease | Feeding problems, vomiting, diarrhea |
| Diabetes (Type I) | Monitoring blood glucose and watching for signs of hypoglycemia (low blood glucose) or hyperglycemia (high blood sugar) | Monitor diet (fruit, protein, and bread exchange) |
| Gastrointestinal disorders | | |
| Gastroesophageal reflux | Aspiration, increased risk for reactive airway disease, partial or total closure of the airway | Discomfort eating, feeding aversion, recurrent pneumonia |

*continued on following page*

Table 11–1 *continued*

| Pediatric Disorders, Deficits, and Influences | Things to Look for Related to Feeding | Effects on Feeding and Nutrition |
| --- | --- | --- |
| Supplemental tube feedings or dependence | Tubes may be placed because of structural abnormalities, inability to eat orally, or unable to get enough nutrition by mouth | Maintain oral feedings, oral simulation, and mealtime interactions |
| Short bowel syndrome | After surgery, receives parenteral nutrition | Transition back to "real" food, diet will be lactose-restricted, low-fat, and low-sugar |
| Metabolic disorders | | |
| Phenylketonuria (PKU) | Test at birth, placed on phenylalanine-restricted diet | Older children have difficulty following diet, food stealing |
| Storage disorders | | |
| Mucopolysaccharidosis (Hurler syndrome) | Short stature, progressive mental retardation, liver and spleen enlargement, full lips | Deteriorating motor and mental skills may affect feeding |
| Intrauterine growth retardation | | |
| TORCH (Toxoplasmosis, syphilis, rubella, cytomegalovirus [CMV], herpesvirus) | The five TORCH infections cause similar defects, including microcephaly, hydrocephalus, mental retardation, or brain damage | Varying effects depending on the degree of mental retardation or brain damage |
| Fetal alcohol syndrome | Cleft palate, low or weak muscle tone, weak suck | Slow postnatal growth, small and tire easy |
| Small for gestational age and prematurity | Immature oral musculature, high risk for BPD, medical complications requiring ventilation and feeding tubes | Sleepy, reduced endurance, aversion to oral feedings |
| Chronic illness | | |
| Cystic fibrosis | Trouble coordinating sucking, swallowing, and breathing, lung difficulties | Higher calorie needs |
| Bronchopulmonary dysplasia | Poor sucking, difficulty coordinating breathing, sucking, swallowing, fluid restriction, low tolerance for volume of foods, medications | Needs more food, but often eats less than other children, increased work of breathing and vulner-ability to fatigue |
| Cognitive or behavioral limitations | | |
| Mental retardation | Feeding difficulties will be varied, depending on degree of delay | Varied |

*continued on following page*

| Autism | May have obsessive rituals, sensory sensitivities that may be apparent orally | Eating at same time every day or eating a restricted diet of foods |
|---|---|---|
| Environmental influences Prenatal exposure to substances | Fussiness, distractibility, poor coordination, sensory defensiveness | Inefficient sucking and poor weight gain, poor persistence with feeding |
| Psychosocial Failure to thrive | Problems sucking, chewing, swallowing, oral hypersensitivity, sensitivity to different textures | Weight gain and growth are below normal levels for age |

Adapted from Batshaw & Perret (1992), Berkow & Fletcher (1992), Klein & Delaney (1994), Singer (1990), Starrett (1991), and Walter (1994).

**Down syndrome.** Down syndrome is a chromosomal abnormality also known as trisomy 21. Characteristics of Down syndrome related to feeding and nutrition are delayed acquisition of motor milestones because of mental retardation, retarded growth, craniofacial abnormalities, and generalized hypotonia (*Stedman's*, 1995). Feeding problems typically associated with hypotonia in children with Down syndrome include delayed development of head control, inadequate lip closure, weak sucking, tongue protrusion, poorly developed swallowing patterns, and decreased jaw stability (Hunt, 1982). Oral-motor problems related to the common craniofacial abnormalities of Down syndrome include open mouth, large tongue, and small oral cavity (Hunt, 1982). These problems in low tone and abnormal structure can led to abnormal variations in oral-motor patterns that lead to difficulties in the feeding process (Caretto et al., 1997). In addition to specific oral-motor problems, children with Down syndrome sometimes demonstrate behavioral feeding difficulties such as food refusal, trouble adjusting to different food textures and solid foods, an aversion to specific food textures, or holding food in the mouth (Spender, Dennis, Stein, Cave, Percy, & Reilly, 1995). Even with these problems, good feeding habits can be obtained through intervention and perseverance (Caretto et al., 1997).

**Fetal alcohol syndrome.** Fetal alcohol syndrome (FAS) is a condition found among children of some mothers who are chronic alcohol users. Specific to oral-motor development and feeding skills, alcohol exposure in utero may cause growth deficiencies, craniofacial abnormalities, seizures, problems in muscle tone, and tremors. Infants with FAS are usually small for gestational age with low birth weight, have slow postnatal growth, and are sometimes classified as failing to thrive (Clarren & Aldrich, 1993). Children with FAS often have problems related to feeding and nutrition because of craniofacial abnormalities (such as cleft palate) and because of low muscle tone, which affects sucking (Klein & Delaney, 1994).

**Prenatal exposure to substances.** As discussed in Chapter 2, substances of abuse are rarely used alone. Thus prenatal exposure often suggests a combination of substances including cocaine, heroin, alcohol, and nicotine. Although some behaviors may be generalized, different substances may have different effects on infants. In general, infants who have been exposed in utero to opiates exhibit fussiness, extreme distractibility, poor coordination, inefficient sucking, and poor weight gain, often as part of a pattern of deficits known as neonatal abstinence syndrome (Klein & Delaney, 1994; Lane, 1996).

Another impact on feeding and nutrition in an infant following prenatal substance exposure may be a vulnerable mother-child relationship, interaction, or bonding (Lane, 1996). Parent characteristics that may interfere with interaction, bonding, and thus the feeding process include inability to read unclear infant cues, inappropriate responses to cues, or parenting skills influenced by the use of substances (Barabach, Glazer, & Norris, 1992). Disruptions in the feeding process may also be caused by the disorganization of the infant, such as poor control of state, continuous crying, poor sucking, abnormal muscle tone, and disorganized patterns of movement. This group of difficulties falls into the behavioral realm of feeding problems and is addressed further below.

**HIV/AIDS.** Children born with the human immunodeficiency virus (HIV) who eventually develop acquired immunodeficiency syndrome (AIDS) may have a number of problems related to feeding and nutrition, such as anemia, diarrhea, thrush, and failure to thrive. Receiving adequate nutrition is a continual challenge. As symptoms change, feeding issues change. Children destined to develop neurological sequelae of AIDS will experience feeding difficulties associated with encephalopathy. These might include reduced head control, tonic bite, tongue thrust, and poor jaw stability, not unlike the problems faced by children with cerebral palsy. Difficulties with sucking may also be related to or be complicated by fatigue, oral sensitivity, and/or stress to put forth high amounts of energy during feeding. Thus, infants with weak sucking patterns may suck for a short time to reduce hunger, and then stop. The calorie intake may be sufficient to satiate extreme hunger but not to support growth and weight gain.

A similar situation may occur when infants have significant oral hypersensitivity; they may eat only enough to take the edge off their hunger and then reject the nipple. As noted above, this will compromise both nutrition and growth. This eating pattern also sets the child up to be hungry very often, as well as irritable. Thus the potential exists for this to interfere with the mother-child relationship and to create a stress around eating time, and behavioral problems can develop. Ongoing problems may require tube feeding to ensure adequate nutrition (Klein & Delaney, 1994).

**Failure to thrive.** Failure to thrive is a condition in which the infant's weight gain and growth are below normal levels for his or her age (*Stedman's*, 1995). The condition can be attributed to organic causes (such as disease or biological factors), to nonorganic causes (psychosocial factors), or to the combination of both organic and nonorganic factors (Dawson, 1992). Oral-motor abnormalities that occur in children who are failing to thrive include problems with sucking, chewing, or swallowing; tongue thrusting; involuntary tonic biting on spoon; excessive drooling; oral hypersensitivity; and an intolerance to different textures of foods (Lewis, 1982).

Behavioral problems related to feeding are often presented within the context of failure to thrive, although as already alluded to, a variety of physical disabilities and feeding problems may lead to behavioral problems around feeding. Behavioral or psychosocial factors related to failure to thrive include setting and duration of feeding, positioning of infant, and tense or disorganized interaction between the infant and caregiver (Mathisen, Skuse, Wolke, & Reilly, 1989; Arvedson, 1997). Psychosocial factors such as frustrations over feeding an infant failing to thrive can exacerbate tension and further threaten the interactions between the child and the caregiver (Mathisen et al., 1989). Environmental factors such as disorganization and time constraints can further intensify the problem. Failure to thrive is a multifaceted condition requiring specific feeding intervention with infants and with caregivers who may have many disadvantages (Mathisen et al., 1989).

**Behavioral issues.** A thorough discussion of the many behavioral issues associated with feeding problems is beyond the scope of this chapter. The reader can find many complete books on the topic, and a recent review is available in Arvedson (1997). For our purposes it is important to keep in mind that any of the previously listed physical limitations or disabilities may lead to or be coupled with behavioral issues. For example, a child tube fed for a lengthy period of time because of prematurity may refuse the transition to oral foods, developing into a child with failure to thrive. In this case, what was a physical or organic problem and basis for feeding difficulties became a nonorganic behavioral problem. Sensory processing difficulties may contribute to behavioral problems with feeding. Poor self-regulation, poor overall sensory modulation, and oral hypersensitivity can also be reflected in behavioral refusal to eat, difficulty making food transitions, or a very limited repertoire of acceptable foods. Environmental factors are a third source of behavioral feeding problems. The absence of a mealtime schedule, disorganized lifestyle, and a home environment characterized by stress and/or danger may all interfere with the feeding process, leading to behavioral problems around feeding. Any or all of the feeding problems noted previously can stress the caregiver-infant relationship, potentially compounding existing feeding problems (Arvedson, 1997). Thus, as we look at oral-motor problems that follow, keep in mind that these may be complicated by behavioral problems. Assessment and intervention must address both aspects feeding.

*Impact on breastfeeding.* All of the above problems can impact the process of breastfeeding, which can add yet another dimension to behavioral complications and difficulties in mother-infant interaction. Poor postural control, difficulty with positioning, a weak suck, or an oral-facial anomaly can all make success in breastfeeding a challenge. Coupling any of these with oral hypersensitivity, behavioral disorganization, and difficulty with interaction and bonding exacerbates the challenge of breastfeeding. For some mother-infant dyads, alternatives to breastfeeding may be a viable option; for others, this will not be the case. In this latter event, the therapist will need to work with the mother to try intervention techniques suggested later in this chapter in order to improve breastfeeding ability.

## COMMON ORAL-MOTOR PROBLEMS

Children may be born with or develop atypical oral-motor patterns. These abnormal patterns may be characterized by deviations in tone and movement patterns and may interfere with the normal development of feeding skills (Morris & Klein, 1987). Atypical patterns may be seen in the child's ability to suck, to swallow, or to coordinate the suck-swallow-breathe process.

**Sucking.** A normal sucking pattern is seen in infants when the tongue forms a groove around the nipple and moves up and down to draw the liquid into the mouth (Copeland & Kimmel, 1989). When abnormal tone exists, the up-and-down tongue movements may be altered. Another oral-motor difficulty that may affect sucking is failure of the infant's lips to close and form a seal around the nipple (Arvedson, 1993; Case-Smith & Humphry, 1996). In fact, difficulties with lip closure are among the most frequent oral-motor problems of children with neurological deficits (Peterson & Ottenbacher, 1986). Difficulties with lip closure may also affect drinking from a cup and removing food from a spoon.

**Swallow.** The swallow involves the following phases: the preparatory phase, the oral phase, the pharyngeal stage, and the esophageal phase. In the preparatory phase of the swallow, the child must be able to manipulate food in the mouth while maintaining closure of the lips. During this phase, the food is prepared for swallowing; it is sucked, chewed, or munched until it forms a bolus. Problems that affect the preparatory phase are difficulties in lip closure, reduced tongue movement, and oral sensitivity (Logemann, 1983).

In the oral phase of the swallow, the masticated food or liquid is moved to the back of the tongue, where the swallow is initiated. Abnormal oral-motor patterns affecting the oral phase of the swallow include jaw thrust, jaw clenching, jaw retraction, jaw instability, tonic bite reflex, tongue retraction, tongue thrust, reduced tongue elevation, reduced anterior to posterior tongue movement, disorganized anterior to posterior tongue movement, and lip retraction and pursing. The preparatory and the oral phases are the only phases the child can control. Intervention to influence these two stages is critical to the development of an efficient swallow (Case-Smith & Humphry, 1996).

In the pharyngeal phase, the bolus moves from the back of the tongue through the pharynx to the opening of the esophagus. Atypical patterns affecting the pharyngeal stage of the swallow include delayed or absent swallowing reflex, reduced laryngeal elevation, and reduced laryngeal closure (Case-Smith & Humphry, 1996). In the esophageal phase, the food or liquid moves through the esophagus. Abnormal patterns affecting the esophageal phase of the swallow are normally handled medically and will not be treated by the therapist (Logemann, 1983).

**Suck-swallow-breathe coordination.** Some children have difficulty smoothly coordinating the functions of sucking, swallowing, and breathing; difficulties with this coordination can cause aspiration of food and swallowing of air, and can affect the efficient intake of nutrients (Wolf & Glass, 1992). It has also been suggested that synchrony of suck-swallow-breathe is critical to speech and language development, the regulation of arousal states, postural control, ego development, and eye-hand coordination (Oetter, Richter, & Frick, 1988). Thus incoordination of these skills may have implications for children with significant oral-motor difficulties, as well as for children with more subtle oral-motor difficulties (such as those seen in a child with a learning disorder).

## GASTROESOPHAGEAL REFLUX

Gastroesophageal reflux (GER) is a condition in which the stomach contents "back up" into the esophagus and/or throat (Klein & Delaney, 1994). GER may be diagnosed by an upper gastrointestinal x-ray series. Reflux is a common problem among a variety of children with feeding and oral-motor difficulties, including children with mental retardation who are nonambulatory and children who have had a feeding tube placed (Starrett, 1991). Symptoms that GER may be occurring include spitting up, chronic vomiting, choking, coughing, difficulties with breathing, recurrent pneumonia, and poor weight gain. Because some children associate discomfort with mealtime, they may refuse to eat, cry, or become irritable (Klein & Delaney, 1994).

## SPECIAL DIAGNOSES: CHILDREN WHO ARE RECEIVING SUPPLEMENTAL TUBE FEEDINGS

Medical and scientific advances have enabled children to receive nutrition through supplemental tube feedings. Tube feedings are typically used with children who might be unable to eat or drink by mouth, who are unable to eat safely orally, or who are unable to take in enough calories by mouth for proper growth (Klein & Delaney, 1994). Tube feedings provide a valuable intervention when nutrition and growth are compromised. There are a number of different feeding tubes, characterized by point of insertion. The nasogastric (NG) tube is inserted into the oropharyngeal area through the nose, down the esophagus, and into the stomach. An NG tube does not require surgery; therefore, it is often used with preterm infants, with children too sick to undergo surgery, or as a temporary measure. The NG tube is kept in place for several days; the child is able to continue sucking and swallowing while the tube is in place. The orogastric (OG), or gavage, tube is inserted through the mouth and down into the stomach. The OG tube is usually removed after feeding. The OG tube has all the benefits of the NG tube, except it is difficult to eat by mouth when the tube is in place (Klein & Delaney, 1994). However, because it is removed following the feeding, oral activity is possible at other times. Both NG and OG tube feeding interventions are likely temporary. Therapeutic intervention during this time should include nonnutritive sucking and oral stimulation.

    A gastrostomy tube, or G-tube, is inserted directly into the stomach, bypassing the mouth. A major advantage of the G-tube is that there is no discomfort in the mouth or throat, and the tube can be used on a long-term basis. Limitations of the G-tube are that placement requires a surgical procedure and that reflux is common. A jejunostomy tube is placed into the beginning of the small intestine past the duodenum; it bypasses the stomach and reduces the risk of reflux (Batshaw & Perret, 1992; Klein & Delaney, 1994). A major disadvantage is that the jejunostomy tube requires a continuous-drip feeding method and pump.

Since children who are receiving their nutrition nonorally do not take foods or liquids through the mouth, they are at risk for failing to develop normal oral-motor feeding skills without specific intervention (Caretto et al., 1997). The chronic presence of an NG feeding tube is aversive to many children, as is the process of placing and removing the OG tube. Children who have received aversive stimulation as a result of tube feedings may also find that this is coupled with the absence of more typical oral stimulation. This combination may lead to sensitivity to touch in and around the mouth. Placement of a feeding tube should not result in cessation of oral stimulation or of the interactive feeding process (Case-Smith & Humphry, 1996).

As we have seen in this section, there are many different types of clinical conditions that result in many different types of oral-motor or feeding difficulties. Because of the many variables, comprehensive information will need to be gathered before planning a specific intervention.

# EVALUATION: ASSESSING NEEDS AND DETERMINING STRENGTHS

The assessment of feeding and nutritional difficulties should always begin by gathering a thorough history of the difficulties. Information can be obtained from a variety of sources and should include family history; prenatal, birth, and perinatal history; history specific to neonatal period (first 28 days); and the child's feeding history (Arvedson, 1993).

There are numerous assessment scales available such as the following scales, profiles, and checklists:

- *The Neonatal Oral-Motor Assessment Scale* (Braun & Palmer, 1986)
- *The Multidisciplinary Feeding Profile* (Kenny et al., 1989)
- *Behavioral Assessment Scale of Oral Functions in Feeding* (Stratton, 1981)
- *Oral-Motor/Feeding Rating Scale* (Jelm, 1990)
- *Pre-Feeding Skills* (Morris & Klein, 1987)
- *Pre-Speech Assessment Scale* (Morris, 1982)

Some of these tools focus on oral-motor issues only, whereas others look at aspects of feeding that relate to context and role performance. Because the feeding and eating processes are an integral part of the infant role and are wedded closely to parent-infant interaction, the therapist will do best to evaluate all aspects of the process, covering performance skills, context, and role. The evaluation of the child's sensory and motor feeding difficulties should be seen as only one step in a larger problem-solving process (Glass & Wolf, 1993). At present, no universally accepted single standard assessment exists for feeding evaluations (Arvedson, 1993).

## THE HOLISTIC FEEDING OBSERVATION

One way to guide the problem-solving process is the use of observation and interview to gather as much information as possible about all aspects of the feeding process. The Holistic Feeding Observation Form in Appendix B at the end of this chapter is one format that may help the team consider all components that might interfere with or have an impact on a child's feeding skills (Lowman & Murphy, 1998). While using the questions on the Holistic Feeding Observation Form as a guide, a therapist can gather information about:

- The family's feeding routine, issues, and cultural implications
- Communication and socialization skills within the feeding process
- Physical development and positioning during feeding
- The presence of any respiratory issues
- The child's sensory and oral-motor development

As can be seen, sections I and II of this tool address issues related to the role of the child as a participant in the eating and feeding process within the context of the family. This information is often missing from other assessment tools. Environment and culture are addressed and information is sought pertaining to motor, sensory, and physiological issues. If additional information is needed pertaining to specific skill components, therapists may want to use other assessment tools to augment the results of this evaluation. The information gathered during this total assessment process can then be used to develop a holistic feeding plan (Lowman & Murphy, in preparation).

# INTERVENTION FROM AN OCCUPATIONAL THERAPY PERSPECTIVE

Numerous books and articles have been written that include specific intervention strategies. Several are listed in the From the Bookshelf box.

## ▌▌▌ FROM THE BOOKSHELF

Critical additions to your professional library should include the following books that present intervention from an OT perspective:

- *Feeding and Nutrition for Children with Special Needs: Handouts for Parents* (Klein & Delaney, 1994).
- *Feeding and Swallowing Disorders in Infancy: Assessment and Management* (Wolf & Glass, 1992)
- *Head-Neck Treatment Issues as a Base for Oral-Motor Function* (Nelson, Meek, & Moore, 1994)
- *Pre-Feeding Skills* (Morris & Klein, 1987)

The next section of this chapter illustrates some general intervention areas and ideas, with an emphasis on problem solving. Feeding intervention involves many skills a typical OT will already have in his or her repertoire, which are then applied to the particular strengths and needs of the child. Because eating is commonly a family affair, we will begin with intervention considerations related to the parents or caregivers. This will include elements of family-centered care, parent-child interactions, and the impact of culture on the feeding interaction. In addition, concepts of intervention related specifically to the child with feeding and nutrition difficulties are covered. These include feeding environment, positioning, oral-motor techniques, food texture and bolus modification, and adaptive equipment (Schuberth, 1994). This section begins with the introduction of a child with feeding difficulties and follows her throughout the intervention process.

## CASE STORY

*Amanda:* Amanda was born to a 24-year-old mother at full term. During the birth process Amanda's mother had a stroke and died. As a result of the stroke and ensuing medical emergency, Amanda experienced severe perinatal asphyxia, leading to brain damage. She spent 4 months in the hospital after birth and is now living at home with an older sister (age 2) and a grandmother as primary caregiver. She was discharged from the hospital with a gastrostomy tube for feeding. At 6 months of age Amanda is referred for a feeding evaluation because her grandmother would like to see if she can be taught to eat by mouth. At this point in time Amanda has muscle tone abnormalities that include spasticity of the extremities and trunk and poor head control. She has a great deal of difficulty handling oral stimulation, demonstrating a strong bite reflex and apparent hypersensitivity to things placed in her mouth.

## FAMILY-BASED INTERVENTION

Feeding is a critical component of parenting behavior and is often a source of pride as parents report on the quantity of formula or milk their children have eaten in a feeding session. Feeding is viewed as one of the few activities of parenthood that *should* be straightforward. When an infant or child has a feeding problem, the ramifications go beyond the immediate and specific needs of the child and extend to the self-esteem of the primary caregiver (often the mother), and the bonding between the mother and the child (Glass & Wolf, 1993). Furthermore, when feeding problems exist, they may be associated with stress for infant and/or caregiver, which may translate to the family if feeding is difficult and/or requires excessive amounts of time. The potential then exists for a vicious cycle to develop in which infant or child feeding difficulties lead to maternal feelings of inadequacy and family stress, which in term further disrupt the fragile feeding skills the infant or child may be developing. Given the potential disruption, when intervening with feeding difficulties, it is imperative to begin from a family focus.

If a tool such as the Holistic Feeding Observation Form has been used to gather information, the therapist will have an idea of the strengths and needs emerging around feeding. Because cultural issues will impact all forms of intervention, the cultural umbrella should cover all aspects of intervening in the feeding process. Although it is beyond the scope of this chapter to delineate cultural mores related to feeding, some general suggestions are in order. Before intervening, be sure to determine the cultural norms for breastfeeding, weaning from the breast or bottle, beginning solid foods, using utensils, talking during mealtimes, or eating with the entire family. Suggesting that the child be included in the family meal to promote socialization is worthless if the cultural habits of the family do not include children at mealtime. Be certain to check all suggestions for intervention with the family first to be sure they are consistent with the family's beliefs and values.

## BEGIN WITH THE FAMILY

The Holistic Feeding Observation Form guides the evaluator first to determine if a feeding routine has been established and then to understand what this routine involves. Keep in mind that if the feeding process already requires a large amount of caregiver time, it is unlikely that increasing the amount of time involved will be viewed as a positive change. Looking at both the specifics of the routine and the satisfaction of the family with this overall process will form a foundation upon which the therapist can base changes. As the therapist gathers information related to the routine, he or she should also find out what aspects the family would like to keep, what they would like to modify, and what they would like to discard. The therapist should look carefully at the pleasurable components of the feeding interaction and be certain *not* to interfere with these, but instead incorporate them into the feeding program and capitalize on their potential positive contributions to the process. For instance, if the caregiver identifies being able to hold the child or infant as a positive aspect of feeding, the therapist had best not recommend that a more stable seating arrangement be found!

> Amanda is currently tube-fed small amounts five times daily. During feedings she is in an infant seat, and her grandmother either sits with Amanda or sets up a mobile for her to watch as the feeding is given. Each feeding requires about 30 minutes, along with setup and cleanup. Because there is another child in the picture, Grandma does not have a great deal of time to spend with Amanda alone. She attempts to feed the sister her meals when Amanda is receiving her breakfast, lunch, and dinner, and then she tries to be alone with Amanda during her other two feedings by giving them when the sibling is either napping or in bed for the night. This allows Grandma some quiet time with Amanda.

The second aspect of the Holistic Feeding Observation Form of interest here is understanding the issues identified by the caregiver. From a family-centered perspective, there are the areas in which intervention should begin. The therapist must look at the priorities set by the family, and when at all possible, establish these as the priorities for the feeding intervention program. There are times when for health or safety reasons this may not be possible, in which case the therapist must address issues with the family and attempt to establish priorities that are safe and promote child health.

> Grandma's priority is to have Amanda be an oral feeder. She does not mind the feeding part, but she does not like having to feed Amanda through the gastrostomy tube.

Collaboration with the family also involves acknowledging and accepting the cultural values of the family. Cultural issues may dictate food type, food preparation, time of meals, and who is involved in the meals, to name just a few areas. The therapist need not agree with these guidelines, but must include them when planning any intervention program.

> There are no specific cultural restrictions for this family in terms of food preparation, food type, or mealtime. In fact, mealtimes, although regular, are not formal and often involve having the TV on. In addition there are times when Amanda's sister brings her tape recorder to the table to listen to music while she eats.

With these caveats for intervention, the therapist can begin to look at ways to intervene with the specific feeding and eating needs of the child and work the intervention program into the actual family milieu.

## INTERVENTION RELATED SPECIFICALLY TO THE CHILD

**The feeding environment.** Although often difficult to truly control, one must look at the feeding environment and determine how well it works for the child and family. If the child spends mealtimes at school or in a program, the therapist must also consider this environment as feeding programs are developed. There is no single correct environment. Some children do best in quiet environments, controlled for the amount of sensory input available; other children thrive on the social stimulation of the cafeteria. Included in Table 11–2 are some common feeding environments and characteristics associated with them. Based on the child's needs, the family preferences, and the actual characteristics of the feeding environment, the therapist can make an informed recommendation (Lane & Cloud, 1988).

> The feeding environment for Amanda is somewhat chaotic, with TV and sometimes music an integral factor. Grandma attempts to pay attention to Amanda and her sister, but generally the sister receives the bulk of the attention when she is present. Grandma reports that Amanda seems to sleep during these feedings. The two feedings done

when Amanda's sister is sleeping are generally quieter, and Grandma reports that Amanda often has her eyes open during these periods. Grandma tries to talk to Amanda during this times, and often strokes her face, arms, and legs. Sometimes it seems that Amanda does not like to have her face stroked. Grandma relishes these quieter times with Amanda.

Table 11–2 **Characteristics of Feeding Environments**

| Environment | People Present | Potential Characteristics |
|---|---|---|
| Home, a family meal | Family members | Moderate noise, potential for startling noise; some potential for disorganization, conversation, potential for socialization with family members |
| Home, meal before or after family meal | Primary caregivers | More controllable noise level, individualized attention, fewer distractions, greater potential to be responsive to communication attempts and choices, less social interaction |
| Cafeteria | Classmates, other classes of children, teachers, aides | High noise level, high degree of sensory input, startling input at some point in the meal likely, some degree of disorganization, potential for distraction, opportunity to socialize with peers, opportunity to be included in regular school activity |
| School, classroom | Feeder, child | Controllable noise level and potentially more organized, individualized attention, fewer distractions, greater potential to be responsive to communication attempts and choices, less social interaction |
| | Feeder, child, a few select peers | All the above, in addition a greater potential for interaction |
| School therapy room | Therapist, child | As with classroom, although potential for more control over other sensory distractors as well |
| | Therapist, child, a few peers | As with above, with greater potential for social interaction |

**Positioning.** One of the first concerns of many therapists involved in feeding intervention is the position of the child. Correct postural alignment for feeding is critical and can be achieved in a variety of positions, depending on the age of the child (Case-Smith & Humphrey, 1996). Without proper alignment of the head and trunk both feeding skill and safety can be compromised (Glass & Wolf, 1993; Macie & Arvedson, 1993; Morris & Klein, 1987). If the child is an infant or still being fed like an infant using a bottle, holding the child in the lap may be very acceptable. In this position there is potential for great sharing of warmth and interaction between the caregiver and the child. If the child is held supine in the lap, facing slightly toward the caregiver, there will be the opportunity for face-to-face interaction and communication. For safe feeding, the child should be held with the head in a neutral or slightly flexed position, and the body should be well supported with some abdominal and hip and knee flexion. If this is the preferred position for the caregiver, make sure the caregiver is seated comfortably, with arms and feet supported, allowing the caregiver to offer the best support to the child.

Children receiving spoon feeding can also be held, but the process becomes progressively more difficult as the child gets bigger. For spoon feeding the child needs to be held more upright than is needed for bottle feeding—the head should be at neutral with hip and knee flexion. It is important here to attend to the position of the shoulders, too; shoulders should be rounded slightly forward, or protracted. The total picture should be a relaxed position in the caregiver's arms. Although many therapists will balk at this position for the older or larger child, some caregivers continue to prefer it. You may find this to be a favorite position of caregivers if the child has a tendency to choke, and the caregiver feels a need to bring the child to a forward sitting position quickly to dislodge food that may be caught. A similar body position can be attained by using an infant seat that holds the infant in a semi-reclined position but does not strap his or her shoulders down. Such seats offer little external support, but they do recline enough that the head can often be maintained in neutral at midline, with shoulders slightly protracted, and the body, hips, and knees in flexion. Using such a seat will also allow the caregiver to be in a face-to-face position with the child. Benefits of this position that can be emphasized to the caregiver include the ability to watch the child for facial reactions, to have both hands free, and to respond appropriately to the child's needs. The face-to-face position often promotes a great deal of socialization. It can also give the child the ability to communicate likes, dislikes, wants, and needs somewhat more effectively than can be done when the child is being held.

The 90-90-90 upright position is usually the most efficient for children of school age. For some children, achieving this position will require the use of specialized seating systems. Key points for seating include having the head upright and at midline; shoulders in neutral or slightly forward; hips, knees, and ankles flexed to approximately 90 degrees; and feet flat on a footrest or the floor. The specifics of seating will not be covered here, but can be found in several resources (e.g., Angelo, 1996).

Morris and Klein (1987, pp. 172–177) present a number of additional seating or positioning options for young children during feeding. Depending on the skills and needs of the child as well as the skills and preferences of the caregiver, alternative positions may be considered. Some children do well eating in a prone stander or prone on a wedge. These somewhat unique positions may be offered to the caregiver as options. It is important to keep in mind with any position that the complete restriction of movement is *not* desirable. Furthermore, feeding position, just like any other position, should be reevaluated at regular intervals to be certain it is still optimal.

Amanda is generally fed in an infant seat, which places her in a semi-reclined, shoulders forward position. Since she is tube fed, Grandma has not paid attention to where her head rests when the feeding process occurs. During observation it appeared that Amanda's head rested to the right side unless Grandma passively brought it back to midline. Grandma has tried to offer Amanda some of her liquid food by mouth using a spoon. When doing this Grandma continues to have Amanda in the infant seat, or she holds Amanda in her lap. When held in Grandma's lap, Amanda's neck is usually slightly extended, as are her hips. Although Amanda's shoulders begin the process in protraction, they do not remain long in this position as Amanda's body assumes a more extended posture. Because Amanda coughs and sputters a great deal during this process, Grandma feels a need to be able to sit her up quickly and pat her back, and the in-the-lap position allows for this. Grandma loves to hold Amanda, but finds it difficult because of Amanda's muscle tone.

**Oral-motor techniques.** Oral-motor techniques can be grouped into six categories: general sensory stimulation, intraoral stimulation, jaw control, sensorimotor techniques, food placement, and thermal stimulation (Schuberth, 1994). These techniques will be embedded in the following discussion of intervention to show the therapist how they need to be integrated into the thinking and planning process in feeding.

You may have carried out the Holistic Feeding Observation evaluation and obtained additional information on motor and sensory issues from other observation or assessment, and should know where to head with these interventions. A good place to begin is to consider the child's reaction to sensory input in the mouth and around the face. Many children with feeding difficulties may show sensory sensitivities to touch, taste, and temperature. The "cause" of such sensitivities is difficult to pin down, but Glass and Wolf (1993) suggest that it is related to a lack of early oral input (as when children are tube fed for long periods of time), unpleasant oral-tactile experiences (as when children are fed with oral-gastric tubes, have experienced mechanical ventilation, have frequent nasal suctioning, etc.), or delayed introduction of oral feeding. Working with the family and child when he or she is very young, and introducing oral input (i.e., nonnutritive sucking) early in the developmental process may forestall the development of oral touch sensitivity and may also make the transition to bottle and solids easier.

Intervention with the child experiencing oral tactile sensitivity can parallel that suggested for tactile defensiveness of the whole child (Ayres, 1979; Royeen & Lane, 1991). This involves preparing the child for the feeding session by using deep touch pressure, proprioception, and possibly vibration; proceed with touch only within the child's tolerance range. Control of input by the child is important. If motor limitations restrict the child from playing in his or her mouth and around the face, then this type of touch can be applied by the caregiver or therapist, but careful attention must be paid to the child's facial and body cues. This puts the child in control.

Since you are specifically concerned with the oral-facial area for feeding problems, you may be tempted to begin here. However, it may be more acceptable to the child to offer input on other parts of the body first, approaching the face and mouth slowly. Some therapists (e.g., Glass & Wolf, 1993; Nelson et al., 1994) recommend that input progress to the cheeks, outer lips, and last into the mouth. All this should be done prior to offering food. In fact, if possible, tactile activities and oral play should take place at times *in addition to* mealtimes. Oral toy exploration is an integral part of development for many typical children. Typical children engage in oral exploration of the hands within the first month of life and expand to oral exploration of the environment throughout the first year of life. It has been suggested that children will obtain significant amounts of information about an object orally until it is too large or too complex for mouthing to be an effective means of information gathering (Ruff, 1984). It behooves OTs to make it a part of the developmental process for children with disabilities as well. Thus, if motor skills limit the child's ability to bring his or her hands to the mouth, the caregiver can do this. Therapists should show caregivers how to move the upper extremities into protraction and flexion to facilitate oral-motor play. This can be done in semireclined or sitting positions, but is also possible in the sidelying or prone positions, where gravity is not a factor. Be cautious with oral exploration when the child exhibits a bite reflex. Toys that do not break when bitten are imperative. Many therapists have found soft squeaky toys to have an interesting appeal both tactually and visually. They are also easy to hold and do not break when bitten. There are a number of teethers available that can be used for this activity as well, and many are firm but not hard plastic, with interesting surface textures. Taste can be added to this process of exploration by dipping the toy in a favorite food or drink, and using the dipped toy in oral play.

---

■ *THERAPEDS POINTER*

Soft oral toys and interesting teethers can be found in local stores in the pet department and can also be obtained from catalogues that specialize in toys for young children. Two catalogue resources are listed below.

PDP Products
12015 North July Ave
Hugo, MN 55038
612-439-8865

Kapable Kids
PO Box 250
Bohemia, NY 11716
800-356-1564

Amanda has oral hypersensitivity. She has not been fed by mouth for several months, and prior to the placement of the gastrostomy tube, Amanda had been fed using an OG tube placed for each meal. In addition, because of difficulty managing her secretions, Amanda is frequently suctioned. She does not engage in oral exploration and in fact cannot get her own hand to her mouth. Subsequently, Amanda's oral experiences have not been pleasant, nor have they been under her own control. Now, when her grandmother attempts to put a spoon in her mouth, or strokes her face, Amanda demonstrates a strong bite reflex and considerable grimacing.

When children are ready to make the transition to solids, food texture becomes an issue. Because many children are sensitive to the textures of food, the therapist should grade textures based on the child's readiness to accept them. Texture gradations include liquid, pureed, chunky, crunchy, and chewy. It is important to note that food items such as soup combine chunks with liquid and can be very difficult for the mouth to handle because of the different textures. When introducing the child to chunky food, it is best to use food that is chunky but uniform in texture, and not chunky mixed with liquid.

Amanda is not ready for oral foods. In fact, she may be dangerously aspirating the liquids being fed to her by spoon because of great difficulty controlling liquid in her mouth. Keeping with Grandma's desire to develop oral feeding skills, intervention may begin with a general program to decrease tactile defensiveness and encourage oral-motor exploration and play. Body massage, deep touch pressure, and neutral warmth may be used to decrease the defensive responses to touch that Amanda demonstrates. Firm touch should be given on trunk, arms, legs, or wherever Amanda best tolerates it. Swaddling Amanda after a body massage will provide neutral warmth, and Grandma can be shown how to swaddle Amanda with her hands at midline. Amanda can be guided to hold a toy and begin to bring it to her mouth and eyes for exploration as tolerated. Putting Amanda's own fingers in her mouth is not recommended because of her bite reflex. Grandma will need to experiment with different types of toys and surface textures to see what Amanda finds enjoyable to both look at and feel on her cheeks and in her mouth. Introducing the toy into the mouth should be done cautiously, and only when Amanda gives cues with her eyes, her muscle tension, or her affect that this is desirable. The therapist must caution Grandma to use toys that will not break or be bitten into pieces should Amanda's bite reflex be elicited during this activity. If tolerated, the toy can be dipped into food that has an appealing taste (often sweet works), so that Amanda can begin to experience taste as she explores the toys. The process will be slow and will require that Grandma pay attention to Amanda's potentially subtle cues. To avoid distraction, Grandma may want to play in this way when Amanda's sister is sleeping. Because the environment will likely play a role in Amanda's acceptance of oral play, Grandma will need to use her judgment about what environment best suits Amanda's needs.

Oral-motor skills can be promoted using a variety of techniques. Following a problem-solving plan, whenever there are oral-motor difficulties, the therapist should look *first* at the feeding environment, the position in which the child is fed, any sensory sensitivity the child may be experiencing, and the general state of the child during the feeding process (the quiet, alert state is desirable for infants). If all of these features are as optimal as is possible and feeding difficulties remain, the techniques listed in Table 11–3 should

**Table 11–3 Interventions to Consider for Specific Oral-Motor Difficulties**

| Oral Difficulty | Interventions to Consider |
| --- | --- |
| Difficulties with suck | Consider nipple qualities and perhaps try a different type of nipple; make sure nipple hole is patent; if liquid seems uncontrollable, make sure nipple hole is not too large; prefeeding oral stimulation to elicit rooting, nonnutritive suck; use nipple to rhythmically stroke infant's tongue down and forward; pull gently on nipple to improve oral grasp; provide external support on jaw and checks for greater stability |
| Poor modulation of jaw movement | Provide external support on jaw and cheeks for greater stability; try a prone position on a stander or wedge; be certain to check for hypersensitivity; incorporate oral play and oral sensory input at times other than during feeding |
| Tongue retraction | Be sure to have the chin slightly tucked and the neck elongated during feeding; stroke down and forward on the tongue with firm pressure; tap under the chin near the root of the tongue; try prone positioning |
| Tongue thrust | Try different textures of food that may not promote thrusting; develop tongue lateralization skills; work on sucking patterns initiated from the lips, not the tongue; press down and inward on the tongue with firm pressure; if the child tolerates it, add vibration |
| Low tone in the face | Be sure to work first on trunk tone and stability; tapping to the lips, tongue, under the chin |
| Difficulty swallowing | Try prone positioning; use externally applied jaw stability techniques; stroke the lips in a circular movement with a wet cotton swab; use of chilled or frozen liquids during a feeding session may improve initiation of swallow |
| Tonic bite reflex | Relax the child prior to feeding; use a coated spoon to decrease the hypersensitivity; include oral play at times other than feeding |

be considered. This list is by no means comprehensive. Many additional feeding difficulties may be encountered by the therapist, and there are many other techniques useful for specific feeding problems. As you consider the suggestions in Table 11–3, keep in mind that if the child's oral difficulties are related to decreased muscle tone in the mouth and face, you can adapt techniques used on the body to increase tone to the face. Tapping, quick stretch, and icing may all be useful ideas. Similarly, if the difficulty relates to hypertonicity, use techniques to decrease tone. If you can work to understand a possible underlying cause of the oral difficulty, you will generate a myriad of intervention strategies that go well beyond those listed in Table 11–3.

There is some information available that specifically addresses the facilitation of oral-motor skills in relation to breastfeeding. The therapist should first work with the mother to determine the most successful position for breastfeeding. For infants with a weak suck, the therapist can teach techniques such as stroking the cheeks toward the lips, brushing the lips, massaging the gums, and rubbing the hard palate (Marmet & Shell, 1984). If the infant has an oral-facial anomaly such as cleft palate, the therapist can help the mother find the most comfortable position of the nipple in the child's mouth (Danner, 1992a). Other interventions can be adapted from the list in Table 11–3.

---

As Amanda begins to tolerate oral exploration more and more, Grandma may be guided to work on various oral-motor skills. As a safety precaution, further assessment may be needed to determine if Amanda will be a functional feeder. The therapist, Grandma, and the physician should discuss this together, and a barium swallow may be recommended to examine suck and swallow skills.

---

**Food texture and bolus modification.** As alluded to above, the altering aspects of the food can make a difference in the child's ability to control the food in the mouth. It can be truly challenging to control a bit of food containing several different textures (e.g., soup with chunks in it), and this type of food is not generally used with children experiencing difficulties with oral-motor skills. Thin liquids may be very difficult if swallowing is an issue, because they are hard to control in the mouth. For children with difficulty in this area you may need to develop a mechanism for delivering liquids in slow, controlled ways. Morris & Klein (1987) describe a pacifier adapted to attach to a syringe that allows the caregiver to offer small amounts of liquid during sucking, thus promoting the sucking movement without overwhelming the oral-motor capabilities of the child. The Haberman Feeder is a nipple-compression device used for feeding infants with cleft palate (Wolf & Glass, 1992). Through valving, nipple compression keeps milk moving into the infant's mouth rather than back into the bottle. Flow of the liquid is controlled by changing the orientation of the slit in the nipple in the baby's mouth (Wolf & Glass, 1992).

To work on improved sucking, thickened beverages may be offered. This increases the resistance to the suck pattern, may facilitate the transition from suckling to sucking, and gives the child a liquid in his or her mouth that is easier to control. Thick liquids are often delivered to the mouth via a Nosey cup or spoon. Thickened liquids also provide a great transition to cup drinking. Liquids may be thickened in different ways, ranging from adding Thickit to the food to blending foods into a puree or adding applesauce. Older children may prefer milk shakes or smoothie-type drinks (Lane & Cloud, 1988; Morris & Klein, 1987).

Foods that break apart readily in the mouth require a great deal of sophisticated tongue movement to form into a bolus in preparation for swallowing. If the child is having difficulty controlling food in the mouth, you may want to avoid these foods until better control is gained. For children with tongue thrust, it may be beneficial to offer foods with smoother characteristics in order to promote food intake while working on tongue mobility in therapy.

As with oral-motor techniques, there are a variety of strategies to consider when working on food texture and bolus. If you use your own problem-solving abilities, you will likely get some ideas as to how the food texture may be interfering with the child's feeding skills, and you will be able to come up with some ideas for adapting this aspect of feeding to meet the strengths and needs of a particular child. (The reader may wish to refer to Glass and Wolf, [1993] or Morris and Klein [1987] for additional specific ideas.)

**Adaptive equipment.** Adaptive feeding equipment or devices may be used to promote and support feeding and are often considered for the child working on self-feeding skills. Adaptive equipment can be broadly defined to include materials such as Dycem (a nonslip material that can be placed under a plate or bowl to stabilize it), as well as specially designed utensils, bottles, nipples, and feeders (Schuberth, 1994). Some adaptive devices are virtually effortless to use, and likely to be met with great acceptance by the caregivers and the child. Some of the more advanced and complex feeding equipment requires setup and training for both caregiver and child. Before recommending any feeding equipment, the therapist must discuss the prospect with the family and caregivers and be sure they are interested and willing to work with it. Although trial and error may be fine for a special cup or spoon, this may not work for an expensive device such as an electronic feeder. Rather than list adaptive equipment here, we have included a table of catalogs to which the therapist can refer for more information.

---

■ *THERAPEDS POINTER*
*Catalogs of Adaptive Equipment*

- adaptAbility Products for Independent Living (Dycem nonslip products)
- Mealtimes: A Resource for Oral-Motor, Feeding, and Mealtime Program (variety of books, spoons, cups, etc.)
- Sammons Preston catalog ("Nosey" cut-out cups and a variety of utensils)
- Sassy, Inc. (Sassy training cup)
- Haberman Feeder

---

## THE HEALTH SERVICES PLAN

Safe feeding is a primary consideration in the development of any feeding intervention plan. Although the Holistic Feeding Observation Form addresses many issues related to the safety of the child, it may not be sufficient to protect the safety of the child and the feeders involved in meeting the daily nutritional needs of children with complex health care needs.

Children with complex healthcare needs are those who require ongoing support or technology to prevent adverse physical consequences. Children with complex healthcare needs may require specialized health-related procedures such as NG feedings, gastrostomy feedings, or oral feedings where a documented risk of aspiration exists (Lowman, 1994; Virginia Departments of Education and Health, 1995). Little has been written about specific litigation surrounding feeding concerns in community settings, such as schools and childcare centers.

The interdisciplinary team's first and foremost responsibility is the protection of the child and of the feeders (Hall et al., 1993). Written policies and procedures of departments of educations in numerous states have begun to specify documentation that needs to be in place to ensure the child's safety and protect the feeders. Oregon's *Guidelines on Safe Feeding Practices for Special Students* (Hall et al., 1992, p. 16) specifies that the following activities be undertaken:

1. Determine the care needed by the student, and specify that care in the student's healthcare plan.
2. Develop prescriptive and therapeutic measures that are correctly planned, executed, and monitored by the appropriate personnel.
3. Make notations of student behaviors relative to feeding and specific responses to feeding events.
4. Maintain current, signed documentation that is recorded by appropriate personnel.
5. Maintain a log of monitoring and training activities carried out by the responsible specialist.

State departments and local school boards have begun to require the development of a Health Services Plan, such as the one presented in this chapter's Appendix C, to document the specific components outlined above (Lowman, 1994; Virginia Departments of Education and Health, 1995).

A critical component in the development of a safe Health Services Plan is training. Training and documentation of training are absolutely essential to the protection of the feeders. In Oregon's guidelines for feeding students in school, it is emphasized that "no person should ever undertake feeding a child with a feeding problem without appropriate training" (Hall et al., 1992, p. 11). Further, in AOTA's Self-Study Series, it is emphasized that "it is important to keep written documentation regarding what techniques were demonstrated and the competency of the person using that technique" (Clark, 1993, p. 22). Documentation checklists, such as the Documentation Checklist for Gastrostomy Bolus Feeding presented in this chapter's Appendix D, are available to describe "prescriptive and therapeutic measures that are correctly planned, executed, and monitored by the appropriate personnel" (Hall et al., 1992). The format of this checklist allows the trainer to document how, when, and by whom each step in the process was trained (Caldwell, Todaro, & Gates, 1989).

In addition to training, another critical component of the Health Services Plan is the development of an emergency plan. This plan should describe how the child typically reacts, what to look for, how to react, and who to call. Examples of an emergency plan related to feeding might be: (1) the signs of possible aspiration or (2) what to do if the feeding tube is pulled out of the stomach. Family members are valuable resources to describe how the child typically reacts. A school administrator and the medical director or school nurse can help specify who to call. A carefully prepared Health Services Plan can help alleviate fear and stress.

# SUMMARY

Feeding is a multifaceted issue facing the therapist. As medical personnel get more skilled at saving the lives of critically ill and fragile infants, therapists will continue to find themselves faced with more challenging feeding issues. No text can offer the therapist all appropriate techniques. Following a holistic assessment process, the therapist can be prepared to intervene. The therapist must be prepared to look at the feeding difficulties from all sides, and pull from his or her repertoire of intervention ideas that are consistent with the physical, psychological, and nutritional strengths and needs of the child, while being respectful of both family and culture.

---

You have followed some of the process with Amanda. Now, at 1 year of age, Amanda is still fed with a gastrostomy tube. Grandma has worked on decreasing tactile defensiveness for the past 6 months and can engage Amanda in oral-motor play using a soft rubber toy. Grandma begins a session with massage of Amanda's arms and legs. At night Grandma then wraps Amanda in a blanket and seats her in her infant seat for some oral play time. During the afternoon Grandma holds Amanda in her lap for the oral play time. Grandma dips a part of the toy in thickened formula and can introduce very small amounts of this food into Amanda's mouth. During this activity Amanda continues to demonstrate occasional grimacing and a bite reflex but also shows some suckling-like tongue movements. Periodically, Amanda swallows after some tongue movement. Grandma sometimes tries larger amounts of liquid during the afternoon session, but Amanda continues to sputter and cough, and there is still some concern about aspiration. Grandma wants guidance on how to increase the amount of food being offered orally and wonders if she should continue to work on the tactile defensiveness and oral hypersensitivity. How would you proceed?

## Real-Life Lab

**1.** Before working with families of children with feeding problems, explore and acknowledge your own beliefs and biases regarding mealtime. Think about your answers to questions such as: Do you believe a child must eat everything on the plate? Do you believe a child's picky eating reflects on parenting?

**2.** For some of the children with whom therapists work, feeding can be an exhausting activity. At times you may need to collaborate with a nutritionist to increase the caloric content of the food a child is eating just to break even between calories expended to eat and calories in the food. If weight gain is an issue, then the food you use for a feeding session must be very high in calories. Look in some nutritional texts for ideas on increasing the caloric characteristics of common foods, and find out what nutritionists recommend as high-calorie yet nutritious foods. Consider when these supplements may be useful in your intervention plan, how they might be incorporated, and what potential implications for oral-motor control they might have.

**3.** Morris and Klein offer suggestions throughout their book on how you, as a relatively intact individual, can experience some of the feeding difficulties our children experience. Look through this book, try some of the activities, and apply some of your intervention ideas to yourself. See what works well and what does not work. This may be best done in conjunction with a colleague.

# References

Alexander, R., Boehme, R., & Cupps, B. (1993). *Normal development of functional motor skills.* Tucson: Therapy Skill Builders.

American Occupational Therapy Association. (1994). Uniform terminology for occupational therapy—Third edition. *American Journal of Occupational Therapy, 48,* 1047–1054.

Angelo, J. (1996). *Assistive Technology for Rehabilitation Therapists.* S. J. Lane (ed.). Philadelphia: F. A. Davis.

Arvedson, J. (1993). Oral-motor and feeding assessment. In J. C. Arvedson & L. Brodsky (Eds.). *Pediatric swallowing and feeding: Assessment and management* (pp. 249–291). San Diego: Singular Publishing Group.

Arvedson, J. (1997). Behavioral issues and implications with pediatric feeding disorders. *Seminars in Speech and Language, 18,* 51–70.

Avery-Smith, W. (1996). Eating dysfunction positions paper. *The American Journal of Occupational Therapy, 50* (10), 846–847.

Ayres, A. J. (1979). *Sensory integration and the child.* Los Angeles: Western Psychological Services.

Barabach, L. M., Glazer, G., & Norris, S. C. (1992). Maternal perception and parent-infant interaction of vulnerable cocaine-exposed couplets. *Journal of Perinatal and Neonatal Nursing, 6*(3), 76–84.

Batshaw, M. L., & Perrett, Y. M. (1992). *Children with disabilities: A medical primer.* Baltimore: Paul H. Brookes.

Bazyk, B. (1990). Factors associated with the transition to oral feeding in infants fed by nasogastric tubes. *American Journal of Occupational Therapy, 44*(12), 1070–1078.

Berkow, R., & Fletcher, A. J. (Eds.). (1992). *The Merck manual of diagnosis and therapy* (16th Ed.). Rahway, NJ: Merck Research Laboratories.

Braun, M. A., & Palmer, M. M. (1986). A pilot study of oral-motor dysfunction in "at-risk" infants. *Physical & Occupational Therapy in Pediatrics, 5*(4), 13–25.

Caldwell, T. H., Todaro, A. W., & Gates, A. J. (Eds). (1989). *Community providers guide: An information outline for working with children with special health care needs.* New Orleans: National MCH Research Center, Children's Hospital.

Caretto, V., Francois, K., & McKinney, C. (1997). *Facilitating oral motor feeding.* Unpublished master's research, Virginia Commonwealth University, Richmond.

Case-Smith, J., & Humphrey, R. (1996). Feeding and oral motor skills. In J. Case-Smith, A. S. Allen, & P. N. Pratt (Eds.). *Occupational therapy for children* (pp. 430–460). St. Louis: C. V. Mosby.

Center on Hunger, Poverty, and Nutrition Policy. (1995). *Statement on the link between nutrition and cognitive development in children.* Boston: Tufts University School of Nutrition.

Clark, G. F. (1993). Oral-motor and feeding issues. In C. B. Royeen (Ed.), *AOTA self-study series: Classroom applications for school-based practice* (Vol. 9). Rockville, MD: American Occupational Therapy Association.

Clarren, S. K., & Aldrich, R. A. (1993). *A concise manual for fetal alcohol syndrome screening.* Washington, D.C.: U.S. Department of Health and Human Services.

Copeland, M. E., & Kimmel, J. R. (1989). *Evaluation and management of infants and young children with developmental disabilities.* Baltimore: Paul Brookes.

Danner, S. C. (1992a). Breastfeeding the infant with a cleft defect. *NAACOG's Clinical Issues in Perinatal and Women's Health Nursing, 3*, 634–639.

Danner, S. C. (1992b). Breastfeeding the neurologically impaired infant. *NAACOG's Clinical Issues in Perinantal and Women's Health Nursing, 3*, 640–646.

Dawson, P. (1992). Should the field of early childhood and family intervention address failure to thrive? *Zero to Three,* June, 20–22.

Glass, R. P., & Wolf, L. S. (1993). Feeding and oral-motor skills. In J. Case-Smith (Ed.). *Pediatric occupational therapy and early intervention* (pp. 225–288). Boston: Andover Medical Publishers.

Hall, S., Yohn, K., & Reed, P. R. (1992). *Feeding students in school: Providing guidelines and information on safe feeding practices for special students.* Salem, OR: Oregon Department of Education.

Horsley, J. W., Allen, E. A., & White, P. A. (1996). *Nutrition management of school aged children with special health care needs.* Virginia Department of Health and Virginia Department of Education.

Hunt, P. J. (1982). Oral motor dysfunction in Down's syndrome: Contributing factors and interventions. *Physical and Occupational Therapy in Pediatrics, 1*(4), 69–78.

Jelm, J. W. (1990). *Oral-motor/feeding rating scale.* Tucson: Therapy Skill Builders.

Kenny, D., Koheil, R., Greenberg, J., Reid, D., Milner, M., Roman, R., & Judd, P. (1989). Development of a multidisciplinary feeding profile for children who are dependent feeders. *Dysphagia, 4*, 16–28.

Klein, M. D., & Delaney, T. A. (1994). *Feeding and nutrition for the child with special needs: Handouts for parents.* Tucson: Therapy Skill Builders.

Lane, S. J. (1996). Cocaine: An overview of use, actions, and effects. In L. S. Chandler & S. J. Lane (Eds.). *Children with prenatal drug exposure* (pp. 15–33). New York: Haworth Press.

Lane, S. J., & Cloud, H. H. (1988). Feeding problems and intervention: An interdisplinary approach. *Topics in Clinical Nutrition, 3*, 23–32.

Lewis, J. A. (1982). Oral motor assessment and treatment of feeding difficulties. In P. J. Accardo (Ed.). *Failure to thrive in infancy and early childhood: A multidisciplinary team approach.* Baltimore: University Park Press.

Logemann, J. A. (1983). *Evaluation and treatment of swallowing disorders.* San Diego: College-Hill Press.

Lowman, D. K. (1994). *Integrating preschoolers with complex health care needs into early childhood special education programs: The teacher's perspective.* Unpublished doctoral dissertation, University of Virginia, Charlottesville.

Lowman, D. K., & Murphy, S. M. (1998). *The educator's guide to feeding children with disabilities.* Baltimore: Paul Brookes.

Macie, D., & Arvedson, J. (1993). *Tone and positioning.* In J. C. Arvedson & L. Brodsky (Eds.). *Pediatric swallowing and feeding: Assessment and management* (pp. 209–247). San Diego, CA: Singular Publishing Group, Inc.

Marmet, C., & Shell, E. (1994). Training

neonates to suck correctly. *MCN: American Journal of Maternal/Child Nursing, 9*(6), 401–407.

Mathisen, B., Skuse, D., Wolke, D., & Reilly, S. (1989). Oral-motor dysfunction and failure to thrive among inner-city infants. *Development Medicine and Child Neurology, 31*, 293–302.

Morris, S. E. (1982). *Pre-speech assessment scale*. Clifton, NJ: J. A. Preston.

Morris, S. E., & Klein, M. D. (1987). *Pre-feeding skills: A comprehensive resource for feeding development*. Tucson: Therapy Skill Builders.

Nelson, C. A., Meek, M. M., & Moore, J. C. (1994). *Head-neck treatment issues as a base for oral-motor function*. Albuquerque: Clinician's View.

Oetter, P., Richter, E. W., & Frick, S. M. (1988). *M.O.R.E. Integrating mouth with sensory and postural functions*. Hugo, MN: PDP Press.

Peterson, P., & Ottenbacher, K. (1986). Use of applied behavioral techniques and an adaptive device to teach lip closure to severely handicapped children. *American Journal of Mental Deficiency, 90*(5), 535–539.

Powers, D. E., & Moore, A. O. (1986). *Food medication interactions, 5th Edition*. Phoenix: F-MI Publishing.

Royeen, C. B., & Lane, S. J. (1991). *Tactile processing and sensory defensiveness*. In A. G. Fisher, E. A. Murray, & A. C. Bundy (Eds.). Sensory integration theory and practice (pp. 108–136). Philadelphia: F. A. Davis.

Ruff, H. A. (1984). Infants' manipulative exploration of objects: Effects of age and object characteristics. *Developmental Psychology, 20*(1), 9–20.

Schuberth, L. M. (1994). The role of occupational therapy in diagnosis and management. In D. N. Tuchman & R. S. Walter (Eds.) *Disorders of feeding and swallowing in infants and children: Pathophysiology, diagnosis, and treatment* (pp. 115–129). San Diego: Singular Publishing Group.

Shelton, T. L., & Stepanek, J. S. (1994). *Family-centered care for children needing specialized health and developmental services*. Washington, D.C.: Association for the Care of Children's Health.

Singer, L. (1990). When a sick child won't— or can't—eat. *Contemporary Pediatrics, 12*, 67.

Spender, Q., Dennis, J., Stein, A., Cave, D., Percy, E., & Reilly, S. (1995). Impaired oral motor function in children with Down's syndrome: A study of three twin pairs. *European Journal of Disorders of Communication, 30*, 77–87.

Starrett, A. L. (1991). Growth in developmental disabilities. In A. J. Capute & P. J. Accardo (Eds.). *Developmental disabilities in infancy and childhood* (pp. 181–187). Baltimore: Paul H. Brookes.

*Stedman's medical dictionary* (26th ed.). (1995). Baltimore: Williams & Wilkins.

Stratton, M. (1981). Behavioral assessment scale of oral functions in feeding. *The American Journal of Occupational Therapy, 35*, 719–721.

Virginia Departments of Education and Health (1995). *Report of the Departments of Education and Health: Report on the needs of medically fragile students to the Governor and the General Assembly of Virginia (Senate Document No. 5)*. Richmond: Commonwealth of Virginia.

Walker, M. (1992). Breastfeeding the premature infant. *NAACOG's Clinical Issues in Perinatal and Women's Health Nursing, 3*, 620–633.

Walter, R. S. (1993). Issues surrounding the development of feeding and swallowing. In D. N. Tuchman & R. S. Walter (Eds.). *Disorders of feeding and swallowing in infants and children: Pathophysiology, diagnosis, and treatment* (pp. 27–35). San Diego: Singular Publishing Group.

Wolf, L. S., & Glass, R. P. (1992). *Feeding and swallowing disorders in infancy: Assessment and management*. Tucson: Therapy Skill Builders.

# *Appendix A*

Normal Development of Sensorimotor Milestones, Oral-Motor Skills, Feeding Skills, and Major Cognitive Milestones Related to Feeding

| Age | Major Sensorimotor Milestones (Related to Oral-Motor and Feeding) | Oral-Motor Skills | Feeding Skills | Major Cognitive Milestones (Related to Oral-Motor and Feeding) |
|---|---|---|---|---|
| Birth to 37–40 weeks' gestation | Physiological flexion dominates<br>Total body moves into extension or flexion<br>In prone, can turn head side to side (protective response)<br>In supine, head is mostly to side<br>During feeding, hands will tend to be fisted and flexed across chest<br>Strong grasp reflex | Strong gag reflex<br>Rooting reflex present<br>Autonomic phasic bite-release pattern<br>Suckles/sucks when hand or object comes in contact with mouth<br>Minimal drooling in supine, increased drooling in other positions | On bottle/breast feeding begins with total sucking pattern<br>Mixture of suckling/sucking on bottle (dependent on head position)<br>Incomplete lip closure<br>Unable to release nipple | Total body involved with vocalizations<br>Respiration is mainly abdominal<br>Quiets to voice<br>Can slowly track moving objects |
| 1 to 2 months | Appears hypotonic as physiological flexion diminishes<br>Practicing extension and flexion<br>Continues to gain control of head<br>In prone, elbows move forward toward shoulders<br>In supine, ATNR with head to side | Strong gag reflex continues<br>Rooting reflex continues<br>Automatic phasic bite-release pattern continues<br>Suckles/sucks when hand or object comes in contact with mouth<br>Drooling increases as jaw and tongue move in wider excursions | May lose coordination of sucking-swallowing-breathing process with increased head movements<br>Opens mouth, waits for food<br>Better lip closure<br>Active lip movement when sucking | All sounds still closely associated with movement<br>Respiration still predominantly abdominal, rhythmical at rest<br>Begins to explore through mouthing of objects<br>Activity stops and breathing patterns |

| 3 to 5 months | Grasp reflex is less strong / Voluntary release not yet present / ATNR and grasp reflex fading out / More balance between extension and flexion / Good head control (centered and upright) / Hands to mouth constantly / In prone, supports on extended arms; props on forearms / In supine, brings hand to feet and feet to mouth / In sitting, props on arms with little support / Tactile awareness develops in hands / Reach more accurate; usually with both hands / Begins transfer from hand to hand / Release not controlled; may use mouth to assist | Rooting reflex and autonomic phasic bite-release pattern diminishes / Strong gag reflex begins to diminish at 5 months / Drooling decreases in positions with greater postural stability / Uses mouth to explore objects / Begins new oral movements in association with increased head and body control and movements | Anticipates feeding; recognizes bottle, mouth ready for nipple / Demonstrates voluntary control of mouth during bottle drinking/breast feeding / Liquid loss from lip corners / May begin receiving solids from a spoon at 5 months / Uses suckling during spoon feeding; gags on new textures / Tongue reversal after spoon is removed ejecting food involuntarily | change while focusing / Visual tracking more smooth / Beginning to put hand to bottle and to find mouth / Moves from watching hands to mouthing hands / Increasing variety of sounds; cry is less nasal / Object permanence: moves from searching for a dropped object to finding partially hidden objects / Pats bottle during feeding |
| 6 months | Head control complete / In prone, shifts weight and reaches with one hand / Begins quadruped / In supine, transfers objects from hand to hand | Rooting reflex and autonomic phasic bite-release pattern not present / Gag reflex diminishes in strength / Maintains lip closure longer | Sucks from bottle/breast with no liquid loss and long sequences of coordinated suck-swallow-breathing / Suckles liquid from a cup with liquid loss | Calls to get people's attention / Repeats own sounds / Uses increasingly varied sounds / Sounds increasingly |

continued on next page

Normal Development of Sensorimotor Milestones, Oral-Motor Skills, Feeding Skills, and Major Cognitive Milestones Related to Feeding *(continued)*

| | Sensorimotor Milestones | Oral-Motor Skills | Feeding Skills | Major Cognitive Milestones |
|---|---|---|---|---|
| | In sitting, reaches with one hand while supporting with other<br>Reaches to be picked up<br>Beginning to use thumb in grasp<br>Beginning to hold objects in one hand<br>Shows visual in small things | in supine, prone, and sitting<br>Drools when babbling, reaching, and teething; drools less during feeding | Coughs or chokes when drinking too much liquid from cup<br>Moves upper lip down so food is scraped off spoon on it and uses suckling with some sucking to move food back<br>Gags on new textures<br>Opens mouth when spoon approaches<br>Uses phasic up/down jaw movements, suckling, or sucking with solids placed in front<br>Moves tongue laterally with solids placed on side biting surfaces<br>Begins finger feeding<br>Plays with spoon | disassociated from movement<br>Means-end: Repeats action on toys, people, and things to make something happen |
| 7 to 9 months | Weight shift and reaches in quadruped<br>Creeps<br>Development of extension flexion, and rotation has expanded what infant can do in sitting<br>May pull to stand and hold on<br>Reaches with supination<br>Uses index finger to poke<br>Voluntary release is appearing | Gag reflex diminishes in strength to a more adult protective gag reflex<br>Uses facial expressions that convey likes and dislikes<br>Uses mouth to investigate new objects in combination with visual examination and hand manipulation<br>Bites on fingers and objects to reduce discomfort of teething<br>Produces more coordinated jaw, tongue, and lip | Suckles liquid presented by cup with liquid loss during cup removal<br>Takes fewer sucks/suckles before pulling away from cup to breathe<br>Independently holds bottle<br>Finger feeds self cracker<br>Holds jaw closed on soft solids until piece is broken off<br>Uses variable up and down movement in chewing; moves tongue laterally and jaw diagonally with solids placed on biting surfaces | Puts objects in container<br>Copies movements such as banging objects together<br>Object permanence: begins to search for object in a container<br>Responds to "no"<br>Through playing with movement, explores spatial concepts such as in-out, on-off |

| | | | | |
|---|---|---|---|---|
| 10 to 12 months | Good coordination in creeping<br>Cruising holding on with one hand<br>Standing independently<br>Learning to walk independently<br>Superior pincer grasp with finger tip and thumb<br>Release now smooth for large objects | movements in supine, prone, sitting, and standing; drooling rarely occurs except when teething<br>Produces more coordinated jaw, tongue, and lip movements when sitting, standing, and creeping on hands and knees; drooling rarely occurs except when teething | Assists with cup and spoon feeding<br>Easily closes lips on spoon, uses upper and lower lips to remove food from spoon<br>Uses controlled, sustained bite on soft cookie or cracker<br>Chews with mixture of up and down and diagonal rotary movements<br>Self-finger feeding independently<br>Likes to feed self but needs assistance with spoon; inverts spoon prior to mouth | Desire for independence seen in motor and in feeding<br>Follows simple directions<br>Uses objects to reach goal in independent problem-solving activities |
| 13 to 18 months | Walking alone<br>Learning to go up and down stairs<br>Grasp and release more precise | Movement in upper and lower lips<br>By 15–18 mos, has excellent coordination of sucking, swallowing, and breathing | Uses an up-and-down sucking pattern to obtain liquid from a cup<br>Well-coordinated rotary chewing by 18 mos.<br>Bite is well controlled and sustained<br>Self-feeding practiced and getting neater<br>Able to hold cup and put cup down without spilling | Problem solves by trial and error<br>Uses objects conventionally and begins to group<br>Uses speech to name, refuse, call, greet, protest, and express feelings |
| 19 to 24 months | Equilibrium reactions in standing and walking<br>Running with more narrow base of support | Uses up-and-down tongue movements and tip elevation<br>Internal jaw stabilization | Efficiently drinks from cup<br>Bite is well graded and sustained<br>From this point on, changes in | Follows two step direction<br>Object permanence is reflected in systematic searching |

*continued on next page*

Normal Development of Sensorimotor Milestones, Oral-Motor Skills, Feeding Skills, and Major Cognitive Milestones Related to Feeding (continued)

| | | emerges | self-feeding represent continued refinement | Speech is becoming very important |
| --- | --- | --- | --- | --- |
| | | Swallows with easy lip closure | | |
| 24 to 36 months | From this point on, skills represent refinement of first 24 months | Uses tongue to initiate swallow rather than tongue protrusion | Circular rotary jaw movements are present | Vocabulary increased to 300–500 words |
| | Jumps in place | | Lip closure during chewing | Generally uses speech to express needs and feelings |
| | Pedals tricycle | | Holds cup in one hand | Names body parts |
| | Scribbles | | Spoon handled with more accuracy | Understands and associates words according to function |
| | Snips with scissors | | Fills spoon with use of fingers | |
| | | | May begin drinking from a straw | |

*Source:* Adapted from Alexander, Boehme, & Cupps (1993); Carretto, Francois, & McKinney (1996); Case-Smith & Humphry (1996); Clark (1993); and Glass & Wolf (1993).

# *Appendix B*

## HOLISTIC FEEDING OBSERVATION FORM

Child's Name:                          Date:

Age:                                   Observers:

The questions provided under each heading are suggestions to help guide your observations.

   I. Collaboration with the Family
      • Has a positive family dialogue been established?
      • What is the feeding routine: at home? in the center?
      • Issues identified by the caregiver:
        What is pleasurable specific to the feeding interaction?
        What is difficult specific to the feeding interaction?
      • What cultural implications are important to consider?
  II. Embedding Communication and Socialization Skills
      • Does the child have the maximum control possible?
      • How does the child indicate hunger: food present? not present?
      • How does the child indicate need for a change of pace or pause?
      • How does the child indicate a choice of food or liquid?
      • How does the child indicate readiness for more?
      • How does the child indicate finished?
      • How does the child indicate desire for social closeness or distance?
 III. Physical Development and Positioning:
      • Is 90-90-90 position achievable?
        Are feet and arms supported by a flat surface (not dangling)?
        Are knees at a comfortable 90-degree angle?
        Are hips resting symmetrically against a supportive surface?
        Is trunk upright and symmetrical?
        Is a neutral head position assured for most effective swallow and eye contact?
  IV. Respiratory Issues:
      • Is the gag reflex present and effective (not overresponsive or underresponsive)?
      • Is the swallow reflex present and effective (not inhibited or delayed, no paralysis)?
      • Is the feeding pace determined by the child (not the feeder)?
      • Is swallowing relaxed and without gagging, coughing, or aspiration?
      • If a respiratory infection is present, is enough extra time allowed for coordination of breathing and swallowing?
      • Is the coordination of breathing, swallowing, and talking difficult?

V. Sensory Development:
- Are any limitations of the sensory modalities present: visual, auditory, tactile, gustatory, olfactory, proprioceptive?
- Which *textures* are most easily tolerated: thick liquids, thin liquids, smooth solids, lumpy solids, chewy solids, crunchy, mixed textures?
- Which *tastes* are most easily tolerated (likes vs. dislikes)?
- What *temperatures* are most easily tolerated (note preferences)?
- What types of *tactile input* are most easily tolerated (arousing vs. calming)?

VI. Oral-Motor Development:
- Has overall muscle tone been determined (normal, high, low)?
- Have tone issues specific to the face and mouth been determined?
- Have needs for oral motor treatment been identified? Some common examples include:
  Jaw—thrust, clenching, retraction, instability
  Tongue—retraction, thrust, limited movement
  Lip and Cheek—low tone, lip retraction
  Palate—nasal reflux, cleft
  Other

VII. Feeding Process and Implementation Plan:
- Have the family, all feeders, and needed specialists participated in the development of this plan?
- Has needed medical information (including physician orders and nutrition requirements) been received and factored into this feeding plan?
- Has needed feeding equipment been identified and obtained?
- Has the most effective sequence been determined?

---

Adapted from Lowman, D. K., & Murphy, S. M. (1998). *The educator's guide to feeding children with disabilities*. Baltimore: Paul Brookes.

# *Appendix C*

## HEALTH SERVICES PLAN

Student: _____

Parents: _____

This Health Services Plan will be in effect from _____ to _____.

This plan should be completed *before* the child comes to school or the center. Because health needs can change frequently, this plan should be developed at a meeting *separate* from the IFSP/IEP meeting.

### Members of Planning Team

Members of the planning team should include the parents or guardian, the child (if appropriate), the service coordinator, the primary teacher, the class paraprofessional, the school administrator, the special education administrator, other related service staff as appropriate (speech-language pathologist, occupational therapist, physical therapist), the school nurse or school health contact person, the transportation director, the transition nurse from the discharging hospital or the local health department, the Medicaid waiver case manager, and the representative from the equipment company.

### Description of Child's Medical Condition

This section should contain a complete description of the child's current medical condition, including relevant medical history and the child's needs for growth and development, and the effect of the medical condition on the child's performance in school.

## Strategies to Support the Child in the School or Center-based Setting

In this section specify activities in which the child may participate as well as any adaptations or modifications that may be needed (e.g., no contact sports, avoid contacts with particles such as sand, powder).

## Feeding and Nutritional Needs

Describe the child's current diet, food allergies, food likes and dislikes, fluid intake requirements, feeding plan, and oral-motor interventions.

## Transportation Arrangements

This section should address whether the child will ride the bus or if special transportation arrangements will be made. Is there a need for an assistant to accompany the student? Does the bus driver need to receive special training?

## Medication to Be Dispensed, Amount, Time, and Person Administering

This section should include the type of medication, the dosage to be dispensed, time, how, and where, who will administer medication, and the effect of the medication on the child's performance in school. Define a procedure for record keeping.

## Procedure(s) to Be Performed By School or Center Personnel

This section should outline the child's needs. The planning team should decide which procedure(s) can and cannot be done in school. Each procedure should be described in detail.

## Where and When the Procedure(s) Should Be Performed

Include the location, frequency, and time of day involved with the procedure(s).

## Who Will Perform the Procedure(s)

What are the qualifications of the individual who should perform the procedure(s)?

## Training That Is to Take Place Prior to the Child Entering Class

List in detail who will be providing the training and how often the training will be monitored and reviewed. Note that the training must be provided by a healthcare provider. The parents and a healthcare provider can work as a team to provide the training.

## Schedule for Review and Monitoring of Training

Include timelines for regular review and retraining of the procedures. This should include a schedule for regular review as well as provisions for retraining if the child's needs change.

## Emergency Procedures

Describe expected emergency in terms of how the child typically reacts, if known. List specifically what to do, who to call, and the order in which people should be notified. Who has a copy of the emergency plan? Where is it filed or posted? Be sure to notify the local rescue squad about procedures and the location of child in the school.

## Plan for Absences

- Outline the plan for dealing with instances when the teacher and/or the paraprofessional are absent, such as specific training of a substitute.
- Outline the plan for home-based instruction if the child becomes too ill to attend school. Be sure to build this plan into the child's IEP.
- Outline the plan for receiving current medical information before the child returns to school from an extended illness/hospitalization.

## Plan for Change

- Plan for change and review frequently.
- Revise plan after a major illness or hospitalization.

Signatures:
We have participated in the development of this Health Services Plan and agree with the contents:

| | |
|---|---|
| Parents/Guardian | Date |
| School Administrator | Date |
| Healthcare Professional | Date |
| Teacher | Date |
| | Date |
| | Date |
| | Date |

Adapted from Lowman, D. K. (1994). *Integrating preschoolers with complex health care needs into early childhood special education programs: The teacher's perspective.* Unpublished doctoral dissertation, University of Virginia, Charlottesville.

# *Appendix D*

## DOCUMENTATION CHECKLIST FOR GASTROSTOMY BOLUS FEEDING

|  | Demo | Return Demonstration | | | | | |
|---|---|---|---|---|---|---|---|
|  | Date | Date | Date | Date | Date | Date | Date |
| A. States name and purpose of procedure | | | | | | | |
| B. Preparation<br>  1. Completes at _____ time(s) | | | | | | | |
|   2. _____ cc's amount<br>    _____ Formula/Feeding<br>    (type of feeding) | | | | | | | |
|   3. Feeding to be completed in _____ minutes<br>  4. Position for feeding _____ | | | | | | | |
|   5. Identifies potential problems and appropriate actions | | | | | | | |
| C. Identifies Supplies:<br>  1. Catheter _____ (size)<br>    _____ (type)<br>    Balloon size _____ cc | | | | | | | |
|     a.  Small port plug | | | | | | | |
|     b.  Feeding port | | | | | | | |
|   2. Clamp and plug | | | | | | | |
|   3. 60-cc catheter-tipped syringe | | | | | | | |
|   4. Formula at room temperature | | | | | | | |
|   5. Small glass of tap water | | | | | | | |
| D. Procedure:<br>  1. Washes hands thoroughly<br>  2. Gathers equipment<br>  3. Positions child and explains procedure<br>  4. Removes plug from feeding tube<br>Child-Specific: Steps 5–11 need to be prescribed for each child<br>  5. Checks for proper placement of tube. Attaches syringe and aspirates stomach contents by pulling plunger back<br>  6. Measures contents<br>  7. Returns stomach contents to stomach<br>  8. If stomach contents are over _____ cc's, subtract from feeding | | | | | | | |

*continued*

| | Demo | Return Demonstration | | | | | | |
|---|---|---|---|---|---|---|---|---|
| 9. If more than _____ cc's, hold feeding<br>10. Pinches or clamps off tube | | | | | | | | |
| | Demo | Date | Date | Date | Date | Date | Date | Date |
| 11. Removes syringe | | | | | | | | |
| 12. Attaches syringe without plunger to feeding port | | | | | | | | |
| 13. Pours formula (room temperature) into syringe (approx. 30–40 cc's) | | | | | | | | |
| 14. Releases or unclamps tube and allows feeding to go in slowly | | | | | | | | |
| 15. When feeding gets to 5-cc marker, adds more formula | | | | | | | | |
| 16. Continues this procedure until the feeding has been completed | | | | | | | | |
| 17. Takes about 30 minutes to complete feeding (the higher the syringe if held the faster the feeding will flow) | | | | | | | | |
| 18. Lowers the syringe if feeding is going too fast | | | | | | | | |
| 19. Makes feeding like meal time. Young children may suck on a pacifier | | | | | | | | |
| 20. Flushes tube with _____ cc's of water when feeding is complete | | | | | | | | |
| 21. Pinches off tubing, removes syringe and closes off clamp | | | | | | | | |
| 22. Allows child to remain in feeding position for minimum of one-half hour after feeding | | | | | | | | |
| 23. Washes syringe with soap and warm water and puts in home container | | | | | | | | |
| 24. Reports any problems to parents | | | | | | | | |
| 25. Documents procedure and problems in log | | | | | | | | |

Checklist Content Approved by:

_____ Date _____
Parent/Guardian Signature

_____ Date _____
Administrator

_____ Date _____

Adapted from Caldwell, T. H., Todaro, A. W., & Gates, A. J. (Eds.). (1989). *Community providers guide: An information outline for working with children with special health care needs.* New Orleans: National MCH Resource Center, Children's Hospital.

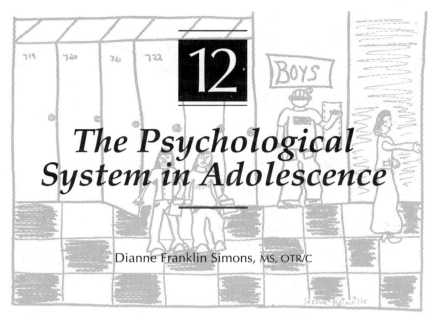

# 12

# The Psychological System in Adolescence

Dianne Franklin Simons, MS, OTR/C

*The essence of our effort to see that every child has a chance, must be to assure each an equal opportunity, not to become equal, but to become different—to realize whatever unique potential of body, mind and spirit he or she possesses.*

—John Fischer

## KEY POINTS

- The developmental tasks of adolescence are primarily psychological and social in nature.
- Developmental delays in these psychological and social tasks are of as much concern to OTs as delays in motor skills are when treating younger children.
- Difficulties in achieving the developmental tasks of adolescence can result in damaging long-term effects upon one's adult life.
- Every child's and adolescent's mental health is important.
- Mental health problems can be recognized and treated.
- Many adolescents have mental health problems that interfere with the way that they feel, think, and act, preventing development of their abilities, limiting their future ability to be productive, and adversely affecting their life satisfaction.
- Children from high-risk environments are at risk for problems of a psychosocial nature during adolescence.
- OTs, with their holistic perspective of human functioning, are excellent

providers of services to adolescents with psychological and social problems.

- Activities that develop new skills or that renew or build upon former skills are a vital part of restoring psychosocial function and occupational performance.

# BEGINNINGS

In this chapter typical developmental tasks of adolescence will be reviewed to provide a foundation for understanding the psychological and social problems that can occur during adolescence. The most commonly made diagnoses for adolescents with psychosocial dysfunction will be discussed in terms of typical clinical pictures, etiology, prevalence, and diagnostic criteria. Characteristic behaviors and functional deficits associated with the various diagnoses will be presented.

The intervention portion of this chapter will focus on restoring function and will not be divided by diagnosis. This decision was made for two reasons: (1) many adolescents with problems in psychosocial areas exhibit behavior for more than one diagnosis (e.g., an adolescent may be depressed *and* addicted to a chemical), and (2) different diagnoses often result in similar problems in functioning (e.g., an adolescent diagnosed with anorexia nervosa *and* an adolescent diagnosed with conduct disorder can both have difficulty in regard to interacting socially with peers).

OTs, because of their emphasis on the treatment of clients from a holistic perspective, recognize that psychological functioning affects one's perception of oneself and of the world. Their concern for the effects of psychological problems on day-to-day functioning, and their treatment focus on the development of the practical skills needed to live a productive and a satisfying life, make OTs well-suited to treating the functional deficits evident in adolescents with psychosocial problems. They contribute in valuable ways to the treatment of adolescents with problems in psychosocial functioning.

# TYPICAL DEVELOPMENT
# OF THE PSYCHOLOGICAL SYSTEM
# DURING ADOLESCENCE

The word *adolescence* is derived from the Latin word *adolescere,* which means "to grow up," "to grow in maturity," or "to grow into adulthood" (Kimmell & Weiner, 1995; Muuss, 1982; Steinberg, 1996). Adolescence is a period of biological, psychological, social, and economic transition. The beginning of adolescence is generally marked by the *biological* changes of puberty. However, it is concluded with the *psychological* and *social* changes brought on by becoming an adult. Attainment of a separate sense of identity, and achievement of adult status and privileges with the acceptance of responsibility for adult work, family, and citizen roles, marks the conclusion of adolescence and the beginning of young adulthood. Nightingale and Wolverton (1993) state that adolescents are defined largely by what they are *not*—"neither child nor adult—legally, in status, role or function" (p. 14). Adolescents frequently regard the "magic age" of 18 with its accompanying privileges, such as the right to vote, to marry without parental consent, or to enlist in the military, as the "official" demarcation point of achieving adulthood. However, most experts regard the passage from adolescence to adulthood as occurring when an individual achieves physical, emotional, psychological, and financial independence from parents or other adult caregivers and through the assumption of independent adult roles (Steinberg, 1996).

Although the beginning of the adolescent period varies with the naturally occurring range of onset of puberty, the transition to adulthood is even more widely variable. Some adolescents enter full-time working roles immediately upon completing high school at age 18 or 19; others may become parents, marry, or become employed full time even before age 18. Other adolescents remain financially dependent upon their parent until well into their middle 20s, postponing their entry into the workforce to pursue graduate education.

## ADOLESCENCE TODAY

*Our youth now love luxury. They have bad manners, contempt for authority; they show disrespect for their elders and love chatter in place of exercise. They no longer rise when others enter the room. They contradict their parents, chatter before company, gobble up their food and tyrannize their teachers.*

Does this describe today's generation of adolescents? It may surprise you that this quotation was not written about today's teens; it was written by Sophocles, a Greek philosopher, about adolescents in the fifth century B.C.! A century later, around 300 B.C., Aristotle wrote that adolescents had "exalted notions, because they have not yet been humbled by life or learnt its necessary limitation. . . . They love too much and hate too much, and the same with everything else. They think that they know everything; and they are always quite sure about it; this, in fact, is why they overdo everything."

Adolescence has always been and continues to be a period of transition. It involves a gradual progression from childhood dependence to independence from the family. Years ago when society was less technologically complex, the period of adolescence was not lengthy in duration. Life spans were shorter. Industrialization created the need for the stage of adolescence because of the need for more education for an industrialized society (Klein, 1990). As we transition from an industrialized society to an information-based society, the need for a protracted period of education will be even greater.

In the United States today, several trends of recent decades have altered the roles of adolescents. Factors such as increased prosperity, increased maternal employment, increased geographical mobility, rapid technological change, and an increased need for academic training and credentialing have resulted in adolescents spending less time with adults, more time with one another, and more time in training (Schulenberg & Ebata, 1994). The high concentration of adolescents in schools and colleges, who are discouraged from "prematurely" entering adult roles as spouses or parents, provides the impetus for a "culture" with its own standards and mores. Other trends that have had an impact on adolescent roles include the shift in the racial and ethnic composition of the U.S. population, resulting in greater cultural diversity and a higher representation of minorities in the adolescent population.

Many adolescents have inadequate family and community support and severely limited prospects. Dryfoos (1990) estimates that one in four adolescents is at risk for continued serious difficulties into adulthood. Approximately one-fifth of the children and adolescents in America live in poverty. African-American and Hispanic children and adolescents are two or three times more likely to be living in poverty than are caucasian children and adolescents (Lipsitz, 1991). Likewise, one-fifth of the children under 18 in America live in single-parent homes, mostly with a mother. The rate of occurrence of single-parent homes is also two to three times higher among minorities than among whites. The poverty rate for those living in female-headed households is 51 percent. Lipsitz (1991) reported that between 1980 and 1988 the Hispanic population grew five times faster (34 percent) than the non-Hispanic population (7%), and that if the population growth is sustained, Hispanics will become the nation's largest minority by the year 2020. These changes in sociocultural diversity will have an effect on education, the workforce, and on occupational therapy practice. OTs are needed to provide services to children and adolescents whose environment has adversely affected their psychosocial development and their resulting mental health. Intervention can help young people develop the abilities to engage in meaningful and satisfying occupation.

## DEVELOPMENTAL TASKS

At the turn of the century, G. Stanley Hall, known as "the father of adolescent psychology," formulated his now famous theory of adolescence that "storm and stress," rebellion, and sexual conflict were a normal part of the developmental process. He identified several "contradicting tendencies" that created turbulent mood swings (Dacey & Kenny, 1997). They included:

- Energy and enthusiasm vs. indifference and boredom
- Gaiety and laughter vs. gloom and melancholy
- Vanity and boastfulness vs. humiliation and bashfulness
- Sensitivity vs. callousness
- Tenderness vs. cruelty

In Western culture, a significant portion of adolescents traverse this period of their life without appreciable turmoil, but most researchers continue to recognize that changes in moods and attitudes such as those identified by Hall are a part of adolescent development.

The developmental challenges or tasks of adolescence have been studied by Erikson (1968), Havighurst (1951), and many others. In 1951, Havinghurst identified a list of developmental tasks of adolescence, which he considered as serving both the needs of the individual and the goals of western society. According to Havighurst, development of the skills, knowledge, functions, and attitudes to accomplish the successful mastery of these nine tasks is essential for success in life. Although written over 40 years ago, Havighurst's list of tasks has held up well to subsequent study and research (Dacey & Kenny, 1997). The tasks Havighurst identified were:

- Accepting one's physique and accepting a masculine or feminine role
- Forming new relations with age mates of both sexes
- Achieving emotional independence from parents and other adults
- Selecting and preparing for an occupation
- Developing intellectual skills and concepts necessary for civic competence
- Desiring and achieving socially responsible behavior
- Preparing for marriage and family life
- Building conscious values in harmony with an adequate scientific view of the world

The cognitive development that occurs during adolescence, identified by the Swiss psychologist Jean Piaget as "formal operational thought," sets the stage for these developmental tasks to be addressed. The intellectual development that occurs during this period results in the adolescent having the ability to engage in abstract thought and metacognition, to take a different viewpoint, to consider hypothetical situations, and perhaps for the first time to become aware of inconsistencies and contradictions in the culture (Dacey & Kenny, 1997). Adolescents are thus able to focus both inward and outward as they define who they are in the world. The cognitive changes of adolescence play an important role in the development of autonomy, which involves making your own decisions. The cognitive changes also provide the logical foundation for changes in thinking about the social, moral, and ethical problems of the world around them.

Theories of adolescent development in western societies have emphasized the goals of identity and autonomy. Erik Erikson (1963), in his conceptualization of psychosocial stages of development, identified the crisis of adolescence to be one of identity vs. identity confusion. Steinberg (1996) states that it is important to bear in mind that healthy adolescent development involves not only the ability to be a successful individual but also the ability to maintain healthy and satisfying attachments with others. In other words, a healthy adolescent must learn to function both independently and interdependently. Occupational therapists Howe and Schwartzberg describe health as involving both a state of independence and capacity for self-direction *and* a state of interdependence and capacity for relatedness (Howe & Schwartzberg, 1995). For the purposes of this discussion, the developmental tasks of adolescence can be clustered into these two primary developmental tasks: achievement of independence through development of identity and autonomy; and achievement of interdependence through the development of intimacy and sexuality. The developmental tasks of adolescence are primarily psychological and social in nature.

## INDEPENDENCE—DEVELOPMENT OF IDENTITY AND AUTONOMY

In his book *Childhood and Society* (1963), Erik Erikson identified the psychosocial crisis that needed resolution during adolescence as identity and repudiation versus identity confusion. Erikson defined identity as a "subjective sense of an invigorating sameness and continuity" and as a "sense of feeling active and alive." When one achieved a state of identity, the various aspects of one's self-image would be in agreement or identical with each other (Erikson, 1963). An essential part of reaching personal identity is repudiating all other possibilities. The task of identity formation has been described by Archer (1990) as one that involves the selection, sorting through, trying on, discarding, reshaping, and ultimate fashioning of a unique sense of self via the integration of values, beliefs, and goals that are self-chosen.

All adolescents are faced with questions of "Who am I?" "What do I believe in?" "Where am I headed?" and "Who will I be?" The task of identity formation takes place over a period of years. The stable commitments required to achieve a sense of identity include deciding upon a set of values and beliefs to guide one's actions, formulating a set of educational and career goals to direct one's efforts in work, and affirming a gender orientation that influences one's acquaintanceship and intimacy with males and females. These three commitments have been identified by Kimmel and Weiner (1995) as an ideological stance, an occupational stance, and an interpersonal stance.

---

### ■ THERAPEDS POINTER

Through the process of *experimentation with new roles and ideologies* and through a broadened range of life experiences, adolescents examine their values, beliefs, interests, and goals. They try new activities not previously available to them, like school clubs, athletic teams, and work. They discover those academic areas to which they are attracted, and for which they have the capabilities. Leadership roles afford young people with the opportunity to assume responsibility and to learn to lead without dominating. Although maintaining or moving away from their prior level of involvement in the family, adolescents typically assume a variety of new roles such as:

- A goal-directed student
- A trusted friend
- A responsible worker
- A contributing club member or leader
- A dedicated teammate
- A committed volunteer
- A caring boyfriend or girlfriend

These roles help them to test their beliefs and values and to confirm them as their own, distinct and separate from those of their parents.

---

The movement from a position where values are prescribed by a social group, whether parents or peers, to a position of formation of a personal value system leads an adolescent to becoming a responsible member of society. Young people successfully negotiating adolescence learn to make choices that provide personal satisfaction and meaning while also satisfying others in their social environment (Barris & Kielhofner, 1985). Acquisition of a set of values to guide adult behavior and the simultaneous development of the self-control to adhere to the value system selected is an important component of self-identity. Development of the desire to be socially responsible and to act in accordance with the laws of the society allows one to see oneself as a part of something greater than the self and to find one's place in the larger world.

According to Bandura (1978), one's view of oneself is learned from the way that one has been treated by others, from one's successes and failures, and from one's views of those experiences. Social learning theorists believe that the self can be influenced greatly by whether an individual believes he or she can succeed or not, and by whether the individual thinks that other people believe in that success. Bandura used the term self-efficacy to describe the beliefs that individuals hold about what they think that they can accomplish as a result of their efforts. He felt that if someone believes he or she will be successful, that person will be more self-confident, will try harder, and will be seen by others as successful and be more available to them.

---

■ *THERAPEDS POINTER*

The Model of Human Occupation, principally developed by Gary Kielhofner, with inspiration from the founders and occupational behavior concepts, is a conceptual practice model that attempts to explain how occupational behavior is motivated, organized, and performed. This model proposes that occupational behavior arises from the interaction of the human system and the social and physical environment. The human system is described as a dynamic, open system composed of three subsystems: *volition, habituation,* and *mind-brain-body performance.* The volition subsystem addresses motivation of occupational behavior by recognizing the impact that an individual's values, interests, and personal causation have upon their choices for occupational activity. The habituation subsystem explains the organizing effect that social roles, patterns, and routine habits have upon occupational behavior. The mind-brain-body performance system recognizes that a number of underlying physical and mental constituents (musculoskeletal, cardiopulmonary, neurological, and symbolic) work in concert to make skilled performance of occupations possible. These three subsystems form a heterarchy in which each subsystem contributes different but complementary functions to the operation of the whole system. At times one subsystem may play a more important role than another subsystem. At other times another subsystem may dominate, and at still other times all three subsystems may exert equal influences. Occupational performance is evident in the perceptual-motor skills, process skills, and communication and interaction skills produced by the human system as it interacts with the physical and social environment. This model asserts that occupational behavior is always a reflection of the complex interplay of our motives, patterns of behavior, capacities, and context (Kielhofner, 1995).

---

Kielhofner (1995) used the term *personal causation* in his conceptualization of the Model of Human Occupation as the collection of beliefs and expectations that a person holds about his or her effectiveness in the environment. Personal causation refers to individuals' personal knowledge of themselves as a cause of change in the environment. The development of personal causation during adolescence involves maintaining confidence in oneself while facing new demands and challenges, acquiring new skills, and experiencing a desire for greater personal control (Barris & Kielhofner, 1985). New settings either demand expanded performance of old skills in new conditions or the acquisition of new skills. In both cases, former successes during childhood provide a foundation for continued development of feelings of competency.

As adolescents age, they become increasingly aware of the presence and influence of time. The future gradually becomes real and comprehensible to them. The relationship of the present to the future takes on newly discovered importance, as the present is understood as a determinant of the future (Barris & Kielhofner, 1985). As they progress through early adolescence, young people begin to entertain ideas of future occupations. As time passes, they begin the process of actively exploring their vocational goals and plans and by late adolescence their vocational plans have become more crystallized. Even if their choice of occupation has not been determined completely, they have narrowed down their choice and their area of interest is more solidly based upon a realistic assessment of their abilities and potentials. Their vocational image of themselves is another component of who they are as persons, further contributing to their self-definition. Their abilities help define who they are; for example, an adolescent may identify that he is good with his hands, or with performing mathematical analysis, or with helping people. A natural part of the process of actively examining types of work, friends, potential mates, and philosophies of life is vacillation for a period of time between what they like and dislike and with whom they want to associate or not associate before making their final choices (Kimmel & Wiener, 1995).

The more developed one's sense of identity, the more fully one appreciates how she is similar to and different from others and the more clearly she recognizes her own assets and limitations. During the process of clarifying one's identity, adolescents begin to recognize the limits of their own power. Their thinking becomes more realistic. As adolescents mature cognitively, they relinquish the adolescent egocentrism that contributes to the two problems in thinking typical of adolescence—the personal fable and the imaginary audience. The personal fable revolves around the adolescent's erroneous belief that he or she is unique or "different," and therefore things that happen to other people cannot or will not happen to them. Their former feelings of omnipotence evolve into a more realistic view of the world and of themselves. They also let go of the imaginary audience belief that everyone else is paying attention to them, scrutinizing them, and that their behavior is the focus of everyone else's concern and attention (Steinberg, 1996). With age and maturity older adolescents begin to recognize that they are merely one of many and that others are not nearly as concerned with their behavior or appearance as they are themselves. The question of "Will I fit in?" that dominates the life of the early adolescent and dictates conformity in dress and behavior for acceptance by a peer group evolves into reliance upon self for security. Although the opinions of others may remain important, the adolescent comes to value his or her own opinion as well.

Issues of identity, which address the question "Who am I?" and self-esteem, which deals with the question "How do I feel about who I am?" are related. Self-esteem is important to adolescent motivation toward success, achievement, and mental health. People with high self-esteem are often good students, do well in sports, are liked by age-mates, are satisfied with their physical appearance, feel in control of their lives, and feel that their successes have resulted from their own efforts (Dacey & Kenny, 1997). Adolescents who feel that their parents, teachers, close friends, and classmates support and approve of them and expect them to succeed develop feelings of high self-esteem. The development of a solid peer group, who have learned to work together cooperatively and respect one another, developed empathy for one another's feelings, and practiced reciprocity in their relationships, provides the nurturing social environment for the adolescent to resolve and move beyond concerns about "fitting in" or being accepted. Young people, who have developed a clear sense of personal identity and who feel good about themselves, work constructively toward well-defined goals, seek out and feel comfortable in close relationships with others, and remain relatively free of emotional distress (Kimmel & Weiner, 1995).

As an adolescent finds satisfactory answers to the questions about whether he or she is lovable, good enough, and capable of being independent, the wide mood swings of early adolescence subside. As an adolescent ages he progresses from having limited skills and abilities to having expanded capabilities. Adolescents discover their strengths and develop a sense of competency and self-efficacy, which contributes further to their consolidated sense of self. As they develop self-motivation, self-determination, and self-direction, feelings of personal control emerge and they feel more responsible for the outcomes of their life. The development of these feelings of self-efficacy and personal control allow them to move from being dependent and reliant upon others to being capable of functioning independently.

## INTERDEPENDENCE—DEVELOPMENT OF INTIMACY AND SEXUALITY

Harry Stack Sullivan (1953) emphasized the social aspects of growth, suggesting that psychological development can best be understood in terms of transformations in relationships with others. In fact, Sullivan viewed not just adolescence, but the entire life cycle, as a developmental process of meeting the challenges of changing interpersonal needs. Sullivan viewed the security that was derived from satisfactory relationships with others as the glue that holds together one's sense of self. He felt identity and self-esteem were developed gradually through interpersonal relationships. The development of independence and interdependence are, therefore, closely connected.

Interdependence is just as important as independence to healthy psychosocial development and maturity. People define themselves as members of social groups. Social groups create a social space or context with a climate of values, interests, boundaries, and structure (Kielhofner, 1995). The various roles one assumes in one's social groups play an integral part of defining an individual's identity. Connection with other people helps with the development of self-identity. Mosey (1970) identified a series of groups that were based upon a developmental sequence, beginning with the parallel group, which she identified as requiring the group interaction skills typical of preschool-age children. The groups progress developmentally through the project group, the egocentric-cooperative group, and the cooperative group, and culminate in the mature group. Each subsequent group requires increasingly more mature group interaction skills. The interaction skills required for a cooperative group are developmentally typical of preadolescents. Group members are able to work cooperatively with others in a group with a homogeneous membership. This level of maturity is typical of the same-sex friendships or chumships of preadolescents. Mosey identified the mature group as typical of the group skills of adolescence. To participate in a mature group, a group member must be able to interact cooperatively in a heterogeneous group. A heterogeneous group may include members of the opposite sex or a socially or culturally diverse membership.

A major challenge of adolescence is making a satisfactory transition from the nonsexual, intimate same-sex friendship roles characteristic of childhood, preadolescence, and early adolescence to the roles created by intimate relationships of late adolescence. Steinberg (1996) identified an intimate relationship as an emotional attachment between two persons characterized by mutual concern for each other's well-being; a willingness to disclose private, sensitive topics of conversation; and a sharing of common interests and activities. Intimacy does not imply a sexual or physical connotation. Adolescent intimate relationships occur most frequently in close friendships, some dating relationships, but they also occur between adolescents and their parents or other significant adults, and between adolescents and their siblings (Steinberg, 1996). These relationships are characterized by higher levels of trust, honesty, and open communication.

The theoretical perspectives of Eric Erikson (1968) on the development of intimacy during adolescence are still respected today. Erikson felt that an individual must establish a sense of identity before being capable of real intimacy. According to Erikson (1968), individuals without a secure sense of identity are afraid and unwilling to make serious commitments to others. He described "pseudointimacy" as a superficial, shallow intimacy that does not involve full disclosure out of fear that complete honesty would result in the loss of the relationship. Pseudointimacy is considered common in this age group because commitment cannot be made before one develops an identity. Erickson identified intimacy versus isolation as the crisis of young adulthood to be addressed once the crisis of identity versus identity diffusion was fully resolved.

The establishment of sexual identity, which includes the acceptance of oneself as a sexually mature human being, leads to the development of meaningful sexual relationships. Coming to terms with one's sexuality contributes to further development of the capacity for intimacy. Healthy sexual relationships involve intimacy and a physical sharing of oneself with a partner. To be sexually intimate an individual has to have mastered the prerequisites of being able to fulfill commitments, to trust others, to have feelings of self-worth and positive self-regard, and to be comfortable with his or her body and sexual identity. Most studies indicate that the majority of dating relationships are not truly intimate until sometime during young adulthood (Steinberg, 1996).

Sexual preference is generally well set by adolescence, but adolescents who are homosexuals may continue to struggle with the reality of their sexual preference during their adolescence. A study of gay men by Rodriguez (1988), reported in Dacey & Kenny (1997), indicated that an awareness of same-sex attraction occurred around age 11, acknowledgment of homosexual feelings occurred around age 16, and self-labeling occurred around age 20. Health-care workers should not assume that adolescents have a heterosexual orientation until it is firmly established via a trusted interview.

Acceptance of oneself as a sexually mature individual leads to the other major question in regard to intimacy and sexuality, which is "With what kind of partner will I want to spend my life?" This question is answered over the course of time. The process of dating is an experimental process of getting to know a variety of people and "ruling-out" and "ruling-in" characteristics that are important in a partner.

Steinberg (1996) reported that adolescents' attitudes toward sex, and toward premarital sex in particular, have become more liberal over the last three decades. Current data indicate that approximately half of all American teenagers have had sexual intercourse by the time that they graduate from high school, with the percentage of boys higher than that of girls. By the end of college the percentages of sexually experienced youth increases to 80 percent (Steinberg, 1996). Research, however, has also indicated that the majority of adolescents believe that openness, honesty, and fidelity are important in sexual relationships. The majority of adolescents also oppose exploitation, pressure, forced sex, sex for physical enjoyment without a personal relationship, and sex between persons who are too young to understand what is involved in a sexual relationship. Although an adolescent may have a series of sexual partners over a period of time, he or she is likely to be monogamous within each relationship. For most adolescents affection, emotional involvement, and commitment to the relationship accompany sexual involvement.

Essential to healthy adolescent psychosocial development is recognition of the importance of others to one's life; the development of mature interaction skills to relate to others who may be different from oneself; the ability to relate intimately to others; and the healthy acceptance of oneself as a social, emotional, and sexual being.

## Delays in Achieving Developmental Tasks

### Independence—Development of Identity and Autonomy

Adolescents who have difficulty mastering the developmental task of creating a stable identity and achieving independence from adult caregivers demonstrate prolonged dependency. They may remain as dependent upon their families as they were in childhood, or they may become prematurely involved in a mutually dependent pseudointimate relationship. They may become dependent upon a group, as many gang members do. Within the gang they may be aggressive and domineering, masking their inadequacy behind a facade of false bravado and toughness.

Adolescents who are confused about their identity may experiment with a variety of identities by becoming involved in different adolescent subgroups. They may even try a series of different subgroups and still fail to find any that suit them. They may lack interest, motivation, or ability to engage in activities or to identify potential vocational pursuits. They frequently have not discovered activities that have any meaning to them nor have they experienced competency from successful performance. School plays a critical role in providing a context for children and adolescents to explore their abilities and to develop their competencies. Adolescents whose lives outside of school have been chaotic may never have had the energy to devote to school and learning. Adolescents with identity confusion may lack any interest in school subjects or activities. They may have experienced "failure" at school either academically, athletically, or socially.

Children who had difficulty competing with other children in elementary school because of an attention deficit disorder or learning disabilities that went undetected carry that deficit self-image into adolescence. Their fledgling identity may be continually bombarded with self-deprecating thoughts and comments. When they lack self-confidence, self-direction, and self-initiative, they just exist day by day with no vision, hopes, dreams, or plans for the future. They may not know who they are or where they are going. They may be excessively self-critical and experience a sense of defectiveness and low self-worth. They may experience confusion about what to value, or they may experience serious value conflicts between what their parents, adult authority figures, and society value and what they themselves value. Value conflict may be demonstrated in angry, oppositional, and delinquent behavior. Self-control may be lacking, resulting in impulsive behaviors with little or no concern for the possible consequences.

Adolescents who are excessively self-critical and feel inferior to others lack the energy to accomplish the developmental tasks of adolescence. They are likely to have difficulty adjusting to a peer-based social system that may be critical and judgmental, further contributing to their sense of inadequacy and low self-worth and fulfilling their self-fulfilling prophecy of rejection by others.

Nearly all adolescents have periodic episodes of self-esteem crisis, but the adolescent who has demonstrated competency in at least some area, whether it be in academics, athletics, or socially, has the "proof" of his or her ability to counteract the fleeting feelings of inadequacy. The adolescent who has no proof of capability, having instead collected proof of failure because of a history of unsuccessful experiences, validates the argument that he or she is without value or worth! To develop esteem, everyone needs to be successful in some area, to experience a sense of competence, and to recognize his or her strengths. Just as resolution of the identity crisis culminates in commitment to a series of occupational and ideological stances, lack of resolution of the identity crisis culminates in the inability to make basic life commitments. The adolescent lacks purpose, meaning, and direction for his or her life.

## Interdependence—Development of Intimacy and Sexuality

In most cases, adolescents with intimacy problems may have never developed a trusting relationship with a peer. They may have never developed close friendships with same-sex peers during childhood and preadolescence. As an adolescent, they may be loners. They have no real friends, although they may have a number of associates. Any relationships that they do have tend to be superficial and not based upon mutual sharing and self-disclosure. Lack of ability to form meaningful relationships results in a lack of ability to make a commitment to another person.

Lack of the development of a supportive peer network can be seen in egocentric behavior, such as self-centeredness, lack of concern or empathy for others, self-absorption, aggressive behavior, violation of other persons or their property, lack of remorse for hurting others, and blatant antisocial behavior. When individuals have not learned to work with peer groups, they lack respect for others as equals. They tend to gravitate to the extremes of passive dependency, passive aggressiveness, or aggressive dominance driven by self-interest and self-protection arising out of lack of trust.

OTs who work with adolescents with psychosocial problems recognize that many of these young people lack the interpersonal skills expected of much younger children for interaction with others in dyads and in groups. They often do not know how to share, ask to borrow, wait their turn, cooperate, show respect for others, or give or receive feedback to others. These young people are delayed in social development. They lack the skills to relate to others and develop meaningful relationships.

Adolescents having difficulty with the developmental task of interdependence often demonstrate extremes of behavior. They may exhibit promiscuous behavior and act out sexually. Young women with self-image deficits often use their bodies to feel loved or approved of, even if only temporarily, by acting out sexually. Adolescents who have a history of sexual abuse will often show promiscuous behavior. At the other extreme, as is seen in cases of anorexia nervosa, young women, in particular, may attempt to cease or reverse the natural course of physical maturation of the body by attempting to keep their bodies as childlike thin and lacking in curves as possible.

Some adolescents, because of their limited social skills and difficulty relating to peers comfortably, fail to recognize the dating process as an opportunity to get to know a variety of personalities. They may not date or they may cling dependently to the first person with whom they develop a relationship, only to be devastated when the relationship does not last. They may commit to one relationship prematurely, even marrying while they are still very young, as happens frequently with children of alcoholics whose early marriages are attempts to escape their home environment. Sexual identity confusion may be another problem that impedes the dating process. Homosexuality is no longer identified as a diagnosis in the fourth edition of the American Psychiatric Association *Diagnostic and Statistical Manual of Mental Disorders*, the *DSM-IV*. Gender identity disorder, however, is recognized as a diagnosis when a strong and persistent cross-gender identification is accompanied by persistent discomfort with one's assigned sex, and there is evidence of impairment in social, occupational, or other important area of functioning (*DSM-IV*, 1994). The process of dating when one is gay or lesbian can create difficulties for the adolescent, because society and adolescent peers are often not accepting. Many homosexual adolescents may choose to hide their true sexuality for fear of the ramifications. The *DSM-IV* states that many individuals with gender identity disorder become socially isolated. Social isolation and ostracism contribute to low self-esteem and may lead to school aversion or dropping out of school. Peer ostracism and teasing are particularly common for boys with this disorder.

## THE DEVELOPMENT OF INDEPENDENCE AND INTERDEPENDENCE THROUGH ROLE PERFORMANCE

It is through the everyday process of engaging in roles that adolescents develop both independence and interdependence. Adolescents' primary occupation is that of a student. Contributions to the developmental tasks of independence and interdependence occur as a result of engaging in the student role. As students, adolescents test their skills and abilities. They learn about themselves as they identify which academic areas interest them and in which areas they have proficiency. This process eventually leads to narrowing their interests in regard to occupational choices. As school becomes increasingly more challenging they are required to assume greater responsibility for studying and performing academically. They are expected to function more independently with each year of progression through the middle and secondary education system. If they choose to go on to college, the demands upon them to be personally responsible for their education are even greater. The student role also provides adolescents with opportunities to develop interdependence as they work collaboratively with other students to accomplish group projects or work in study groups. They may have to work out differences when group members fail to assume sufficient responsibility to make the workload equitable. In co-ed schools, boys and girls learn to work as academic partners and to relate to one another in a different way than friendship or dating roles provide.

Adolescents' participation in school provides them with opportunities to engage in roles other than that of student. Related roles that can occur within the context of the school environment include those of a friend, club, or organization member, and teammate. A boyfriend or girlfriend role might also occur in part within the context of school. These roles involve significant task components that contribute to identity. The students may develop talents as singers, musicians, actors, writers, or athletes. Within the context of these roles, they may develop leadership skills or test potential vocational interests. Although task activities are a component of these roles, all of these roles are largely social in nature. Interacting socially with peers between classes, after school, in meetings, on stage, in locker rooms and on fields, courts, and tracks develops interdependence. The school, through its support of extracurricular activities, provides the opportunity for adolescents to engage in roles that contribute to their healthy development.

These roles may also occur outside the context of school. Friendships and dating relationships blossom from personal contact in the community at large. Friends may be made at workplaces, in neighborhoods, and through mutual acquaintances. Likewise, organization and team activities take place outside of school. Adolescents participate in church- and civic group-sponsored organizations including church youth groups, boy and girl scouting, and community-based athletic organizations. School, church, and community organizations may open doors for adolescents to fill the additional role of a volunteer in the community. Adolescents volunteer in programs such as meal delivery for the homebound, home or lawn maintenance for those who need assistance, and assisting with community activities and fund-raisers. Whether these social roles occur as extracurricular activities or independent of the school, adolescents engaged in social contact with peers, sponsors, adult leaders, coaches, parents, and members of the community develop interpersonal relationships that contribute to their maturity.

The role of the friend deserves special consideration because of the importance of peer relationships during this time of life. Peer relationships provide the social context for learning about communication, trust, and intimacy. Through the process of forming and sustaining friendships, selecting dating relationships, and terminating friendships and dating relationships, adolescents confirm and "rule out" aspects of their identity. Experimentation and trial and error are natural ways to learn about oneself and others during this period of life.

Adolescents may also have roles as paid workers. Many adolescents today work part time or full time to provide themselves with money to pay for clothes, CDs, video games, to go out themselves or with dates, or to pay for cars, gas, or insurance premiums. Even if they received allowances and had money to spend before getting a job, being paid and making your own money adds to feelings of independence. Through acceptance of job responsibilities, working adolescents develop autonomy and integrate work experiences into their developing identity. If they are able to work in areas that hold potential vocational interest for them, they may confirm vocational interests with exposure to the work. However, most of the jobs that adolescents fill are not jobs that require a high level of skill or education. Jobs in the fast food industry, hostessing or waitressing at a restaurant, stocking, bagging, or cashiering at a grocery store, working sales in a retail store, or providing labor at a construction site provide adolescents with the opportunity to learn about meeting employer expectations in regard to job performance, punctuality, dress, grooming, and hygiene. They may have an interest in continuing work in these industries, but many adolescents consider their adolescent work experience strictly as temporary employment to earn spending money. Most jobs also involve social contact with coworkers. Coworkers may be peers or adults. Many of the jobs held by teenagers also involve interaction with the public. These interpersonal contacts are important contributors to the development of the interpersonal skills necessary for interdependence.

Although adolescents are less dependent on the family than they were as children, their roles as family members are still essential in the development of their independence and interdependence. Holding adolescents accountable for routine tasks such as yard maintenance, pet care, taking out the trash, washing the dishes, keeping their rooms clean, laundering their clothes, or assisting with meal preparation teaches them the skills that they will need once they leave home to live on their own. It also teaches them that every family member shares in the responsibility of maintaining a communal living space. Acquiring these independent living skills contributes to a sense of autonomy and independence. Remaining an active member of the family by taking part in family meals and activities while also engaging in activities with peers helps adolescents to have a range of interpersonal interactions. Sibling relationships also help the adolescent learn about living with and understanding others. Connection with family and family support of teens' activities contribute to healthy independence and interdependence as teens "tests their wings" with the support of the family.

Successful involvement in a variety of roles provides adolescents with the opportunities for these developmental tasks to be accomplished. In the next section, we will discuss a variety of psychosocial dysfunctions that adversely affect the development of independence and interdependence. A series of tables will contrast typical adolescent role performance with role performance affected by various types of psychosocial dysfunctions.

## ◢◣◥ FROM THE BOOKSHELF

Csikszentmihalyi, M., & Larsan, R. (1984). *Being adolescent: Conflict and growth in the teenage years.* New York: Basic Books. Although written over a decade ago, this text is highly informative about the daily lives of adolescents. Two psychologists gave beepers to 75 adolescents in a heterogeneous community bordering Chicago. Over the course of a week's time, they were signaled at random and asked to record their thoughts and feelings. The result was a glimpse of the day-to-day world of average American teens.

Wexler, D. B. (1991). *The adolescent self.* New York: Norton. This text presents an innovative 16-group treatment program to promote the development of self-esteem, self-regulation, self-management, self-soothing, self-stimulation, self-control, and self-efficacy.

Wexler, D. B. (1991). *The prism workbook.* New York: Norton. This workbook is designed for use with the 16-group program presented in *The Adolescent Self.*

Pipher, M. (1994). *Reviving Ophelia: Saving the selves of adolescent girls.* New York: Ballantine Books. This book, which has been #1 on the *New York Times* Bestsellers list, uses case histories of adolescent girls who have struggled to find and maintain a sense of self. It closely examines the damage imposed by contemporary culture upon young girls and offers strategies that adults can use to help the adolescent girls they care about to regain their sense of self.

## ADOLESCENTS WITH PSYCHOLOGICAL AND SOCIAL PROBLEMS

Estimates over the last few decades indicate that approximately 20 to 25 percent of American adolescents have serious psychosocial and behavioral problems (Hurrelmann, 1994). Several diagnoses from the *DSM-IV* (1994) make up the majority of diagnoses that will be seen on any regular basis when working with adolescents with psychological and social problems. Because of their prevalence, each of these will be discussed individually. The diagnoses that will be covered in this section are major depressive disorder, dysthymia, bipolar disorder, cyclothymic disorder, conduct disorder, anxiety disorders, substance use disorders, and eating disorders.

Many of the adolescents with these disorders are seen by OTs working in a medical setting. The setting may be an acute inpatient one at a psychiatric hospital or general hospital with a psychiatric unit or service, a partial hospitalization "day treatment" program, or a residential treatment program. Before making a referral for occupational therapy, a psychiatrist or psychologist will generally have conducted a thorough assessment and made a diagnosis. This assessment generally includes taking a history of the present condition; a history of past psychiatric hospitalization and treatment; a medical history; a developmental history; a sexual history; and a history of alcohol, tobacco, and drug use (Harrison & Newcorn, 1996). They will generally include at least a brief school and family history, but if the facility has a social worker on staff, he or she will collect more extensive information in this area. In addition, the psychiatrist or psychologist will have conducted a mental status exam, which includes appearance, behavior, relatedness, speech and language, mood and affect; thought process and content, and a cognitive and developmental assessment. Most psychiatrists and psychologists find it is advantageous to confirm the self-report of the adolescent by taking histories from the parents, caregivers, caseworkers, or any other adult who has knowledge of the adolescent, if it is at all possible. This is of particular importance if the adolescent is resistant to the assessment process. When sufficient information is obtained from the adolescent and knowledgeable adults to determine the presence or absence of diagnostic criteria, as delineated by the *DSM-IV* (1994), a diagnosis is formulated. Diagnosis formulation is the jurisdiction of a psychiatrist or psychologist. When preparing for an occupational therapy evaluation, a chart review of the information collected by psychiatrists, psychologists, and social workers is an important preliminary step. *Be mindful when acquiring information from a medical record that this information is confidential and be aware of maintaining that confidentiality.* The histories taken provide valuable information from which OTs can progress to investigate the effects of the psychosocial disorders upon daily functioning in occupations.

Adolescents are more aware of their feelings than children and can be good self-reporters, when they are willing to talk. A resistant adolescent or an adolescent who sets out intentionally to sabotage the treatment process may either refuse to talk or may deliberately provide false information. To engage an adolescent successfully in an open dialogue about his or her life requires skill and experience. Adolescents are much more likely to feel comfortable sharing openly  and honestly about themselves when they feel that the person helping them is accepting and nonjudgmental. The evaluation interview is often the key in convincing the young person that your role as an OT is to help him or her achieve greater satisfaction with life. After the occupational therapy evaluation, if additional information surfaces that would affect the diagnosis, the therapist should bring this information to the attention of the member or members of the treatment team responsible for diagnosis. In the next section of this chapter we will examine the most frequently made diagnoses for adolescents with psychosocial dysfunction.

# MOOD DISORDERS

Although mood disorders do exist in prepubescent children, rarely do these disorders present in their full form until after puberty. After puberty adolescents often manifest the same symptoms as adults. Mood disorders are serious in children and adolescents. Estimates of the occurrence of depression, from studies conducted by federal agencies within the Department of Health and Human Services, indicate that 6 out of 100 children and adolescents are depressed (1996). Studies of child and adolescent depression have resulted in varying ranges because of differences in the measures used, ages studied, and the manner in which the variable depression was operationalized. In the general population incidence of depression in adolescents is reported to range from 1 to 2 percent, but up to 12 to 14 percent of high school students have demonstrated substantial depressive symptoms on self-report measures (Kowatch, Emslie, & Kennard, 1996). Studies using self-report measures have also reported greater levels of depressive symptoms in African-American students, girls, and particularly Hispanic girls (Kowatch et al., 1996).

The *DSM-IV* divides mood disorders into four categories: the depressive disorders, the bipolar disorders, and two disorders based upon etiology—mood disorder arising from a general medical condition and substance-induced mood disorder. For the purposes of this chapter, we will focus on the depressive disorders and on the bipolar disorders. There are three depressive disorders—major depressive disorder, dysthymic disorder, and depressive disorder not otherwise specified, abbreviated NOS. There are four bipolar disorders—bipolar I disorder, bipolar II disorder, cyclothymic disorder, and bipolar disorder NOS. To facilitate diagnosis, the *DSM-IV* identifies four episodes: major depressive, manic, mixed, and hypomanic. Identification of the occurrence of one or more of these episodes forms the basis of the diagnosis of a depressive or bipolar disorder.

## *Major Depressive Episode*

According to the *DSM-IV* (1994), identification of a *major depressive episode* requires that at least five of the nine symptoms listed in Box 12–1 be present during the same 2-week period, that at least one of the symptoms is either a depressed mood or a loss of interest or pleasure, and the symptoms must represent a change from previous functioning. The symptoms may not meet the criteria for a mixed episode and they must cause clinically significant distress or impairment in social, occupational, or other important areas of functioning. They may not be a result of the direct physiological effects of a substance, such as a side effect of a medication, as a result of drug abuse, or be attributable to a general medical condition like hypothyroidism.

## *Manic Episode*

The *DSM-IV* (1994) defines a *manic episode* as "a distinct period of abnormally and persistently elevated, expansive or irritable mood, lasting at least one week (or any duration if hospitalization is necessary)." During the episode the individual must exhibit at least three of the symptoms listed in Box 12–2.

---

**Box 12–1**

Symptoms That May Be Present During a Major Depressive Episode

- Depressed or irritable mood most of the day, nearly every day, as indicated by either subjective report or observation made by others

*or*

- Marked diminished interest or pleasure in all, or almost all, activities most of the day, nearly every day

*and*

- Significant weight loss when not dieting or weight gain, decrease or increase in appetite nearly every day, failure to make expected weight gains
- Insomnia or hypersomnia nearly every day
- Psychomotor agitation or retardation nearly every day (observable by others)
- Fatigue or loss of energy nearly every day
- Feelings of worthlessness or excessive or inappropriate guilt nearly every day
- Diminished ability to think or concentrate, or indecisiveness, nearly every day
- Recurrent thoughts of death, recurrent suicidal ideation without a specific plan, or a suicide attempt or a specific plan for committing suicide

---

**Box 12–2**

Symptoms That May Be Present During a Manic Episode or Hypomanic Episode

- Inflated self-esteem and grandiosity
- Decreased need for sleep (e.g., feels rested after only 3 hours of sleep)
- More talkative than usual or pressure to keep talking
- Flight of ideas or subjective experience that thoughts are racing
- Distractibility (i.e., attention too easily drawn to unimportant or irrelevant external stimuli)
- Increase in goal-directed activity (either socially, at work or school, or sexually) or psychomotor agitation
- Excessive involvement in pleasurable activities that have a high potential for painful consequences

---

Like the major depressive episode, this mood disturbance must be sufficiently severe to cause marked impairment in occupational or social functioning or to require hospitalization to prevent harm to self or others. Psychotic features may be present during manic episodes.

## Mixed Episode

The criteria for a *mixed episode* are that the criteria for both a major depressive episode (except for the duration) and for a manic episode are met over the course of at least a 1-week period, nearly every day. Like the other mood disorder episodes, the disturbance in mood must be of sufficient severity to cause marked impairment in occupational or social functioning and hospitalization is often necessary to prevent harm to self or others, or for treatment of psychotic features.

## Hypomanic Episode

The *hypomanic episode* as defined by *DSM-IV* is "a distinct period of persistently elevated, expansive, or irritable mood, lasting throughout at least 4 days, that is clearly different from the usual nondepressed mood" (p. 338). For this episode to be identified, three or more of the symptoms from Box 12–2 must be met. The episode must be associated with a change in functioning. Both the disturbance in mood and the change in functioning need to be observable to others. Unlike the other three episodes, the hypomanic episode is not severe enough to cause marked impairment in social or occupational functioning, or to necessitate hospitalization, and there are no psychotic symptoms present.

With awareness of the four episodes that may present in adolescents with mood disorders, we will move our discussion to the actual diagnoses of the depressive and bipolar disorders.

## DEPRESSIVE DISORDERS

### Major Depressive Disorder

The suicide rate for adolescents has increased 200 percent over the last decade (Offer & Schonert-Reichl, 1992). The vast majority of these young people have a major depressive disorder. The essential feature of *major depressive disorder* is the presence of one or more major depressive episodes with no history of a manic, hypomanic, or mixed episode. Diagnostic specifiers indicate whether the major depressive disorder is occurring for the first time, in which case it is labeled as a single episode, or whether it is recurrent. Diagnostic specifiers also indicate the current state of the disturbance. An episode is considered ended when the full criteria have not been met for two consecutive months. The major depressive disorder can be coded as mild, moderate, severe with psychotic features, severe without psychotic features, in partial remission, and in full remission.

Weinberg (1973) has modified the diagnostic criteria for major depressive disorder for adults for the purposes of research with children and adolescents. Box 12–3 lists the signs and symptoms of depression as identified by Weinberg.

Symptoms usually develop over days to weeks. A prodromal period may last weeks to months before the onset of a full major depressive episode. The duration of a major depressive episode is variable. An untreated episode typically lasts for 6 months or longer. In as many as 25 percent of clinical cases major depressive disorder was preceded by dysthymic disorder, which takes place over a period of at least a year (*DSM-IV*, 1994). Studies of recovery in adolescents treated for major depressive disorder (Kovacs & Goldston, 1991;

---

**Box 12–3**

Symptoms of Depression in Children and Adolescents

- Depressed mood characterized by sadness, loneliness, unhappiness, hopelessness, mood swings, irritability, hypersensitivity, a negative attitude and being difficult to please.
- Self-deprecatory ideation manifest by feelings of worthlessness, stupidity, ugliness, guilt, or feelings of persecution or rejection by others, death wishes or suicidal ideation.
- Agitation leading to oppositional and defiant behavior at home or at school may arise from irritability and result in fighting, disrespect for authority, quarreling, and excessive hostility.
- Sleep disturbances are seen in the form of initial, middle, or terminal insomnia, difficulty awakening in the morning, excessive sleepiness and hypersomnia.
- Change in appetite or weight is seen in adolescents who become "picky" eaters, craving sweets or snack foods, or who become voracious eaters. Failure to gain weight as developmentally appropriate is common in children and adolescents depression.
- Diminished socialization with a decline in group participation or changing to a less socially desirable peer group and a decreased interest in seeking out friends. There may also be increased conflict with peers and siblings.
- Change in school performance with lowered grades that teachers may attribute to daydreaming, poor concentration, poor motivation, loss of interest in school, and incomplete schoolwork and homework.
- Change in attitude toward school that may relate to a diurnal mood variation with increased depression in the morning, but generally has to do with a loss of interest in the pleasure of school and its activities.
- Somatic complaints particularly, headaches and stomachaches whose degree of disabling is clearly in excess of medical cause.
- Loss of usual energy resulting in complaints of tiredness, easy fatigue, less energy, boredom during previously enjoyable activities and diminished participation.

*Source:* Weinberg, 1973.

---

McCauley et al., 1993; Strober et al., 1992) demonstrate that depression is a treatable illness. Research studies have indicated that 60 to 80 percent of adolescents treated for major depressive disorder have recovered within a year of admission, and 92 to 98 percent have recovered within 18 months to 2 years after. Recovery is defined as being asymptomatic for two consecutive months. However, it is also important to know that major depressive disorder tends to be episodic. A recent study by Emslie, Rush, Weinberg, Gullion, Rintelman, and Hughes (1997) indicates that episodes may be briefer but more frequent in children and adolescents than in adults. In 20 to 30 percent of the cases some depressive symptoms remain, and in 5 to 10 percent of the cases the full criteria for a major depressive episode continues to be met for 2 years of more. The *DSM-IV* (1994) indicates that in approximately 50 to 60 percent of individuals with major depressive disorder, a single episode can be expected to be followed by a second episode within 5 years. A study by

Kovacs and Goldston (1991) of children and adolescents with major depression reported a 72 percent rate of reoccurrence within 5 years. The majority of those with a reoccurrence had them within 1 to 2 years (Emslie et al., 1997). Individuals who have had a second episode have a 70 percent chance of having a third episode, and individuals who have had a third episode have a 90 percent likelihood of having a fourth episode (*DSM-IV*, 1994). The severity of the first major depressive episode appears to predict the persistence of the disorder. Major depressive disorder is twice as common in adolescent girls as in adolescent boys. Prevalence rates are unrelated to ethnicity, education, income, or marital status (*DSM-IV*).

Single events have not been found to exert much risk on subsequent psychopathology, but a pattern of adverse life experiences, particularly when combined with recent life events, exerts a range of effects on subsequent behavior, thus determining the degree of risk, through their impact on affective-cognitive and physiological processes (Goodyer, 1996). Bonder (1995), states that "Life events alone do not cause depression. There seems to be an interaction between undesirable life events and inadequate coping responses in people who are biologically prone to depression" (p. 110). Research has indicated that a combination of negative life events, particularly family conflict and academic failure, and less constructive perceived problem-solving alternatives are associated with depression and suicidal ideation in adolescents (Adams & Adams, 1996). Adolescents with depressed mood have been found to be less intimate with both parents, to feel less social support, and to have lower self-esteem than their peers (Lasko, Field, Gonzalez, Harding, Yando & Bendell, 1996). There is a familiar pattern to depression. Major depressive disorder is one and a half to three times more common in first-degree biological relatives of persons with the disorder than among the general population (*DSM-IV*). Adolescents who perceived either of their parents as unhappy also reported less intimacy with both parents and less social support (Lasko et al., 1996). Social support serves as a valuable coping strategy. Its absence leaves individuals feeling totally alone to face their problems. Some of the stressors associated with adolescent depression are listed in Box 12–4.

It is also important to note that researchers have learned more about the neurophysiological basis of depression than they knew several years ago. PET scans have allowed scientists to identify that persons with hereditary depression have decreased size (39 to 48 percent less brain tissue) and less activity in the subgenual prefrontal cortex, which has been recognized for some time as playing an important role in the control of emotions (*Time*, May 5, 1997).

## Dysthymic Disorder

*Dysthymic disorder* refers to a chronically depressed or dysphoric mood that although less intense than major depressive disorder has no prolonged well states (Kowatch, Emslie, & Kennard, 1996). The features of dysthymic disorder in adolescents are similar to those of major depressive disorder—a depressed mood for most of the day, for more days than not, but in the case of dysthymic disorder, the duration of the mood disturbance must be for at least 1 year. In addition to the prolonged depression, the presence of two or more symptoms listed in Box 12–5 must be present.

**Box 12–4**

Stressors Associated with Adolescent Depression

Death of a loved one (parent, close family member, friend, pet)
Separation from a loved one (parental separation/divorce, break-up of a relationship, move, separation from parent because of work, military assignment, incarceration, separation from sibling because of college, marriage, move)
Loss of a friendship (move, disagreement, replacement)
Loss of a familiar way of being (change in school, loss of dependency, childhood simplicity, move)
Loss of respect (inability to live up to parental or personal expectations, sibling rivalry)
Loss of self-esteem (physical awkwardness or unattractiveness, failure in academics or athletics, lack of praise or support, target of teasing, put-downs, criticism)
Loss of boundaries and guidelines (excessive permissiveness, lack of rules, support, caring)
Loss of attention (diversion of parental attention because of addiction, divorce, illness, single parenting, dual careers, working two or three jobs to make ends meet, parental workaholism)
Loss of sense of security
Loss of normality or health (disability, chronic illness)
Learning disabilities
Loss of goals
Parental depression or addiction
Family conflict
History of physical, emotional, mental, or sexual abuse

**Box 12–5**

Criteria for Dysthymic Disorder

- Depressed mood for most of the day, for more days than not, as indicated either by subjective account or observation by others, for at least 1 year

*and* two or more of the following:

- Poor appetite or overeating
- Insomnia or hypersomnia
- Low energy or fatigue
- Low self-esteem
- Poor concentration or difficulty making decisions
- Feelings of hopelessness

During the 1-year period the adolescent has not been without these symptoms for more than 2 months at a time.

Adolescents with dysthymic disorder may have a good day or a mixed day, but they have no good weeks. Often adolescents with this disorder have experienced symptoms since early childhood (Kowatch et al., 1996). The most common symptoms of dysthymic disorder are:

- Feelings of inadequacy
- Generalized loss of interest or pleasure
- Social withdrawal
- Feelings of guilt or brooding about the past
- Feelings of irritability or anger
- Decreased activity, sense of effectiveness, and productivity

Adolescents with dysthymic disorder are generally cranky and irritable as well as depressed. They have low self-esteem and poor social skills and are generally pessimistic. They often have impaired school performance and social interaction. The *DSM-IV* (1994) reports that this disorder occurs equally in boys and girls, and that its lifetime prevalence is estimated at 6 percent. Like other mood disorders, dysthymic disorder is more common among first-degree biological relatives with major depressive disorder than among the general population. The term used to describe the condition when an adolescent, during the course of a dysthymic disorder, experiences a major depressive disorder is *double depression.*

### Depressive Disorder NOS

*Depressive disorder NOS* is also an episodic disorder, but the episodes are below the criteria for major depressive disorder. The symptoms are either fewer or of a shorter duration. This disorder, sometimes referred to as minor depression, may be a precursor to major depressive disorder or may occur independently. An episode of depressive disorder NOS will cause less dysfunction than a major depressive disorder.

## BIPOLAR DISORDERS

Bipolar disorders in adolescents are characterized by exaggerated mood swings between depressive lows and markedly excited highs. Periods of moderate mood may occur in between the extremes of mood. Adults with bipolar disorders report experiencing their first symptoms during adolescence.

### Bipolar Disorder I

The essential feature of *bipolar disorder I* is the occurrence of one or more manic or mixed episodes. Often individuals have also had one or more major depressive episodes. The specific diagnosis will identify the current or most recent episode as either manic, mixed, hypomanic, or major depressive. The same specifiers as for major depressive disorder (mild, moderate, severe with psychotic features, severe without psychotic features, in partial remission, and in full remission) are used to describe the current manic, mixed, or major depressive episode. Violent behavior, school truancy, school failure, occupational failure, and antisocial behavior are associated problems with this disorder.

Bipolar I is a recurrent disorder. More than 90 percent of the individuals who have a single manic episode will go on to have future episodes. Some 60 to 70 percent of manic episodes occur either immediately before or immediately following a major depressive disorder. Approximately 10 to 15 percent of adolescents with recurrent major depressive disorder will go on to develop bipolar disorder I. This disorder is equally common in boys and girls. The first episode in boys tends to be a manic episode, whereas the first episode in girls is more likely to be a major depressive episode. Although the majority of individuals with bipolar disorder I return to a fully functional level between episodes, approximately 20 to 30 percent continue to exhibit mood lability and to have interpersonal and occupational difficulties. As in the mood disorders previously mentioned, first-degree biological relatives of individuals with mood disorders have elevated rates of mood disorders.

## Bipolar Disorder II

*Bipolar disorder II* is characterized by the occurrence of one or more major depressive episodes accompanied by at least one hypomanic episode. The presence of a manic or a mixed episode precludes a bipolar II diagnosis. Because individuals in a major depressive episode have difficulty recalling periods of hypomania, information from close friends and relatives is often essential in the diagnostic process. The current or most recent episode, whether hypomanic or depressed, is specified as part of the diagnosis. Like bipolar I, school truancy, school failure, and occupational failure are frequently associated with this disorder. Bipolar II is more common in females and occurs either before or after a major depressive episode 60 to 70 percent of the time.

## Cyclothymic Disorder

The essential feature of *cyclothymic disorder* in adolescents is a "chronic, fluctuating mood disturbance involving numerous periods of hypomanic symptoms and numerous periods of depressive symptoms" over a period of at least 1 year (p. 363). The hypomanic symptoms are of insufficient number, severity, pervasiveness, or duration to meet full criteria for a manic or mixed episode, and the depressive symptoms are of insufficient number, severity, pervasiveness, or duration to meet full criteria for a major depressive episode. During the 1-year period, any symptom-free interval cannot have lasted more than 2 months.

## Medical Treatment of Mood Disorders

In most cases medical treatment of mood disorders consists of a combination of psychopharmacological treatment and psychotherapy. Although research data has been inconclusive in regard to the effectiveness of antidepressant treatment in adolescents, on an individual basis clinicians have found antidepressants to be effective, particularly in cases where psychosocial interventions have been ineffective or when a family history of depression or anxiety disorders exists (Carrey, Wiggins, & Milin, 1996). In recent years the selective serotonin reuptake inhibitors, or SSRIs (e.g., fluoxetine, fluvoxamine, setraline, and paroxetine), have become well accepted because of their positive effect on mood and reduced side effects in comparison with the first-generation antidepressants, the tricyclic antidepressants (e.g., imipramine, clomipramine, desipramine, nortriptyline). The SSRIs have the advantage of being safe in an overdose, which is of particular importance with the risk for suicide in depressed individuals. The tricyclics are still used, particularly imipramine and nortriptyline, but their adverse side effects, like dry mouth, tremor, sedation, constipation, weight gain, blurred vision, headaches, and anxiety often interfere with medication compliance. They are generally reserved for patients whose disorders are more difficult to treat. Sometimes the tricyclics are used in combination with an SSRI medication (Parmelee, 1996). Individual case studies (Carrey et al., 1996) and a double-blind, placebo-controlled trial (Emslie, 1996) have indicated that fluoxetine (Prozac) has been useful in treating depression in children and adolescents. Headache, dry mouth, and gastrointestinal problems are reported side effects of SSRIs, but these symptoms tend to be transient and to resolve within the first few weeks of treatment. Insomnia associated with SSRIs is usually alleviated with the addition of small doses of trazodone. Monoamine oxidase inhibitors (MAOIs), phenelzine or tranylcypramine are occasionally used with adolescents, but because they can trigger hypertensive crises, they are considered more risky to use and may only be tried when other drugs have not been effective (Hodgman, 1996).

For bipolar disorder in which a definite mania has occurred, lithium has been the drug of choice for some time. Carlson (1990) recommended the use of lithium in severe cases of mania, in which there has been a history of severe depression with a family history of mood disorder, an acute psychotic episode, or a disruptive behavior disorder with a family history of mood disorder. Adverse side effects of taking lithium include nausea, vomiting, diarrhea, fine tremor, increased thirst and urination, and weight gain. Possible long-term effects, after 6 months to a year of use, are hypothryoidism and kidney damage. Recently, valproic acid (Depakote), which is an anticonvulsant medication, has been found to be an effective replacement for lithium in the treatment of the acute phase of mania in adolescents, and its side effects are better tolerated. Carbamazepine, another anticonvulsant medication, has also been found to be useful with adolescents with lithium-resistant mania and aggressive or explosive behavior (Carrey et al., 1996). Lithium, valproic acid, and carbamazepine all require regular monitoring of blood levels (Parmelee, 1996).

Psychopharmacological treatment is rarely used without being accompanied by psychotherapy. A study comparing psychotherapy in adolescents with major depression found cognitive-behavioral therapy that taught patients to monitor and correct automatic thoughts and helped them to develop problem-solving skills was more effective than either family or supportive therapy that focused on expression of feelings. Seventy-three percent of those who received cognitive-behavioral therapy recovered and tended to recover sooner (Brent, Holder, & Kolko, 1997).

## Mood Disorders and Development

Mood disorders interfere with the process of developing independence and interdependence by affecting an adolescent's routine pursuit of social and occupational roles. Table 12–1 contrasts a typically developing adolescent with an adolescent with a mood disorder.

**Table 12–1** **Comparison of Social and Occupational Roles of a Typically Developing Adolescent with Those of an Adolescent with a Mood Disorder**

| Social and Occupational Roles | Typically Developing Adolescent | Adolescent with a Mood Disorder |
|---|---|---|
| Student | Exploring areas of interest and testing capabilities<br><br>Developing habits of self-discipline, self-control, and organization<br><br>Experiencing success and competency<br><br>Defining who he or she is, including skills and abilities (identity)<br><br>Answering identity question—What do I want to do in the future?<br><br>Working collaboratively in study or project groups (interdependence) | Loss of interest, loss of motivation<br><br>Loss of attention, distractible<br><br>Minimal exploration preventing the ruling-in and ruling-out process that identifies capabilities<br><br>Lack of adaptive habit development<br><br>Experiencing failure resulting in feelings of inadequacy, inability and incompetency<br><br>Lack of academic and occupational goals |
| Friend | Development of meaningful intimate same sex and opposite sex relationships that involve trust and ability to confide in others (interdependence)<br><br>Discovery of new interests through association with others<br><br>Development of interpersonal skills, ability to communicate and relate to others<br><br>Development of an understanding of multiple viewpoints and individual differences<br><br>Experiencing security from acceptance, support, and encouragement of others | Social withdrawal, disengagement from others or driving other people away due to depressed or manic behavior<br><br>Lack of stimulation from others stunts exploration of new interests and ideas<br><br>Lack of interpersonal skill development<br><br>Difficulty relating to others<br><br>Difficulty expressing ideas and feelings<br><br>Difficulty assuming a different perspective or recognizing the value in diversity<br><br>Alone, isolated and without support |
| Family member | Mutual respect and support between all members of the family (interdependence)<br><br>Acceptance of responsibility for chores and adherence to rules<br><br>Increasing freedom within limits (independence)<br><br>Open communication including a willingness to confront and deal with conflict | Withdrawal from family<br><br>Disrespect for parents, caregivers, siblings<br><br>Lack of energy to put toward contributing to the family<br><br>Lack of willingness to accept responsibility for chores, family member tasks<br><br>Lack of communication with others in the family<br><br>Little expression of feelings with the exception of anger<br><br>May be hostile and aggressive or passively resistant |

| | | |
|---|---|---|
| Worker | Development of a relationship with an employer that requires commitment and dependability<br>Assumption of responsibility<br>Development of work skills<br>Development of co-worker relationships (interdependence)<br>Increased autonomy by making his or her own money (independence)<br>Exploring the world of work, answering identity questions—To what kind of work am I attracted? (identity) | Lack of commitment to job responsibilities<br>May not have the energy, desire, or concentration level to work<br>If working, is likely to do the minimum and experience poor evaluation ratings<br>Disinterest in developing work skills or developing relationships with others on the job<br>Critical of job, work, employer, coworkers |
| Boyfriend or girlfriend | Developing intimate trusting relationships with another person (interdependence)<br>Answering questions of identity—To what kind of person am I attracted? (identity) | May withdraw from all relationships or may be involved in a highly dependent relationship where the adolescent is looks to another person to fill his or her emptiness and make them whole<br>May engage in sexual relationships without intimacy or commitment |
| Club or Organization Member | Exploring group membership, working collaboratively with others and contributing to group success<br>Learning to accept and respect differences of opinions and ideas (interdependence)<br>Developing new skills<br>Testing leadership abilities (independence) | May reject social groups avoiding all opportunities to interact with others<br>May project blame on groups and members of groups as being exclusionary or elitist<br>No opportunity to develop member or leadership skills |
| Teammate | Developing talents and abilities (identity)<br>Developing relationships with others that involve mutual commitment and responsibility to the entire team (interdependence)<br>Interacting with coaches | Discomfort with making commitments to others<br>Loss of opportunities to develop skills and relationships |
| Volunteer | Developing the altruistic value of helping/serving others<br>Exploring service occupation | Lack of energy to serve others perpetuates self-absorption |

# DISRUPTIVE BEHAVIOR DISORDERS

The two diagnoses discussed in the section are listed under the category of "Usually First Diagnosed in Infancy, Childhood, or Adolescence" in the *DSM-IV*. Conduct disorder is one of the most frequently diagnosed conditions in inpatient and outpatient mental health facilities for children and adolescents. Conduct disorder causes adolescents to act out their feelings and impulses toward others in destructive ways.

## *Conduct Disorder*

A repetitive and persistent pattern of behavior in which the basic rights of others or major age-appropriate societal norms or rules are violated is the essential criterion of *conduct disorder*. In addition, three or more criteria listed in Box 12–6 must have been met within the last 12 months, with at least one of those having occurred within the last 6 months in order to make the diagnosis. The 15 criteria are clustered into four categories—aggression to people or animals, destruction of property, deceitfulness or theft, and serious violation of rules. The disturbance in behavior must cause significant impairment in social, academic, or occupational functioning. The diagnosis is specified as either childhood-onset or adolescent-onset, depending upon whether at least one criterion was met prior to age 10. The severity of the conduct disorder diagnosis (mild, moderate, or severe) is made based on the number of conduct problems and the effect of harm upon others.

Adolescents with conduct disorder often initiate aggressive behavior toward others, provoke others, and react aggressively in response to others. Deliberate destruction of property and lying and deceitfulness are common. There are generally also serious violations of parental, school, and societal rules. Individuals with conduct disorder may have little empathy or concern for the feelings, wishes, or well-being of others. They often misperceive the intentions of others as hostile and aggressive and respond in kind. They may be callous and lack remorse or any reasonable guilt for their actions. They often have low self-esteem, poor frustration tolerance, and place blame on others. They tend to be highly irritable, to have temper outbursts, and to be reckless, leading to accidents. Early onset of sexual behavior, drinking, smoking, use of illegal substances, and risk-taking behavior are associated with this diagnosis. Conduct disorder behavior may lead to school suspension or expulsion, problems in adjusting to work, legal difficulties, sexually transmitted diseases, unplanned pregnancies, and physical injury from accidents or fights. Suicidal ideation, attempted suicide, and completed suicide all occur at a higher rate than in the general population in adolescents with conduct disorder. Conduct disorder is often associated with lower intelligence and with learning disorders and communication disorders. Attention deficit hyperactivity disorder is also common in adolescents with this diagnosis. Family rejection and neglect; difficult infant temperament; inconsistent child-rearing practices, particularly with harsh discipline; physical or sexual abuse; lack of supervision; early institutional living; frequent changes of caregivers; large family size; association with a delinquent peer group; and family pathology are considered factors that predispose an adolescent to the devel-

**Box 12–6**

Criteria for Conduct Disorder

- A repetitive persistent pattern of behavior in which the basic rights of others or major age-appropriate societal norms or rules are violated

*and* three or more of the following criteria within the last 12 months, with at least one within the last 6 months:

**Aggression to people or animals**

- Often bullies, threatens, or intimidates others
- Often initiates physical fights
- Has used a weapon that can cause serious physical harm to others (e.g., bat, brick, broken bottle, knife, gun)
- Has been physically cruel to people
- Has been physically cruel to animals
- Has stolen while confronting a victim (e.g., mugging, purse snatching, extortion, armed robbery)
- Has forced someone into sexual activity

**Destruction of Property**

- Has deliberately engaged in fire setting with the intention of causing serious damage
- Has deliberately destroyed others' property (other than by fire setting)

**Deceitfulness or theft**

- Has broken into someone's house, building, or car
- Often lies to obtain goods or favors or to avoid obligations (i.e., "cons" others)
- Has stolen items of nontrivial value without confronting a victim (e.g., shoplifting, but without breaking and entering; forgery)

**Serious violation of rules**

- Often stays out at night despite parental prohibitions, beginning before the age of 13 years
- Has run away from home overnight at least twice while living in parental or parental surrogate home (or once without returning for a lengthy period)
- Is often truant from school, beginning before age 13 years

The disturbance in behavior causes clinically significant impairment in social, academic, or occupational functioning.

opment of conduct disorder. The prevalence of conduct disorder appears to have increased over the last decades and is more prevalent in urban than in rural settings. Conduct disorder is much more common in males. Rates of prevalence for males range from 6 to 16 percent, depending upon the population sampled, and for females the projected rate of conduct disorder is 2 to 9 percent. Conduct disorder has both genetic and environmental components. The disorder is more common in children of biological parents with alcohol dependence, mood disorders, or schizophrenia or who have a history of attention deficit hyperactivity disorder or conduct disorder. Although onset may occur as early as age 5 to 6, onset usually occurs in late childhood or early adolescence and rarely after age 16. Many individuals with adolescent-onset conduct disorder achieve adequate social and occupational adjustment as adults. Early onset predicts a worse prognosis.

## Oppositional Defiant Disorder

*Oppositional defiant disorder* is characterized by a recurrent pattern of negativistic, defiant, disobedient, and hostile behavior toward authority figures that must persist for at least 6 months. Four or more of the behaviors listed in Box 12–7 must be present to make this diagnosis, and the behavior disturbance has to be sufficiently severe to cause clinically significant impairment in social, academic, or occupational functioning. In addition, the behaviors cannot have occurred during the course of a mood disorder or psychotic disorder. If the child's or adolescent's behavior meets the criteria for a conduct disorder, that diagnosis would take precedence.

Generally, the defiant behaviors seen in adolescents with this disorder include persistent stubbornness; resistance to following directions; an unwillingness to compromise, give in, or negotiate; deliberate testing of limits; arguing; and failing to accept blame for misbehavior. Symptoms of this disorder are typically more evident in interactions with adults or those the adolescent knows well, thus it occurs mostly in the home and may not be evident in the school or community. It is associated with low self-esteem; mood lability; low frustration tolerance; swearing; and use of alcohol, tobacco, and illicit drugs. This disorder is more prevalent in families with a succession of care providers or in families in which harsh, inconsistent, or neglectful child-rearing practices are common. It is also associated with learning disorders and communication disorders.

## Medical Treatment
## of Disruptive Behavior Disorders

These disorders, like the mood disorders, are generally treated with a combination of psychopharmacology and psychotherapy treatment. Often ado-

---

**Box 12–7**

Criteria for Oppositional Defiant Disorder

A pattern of negativistic, defiant, disobedient, and hostile behavior lasting at least 6 months, during which four (or more) of the following are present.

- Often loses temper
- Often argues with adults
- Often actively defies or refuses to comply with adults' requests or rules
- Often deliberately annoys people
- Often blames others for his or her mistakes or misbehavior
- Is often touchy or easily annoyed by others
- Is often angry and resentful
- Is often spiteful or vindictive

lescents with disruptive behavior disorders have concomitant diagnoses of a mood disorder or a substance disorder or both. For this reason it is not uncommon to see SSRIs prescribed. Carbamazepine (Tegretol) and valproic acid (Depakote), both anticonvulsant medications, have also been found to be useful in adolescents with aggressive or explosive behavior (Carrey et al., 1996). When there is evidence of some organic impairment, a depressive disorder, or a psychotic disorder in addition to the disruptive behavior disorder, an antipsychotic such as haloperidol (Haldol), chlorpromazine (Thorazine), thioridazine (Mellaril), or risperidone (Risperdal) may be prescribed (Parmelee, 1996).

## *Disruptive Behavior Disorders and Development*

Disruptive behavior disorders, like mood disorders, interfere with the developmental process of developing independence and interdependence by affecting an adolescent's routine pursuit of social and occupational roles. Table 12–2 contrasts a typically developing adolescent with an adolescent with a disruptive behavior disorder.

## SUBSTANCE-RELATED DISORDERS

Substance disorders are an all too common problem in adolescents. Risk factors identified by the National Center on Addiction and Substance Abuse at Columbia University include poor school performance, involvement in deliquent behavior, sexual promiscuity, involvement in a peer group that uses drugs, parental abuse or tolerance of use, inadequate parental guidance, high levels of family conflict, poverty, disconnected communities, genetic predisposition, developmental disorders like ADHD and learning disabilities, and psychological disorders.

The substance-related disorders deal with disorders related to the taking of a drug of abuse. Substances are grouped into 11 classes: alcohol; amphetamine; caffeine; cannabis; cocaine; hallucinogens; inhalants; nicotine; opioids; phencyclidine (PCP); and sedatives, hypnotics, or anxiolytics. The substance-related disorders are divided into two groups: the substance use disorders, which include substance dependence and substance abuse, and the substance-induced disorders, which diagnose substance intoxication, withdrawal, delirium, dementia, and others. We will address substance use disorders in this chapter, since they are the most prevalent in adolescents.

## *Substance Abuse*

The essential feature of *substance abuse* is a maladaptive pattern of substance use, demonstrated by recurrent and significant adverse consequences related to the repeated use of substances. At least one of the four criteria listed in Box 12–8 must have occurred within a 12-month period for a diagnosis to be made.

Table 12–2 **Comparison of Social and Occupational Roles of a Typically Developing Adolescent with Those of an Adolescent with a Disruptive Behavior Disorder**

| Social and Occupational Roles | Typically Developing Adolescent | Adolescent with a Disruptive Behavior Disorder |
|---|---|---|
| Student | Exploring areas of interest and testing capabilities | Disinterest in school and learning |
| | Developing habits of self-discipline, self-control, and organization | Loss of attention, distractible Hostility and fighting with peers |
| | Experiencing success and competency | Not exploring or defining academic capabilities |
| | Defining who he or she is, including skills and abilities (identity) | Lack of adaptive habit development |
| | Answering identity question—What do I want to do in the future? | Experiencing failure resulting in feelings of inadequacy, inability and incompetency |
| | Working collaboratively in study or project groups (interdependence) | Lack of academic and occupational goals |
| Friend | Development of meaningful intimate same-sex and opposite-sex relationships that involve trust and ability to confide in others (interdependence) | Few if any friends, may have "associates," people they spend time with but with whom they have no real trust |
| | Discovery of new interests through association with others | Lack of constructive stimulation from others and |
| | Development of interpersonal skills, ability to communicate and relate to others | May be subject to destructive influences from others Lack of interpersonal skill development |
| | Development of an understanding of multiple viewpoints and individual differences | Difficulty expressing ideas and feelings Lack of regard for others No development of reciprocity |
| | Experiencing security from acceptance, support, and encouragement of others | Difficulty assuming a different perspective or recognizing the value in diversity |
| Family member | Mutual respect and support between all members of the family (interdependence) | Frequently come from families with family conflict |
| | Acceptance of responsibility for chores and adherence to rules | Lack of communication or support from others in the family |
| | Increasing freedom within limits (independence) | Little expression of feelings with the exception of anger |
| | Open communication | May be hostile and aggressive |

| | | |
|---|---|---|
| | including a willingness to confront and deal with conflict | May intentionally or unintentionally sabotage relationships |
| Worker | Development of a relationship with an employer that requires commitment and dependability<br>Assumption of responsibility<br>Development of work skills<br>Development of co-worker relationships (interdependence)<br>Increased autonomy by making his/her own money (independence)<br>Exploring the world of work, answering identity questions—To what kind of work am I attracted? (identity) | If working, is likely to do the minimum, have difficulty getting along with co-workers and may even become aggressive on the job<br>Disinterest in developing work skills<br>May lack family or community role models that value work |
| Boyfriend or girlfriend | Developing intimate trusting relationships with another person (interdependence)<br>Answering questions of identity—To what kind of person am I attracted? (identity) | May be involved in a highly dependent relationship<br>May seek a relationship to "feel loved" and "cared for" in response to unmet needs to be nurtured<br>May be in an abusive relationship, as the abuser or the abused<br>May act out aggressively via sexual relationships |
| Club or organization member | Exploring group membership, working collaboratively with others and contributing to group success<br>Learning to accept and respect differences to opinions and ideas (interdependence)<br>Developing talents and abilities (identity)<br>Testing leadership abilities (independence)<br>Interacting with adult advisers, sponsors, directors, or coaches | May reject socially acceptable groups choosing nonsocially acceptable (e.g., gang) group membership in its place<br>May acquire deviant skills from others (e.g., how to hot-wire a car, break and enter a building, shoplift) |
| Teammate | Developing talents and abilities (identity)<br>Developing relationships with others that involve | Loss of opportunities to develop skills and build camaraderie with peers in a constructive |

*continued on next page*

Table 12–2 *continued*

| Social and Occupational Roles | Typically Developing Adolescent | Adolescent with a Disruptive Behavior Disorder |
|---|---|---|
| | mutual commitment and responsibility to the entire team (interdependence) Interacting with coaches | environment with adult supervision |
| Volunteer | Developing the altruistic value of helping/serving others Exploring service occupations | No interest in serving others |

---

**Box 12–8**

Criteria for Substance Abuse

A maladative pattern of substance use, leading to clinically significant impairment or distress, as manifested by one (or more) of the following, occurring within 12-month period:

- Recurrent substance use resulting in a failure to fulfill major role obligations at work, school, or home (e.g., repeated absences or poor work performance related to substance abuse; substance related absences, suspensions, or expulsions from school)
- Recurrent substance use in situations in which it is physically hazardous (e.g., driving an automobile)
- Recurrent substance-related legal problems
- Continued substance use despite having persistent or recurrent social or interpersonal problems caused or exacerbated by the effects of the substance

Symptoms do not meet the criteria for a diagnosis of substance dependence.

---

## Substance Dependence

The essential feature of *substance dependence* is a cluster of cognitive, behavioral, and physiological symptoms indicating that the individual continues to use the substance despite significant substance-related problems. The diagnosis can apply to every class of substance listed above, with the exception of caffeine. The *DSM-IV* criteria for a diagnosis of substance dependence are provided in Box 12–9.

## Classes of Substances and Adolescent Use

Alcohol is the leading substance abused by adolescents. Depression, conduct disorder, and eating disorders often co-occur in adolescents with alcohol abuse or dependence. Alcohol abuse and alcohol dependence is 5 times greater in males than in females. Lifetime prevalence is 8 percent for alcohol dependence and 5 percent for alcohol abuse. Treatment for alcohol depen-

---

**Box 12–9**

Criteria for Substance Dependence

A maladaptive pattern of substance use, leading to clinically significant impairment or distress, as manifested by three (or more) of the following occurring at any time in the same 12-month period:

- Tolerance, as defined by either of the following:
  - A need for markedly increased amounts of the substance to achieve intoxication or the desired effect
  - Markedly diminished effect with continued use of the same amount of the substance
- Withdrawal, as manifested by either of the following:
  - The characteristic withdrawal syndrome for the substance
  - The same or closely related substance is taken to relieve or avoid withdrawal symptoms
- The substance is often taken in larger amounts or over a longer period of than was intended.
- There is a persistent desire or unsuccessful efforts to cut down or control the substance use.
- A great deal of time is spent in activities necessary to obtain the substance, use the substance, or recover from its effects.
- Important social, occupational, or recreational activities are given up or reduced because of substance use.
- The substance use is continued despite knowledge of having a persistent or recurrent physical or psychological problem that is likely to have been caused or exacerbated by the substance.

---

dence is much more effective than once thought. The results of follow-up studies of high-functioning individuals indicate a 65 percent 1-year abstinence rate following treatment, and it has been estimated that perhaps 20 percent of individuals with alcohol dependence achieve lifelong sobriety even without treatment. Alcohol dependence has a familial pattern. Twin and adoption studies have shown that at least some of the transmission can be traced to genetic factors. The risk is three to four times higher in close relatives of persons with alcohol dependence. Genetic factors, however, only account for part of the risk. A significant part of the risk comes from interpersonal and environmental factors that include cultural attitudes, exposure, and stress.

Cannabis is among the first drugs of experimentation for teenagers. Cannabis is often used in conjunction with other substances, particularly nicotine, alcohol, and cocaine. This "gateway drug" is often later mixed with opioids, phencyclidine, or other hallucinogens. Cannabis use disorders are most commonly seen in males. Studies of 12th grade students have indicated that 25 percent of them use marijuana and other drugs (The National Center on Addiction and Substance Abuse at Columbia University, 1997). The psychoactive effects of cannabis are caused by the cannabinoid, delta-9-tetrahydrocannabinol, or THC. The THC content of illicit marijuana has increased significantly since the 1960s from an average of 1 to 5 percent to as high as 10 to 15 percent, making today's marijuana much more potent and addictive.

Cocaine hydrochloride powder is usually "snorted" through the nostrils or dissolved in water and injected intravenously. A commonly used form of cocaine in the United States is "crack," a cocaine alkaloid that is extracted from powdered hydrochloride salt by mixing it with sodium bicarbonate and allowing it to dry into small "rocks." Crack is easily vaporized and inhaled and thus has an extremely rapid effect. Cocaine has very potent euphoric effects and individuals can develop dependence in a short period of time. Individuals with cocaine dependency can spend large amounts of money on the drug very quickly, and because the effects are short-lived, frequent dosing is required to maintain a "high."

Hallucinogenic substances include lysergic acid diethylamide (LSD), morning glory seeds, psilocybin (mushrooms), mescaline, and MDMA or "ecstasy." Tolerance to the euphoric and psychedelic effects of hallucinogens occurs rapidly. Because these drugs have a long half-life, individuals with hallucinogen dependence spend days using and recovering from the effects. Hallucinogenic intoxication usually first occurs during adolescence. Lifetime prevalence has been reported (1991) at 8 percent. Hallucinogen use appears to decrease with age, with the most regular use demonstrated by the 18- to 25-year-old cohort, in which 2 percent showed use within the last month.

Inhalants are often abused by adolescents. This disorder is induced by the inhaling of aliphatic and aromatic hydrocarbons found in substances like gasoline, glue, paint thinners, spray paints, or halogenated hydrocarbons found in cleaners, correction fluid, and spray can propellants, and other volatile compounds that contain esters, glycols, or ketones. The most common means of inhaling the intoxicating vapors is to apply a rag soaked with the substance to the nose and mouth, and breathe the vapors in. Breathing the vapors from a paper or plastic bag containing the substance is another common method. Substances can also be inhaled directly from the containers or aerosols can be sprayed directly into the mouth or nose. Onset is rapid. The substances reach the lungs and bloodstream within minutes. Most compounds that are inhaled are a mixture of several substances, making it difficult to determine the exact substance. For this reason the general term *inhalant* is used in most cases in recording the diagnosis. With the low cost and ready availability, inhalants are often one of the first drugs with which adolescents experiment. Inhalant use may begin as early as age 9 and generally peaks in adolescence. Younger children diagnosed with inhalant dependence use inhalants several times a week, with this use occurring most frequently on weekends and after school. Inhalants are most commonly used by adolescents in groups. Inhalant use is associated with truancy, poor grades, dropping out of school, family conflict, unemployment, and delinquency. Males account for 70 to 80 percent of the emergency room visits caused by inhalant use.

Amphetamine and amphetamine-like substances such as methamphetamine, commonly known as "speed," and substances that are structurally different but act like an amphetamine as "diet pills" do are substances that adolescents abuse and can become dependent upon. A very pure form of methamphetamine, called "ice," can be smoked like crack cocaine for an immediate stimulant effect.

Opioids, like morphine and heroin, and synthetic opioids, like codeine, methadone, and fentanyl, are abused by some adolescents. Use of opioids is rare before the later teens, as it generally takes a period of experimental and regular use of other illicit drugs, such as marijuana, PCP, and cocaine before use of opioids is begun. Individuals with opioid dependence develop such patterns of compulsive drug use that their daily life activities revolve around their drug use. Opioid dependence is associated with drug-related crime, such as possession and distribution of drugs, burglary, larceny, robbery, and receiving stolen goods. The presence of conduct disorder is considered a risk factor for all substance-related disorders, but especially for opioid dependence. There is a 3 or 4:1 male to female ratio for opioid dependence.

PCP is a frequently abused drug by adolescents. PCP or angel dust and other similarly acting substances can be taken orally, smoked, or injected intravenously. Intoxication can cause agitated, bizarre, confused psychotic and aggressively violent behavior. Conduct disorder is associated with PCP use. Prevalence appears to be 2:1 in males compared to females.

Sedatives, hypnotics, and anxiolytic substances, which comprise the benzodiazepines, carbamates, barbiturates, and barbiturate-like hypnotics, includes all prescription sleeping medications and most antianxiety medications. Very significant physiological dependence, noted by increased tolerance and withdrawal symptoms, can develop with these medications. Sedative, hypnotic, or anxiolytic dependence or abuse is often associated with dependence and abuse of other substances such as alcohol, cannabis, cocaine, heroin, and amphetamines. Sedatives are often used to counteract the undesired effects of the other substances. Accidental overdoses are common, particularly when alcohol and benzodiazepines or barbiturates and nonbarbiturates, like methaqualone, are combined. Teens use these drugs to achieve a deliberate high. These prescription medications are widely available, because 90 percent of hospitalized patients are prescribed them in conjunction with medical and surgical treatment.

## Medical Treatment
## of Substance-related Disorders

Substance-related disorders often coexist with other disorders like mood, conduct, and eating disorders. In a study of teens who committed suicide during a 2-year period, 45 percent had been abusing alcohol at the time of their deaths (Shaffer, 1995). Successful treatment of substance-related disorders in children and adolescents begins with abstinence and addresses concurrent psychopathology by treating family problems, depression, anxiety, and other disorders with psychotherapy or counseling and self-help group involvement (Mann, 1998). Substance-related disorders are often treated with psychopharmacology. The selective serotonin reuptake inhibitors (SSRIs) have found favor with physicians treating adolescents for substance-related disorders.

## Substance-related
## Disorders and Development

Substance-related disorders interfere with the developmental process of developing independence and interdependence by affecting an adolescent's routine pursuit of social and occupational roles. Table 12–3 contrasts the roles of a typically developing adolescent with an adolescent with a substance-related disorder.

Table 12–3  **Comparison of Social and Occupational Roles of a Typically Developing Adolescent with Those of an Adolescent with a Substance Abuse Disorder**

| Social and Occupational Roles | Typically Developing Adolescent | Adolescent with a Substance Abuse Disorder |
| --- | --- | --- |
| Student | Exploring areas of interest and testing capabilities<br><br>Developing habits of self-discipline, self-control, and organization<br><br>Experiencing success and competency<br><br>Defining who he/she is, including skills and abilities (identity)<br><br>Answering identity question—What do I want to do in the future?<br><br>Working collaboratively in study or project group (interdepedence) | Loss of interest in school and loss of motivation for learning<br><br>Loss of attention, distractible<br><br>Not exploring or defining academic capabilities or future interests<br><br>Lack of adaptive habit development<br><br>Experiencing failure resulting in feelings of inadequacy, inability and incompetency<br><br>May have a history of ADD or learning disabilities that have undermined confidence in ability to learn |
| Friend | Development of meaningful intimate same sex and opposite sex relationships that involve trust and ability to confide in others (interdependence)<br><br>Discovery of new interests through association with others<br><br>Development of interpersonal skills, ability to communicate and relate to others<br><br>Development of an understanding of multiple viewpoints and individual differences<br><br>Experiencing security from acceptance, support, and encouragement of others | Few if any friends, may have "associates" with whom they spend time using substances but with whom they have no real trust<br><br>Lack of constructive stimulation from others<br><br>May be subject to destructive influences from others<br><br>Lack of interpersonal skill development<br><br>May have used substances initially to overcome insecurities interacting with others especially in dating situations and never developed the skills while sober<br><br>Difficulty expressing ideas and feelings<br><br>Relationships become increasingly less important as relationship with substance(s) becomes the sole preoccupation<br><br>Relationship with a substance or substances eventually eventually replaces relationships with people |

| Family member | Mutual respect and support between all members of the family (interdependence)<br>Acceptance of responsibility for chores and adherence to rules<br>Increasing freedom within limits (independence)<br>Open communication including a willingness to confront and deal with conflict | Often a family history of substance abuse or dependence and a family system laden with conflict<br>Physical, mental, emotional, and/or sexual abuse may be present in the family<br>Parenting styles are often rigid and strict or excessively lenient<br>Lack of communication or support from the family<br>Little expression of feelings with the exception of anger |
|---|---|---|
| Worker | Development of a relationship with an employer that requires commitment and dependability<br>Assumption of responsibility<br>Development of work skills<br>Development of co-worker relationships (interdependence)<br>Increased autonomy by making his/her own money (independence)<br>Exploring the world of work, answering identity questions—To what kind of work am I attracted? (identity) | If working, is likely to do the minimum<br>May have difficulty interacting cooperatively with co-workers and may even be prone to sudden emotional outbursts<br>Disinterest in developing work skills<br>No developing sense of responsibility and contribution<br>May not have any family or community role models that value traditional work roles<br>May be involved in deviant work roles (e.g., dealing drugs) |
| Boyfriend or girlfriend | Developing intimate trusting relationships with another person (interdependence)<br>Answering questions of identity—To what kind of person am I attracted? (identity) | Is likely not to be involved in a boyfriend or girlfriend relationship unless that person is also substance-dependent<br>Preoccupation with the substance ultimately replaces any human relationship |
| Club or organization member | Exploring group membership, working collaboratively with others and contributing to group success<br>Learning to accept and respect differences of opinions and ideas (interdependence) | Disinterest in constructive, task-focused group activity |

*continued on next page*

Table 12–3 *continued*

| Social and Occupational Roles | Typically Developing Adolescent | Adolescent with a Substance Abuse Disorder |
|---|---|---|
| | Developing talents and abilities (identity) Testing leadership abilities (independence) Interacting with adult advisers, sponsors, directors, or coaches | |
| Teammate | Developing relationships with others that involve mutual commitment and responsibility to the entire team (interdependence) Developing talents and abilities (identity) Interacting with coaches | Disinterest in any activities other than abusing substances All person-person relationships are replaced by the person-substance relationship |
| Volunteer | Developing the altruistic value of helping/serving others | Concern is with self and substance No concern for others |

## ANXIETY DISORDERS

Anxiety disorders are the most common of childhood and adolescent disorders. The U.S. Department of Health and Human Services Center for Mental Health Services (1996) estimates that anxiety disorders affect 8 to 10 percent of children and adolescents. Among adolescents, more girls are affected than boys. Other mental or behavioral disorders, like major depressive disorder, often co-occur with anxiety disorders. A number of disorders are identified by the *DSM-IV* as anxiety disorders, including panic disorders, phobias, obsessive-compulsive disorder, posttraumatic stress disorder, and generalized anxiety disorders. Onset of *panic disorder* is frequently late adolescence. The essential feature of panic disorder is the presence of terrifying recurrent, unexpected panic attacks that include physical symptoms, such as rapid heartbeat, sweating, nausea, and dizziness, followed by at least a month of persistent worry about having another panic attack, worry about the possible implications or consequences of the panic attacks, or significant behavior change related to the panic attacks (e.g., going to great lengths to avoid any situation that might seem likely to bring on a panic attack). An adolescent with panic disorder may not want to go to school, date, or drive a car. The criteria for a panic attack are listed in Box 12–10.

*Specific phobias* are intense and unrealistic fears of something in particular such as animals, storms, water, heights, injections, bridges, flying, or being in an enclosed space. Specific phobias tend to peak in childhood and again in early adulthood, but they are occasionally seen in adolescents. *Social phobias* also tend to have an onset in childhood, but there have been cases of ado-

---

**Box 12–10**

Criteria for Panic Attack

A discrete period of intense fear or discomfort, in which four (or more) of the following symptoms developed abruptly and reached a peak within 10 minutes:

- Palpitations, pounding heart, or accelerated heart rate
- Sweating
- Trembling or shaking
- Sensations or shortness of breath or smothering
- Feeling of choking
- Chest pain or discomfort
- Nausea or abdominal distress
- Feeling dizzy, unsteady, lightheaded, or faint
- Derealization (feelings of unreality) or depersonalization (being detached from oneself)
- Fear of losing control or going crazy
- Fear of dying
- Paresthesias (numbness or tingling sensations)
- Chills or hot flushes

---

lescent onset. In these cases, both social and academic performances deteriorate. Common associated features of social phobias include hypersensitivity to criticism, negative evaluation, difficulty with being assertive, low self-esteem, and feelings of inferiority. Adolescents with social phobia fear evaluation by others. They are terrified of being criticized or judged harshly by others. They have poor social skills, generally have observable signs of anxiety, such as cold, clammy hands, tremors, and shaky voices. They often underachieve in school because of test anxiety and avoidance of classroom participation. They lack a social support network, often having no friends or clinging to an unfulfilling relationship. They may not date, never marry, and remain with their family of origin into adulthood.

*Obsessive-compulsive disorder* usually begins in adolescence, but it can also have a childhood onset. Onset is usually gradual. Washing, checking, counting, and ordering rituals are particularly common in children and adolescents. Schoolwork generally declines because of difficulties with concentration. Exacerbation of symptoms may be related to stress. Diagnostic criteria are listed in Box 12–11.

*Posttraumatic stress disorder* occurs in children and adolescents who have experienced severe psychologically distressing events such as physical or sexual abuse; being a victim or witness of violence; being involved in serious automobile or airplane accidents or devastating tornadoes, hurricanes, or floods. It has also been reported in children and adolescents who have emigrated to the United States from areas of considerable social unrest and civil conflict. The severity, duration, and proximity of an individual's exposure to the traumatic event are the most important determining factors as to likelihood of developing this disorder. Children and adolescents with this disorder experience the event again and again in strong memories, flashbacks, nightmares, and troublesome thoughts. They may overreact when startled or touched and have difficulty sleeping.

---

**Box 12–11**

Criteria for Obsessive-Compulsive Disorder

Presence of either obsessions or compulsions, or both
**Obsessions:**

- Recurrent and persistent thoughts, impulses, or images that are experienced, at some time during the disturbance, as intrusive and inappropriate and that cause marked anxiety or distress
- The thoughts, impulses, or images are not simply excessive worries about real-life problems
- The person attempts to ignore or suppress such thoughts, impulses, or images, or to neutralize them with some other thought or action
- The person recognizes that the obsessional thoughts, impulses, or images are a product of his or her own mind (not imposed from without as in thought insertion)

**Compulsions:**

- Repetitive behaviors (e.g., hand washing, ordering, checking) or mental acts (e.g., praying, counting, repeating words silently) that the person feels driven to perform in response to an obsession, or according to rules that must be applied rigidly
- The behaviors or mental acts are aimed at preventing or reducing distress or preventing some dreaded event or situation; however, these behaviors or mental acts either are not connected in a realistic way with what they are designed to neutralize or prevent or are clearly excessive.

At some point during the course of the disorder, the person has recognized that the obsessions or compulsions are excessive or unreasonable. The obsessions or compulsions cause marked distress, are time consuming (take more than an hour a day), or significantly interfere with the person's normal routine, occupational or academic functioning, or usual social activities or relationships.

---

With *generalized anxiety disorder*, the extreme unrealistic worries may not be related to any recent event. However, anxieties may be in relation to the quality of their performance or competence at school or in athletic events, or about punctuality. Adolescents with this disorder tend to be highly self-conscious, always tense, overly conforming, perfectionistic, and unsure of themselves. They often redo tasks because of excessive discontent with any performance that is less than perfect. They are typically overzealous in seeking approval from others and they require an inordinate amount of reassurance that their performance is satisfactory and that their worries are unfounded or unnecessary. Stomachaches and other physical discomforts are frequent complaints. Anxiety as a trait has a familial pattern.

## Medical Treatment of Anxiety Disorders

Hodgman (1996) states that the psychopharmacologic treatment of anxiety often involves the element of suggestion, implying that the effectiveness of antihistamines may be as much in their placebo effect as in their sedation effect. Diphenhydramine (Benadryl) and hydroxyzine (Vistaril) are the most commonly prescribed antihistamines for this purpose. Benzodiazepines are anxiolytic, but they run the risk of abuse so they are used with caution for short periods of time in only the most responsible adolescent patients. Buspirone (Buspar), a relatively new anxiolytic, has been reported to cause less sedation, to not interfere with cognitive functioning, and to have a reduced potential for causing physiological dependence. Conclusive studies have indicated that buspirone is effective for treatment of adults with anxiety, but there have not been any controlled trials with children or adolescents as of yet (Carrey et al., 1996). Nevertheless physicians rarely wait to treat adolescents until conclusive studies are conducted; they generally begin treatment with reduced dosages. Phenothiazines and other major tranquilizers have no abusive value and are safe in overdose, so they may be used in less-reliable patients. Tricyclic and SSRI antidepressants are also often used in the treatment of anxiety disorders. Clomipramine, a tricyclic antidepressant, and the SSRIs have been found to be especially effective in the treatment of obsessive-compulsive disorder.

## *Anxiety Disorders and Development*

Anxiety disorders interfere with the developmental process of developing independence and interdependence by affecting an adolescent's routine pursuit of social and occupational roles. Table 12–4 contrast a typically developing adolescent with an adolescent with an anxiety disorder.

## EATING DISORDERS

The symptom that characterizes eating disorders is a severe disturbance in eating behavior. A disturbance in perception of body weight and shape is also a feature of both anorexia and bulimia. A study in the Journal of Abnormal Psychology (Lowe et al., 1996) found that distant, critical fathers who avoid closeness and criticize their daughters' weight may be agents in their daughters' eating disorders. Eating disorders are believed to involve biological, social, individual, and familial factors. Eating disorders can be life-threatening. Anorexia nervosa is characterized by a refusal to maintain a minimally normal body weight, and bulimia nervosa is characterized by repeated episodes of binge eating followed by inappropriate purging behaviors, such as self-induced vomiting, laxative misuse, or diuretic or enema use. Persons with bulimia nervosa also fast and exercise excessively.

**Anorexia Nervosa.**  The essential features of *anorexia nervosa* are the refusal to maintain a minimal body weight, an intense fear of gaining weight, and a significant perceptual distortion regarding the shape and size of one's body. Anorexia rarely develops before puberty. Postmenarcheal females with this disorder are amenorrheic. More than 90 percent of the cases of anorexia nervosa are in females, and the U.S. Department of Health and Human Services reports that anorexia nervosa affects 1 in every 10 to 20 adolescent girls. The disorder is far more prevalent in industrialized societies where there is an abundance of food and thinness is equated with attractiveness in females.

Table 12–4 **Comparison of Social and Occupational Roles of a Typically Developing Adolescent with Those of an Adolescent with an Anxiety Disorder**

| Social and Occupational Roles | Typically Developing Adolescent | Adolescent with an Anxiety Disorder |
|---|---|---|
| Student | Exploring areas of interest and testing capabilities | Performance anxiety results in a loss of capacity to perform and thus with decreased satisfaction with school and learning |
| | Developing habits of self-discipline, self-control, and organization | |
| | Experiencing success and competency | |
| | Defining who he or she is, including skills and abilities (identity) | Anxiety interferes with attention |
| | Answering identity questions—What do I want to do in the future? | Lack of successful opportunities to explore capabilities and develop a sense of competency |
| | Working collaboratively in study or project groups (interdependence) | Lack of adaptive habit development |
| | | Experiencing academic failure resulting in feelings of inadequacy, inability and incompetency |
| Friend | Development of meaningful intimate same sex and opposite sex relationships that involve trust and ability to confide in others (interdependence) | Anxiety interferes with the initiation and maintenance of friendships |
| | | Limited number of friends, if any |
| | Discovery of new interests through association with others | Lack of interpersonal skill development |
| | Development of interpersonal skills, ability to communicate and relate to others | Difficulty communicating ideas and feelings to others |
| | Development of an understanding of multiple viewpoints and individual differences | Development of feelings of inadequacy in relationships |
| | Experiencing security from acceptance, support, and encouragement of others | Self-devaluation |
| | | Isolation |
| Family member | Mutual respect and support between all members of the family (interdependence) | Often come from families with history of anxiety disorders |
| | Acceptance of responsibility for chores and adherence to rules | May be criticized, belittled or embarrassed by family members |
| | | May be compared to |

| | | |
|---|---|---|
| | Increasing freedom with limits (independence) Open communication including a willingness to confront and deal with conflict | more competent siblings Family communication is generally poor Around family and home may be the only environment where the adolescent feels safe (dependent) |
| Worker | Development of a relationship with an employer that requires commitment and dependability Assumption of responsibility Development of work skills Development of coworker relationships (interdependence) Increased autonomy by making his/her own money (independence) Exploring the world of work, answering identity questions—To what kind of work am I attracted? (identity) | Likely not to be working but, if working, may be a perfectionist and a "worrier" that strains relationships with co-workers and employer. May be fired, resulting in further feelings of failure and inadequacy |
| Boyfriend or girlfriend | Developing intimate trusting relationships with another person (interdependence) Answering questions of identity—To what kind of person am I attracted? (identity) | Is likely not to be involved in a close dating relationship but if attemping to date, their anxiety symptoms will often drive others away |
| Club or organization member | Exploring group membership, working collaboratively with others and contributing to group success Learning to accept and respect differences of opinions and ideas (interdependence) Developing talents and abilities (identity) Testing leadership abilities (independence) Interacting with adult advisers, sponsors, directors, or coaches | Anxiety will generally prevent pursuit of group activities but if he or she does belong to a club or organization their perfectionism and rigidity will interfere with group relations |

*continued on next page*

Table 12–4 *continued*

| Social and Occupational Roles | Typically Developing Adolescent | Adolescent with an Anxiety Disorder |
|---|---|---|
| Teammate | Developing talents and abilities (identity) | |
| | Developing relationships with others that involve mutual commitment and responsibility to the entire team (interdependence) Interacting with coaches | If involved, performance is paramount, worry and performance anxiety will limit success and excessive self-criticism is likely to follow |
| Volunteer | Developing the altruistic value of helping/serving others Exploring service occupations | Unlikely to be involved but if involved, the experience is upsetting and anxiety provoking |

The onset of illness is often associated with a stressful life event. Mortality from anorexia nervosa is over 10 percent. When seriously underweight, the individual with anorexia nervosa may show a depressed mood, social withdrawal, irritability, insomnia, and diminished interest in sex. There may be problems with constipation, abdominal pain, cold intolerance, lethargy, and excess energy. They may have hypotension, bradycardia, peripheral edema, and hypertrophied salivary glands. They may meet the criteria for major depressive disorder, but the *DSM-IV* warns that these symptoms are consistent with persons experiencing semistarvation. Most persons with anorexia nervosa are preoccupied with thoughts of food. Some collect recipes or hoard food. The obsessions are likely also to be caused by malnutrition. Feelings of ineffectiveness, a strong need to control one's environment, inflexible thinking, limited social spontaneity, and overly restrained initiative and emotional expression are all associated with this disorder.

**Bulimia nervosa.**   The essential features of *bulimia nervosa* are binge eating, an inappropriate compensatory method to prevent weight gain at least twice weekly for a period of at least 3 months. A binge involves eating, within a discrete period of time, usually less than 2 hours, an amount of food that is greater than would normally be consumed in that time. Individuals with bulimia nervosa are generally ashamed of their eating disorder and attempt to hide their symptoms from others. Binges are usually done in secrecy or very inconspicuously. Binge eating is often triggered by a dysphoric mood, interpersonal stressors, intense hunger following dietary constraint, or in response to feelings about body weight or body shape. Binging usually continues until the person is painfully full. Binging may temporarily decrease the dysphoria, but once the binge is completed, extreme self-criticism contributes to the return of the depressed mood state. Binge eating is typically accompanied by a sense of loss of control. Of persons with bulimia nervosa, 80 to 90 percent use self-induced vomiting to prevent weight gain from their binges. Approximately a third misuse laxatives and diuretics to prevent weight gain. Some individuals with this disorder will use excessive exercise to control their weight. Excessive exercise either significantly interferes with important activities, occurs at inappropriate times or in inappropriate settings, or occurs despite injury or medical contraindications. At least 90 percent of persons with bulimia nervosa are female. Prior to onset, persons with this disorder tend to be slightly overweight. There is an increased incidence of major depressive disorder, dysthymia, anxiety disorders, and substance abuse or dependence, particularly involving alcohol and stimulants. Between one-third and one-half of persons with eating disorders meet the criteria for at least one personality disorder, most frequently borderline personality, which will be discussed next. Individuals with bulimia nervosa place excessive emphasis on body shape and weight in their self-evaluations. Their dissatisfaction with their bodies results in low self-esteem. Frequent vomiting results in loss of tooth enamel, dental caries, and enlarged salivary glands, particularly the parotid gland. Fluid and electrolyte imbalances are sometimes so severe that they create medical problems. Cardiac arrhythmias are also a potentially serious problem. The prevalence of bulimia nervosa among adolescent and young adult females is reported at 1 to 3 percent.

## *Medical Treatment of Adolescents with Eating Disorders*

The SSRIs have been used effectively in the treatment of eating disorders. There is often a concomitant mood or substance-related disorder in adolescents with eating disorders. Like all of the other orders discussed thus far, treatment is generally a combination of psychopharmacology and psychotherapy. Family therapy is also an important part of the treatment plan.

## *Eating Disorders and Development Disorder*

Eating disorders interfere with the developmental process of developing independence and interdependence by affecting an adolescent's routine pursuit of social and occupational roles. Table 12–5 contrasts a typically developing adolescent with an adolescent with a eating disorder.

## BORDERLINE PERSONALITY DISORDER

*Borderline personality,* is one of the 10 personality disorders presented in Axis II. A personality disorder is an enduring pattern of inner experience and behavior that deviates markedly from the expectations of the individual's culture, is pervasive and inflexible, has an adolescent or early-adulthood onset, is stable over time, and leads to distress or impairment. Borderline personality is included in Cluster B, which also includes the antisocial, histrionic, and narcissistic personality disorders. For the purposes of this chapter, borderline personality disorder will be the only personality disorder discussed. This is because it is frequently apparent in adolescents receiving psychosocial treatment and therapists should be familiar with the disorder and its treatment. Persons with any of these disorders often appear excessively dramatic, emotional, or erratic. In borderline personality disorder there is a pattern of instability in interpersonal relationships, self-image, and affects. There is also

## Table 12–5 Comparison of Social and Occupational Roles of a Typically Developing Adolescent with Those of an Adolescent with an Eating Disorder

| Social and Occupational Roles | Typically Developing Adolescent | Adolescent with an Eating Disorder |
| --- | --- | --- |
| Student | Exploring areas of interest and testing capabilities<br>Developing habits of self-discipline, self-control, and organization<br>Experiencing success and competency<br>Defining who he or she is, including skills and abilities (identity)<br>Answering identity question—What do I want to do in the future?<br>Working collaboratively in study or project groups (interdependence) | Often a perfectionist<br>Even if a good student generally highly self-critical and discontented with his or her performance<br>Set unrealistic expectations for themselves |
| Friend | Development of meaningful intimate same sex and opposite sex relationships that involve trust and ability to confide in others (interdependence)<br>Discovery of new interests through association with others<br>Development of interpersonal skills, ability to communicate and relate to others<br>Development of an understanding of multiple viewpoints and individual differences<br>Experiencing security from acceptance, support, and encouragement of others | Few, if any friends<br>May have one close friend who is mutually dependent and may also have an eating disorder<br>Difficulty trusting others<br>Lack of interpersonal skill development<br>Difficulty expressing ideas and feelings |
| Family member | Mutual respect and support between all members of the family (interdependence)<br>Acceptance of responsibility for chores and adherence to rules<br>Increasing freedom within limits (independence)<br>Open communication including a willingness to confront and deal with conflict | Often enmeshed with family<br>Often come from families with a distant, critical father<br>Lack of communication in the family<br>Little expression of feelings |

| Worker | Development of a relationship with an employer that requires commitment and dependability<br>Assumption of responsibility<br>Development of work skills<br>Development of co-worker relationships (interdependence)<br>Increased autonomy by making his/her own money (independence)<br>Exploring the world of work, answering identity questions—To what kind of work am I attracted? (identity) | More than likely not working but if working, may work in food preparation (e.g., cake decoration) |
|---|---|---|
| Boyfriend or girlfriend | Developing intimate trusting relationships with another person (interdependence)<br>Answering questions of identity—To what kind of person am I attracted? (identity) | Generally disinterested in dating<br>Self-criticism, devaluation, and feeling unworthy to engage in a relationship |
| Club or organization member | Exploring group membership, working collaboratively with others and contributing to group success<br>Learning to accept and respect differences of opinions and ideas (interpendence)<br>Developing talents and abilities (identity)<br>Testing leadership abilities (independence)<br>Interacting with adult advisers, sponsors, directors, or coaches | May belong to a group like a sorority or a ballet troupe with focus exclusively on the task<br>Generally a follower rather than a leader |
| Teammate | Developing talents and abilities (identity)<br>Developing relationships with others that involve mutual commitment and responsibility to the entire team (interdependence)<br>Interacting with coaches | May be on a team (i.e., gymnastics) but preoccupation with food and weight keeps the focus on themselves as opposed to the team<br>May be highly competitive |
| Volunteer | Developing the altruistic value of helping/serving others<br>Exploring service occupations | Unlikely to be involved, but if required will focus on the task and devalue contribution |

---

**Box 12–12**

Criteria for Borderline Personality Disorder

A pervasive pattern of instability of interpersonal relationships, self-image, and affect, and marked impulsivity beginning by early adulthood and present in a variety of contexts, as indicated by five (or more) of the following:

- Frantic efforts to avoid real or imagined abandonment
- A pattern of unstable and intense interpersonal relationships characterized by alternating between extremes of idealization and devaluation
- Identity disturbance: markedly and persistently unstable self-image or sense of self
- Impulsivity in at least two areas that are potentially self-damaging (e.g., spending, sex, substance abuse, reckless driving, binge eating)
- Recurrent suicidal behavior, gestures, or threats, or self-mutilating behavior
- Affective instability due to a marked reactivity of mood
- Chronic feelings of emptiness
- Inappropriate, intense anger or difficulty controlling anger
- Transient, stress related paranoid ideation or severe dissociative symptoms

---

marked impulsivity that manifests in a variety of contexts. The diagnostic criteria are listed in Box 12–12.

Persons with borderline personality disorder are extremely sensitive to environmental circumstances. They experience intense fears of abandonment and inappropriate anger when faced with realistic time-limited separation or an unavoidable change in plans. They have an intense intolerance of being alone and an insatiable chronic need to have other people around them. Their self-mutilating and suicidal behaviors are frantic behaviors to prevent others from leaving them alone. Persons with borderline personality disorder are prone to very sudden and dramatic shifts in their view of others. This is often problematic in the therapy process, because their view often shifts from idealizing the therapist as supportive and nurturing to viewing him or her as cruel and punitive. The unstable self-image results in sudden and dramatic shifts in life goals, values, career goals, occupational plans, sexual identity, or choice of friends. Although they may perform well in structured work or school tasks, performance deteriorates dramatically in unstructured situations. Their basic mood is generally dysphoric, which is interrupted by episodes of bitterness, anger, or panic. They often feel empty and rarely experience feelings of well-being or satisfaction. They may have a pattern of undermining themselves on the brink of fulfilling a goal. Mood disorders, substance-related disorders, eating disorders, posttraumatic stress disorder, and other personality disorders often co-occur with borderline personality disorder. This disorder is diagnosed 75 percent of the time in females. Estimates of prevalence is 2 percent in the general population, 10 percent of outpatient mental health clinics and 20 percent of hospitalized psychiatric inpatients. As with mood and substance-related disorders, there is increased familial risk for borderline personality disorder. It is about five times more common among first-degree biological relatives than in the general population.

## Medical Treatment
## of Borderline Personality Disorder

This disorder is rarely observed without concomitant diagnoses. Most commonly those diagnoses are a mood disorder or a substance-abuse disorder. Therefore, the physician prescribes psychopharmacological treatment for those disorders.

## Borderline Personality
## Disorder and Development

Personality disorders interfere with the developmental process of developing independence and interdependence by affecting an adolescent's routine pursuit of social and occupational roles. Table 12–6 contrasts a typically developing adolescent with an adolescent with a borderline personality disorder.

# EVALUATION

Adolescents being treated for the disorders that have been described in this chapter are most frequently seen by OTs working in a hospital, residential treatment center, juvenile correction facility, or day treatment setting. Those who have worked with these groups of young people know that many of the problems addressed in treatment remain as issues for adolescents once they leave the treatment facility and re-enter the school system. A review of the literature, however, indicates that school system therapists have not been providing services to this group. Dr. Sally Schultz, in her 1997 AOTA Institute entitled "Treating Students with Behavioral Disorders: Occupational Adaptation Model" reported that she had initially obtained grant funding and later received funding from the school system to provide occupational therapy services to children with behavioral disorders because these students were not being served by the therapists working in the schools (Schultz, 1997). Hopefully, this will change as OTs realize that occupational therapy in the school system can be expanded to serve the needs of children and adolescents with a variety of psychosocial as well as physical disability disorders.

For the purposes of the remainder of this discussion, the focus will be on OTs' contributions in the more traditional settings. OTs in these settings will generally contribute to the adolescent's treatment as a member of the treatment team. The treatment team might include a psychiatrist, a psychologist, a social worker, a nurse, a recreational therapist, a rehabilitation or substance abuse counselor, and a variety of unit staff such as mental health workers or residential or cottage staff persons. A teacher or educational specialist is generally also a part of the team. A caseworker may also be a member. This collection of team members will each bring to the team a unique professional perspective. OTs generally operate on the basis of referrals and will not be the first professionals to evaluate the client. Therefore, it is important that the OT consult the adolescent's chart prior to initiating the evaluation so that data gathering is not unnecessarily repeated. A thorough chart review will involve

Table 12–6   **Comparison of Social and Occupational Roles of a Typically Developing Adolescent with Those of an Adolescent with a Borderline Personality Disorder**

| Social and Occupational Roles | Typically Developing Adolescent | Adolescent with a Borderline Personality Disorder |
|---|---|---|
| Student | Exploring areas of interest and testing capabilities<br>Developing habits of self-discipline, self-control, and organization<br>Experiencing success and competency<br>Defining who he or she is, including skills and abilities (identity)<br>Answering identity question—What do I want to do in the future (identity)<br>Working collaboratively in study or project group (interdependence) | Performance is erratic<br>May be quite capable of performing and still perform poorly<br>Peer relationships are often confictual, may result in hostility and fighting<br>Loss of attention, distractible<br>Not exploring or defining capabilities<br>Lack of adaptive habit development<br>Experiences of failure result in feelings of inadequacy, inability, and incompetency |
| Friend | Development of meaningful intimate same-sex and opposite-sex relationships that involve trust and ability to confide in others (interdependence)<br>Discovery of new interests through association with others<br>Development of interpersonal skills, ability to communicate and relate to others<br>Development of an understanding of multiple viewpoints and individual differences<br>Experiencing security from acceptance, support, and encouragement of others | Few if any friends<br>Relationships are highly unstable<br>People are labeled either good or bad<br>Lack an understanding of "gray" areas, that people can be both good and bad<br>Difficulty with intimacy because of lack of ability to share and to trust another person<br>Lack of interpersonal skill development<br>Highly volatile emotions<br>Self-focused and self-centered<br>Lack of regard for the needs and feelings of others<br>Unforgiving |
| Family Member | Mutual respect and support between all members of the family (interdependence)<br>Acceptance of responsibility for chores and adherence to rules<br>Increasing freedom within limits (independence)<br>Open communication | Often come from families with intense family conflict<br>May have experienced severe neglect<br>Lack of communication within the family system<br>Little expression of feelings with the exception of anger<br>Unresolved anger over feelings of abandonment |

|  | including a willingness to confront and deal with conflict | as a child limits relationship with the family |
|---|---|---|
| Worker | Development of a relationship with an employer that requires commitment and dependability<br>Assumption of responsibility<br>Development of work skills<br>Development of co-worker relationships (interdependence)<br>Increased autonomy by making his/her own money (independence)<br>Exploring the world of work, answering identity questions—To what kind of work am I attracted? (identity) | If working, is likely to have difficulty getting along with coworkers and may even become abusive or aggressive on the job |
| Boyfriend or girlfriend | Developing intimate trusting relationships with another person (interdependence)<br>Answering questions of identity—To what kind of person am I attracted? (identity) | May be involved in a highly volatile dating relationship<br>May seek a relationship to "feel loved" and "cared for" in response to unmet needs to be nurtured<br>May be involved in homosexual and/or heterosexual relationship |
| Club or organization member | Exploring group membership, working collaboratively with others and contributing to group success<br>Learning to accept and respect differences of opinions and ideas (interdependence)<br>Developing talents and abilities (identity)<br>Testing leadership abilities (independence)<br>Interacting with adult advisors, sponsors, directors, or coaches | If a member of a club or organization may create tension between other members<br>May attempt to sabotage individuals |
| Teammate | Developing talents and abilities (identity)<br>Developing relationships with others that involve mutual commitment and responsibility to the entire team (interdependence)<br>Interaction with coaches | If a member of a team, which is unlikely, may create tension between teammates by turning one against the other |

*continued on next page*

Table 12–6 *continued*

| Social and Occupational Roles | Typically Developing Adolescent | Adolescent with a Borderline Personality Disorder |
|---|---|---|
| Volunteer | Developing the altruistic value of helping/serving others<br>Exploring service occupations | Unlikely to participate in volunteering because own needs are sole concern |

reviewing the admitting physician's admission note, the history and physical, the nursing evaluation, the prescribed medications, and any initial progress notes that might be recorded. School and family histories are also sources of valuable information, if they have been completed. If psychological testing or educational testing has been done, this information can be helpful as well. In some cases, the adolescent may have been treated previously, in which case it is helpful to consult previous psychological, social, and educational reports. In some facilities prior chart records are added to the new chart, generally at the back of the chart. In other facilities the records from previous admissions are kept separate but made available. Adolescents in residential treatment or in correctional facilities will often have lengthy charts that should be scanned for changes in the adolescent's behavior and treatment over time. It is important for therapists to formulate a preliminary picture, but not to begin making assumptions based upon the observations and reporting of others. OTs often obtain information that "sheds new light" on prior reports. Being familiar with the client's history is very helpful in assuring that clients remain truthful and not fabricate or manipulate their stories to make them more "palatable" when they are interviewed. If the adolescent's story deviates in some significant way from what has been reported in their chart or record, the discrepancy can be confronted as it occurs. Lack of preparation can result in naively being deceived by the manipulating adolescent who prides himself or herself in an ability to "pull the wool over" the eyes of adults!

With this preliminary information gathered, the OT begins to generate questions in regard to the client. OTs have several frames of reference or models to use to help guide their thinking and assessment process. There are, however, several universal questions that therapists, regardless of theoretical orientation, ask, such as:

- How do they routinely spend their time?
- What do they like to do?
- How well do they feel that they are able to do the things they routinely do?
- When did they start to feel or act differently?
- What were they like before that time?
- What kind of family and friendship support do they have?
- How satisfied are they with their life?
- Do they want to make changes in their life? If so, what kind?

- Are they ready to make changes? To what extent is their current psychiatric condition interfering with their ability to initiate changes.

These questions are guided by core beliefs of occupational therapy that people are active beings who find meaning and life significance through engagement in occupation that is intrinsically motivated. Through this process of engaging in occupation people are able to influence their physical and mental health and their physical and social environment. Human life involves a process of ongoing biological, psychological, and environmental adaptation.

To gain an understanding of someone's current level of occupational functioning, a therapist must understand how his or her adaptation process has been impaired. Adolescents are often distrusting of adults, even young adults, especially if the adult projects an impression of self-righteousness or a "know-it-all" attitude. The experienced therapist knows the importance of establishing rapport and a basic level of trust from the outset of the therapist-client relationship. This is best accomplished in a private one-on-one interview session. Although there are a number of appropriate assessment instruments, nothing is as effective as a good interview that involves using yourself as the primary instrument and therapeutic use of self throughout the interview. Some young people are difficult to reach, especially those whose problems are a result of years of pain and suffering, but consistent, sincere caring; patience; and a genuine desire to help them help themselves can go a long way to softening even the most hardened defenses.

Preface your interview by letting the adolescent know that you have reviewed his or her chart and that you are interested in learning more about his or her everyday life. As stated previously, having a basic familiarity with the person's condition, by having read the chart first, prevents the client from withholding key information and allows the therapist to question contradictions or confront obvious inconsistencies, if they arise during the interview.

The *Occupational Performance History Interview (OPHI)*, developed by Gary Kielhofner, Alexis Henry, and Deborah Walens with a grant from the American Occupational Therapy Association, provides therapists with a standardized interview procedure with established reliability and validity (Kielhofner, Henry, & Walens, 1989). This instrument assesses content in five areas: organization of daily living routines; life roles; interests, values, and goals; perceptions of control and ability; and environmental influences. This interview does not specify each question to be asked. Instead this instrument provides "yields" or information that you want to come away from the interview knowing. The *OPHI* recommends some questions that might be asked to arrive at the yields, but the therapist is free to obtain the information by asking any relevant questions that will result in the yields. Preparation by the therapist is required prior to administering this interview. Therapists should review the yields, recommended questions, and generate questions that may be specific to the client. Sample interview questions based on this instrument are listed in Box 12–13.

By the end of the interview, the therapist should have a well-formed clinical picture of the adolescent's current and previous level of occupational functioning. As a result of gathering a collection of small pieces of informa-

**Box 12–13**

Possible Questions for an Adolescent Interview Based upon the Occupational Performance History Interview

### Organization of Daily Living Routines

**Daily**
I'd like to know about how you routinely spend your time. Let's start with a school day. Can you tell me about what a typical school day is like for you from the time you get up in the morning? (*Do they have a morning hygiene routine? Do they eat breakfast? Do they go to school most days? What structure does the school day have? Is it the same everyday or do they have block scheduling?*)
What do you do at the end of the school day? Do you generally go home or go somewhere else after school? (*If they go somewhere else, where do they usually spend their afternoons? How long do they stay and who is with them?*)
What time do you generally get home? Who else is usually home at that time?
How do you spend most of your evenings? Do you usually eat dinner at home? Does your family eat dinner together? What do you do after dinner? (*If they are not at home most evenings, when do they generally come home on school nights?*)
What time do you generally go to bed on school nights?
Do you have any assigned responsibilities or chores to do at home? What are they? Do they have to be reminded to do them, or do you do them without being reminded?
Do you ever need to be reminded to take a bath/shower, or to brush your teeth, or do you generally do those daily hygiene activities without reminders?

**Weekly**
How do you spend your time on weekends? What is a typical weekend like for you? Does it vary depending upon the time of year?
Do you generally have a plan for what you intend to do most weekends or do you just let things sort of happen?
Do you have the transportation to get to the places where you want to go on weekends?

**Monthly/Seasonally**
Do you have any activities that you don't do every week but that you do every few weeks or monthly?
Are there activities that you do only in certain seasons? What are they?
How do you spend your time when you are out of school for the summer?

**Adaptability**
How do you handle changes in your routine? Does it bother you when things don't run on schedule or go as planned?

*After having the "big picture" explore each of the social and occupational roles that surfaced during the questioning on daily routines. Discussion of life roles will reveal information about interests, values, goals, perception of abilities and assumption of responsibility.*

### Life Roles

**Student**
Tell me a little more about school. What grade are you in? What do you like about school? Do you have any favorite subjects?

How well do you get along with your teachers? Have you ever had a favorite teacher or a teacher that you particularly admired or were inspired by? What made him/her special to you?

What do you dislike about school? Is there a subject or are there certain subjects that are more difficult for you or that have caused you particular problems?

How well do you do in school? How important is doing well in school to you?

Are you satisfied with your grades? Do you think that you could do better in school than you are doing presently? How? Do you usually follow your teacher's suggestions on how to improve?

In most cases, do you feel that your teachers' and parents' expectations of you, as a student, are fair and reasonable?

Do you have homework most nights? Do you have a regular time and routine for doing your homework? Do you have friends or people in your family who help you with your homework when you need them?

## Worker

Do you work or have you worked before? What jobs have you had in the past?

Do you like working? Why or why not?

Do you consider yourself a "good employee?" Why or why not?

What kind of work habits have you had to develop to meet the expectations of your employer?

When you think about the future, what kind of work do you see yourself doing someday?

What interests you about being a (job title of desired future work)?

Do you know what kind of education and/or training is necessary to be a (job title)?

What skills do you have that are important for a (job title) to possess?

What makes you think that you would make a good (job title)? Have you ever had any experience with (associated task)?

## Family Member

Who do you live with? [*Mother, father, brother(s), sister(s), extended relative(s)*]?

Are other members of your family, like older siblings or half-brothers or half-sisters, that don't live with you? Where do they live?

Do you enjoy spending time with your family? Do you routinely do things together as a family?

What is your favorite thing to do with them?

How well do you get along with _____ (*take each family member separately*)?

Do you feel comfortable expressing your feelings directly to your fellow family members?

How do members of your family handle conflict that arises between them?

When we talked about your normal routine you said that you have (or don't have) certain responsibilities or chores to do at home. What other kinds of expectations does your family place on you? Has your family set any rules that they expect you to follow? Do you think these expectations are fair?

Do you generally meet the family's expectations of you? What happens when you break one of those rules?

How do you get money to spend? How do you spend the money you get?

Do you buy your own clothes? Are you able to dress the way that you would like?

Do you save any money? Are you saving your money for anything in particular?

**Player, hobbyist, team member, organization participant.**
Let's talk about some of the things that you like to do for fun.
Are you now or have you ever been a part of any group, club, or athletic team?
Do you enjoy being part of a group or team?
What are activities that you enjoy doing in the community? (*i.e., parks, library, video arcade, putt-putt, bowling alley, roller/ice skating, sporting events, museums*)
Are there special activities that you enjoy doing every once in a while?
Are there other activities that you would like to do, if you could? What else would you like to be able to do? What prevents you from doing those things?

**Friend**
What kinds of things do you like to do with your friends? How do you spend your time together when you are with your friends?
Do you have any close friends or a best friend? How long have you all been good friends? What makes (*name*) special as a friend?
Do you trust your friends enough to confide your feelings to them?
Do you consider yourself a "good friend"? What do you think that your friends like about you?
What do your friends expect from you as their "friend"?
When there are no friends around, how do you spend your time alone?

**Boyfriend/Girlfriend**
Do you have a regular boyfriend/girlfriend? How long have you been involved in the relationship?
Do you consider yourself a good "boyfriend/girlfriend"? Why or why not?
What does it mean to you to be a "boyfriend/girlfriend"?
How important is this relationship to you?

**Adaptability**
What do you do when things don't work out the way you would like? What is the biggest disappointment that you have had to deal with so far? How did you handle it?

**Environmental Influences**

Where do you live? Do you live in a house, apartment, trailer? How do you like where you live?
Do you have your own room?
Are you satisfied with your home? School? Neighborhood/Community? (*Listen for satisfaction with both the physical/spatial (non-human) and social (human) environments*)
What are your most prized possessions? What did you ask for during the last holiday that you received gifts (Christmas, Hanukah, birthday)?
Do you have the supplies, equipment and financial resources you need to pursue the activities that interest you?
To whom do you turn when you need support, advice, understanding and/or encouragement? (*May have been revealed in roles discussion.*)

**Closure**

You've told me about your capabilities in _____, _____, _____ and _____ and your difficulties with _____, _____, _____ and _____. Is there anything else

that we haven't discussed that you think might help me to know you better? Is there anything more that you would like to tell me about yourself?
Is there anything else in your life that we haven't discussed that is causing problems?
Overall, are you generally content and satisfied with your life or are there things about your life that you would like to be different, that you have some ability to change? What would you like to be different about your life?
If your future could be whatever you wanted it to be, what would you want for your life five or ten years from now? Do you ever dream about that happening?
It sounds like .......... (*draw some conclusions and send up a "trial balloon" to test it out*)
Attempt to move right into joint treatment planning, allowing the adolescent to guide the process as much as possible. What are they willing to do in order to make their lives more meaningful and satisfying to them?

tion about this individual, the resulting mosaic should reveal whether the adolescent has:

- A balance of work (school, job, household chores) play, and self-care activities (performance areas)
- Well-developed, organized, and adaptable routines and habits
- Satisfying social and occupational life roles and a balanced pattern of role involvement
- The necessary skills (performance components) to perform the occupational tasks of his or her life roles
- A range of interests that are socially appropriate and age appropriate
- A sense of competency and confidence in his or her capabilities to perform in his or her life roles
- A sense of effectiveness
- A sense of enjoyment, satisfaction, and meaning in the occupation of his or her life
- Anticipation of future success
- Realistic expectations of himself or herself in his or her various roles
- Goals that are guided by interest and competence
- Any experience with the occupational choice process
- A good person-environment fit (a match between the demands and expectations of the environment and the individual's capabilities)
- The necessary physical and social support of the environment to perform his or her life roles
- A sense of responsibility
- A sense of independence
- A sense of interdependence

Some of the information that is gathered by the *OPHI* can be compiled in other ways. *The Role Checklist* (Oakley, Kielhofner, Barris, & Reichler, 1986) can be used as a means of having the adolescent begin to identity his or her various life roles and the extent to which he or she values those roles. The *Interest Checklist* (Matsutsuyu, 1969) can be used for the identification of interests using recognition skills rather than relying on recall. The *Occupational Question-*

*naire,* which was developed by Riopel in 1981, has the respondents record their daily activities in half-hour increments and then rate each of the activities in which they engage as a work, rest, play, or self-care activity. The respondents also record their feelings of competency performing each of their daily activities and assign a value of importance to each activity. Certainly all of the information these instruments are designed to collect contribute to the assessment. Self-report instruments, however, are only as good as the information that the respondent is willing to report. Some adolescents may be accurate self-reporters, but many will not be. My experience with attempts to use self-report instruments with adolescents has been that generally the information is very sketchy and always requires extensive follow-up questioning. If self-report instruments are used, they should definitely be reviewed with the client to ensure thoroughness and accuracy of responses and to ensure that any interpretation by the therapist is correct. If self-report instruments are used, the interview can proceed naturally from the discussion of responses on the instruments, being absolutely sure to cover any interview questions that were not fully addressed on the self-report instruments. At the conclusion of the interview, a therapist using the Model of Human Occupation may want to use the *Self-Assessment of Occupational Functioning—Children's Version* (Curtain & Baron, 1990) to enlist the adolescent's participation in a joint treatment planning process. The children's version of this instrument uses language that is simpler and less intimidating to an adolescent than that used in the adult version. The adolescent client may not recognize the need for change or may not be interested in working in treatment. Collaborating with the client from the start will help therapists recognize the adolescent's attitude in regard to therapy and will help the therapist to set realistic goals.

Like information provided on other self-report instruments, an adolescent's self-assessment of his or her capabilities is not always accurate. Adolescents may overevaluate or underevaluate themselves. They might grossly undervalue their abilities, viewing themselves as incapable and ineffective when indeed they have skills that they refuse to recognize or they describe themselves as extremely capable and competent when in truth they are severely lacking in skills. For this reason, it is always valuable to assess task skills and interpersonal skills by observation of performance in addition to self-report. The ability to process and follow oral instructions and written directions, to use tools properly, cooperate, share materials, and engage in conversation with peers can easily be observed in a task group. This can be done informally or the *Comprehensive Occupational Therapy Evaluation (COTE)* Scale (Brayman & Kirby, 1982) can be used for this purpose. The *Assessment of Communication and Interaction Skills (ACIS)* (Salamy, Simon & Kielhofner, 1993) requires observation of individuals acting within social groups. Since communication and interaction skills are often negatively affected by psychosocial disorders, this instrument could be useful provided there is sufficient time for making several observations in several different settings.

If the adolescent's processing skills are in question, or if disposition is an issue with the adolescent, OTs who have been trained and calibrated the *Assessment of Motor and Process Skills (AMPS)* (Fischer, 1994) may wish to administer this instrument. It is important to note that this tool requires that the therapist be trained before it can be used. The *AMPS* examines motor skills and process skills. The *AMPS* assesses the motor skill domains of posture, mobility, coordination, strength and effect, and energy and the process skill domains of energy, knowledge, temporal organization, organizing space and objects, and adaptation. These motor and process skills are within the context of performance of instrumental tasks of daily living. There is not generally a problem identifying two to three tasks that the adolescent has a history of performing and is willing to do for the purpose of evaluation from the lengthy list of possible tasks that can be used for the *AMPS* (e.g., making a bed, making a sandwich, washing dishes, setting a table, polishing shoes).

Typical problems identified as a result of OT evaluation include a lack of balance of roles. Often roles lose meaning and are relinquished as dysfunction progresses. Neither the task component nor the social component of any remaining roles provides a sense of satisfaction or accomplishment. Habits may deteriorate completely or become rigid around dysfunctional activities such as alcohol or drug use, eating binges, or compulsive behaviors. Lack of active engagement in the roles that typically test interests and develop problem-solving and interpersonal skills means that these skills are not acquired. Feelings of competency in these abilities are not added to what should be a growing repertoire of competencies. Likewise, repeated failure prevents adolescents from seeing themselves as effective. The adolescent often views himself or herself as defective and incapable of success in the future. Goals are nonexistent because the adolescents fail to recognize that their lives could be better in the future. This may result from exposure to environments where opportunities are limited and life holds little promise. In family systems where parents or caregivers are so occupied with their own concerns, adolescents are often neglected and left unsupervised to "fend for themselves." Opportunities to experience success in accomplishing academic, work, and play tasks that contribute to the development of identity and autonomy are missing from the adolescent's experience. Also missing are the successful experiences of interacting socially with peers and adults that help to develop interdependence.

In summary, a thorough assessment that includes an interview and observation of an adolescent's motor, processing, and interpersonal skills is essential to quality treatment planning and intervention. The adolescent will benefit the most when he or she is an active participant in the planning process. Commitment to helping themselves is essential to adolescents' recovery. Even extremely sad and angry adolescents will tell you the way that they would like for things to be if you listen long enough in a sensitive, caring way. There is time to do reality testing later in the relationship after rapport has been established. A critical and judgmental attitude on the part of the therapist will prevent a trusting relationship from developing. Listen before confronting and recognize that behavior and attitudes generally reflect prior experiences. The therapist's role might well be to provide the adolescent with a different context that confronts maladaptive, old ideas and attitudes and fosters new, more adaptive ones.

# INTERVENTION

With the client evaluated and the collaborative goals at least partially set, the therapist completes the documentation process and writes this treatment plan. Next we will look at the types of problems that might be present with adolescents with the types of psychosocial dysfunction that were discussed earlier in the chapter. This section of the chapter will not look separately at problems by diagnoses, as many of these problems co-occur in adolescents receiving treatment. We will begin with a brief discussion of the treatment that is likely to be provided by other professionals on the treatment team who may be working with the adolescent. A knowledge of the contributions of other members of the team helps us to recognize the unique contributions that are provided by occupational therapy practitioners working with these young people. At that point, we will be prepared to examine intervention from an occupational therapy perspective.

Adolescents being treated for diagnoses of mood disorders, anxiety disorders, conduct disorders, substance-related disorders, and eating disorders will, in most cases, be receiving individual psychotherapy (Brent & Kolko, 1998; Mufson & Fairbanks, 1996). Psychotherapy may be provided by a psychiatrist, a psychologist, or a clinical social worker. In some cases, this therapy takes the form of cognitive-behavioral treatment, which aims at changing how people think and behave. It is focused on the internal dialogue that takes place in the person's mind and what he or she can do in the present to help change the way that he or she is feeling (Beck, 1997). Other times, interpersonal therapy may be the focus and the client will discuss social relationships and how to improve them. Sometimes individual therapy is targeted on developing insight into one's current problems by exploring past influences (Garner et al., 1993). With the growing influence of managed care, the number of approved visits for therapy has decreased and amount of time therapists are spending with clients has decreased, causing therapists to focus more on immediate behavioral changes and increased reliance on psychopharmacologic treatment (Sourander et al., 1969).

Other forms of therapy are also a part of adolescent treatment programs. Group therapy and family therapy sessions may also be provided by a psychologist, social worker, or in some cases a licensed professional counselor who may have a background in rehabilitation counseling and substance abuse counseling (Hoag & Burlingame, 1997). Some programs offer "multi-family therapy" sessions that allow parents to find consolation, support, and hope from other parents who have dealt with similar problems (Brent et al., 1997). The effects of managed care have also had the influence of trying to maximize the benefits while containing or reducing costs. Group therapy is valued for these reasons. Most programs also recognize the importance of helping the adolescent restructure leisure time use. In many residential, inpatient, and outpatient programs, *Certified Therapeutic Recreation Specialists* (CTRS) provide leisure activities, offer leisure education groups, and take adolescents on leisure outings in the community. In some cases, OTs and recreation therapists team up to help adolescents develop play and leisure skills. Some programs offer a variety of "expressive therapies," like art and music therapy (Berry & Pennebaker, 1993; Zonnaveldt, 1969). Some hospital, residential, correctional and day treatment programs offer programs, such as rope and initiative courses, that require individuals to work cooperatively with their peers as a group to accomplish physical and emotional challenges. These programs foster participant's abilities to engage in cooperative activity and dialogue, skills that are often missing from many adolescents with psychosocial problems. Some residential and juvenile corrections facilities include outdoor activities like hiking, backpacking, and rock climbing as part of their programming (Kimball, 1986). Like ropes courses, these activities provide adolescents with successful experiences that send them clear messages that they are capable and valuable members of the group. With a network of physicians, nurses, social workers, individual and group therapists, and recreation and expressive therapists all providing services to adolescents with problems, what unique contribution does occupational therapy have to add to an adolescent's treatment? This will be the topic of the next section.

## INTERVENTION SPECIFICALLY
## RELATED TO THE ADOLESCENT

Intervention will, of course, be based upon the results of the evaluation and, hopefully, the goals of the adolescent. In most cases, adolescents with depression, eating disorders, substance abuse problems, conduct disorders, or anxiety disorders have little sense of confidence in their abilities (Barris et al., 1986). Their self-assessments are generally filled with a great deal of self-criticism. They frequently make self-depreciating comments ("I stink at this. I can't do this. There's no point in even trying. It's hopeless. I'm just not smart enough, artistic, likeable, etc.") and any praise they receive is taken skeptically and regarded as a manipulative ploy ("She doesn't really mean that, she's just saying that to keep me from leaving the group"), or as untrue and only given for therapeutic purpose ("You are just saying that because you are a therapist"). Adolescents with a severely damaged sense of self-efficacy cannot be convinced otherwise by words. More than likely, they have experienced numerous failures or been told on many occasions that they were not able or capable of being successful (Barris et al., 1985). The ultimate goal of the therapist is to help the adolescent re-establish a sense of control and direction for his or her own life or, in Model of Human Occupation terms, to develop feelings of "personal causation." A therapist will contribute tremendously to an adolescent's treatment if he or she can creatively structure occupations so that the adolescent begins to feel capable and effective. Occupational therapy has emphasized learning by doing throughout its history. Most adolescents with psychosocial problems, for one reason or another, have not learned that they have abilities that are of value to the world. In many cases, adolescents with psychosocial problems come from environments where they were not supported or encouraged, and where interpersonal skills were not taught. We can only develop a sense that we have an impact on the world when we have the skills to have an impact on the world. If an adolescent has had a history of failing and being unsuccessful, it may have been because they lacked a skill necessary to be successful. If the reason that an adolescent feels incapable is because he or she lacks the skills to have a positive effect, then those skills need to be developed. Skill training has also been an important contribution of occupational therapy since its beginnings (Howe & Schwartzberg, 1994). It takes many different types of skills for an adolescent to be successful in his or her world, including many educational skills, like reading and the ability to do mathematics. Problems with auditory and visual perception can severely affect a child or adolescent's ability to be successful in school. Failure at school leads to generalized feelings of inadequacy, devaluing, and low self-esteem. OTs can assist their clients by identifying and treating underlying perceptual, gross motor, or fine motor deficits that interfere with success in activities of meaning to the individual. If deficits are not remediable, then compensatory methods may be of help.

Ultimately a goal of occupational therapy with adolescents is to empower individuals with the skills that will contribute to their sense of being an actor in their own life, to inspire them to be able to chart their own direction for their life, and to instill in them the ability to find meaning in their life through the pursuit of occupations that provide them with a personal sense of meaning and purpose (Kielhofner, 1995). When adolescents without psychosocial dysfunction are compared to those with dysfunction, the overriding difference is that adolescents without dysfunction have developed the self-direction to seek and pursue occupations that have meaning to them. Whether that pursuit occurs in the classroom, on an athletic field, in the lunchroom, at work, on a date, or anywhere else in the adolescent's world, the resulting feelings of competency and capability contribute to that person's belief that he or she can have a desired effect on the world by his or her own actions (Baron, 1987). Because most of an adolescent's life roles involve a social component, having the interpersonal or interactional skills to relate to others is an essential skill for life satisfaction (Pezzuti, 1979).

Occupational therapy practitioners can teach adolescents how to relate in healthy ways to peers and adults. Communication styles, such as aggressiveness, passivity, and passive-aggressiveness are most often learned in the family. Most adolescents fail to recognize that they have a choice in how they communicate. They view their communication style as an unchangeable part of who they are rather than seeing it as learned behavior. Assertiveness skills are valuable skills for adolescents to learn (Thompson et al., 1996; Thompson et al., 1995; Wise et al., 1991). OTs, with their commitment to active doing have adolescents engage in role playing and "trying new behaviors on for size" (Brown & Carmichael, 1992). Development of processing skills is another area on which occupational therapy practitioners can focus. Many adolescents with psychosocial problems lack healthy role models and therefore fail to observe healthy problem solving and decision making. If children and adolescents live in homes where adults cope with life problems by using alcohol or drugs, being violent, blaming others, or by withdrawing and being silent, they have not had healthy coping with life's problems modeled for them (Williamson et al., 1993). Adolescents can be presented with sample problems and work together to generate alternative ways to deal with the problems. The advantages and disadvantages of each alternative lead to the selection of the best alternative.

Like assertiveness skills, coping skills can be learned (Seiffge-Krenke, 1993). Engaging in scenarios and discussions of real-life dilemmas and working together to learn how to cope in ways that have long-term positive results helps adolescents realize that alternative actions exist. Once they are aware of alternative behaviors they cannot return to their former limited perspective. Their behavior may or may not change immediately, but they have acquired knowledge that requires that they at least acknowledge that they are making a choice where previously they recognized no options. Being successful in having an effect leads to further attempts and additional successes (Schinke et al., 1987). Treatment focused on these two major skill areas, interpersonal skills and processing skills, has the potential to alter an adolescent's feelings of competency and self-direction (Johnson & Hayworth, 1992). Successful involvement in meaningful occupations that build skills, whether it is via a cooking activity, involvement in a game, craft activity, or a role-playing session enhances the participant's feelings of efficacy and establishes a foundation of hope for the future.

For therapists working with adolescents with psychosocial dysfunction much of the challenge is *creating the environment that will stimulate the adolescent to explore occupations*. Again, the wisdom of the founders of the profession guide us in this regard. For an occupation to be therapeutic it must be intrinsically motivating (Barris et al., 1983). Adolescents who have had no success in occupations in the past are likely to comment that anything suggested "is boring." Many adolescents became depressed or started using alcohol and drugs in their early teens right about the time when their interests would normally have evolved from childhood interests to teenage interests. Past interests may not be helpful in guiding treatment if they were activities such as collecting baseball cards or playing with dolls. Lack of interest in pursuing pleasurable activities, excessive sleeping, and spending time "getting high" interferes with the typical developmental sequence of experimenting with work and leisure activities and the "ruling in/ruling out" process that occurs as a result of "trying activities on for size," that is, finding matches between one's interests and abilities and the demands of different activities. Not all activities are going to be a match for one's interests and capabilities. What is meaningful for one person may not be at all meaningful to another. Finding occupations of meaning is an experimental process. Adolescents who have missed this process have to start the process of experimenting and trying out new things. For this reason, *exploration of possible interests* is an important intervention with this group. The therapist needs to understand that not all of the occupations that an adolescent tries will be a good match. If the process can be guided by the adolescent saying "I'd like to give such and such a try," the therapist can help make the experience successful by supporting the exploratory approach. If the occupation proves to be meaningful for the adolescent, and he or she is motivated to continue involvement in the occupation, the therapist can grade the complexity of the task to structure the task at the ever-changing "just right" challenge level. (Ayres, 1972). Occupations that have meaning to individuals and are in concert with their value system and culture will have the greatest likelihood of being generalized beyond supported performance in treatment. Experimentation takes time. It takes some time for someone to try an activity to which they are attracted, but which requires a level of skill that they have yet to develop, to engage in that activity with sufficient skill to be successful at it. Adolescents should be encouraged not to give up too quickly. It is helpful for them to hear stories about the amount of practice that it took for athletes, skilled craftspeople, or others that they admire to develop their skills. If the adolescent can be provided with a series of successful experiences that increasingly approximate involvement in the full activity, he or she is likely to sustain interest and not give up.

The majority of adolescents with the disorders discussed in this chapter live day to day with no real plans for the future. In fact, many adolescents diagnosed with depression or substance abuse do not anticipate even being around in the future. As chemical dependency develops, the identity of a young addict becomes that of a "user" only. If he ever had dreams of being a pilot, or a mechanic, or a teacher, or television personality, his dreams have fallen by the wayside and he does not see himself as anything other than a drug addict or alcoholic. Severely depressed adolescents with suicidal ideation or prior suicidal attempts do not expect to be alive in the future. *Establishment of a vision of the future* is another important contribution of occupational therapy. One-to-one collaboration on goal setting for the immediate and distant future is begun at the time of the initial evaluation and is an important part of ongoing treatment (Lloyd, 1986; Scott, 1984). Goals change as attitudes and visions change. The adolescent in treatment has the entire treatment team working with him or her. The influences of team members can at different times bring about changes in goals. The OT will focus on the individual's goals to re-engage in meaningful occupation and to build the skills to engage successfully in those occupations of choice. OTs are well trained in writing goals that are behaviorally based and therefore observable and measurable. They have the skills to help their clients write specific, clear goals that leave no doubt as to whether they were accomplished. The process of developing goals that reach further into the future is tied to instilling hope (Yalom, 1970). When an adolescent can begin to see himself or herself in the future and to see that the future is not a mere continuation of days like those in the past, but that it holds promise for a different life, then true progress has been made. OTs, because of their concern for their clients' day-to-day functioning, are often inspirational in instilling hope.

The process of experiencing success and competency as a result of engaging in an occupation with meaning results in feelings of empowerment that one can choose to change his or her life. When feelings of empowerment are supported by an awareness of one's abilities and a sense of accomplishment from the achievement of personal goals, a transformation takes place. The adolescent becomes self-directed, guided by personal vision, and energized by intrinsic motivation. Since the goal of therapy is to see the client taking charge of his or her own life without the help of the therapist, it is extremely gratifying to witness a young person rediscover that life is worth living.

Adolescents in treatment also frequently present with problems organizing their time and routines. If they have not been encouraged to develop habits at home, to adhere to any routines in regard to grooming and hygiene, to care for their own clothes, to assume any responsibility for work around the house, to manage their own money, to follow family rules, or to show mutual consideration and respect for others, then the structure of a treatment program may be a new experience for them. OTs understand the organizing effect of daily habits and routines. They can exert influence on program directors, convincing them of the importance of building habit structure into the daily schedule. Many treatment programs have a behavioral orientation. Level systems of points are frequently used. As adolescents accumulate points for "positive behavior" they are granted privileges. It is very easy for these reward systems to remain focused on extrinsic motivation and for intrinsic motivation to be lost in the process. It is important for OTs to stress to their administrators and fellow team members the importance of helping adolescents recognize how much better they feel when they make conscious choices to take responsibility for themselves. This, of course, would require decreasing external structure while maintaining the necessary scaffolding that holds the adolescent responsible for fulfilling personal responsibilities without cueing or external reinforcers. OTs can work with the adolescent to structure and balance his or her time within the structure of the treatment schedule as a first step to taking personal responsibility even within a controlled situation. They can revisit the topic of managing and balancing one's time prior to discharge. Although it is unlikely that any schedule will be followed verbatim, it is still important to plan for structuring a routine once the adolescent leaves treatment. This can be done as an individual or a group activity. If it is done as a group activity, the group should be small, five people or fewer, in order to allow everyone sufficient attention. As with any schedule, the more specific to the person's life it is, the greater the likelihood that it will be followed. A treatment idea that has worked well for adolescents involves having them compose a letter to themselves that outlines their intentions for daily routines and goals for the first couple of months following discharge. They complete a self-addressed envelope and the therapist mails it to them 30 days after their discharge date as a reminder to themselves of the structure and plans they made for themselves while in treatment.

It is important for therapists working with adolescents with psychosocial problems to realize that these youths may not be physically, cognitively, emotionally, or socially capable of engaging in treatment at times. Positive emission tomography (PET) scans have revealed that persons with depression have a reduced capacity to process information in the frontal lobes of the brain. Executive problem-solving functions take place extensively in the frontal lobes (Gorman, 1997). The implications of this might be that when a client has difficulty solving problems that there may very well be a physiological basis for the problem. Antidepressant medications increase the level of processing activity in the frontal lobes, but even with medication, processing may be limited and slower in an individual with depression. This is mentioned so that therapist's expectations are achievable and not based upon unrealistic goals. Research is increasingly revealing the role that neuroscience plays in psychosocial disorders. Recognition of a biological basis of these disorders should reduce the stigma associated with mental illness and hopefully reduce the numbers of persons who suffer unnecessarily with disorders that are treatable.

Adolescents who have problems with psychosocial functioning may have no motor problems. Others may have a history of sensorimotor problems that were not addressed when they were younger. Many of the adolescents processed in the juvenile correction system and who have never been identified for special education services have perceptual-motor, fine-motor, and gross-motor deficits sufficient enough to qualify them for special education services. Unfortunately, by the time they enter the juvenile correction system, many of these children have experienced such failure in school that identification occurs too late to alter the adolescents' attitudes about themselves or about the value of an education. Research has shown that a higher than normal percentage of adolescents with disruptive behavior disorders have learning disabilities (Scheffel, 1996).

In addition to sensorimotor and cognitive deficits, adolescents diagnosed with depression, substance abuse, conduct disorders, eating disorders, and other disorders nearly always have problems with interpersonal skills. Interpersonal skill development is a part of the socialization process. Children who come from living environments where they were not provided with opportunities to learn to give and receive respect or learn to express themselves assertively may have developed survival patterns of passivity or aggression. These patterns have become familiar and are often absorbed into their identity of who they are as a person. *OTs can address how communication styles are learned and how dysfunctional patterns can be changed with practice.* Intervening at the skills level with teaching communication, social skills, and assertiveness training is an important area for most therapists working with this age group (Temple & Robson, 1991). Personal effectiveness training, although developed a number of years ago, is still an effective method to utilize with adolescents today. In this intervention persons select someone in the group to play someone with whom they have problems interacting. It is often a family member, but it could be a teacher, co-worker, boss, friend, or anyone else with whom they need to learn to communicate more effectively. They give the actor enough information about this person to play the role and then use the new skills that they have learned to test new ways of interacting with them.

---

■ *THERAPEDS POINTER*

There are several key factors that make Personal Effectiveness Training a useful intervention. The first is the client's designing of the role-plays. This makes the role-plays relevant to the individual and increases the chances of generalizability. A second factor is that the client then has a choice of the group member or leader that he or she would like opposite him or her in the role-play. Once this person is chosen the client takes time to prepare the chosen group member or leader about how the individual should "act" to make the role-play as realistic as possible. The final factor that makes this technique effective is the active coaching process that the group leader takes. This process is very similar to drama coaching, where suggestions are made on an ongoing basis throughout the role-play. Role-plays are rehearsed and repeated until certain skills are incorporated. The level of involvement and requisite expertise of the group leaders require that therapists be knowledgeable and confident in their skills. This is a very practical technique, which can be very effective in helping adolescents with varying levels of social skills. Role-plays afford participants opportunities to improve their abilities to express themselves to family members, friends, and adults and to persons in authority. They practice social skills such as how to introduce themselves, make new friends, say "no," maintain a conversation, interview for a job, and deal with an aggressive peer. Some groups may find videotaping their role-plays very helpful. Much can be learned from observing yourself as others see you. Comparison of role-plays over time can also serve to demonstrate the progress group members have made. If videotaping is used, take care that releases are signed and that the taping process is as inconspicuous as possible.

---

Another skill that is frequently the focus of adolescent treatment involves development of *stress management* or *coping skills* (Kinsella et al., 1996). The purpose of this treatment is generally to educate clients in regard to healthy coping strategies (Courtney & Escobedo, 1990). The interventions mentioned previously, such as helping the client discover meaningful occupation, building daily routines that reflect a balance of productive time and leisure time, and fostering the development of skills to get along with others and get your needs met, are all effective coping methods. Relaxation techniques like progressive muscle relaxation, autogenic relaxation (a technique in which the client repeats relaxation-inducing phrases that emphasize feelings of heaviness and warmth), and guided imagery, all of which take some time, may be interesting to some adolescents, but most do not find them suitable for general use (Payne, 1995). The skills that are most useful to the adolescent in his or her life after leaving treatment are the skills that the OT should concentrate upon. For this reason, simple methods like deep breathing or self-talk to calm oneself may be a better use of therapy time. Time is well spent helping the adolescent sort through problems and generate alternative ways to deal with them. Brainstorming is a highly effective way of having adolescents recognize that often the first solutions that come to mind are frequently not the optimal ones to choose to carry out!

Of course, intervention as addressed here suffers from having to approach it generically. Intervention is a highly individual process. Each of the areas mentioned in this discussion need to be individualized and customized to match to needs of the particular client. The challenge for any therapist is to "connect" with the client temporarily, to travel side-by-side for a time, and through therapeutic use of self and the use of carefully chosen occupations to help the client rediscover his or her abilities and potential. As they gain confidence in their ability to act on their own behalf and make decisions that help them feel more capable and competent, they gain the ability to guide their lives in more satisfying and fulfilling directions. This is satisfying with any client but it is particularly gratifying when a child or adolescent discovers his value and uniqueness as a human being and gets back on track toward achieving the developmental tasks of independence and interdependence that lay the foundation for a satisfying adulthood.

| Adolescent Characteristic | Seen As | In This Setting | Possible Solution or Strategy |
|---|---|---|---|
| 15-year-old boy who has lost interest in school and extra-curricular activities | Drop in grades Dropping out of the school play; spending a lot of time alone in his room sleeping or listening to music; talking of being of no value to anyone | School and home | 1. Creation of a personal narrative that reveals the life events that occurred around the time that his interests waned 2. Joint goal setting for treatment 3. Development of a plan to increase participation in occupations that have meaning to him 4. Development of skills to express feelings and needs to others 5. Develop a list of routine problems and a |

| | | | |
|---|---|---|---|
| | | | list of alternatives for coping with those problems |
| 14-year-old girl who has lost 20 lb by refusing to eat and now weighs 85 lb | Staunch refusal to eat any foods containing fat or sugar; excessive exercising | At school and at home | 1. Engage in exploratory activities with no risk of failure and no competition<br>2. Joint treatment planning and goal setting that provides client with an area other than food to experience a sense of control<br>3. Develop a schedule that promotes a balance between productivity, play, and rest.<br>4. Include in Personal Effectiveness Training group to encourage expression of feelings |

# INTERVENTION CONSIDERATIONS RELATED TO THE PARENTS OR CAREGIVERS OF THE ADOLESCENT

Adolescents need the support of an environment that nurtures them in their progress toward achievement of their developmental tasks. Parents and caregivers contribute significantly to adolescents' establishment of their identity, to their development of self-esteem, and to the healthy adjustment to their sexuality. Adolescent treatment programs recognize the need for family and/or caregiver involvement in an adolescent's treatment. Most programs strongly encourage, if not require, family therapy. Some programs have special family weekend programs. OTs can provide services to the families or caregivers in the form of parent effectiveness training, or in speaking to parents about the important role they play in supporting their son or daughter's involvement in meaningful activity that allows their child to feel good about himself or herself. They should also be educated about the importance of setting and enforcing reasonable limits and the adolescent's need for structure and responsibility. Separate parent and child groups and joint groups can examine mutual expectations. For more intense programming a group protocol could be developed for a group experience that allowed adolescents to engage in experiences that promote self-discovery, while the parents engage in activities that allow them to revisit their own adolescence experience. The programs would culminate with reconnecting the adolescents and parents to share the insights they had gained of their similarities and differences.

Programs with ropes and initiatives components offer family experiences using those media. Adolescents and their parents can learn to relate to each other in ways that they never have before. There seems to be nothing like the woods and being free of distractions of the "real world" to get people of all generations to look at each other and talk honestly to one another. Even in less intense structured experiences, with programming occurring on the weekend, visiting parents can be invited to participate in certain groups, like task groups, games, and physical activities. Families should be encouraged to enjoy each other's company by discovering activities that they like doing together. There are a number of community resources available to parents. Distributing a list of these local contacts and telephone numbers is helpful to parents desiring ongoing support. Discharge planning sessions can be organized with the adolescent and his or her family, making plans for daily, weekly routines, and special occasions.

It is important for OTs treating adolescents in traditional settings to make a point of seeing the adolescent in the context of his or her family, and if intervention is possible with the family, to include it as a part of the treatment plan. If an adolescent is being discharged to a foster situation or a group home, the OT may be able to schedule a site visit or a session or two with the foster parents to discuss the structure and limit setting needed by the adolescent to help him achieve his goals. The interpersonal and processing changes that have occurred within the adolescent responding to treatment are difficult to maintain unless the ongoing environment continues to nurture those skills. Just as the therapist designs a therapeutic environment for change to take place in treatment, careful attention to the environment where the adolescent will live after treatment is concluded is essential to sustaining any gains made in treatment.

## INTERVENTIONS RELATED TO THE ENVIRONMENT OF THE ADOLESCENT

The environment plays an integral part in an adolescent's ability to engage in meaningful occupation. If the environment blocks any opportunities for a young person to experience a sense of ability and success, then that child experiences a life of frustration and anger. Very often treatment opens new doorways for young people to see the opportunities that a different environment can offer. In these cases, the adolescent has to be taught that she can have an effect upon her environment by her own actions. The adolescent may also need to develop enough personal resolve so as not to succumb to pressure to return to his old way of being.

At times, intervention needs to be addressed to the environment. That may mean a change in schools or friends to help the adolescent solidify the positive changes he or she has made. Change is difficult enough without having to deal with an environment that is pressing for a return to past behaviors. At times a "fresh start" can be a helpful step in making changes. Adolescents who have a history of substance abuse are counseled to stay away from "slippery places" where they might find themselves around people using drugs. Similar advice can be given to young people who have friends who are also depressed, suicidal, or who routinely engage in behavior that violates the rights of others. If an adolescent wants to alter the course and direction of her own life, she has to make choices to change the group with whom she associates and to develop new relationships with persons who support recovery and a healthier way of being. This is difficult for many adolescents; even those who don't want to return to the way they were living before treatment have difficulty giving up their prior peer relationships. They want to believe that it is possible to associate with their friends without engaging in the other behaviors. It often takes the "proof" of returning to those situations and not being able to handle them as they thought they could for some to realize that they were wrong and to begin the process of building a new circle of friends. Adolescents who have dressed in a style that identifies them as associating with a certain group known to use drugs or to engage in illegal activity are also counseled to change their image by changing their dress. This suggestion frequently also meets with resistance, but experience is an excellent teacher in these situations as well. If the adolescent wants to change, he will begin to recognize that the way he dresses and the persons with whom he associates determine how he is regarded and treated by others.

## CASE STORY

One of the most serious problems facing our society today is youth violence and crime. Some youths are at high risk for drug use, delinquency, dropping out of school, gang membership, teen pregnancy, and premature death. Occupational therapy, with its focus on engagement in meaningful occupation that fosters feelings of self-worth and value, has much to offer this group of young people, many of whom have never experienced feelings of personal success and accomplishment.

Imagine that you are an OT (you can be an OTR or COTA) working in an urban public school system. You most frequently work with the younger children in three elementary schools. An occupational therapy faculty member at the local university, Dr. Lovett, has received funding to provide occupational therapy services to youth at the high school in the inner city that has been designated to provide an educational program for at-risk students. These students are considered at risk for academic failure because of prior aggressive behavior, known drug use, or a history of family dysfunction. The program is currently above capacity, serving 180 students. The OT faculty member will be using the group sessions as an opportunity to train students. Your supervisor wants to promote connections between the university and the therapists in your school division. She has chosen you to work collaboratively with the faculty member and the occupational therapy students on this project. You, however, are not so sure about this new assignment. This type of occupational therapy is definitely outside of your "comfort zone." You have never before considered offering occupational therapy services to the students at this alternative school, even though there is a high population of them identified and eligible for special education services because of learning disabilities or behavioral disorders.

This idea for this program began when the occupational therapy students conducted a needs assessment during the first month of the fall semester. They conducted interviews of students, teachers, parents, caseworkers, probation officers, and potential employers to determine the lifeskill needs of this group of young people. The results of their interviews indicated that these high school students would benefit from occupational therapy services and that small-group work would be a valuable addition to the educational program. The students interviewed ranged in age from 15 to 18 years old. Some were on grade level for their age, but most were 1 to 2 years behind in school. Many were at reading levels 4 or more years below their grade level. African-American, Hispanic, Caucasian, and Asian ethnic groups were included in the representative sample. A large number were from homes with a single head of household, most frequently a mother. Some were living with a parent and stepparent. Family systems ranged from functional to highly dysfunctional.

Grant funding was received to provide occupational therapy services to 12 to 16 students (two groups of 6 to 8 students) 2 days per week from January until the end of May (15 weeks). Thirty group meeting times were believed to be sufficient to demonstrate positive change as a result of the intervention. The plan was for you to facilitate one group with two student assistants while Dr. Lovett facilitated the other group with two student assistants.

You are scheduled to meet with Dr. Lovett next week. You decide to do some research of your own to prepare yourself for the meeting.

1. Find an article on working with at-risk youth. Do not limit yourself to looking only at occupational therapy literature. What recommendations does it suggest for working with adolescents at-risk for psychosocial problems?

2. a. If you are an occupational therapy student, what theoretical frames of reference or models for practice (developmental; model of human occupation; role acquisition; sensory integration; occupational adaptation; coping; others) might you consider using with this population? (*Hint:* A case could be made for any of these frames of reference to be used). What is your preference and why?
   b. If you are an OTA student, imagine that Dr. Lovett has selected the model of human occupation as the theoretical model that will be used for these groups; what instruments might you be able to administer to assist Dr. Lovett in evaluating the specific students who will be in your group?

3. a. If you are an occupational therapy student, your choice of theoretical frame or frames of reference determines what and how problems are assessed. Problem finding is closely related to what is evaluated. Using your theoretical frame or frames of reference of choice, what problems might you anticipate seeing in this group of students?
   b. If you are an OTA student, Dr. Lovett and her students have identified a list of problems that includes the following: lack of confidence in abilities; anticipation of failure in school and work; undefined occupational interests; limited leisure interests; lack of recognition of the rights of others; lack of an organized daily routine; lack of work habits; no meaningful work or volunteer role; limited skills for interacting pro-

ductively with peers and adults in authority; difficulty controlling impulses; lack of work skills; and limited problem-solving skills. Do these problems "fit" with what you know about problems that might be seen in this population? Are there others that you might expect that were not identified? How would you deal with the situation of an undetected problem by the OTR with whom you are working?

4. What assets or strengths would you look for in this group of young people?

5. You know that goals for the group will initially be set by you and Dr. Lovett and then modified to meet the specific needs of the group. What goals might you consider in developing a group plan protocol for this group?

6. Although the needs assessment was conducted in the fall, the plan is for members of each group to have the opportunity to set group goals specifically for their group. How might you go about organizing the first session to allow them to develop these goals among themselves with your guidance? What kind of an activity might be designed for this purpose?

7. How do you *feel* about working with this group? Do you believe in the value of occupational therapy with this population? Why or why not?

8. As was mentioned in the chapter, OTs in most school systems are not providing occupational therapy for students with psychosocial disorders, and particularly not for older children middle-school and high-school aged? Why do you think this is and what can be done about it?

9. What factors might you need to be aware of when working in this environment (e.g., safety, confidentiality)?

10. Adolescents need clear, consistent limit setting. What might you propose to Dr. Lovett in regard to setting limits within the group to ensure that there is as much consistency between the two groups as possible?

11. You have discovered that many of these adolescents come from very stressful home and community environments where they receive little support or nurturing. You are aware that survival defenses often result in an adolescent developing a "hardened" protective shell that masks an underlying need for love and caring. When they begin to shed the shell, they become vulnerable, which can be very frightening to them. Think about how you might help these young people to recognize their needs to be nurtured, cared for, and to feel good about themselves. How can you help these students to learn to meet these needs in socially appropriate ways? Also think about how you can provide care for the emotional health of these teens, without feeling sympathy for these young people and losing focus of your purpose for being there.

12. What suggestions might you make to the teachers who are working with the students who are participating in these two therapy groups that would help the teachers to reinforce what you are attempting to accomplish with the student in therapy?

13. Which of the following modalities would you recommend using for this group? Why or why not?
    a. Crafts (e.g., woodworking, leather, copper tooling, ceramics, tile trivets)
    b. Personal narratives, pictorial autobiographies
    c. Problem-solving mock situations
    d. Personal effectiveness training (role playing)
    e. Vocational interest testing (e.g., Holland's Self-Directed Search)
    f. Money management
    g. Trust activities
    h. Games
    i. Meal planning and preparation
    j. Job application and interviewing skills
    k. Goal setting
    l. Group projects (e.g., plays, talent show, talk show)
    m. Fieldtrips (e.g., restaurant, hiking, biking, beach, museums)
    n. Expressive activities (e.g., mask making, collages, drawing, painting)
14. What might you suggest as a possible culminating activity at the conclusion of the last group session?
15. A large study by Masse and Tremblay (1997) indicated that high novelty-seeking behavior, which refers to a heritable tendency toward exploratory activity and exhilaration when presented with novel stimuli, and low harm-avoidance behavior, which refers to the heritable tendency to not react intensively to aversive stimuli, in kindergarten-aged boys predicted early onset of substance abuse in adolescence. The authors concluded that preventive efforts were called for. Do OTs have a role in preventing problems in adolescence by targeting children at high risk for later dysfunction?

## Real-Life Lab

**1.** You are a staff OTR or COTA in a partial hospitalization program for adolescents. You have been asked to contribute to a weekend family program that will be offered to patient's parents and/or caregivers one weekend each month. This is your opportunity to have an impact upon the home environments of the young people with whom you work. The first day is for parents and caregivers only. The second day adolescents in the partial program and any siblings are invited to attend. The clinical social worker will be responsible for scheduling opening and closing multifamily group sessions each morning and afternoon and a didactic session each day from 1 to 2 PM. The certified therapeutic recreation specialist will coordinate an hour of experiential therapy on the hospital's ropes course on Saturday (11 AM to 12 PM) and 2 hours on Sunday (2 to 4 PM). You have been asked to plan for 4 hours over the course of the 2 days (Saturday 10 to 11 AM and 2 to 3 PM and Sunday 10 AM to 12 PM). The goals of the family weekend are to enhance communication between the adolescent and their families, particularly their parents. The social worker addresses feelings that have formed barriers to communication between family members. You are considered the "expert" who uses activities to educate families about setting reasonable expectations, setting limits, disciplining with love, and planning time "to be and do things" as a family.

   **a.** Four hours is not a long time to accomplish these goals; how can this time be best utilized? The program director wants write "something" in for those times on the letter that she is composing to send out to the parents. What will you tell her to put in each of the three time slots?

      **a.** Sat. 11 AM–12 PM-_____

      **b.** Sat. 2–3 PM-_____

      **c.** Sun. 10–12 PM -_____

   **b.** What activities might you select for the parents or caregivers to accomplish the goals that have been set for these sessions?

   **c.** You have decided to use one of the hour sessions on Saturday to discuss community resources. Research and compile a list of resources in your community (from leisure opportunities to support groups) that could be used if you were offering a group of this type in your community. Be specific and complete. Give addresses and telephone numbers if possible.

**2.** You are a therapist in private practice. You have just received a call from Mr. and Mrs. Hoffman, the parents of 16-year-old Michael Hoffman, who is scheduled for discharge from a chemical dependency treatment center in Minnesota this weekend. They heard through friends that you had excellent skills for helping young people learn to organize and plan their time. They are willing to pay "out-of-pocket" to have you work with their son to help him reorganize his life, explore new interests, and investigate potential college and career choices. The parents assure you that this young man is committed to a recovery program. The parents have made arrangements for Michael to see a social worker, whose specialty is in working with persons in recovery, once a week. He will also attend either Alcoholics Anonymous or Narcotics Anonymous daily for the first 3 months he is home. Mr. and Mrs. Hoffman would like for you to work with Michael two afternoons a week after school. They would like to contract you initially for four sessions. They have implied that if things go well and they feel that Michael is benefiting from the sessions, they would like the option to extend the sessions for an additional 2 to 3 weeks.

   **a.** The parents inform you that Michael has an interest in computers. You use a laptop computer routinely for documentation. As you think about working with this young man, you consider the idea of having him use a computer program to organize his daily schedule.

Visit two software retailers and investigate software that might be used for this purpose. While you are there, investigate software for career exploration. If the retailer allows you to try out the software, test it to see whether it would serve your purposes with this client and whether or not it would be appealing to a 16-year-old boy.

**b.** Do a search on the World Wide Web for information on the programs of study offered by colleges in your state. How could you help Michael begin the process of looking at colleges and determining whether he has the credentials (grade point average and SAT scores) to be considered by certain schools?

**c.** What are some activities that you could have Michael do:

• to rebuild his self-confidence?

• to explore new interests or to become reinvolved in interests he abandoned when he began using drugs regularly?

• to find new ways to cope with disappointment, frustration, and anger when things don't go as he would like them to?

• to learn to accept his feelings and express them openly and honestly rather than denying, minimizing, or masking them?

# References

Alexander, N. (1986). Characteristics and treatment of families with anorectic offspring. *Occupational Therapy in Mental Health, 6*(1), 117–135.

Allen, C. K. (1985). *Occupational therapy for psychiatric diseases: measurement and management of cognitive disabilities.* Boston: Little, Brown.

Ambrosini, P. J., et al. (1993). Antidepressant treatments in children and adolescents. I. Affective disorders. *Journal of the American Academy of Child and Adolescent Psychiatry, 32* (1), 1–6.

American Psychiatric Association. (1994). *Diagnostic and statistical manual for mental disorders* (4th ed.). Washington, D.C.: Author.

Ayres, A. J. (1972). *Sensory integration and learning disorders.* Los Angeles: Western Psychological Services.

Bailey, G. (1989). Current perspectives on substance abuse in youth. *Journal of the American Academy of Child and Adolescent Psychiatry, 28*(2), 151–162.

Bailey, M. K. (1986). Occupational therapy for patients with eating disorders. *Occupational Therapy in Mental Health, 6*(1), 89–117.

Baron, K. B. (1987). The model of human occupation: A newspaper treatment group for adolescents with a diagnosis of conduct disorders. *Occupational Therapy in Mental Health, 7*(2), 89–104.

Baron, K. B., & Curtin, C. (1990). *A manual for use with self assessment of occupational functioning.* Chicago: Model of Human Occupational Clearinghouse, University of Illinois at Chicago.

Barris, R. (1986). Occupational dysfunction and eating disorders: Theory and approach to treatment. *Occupational Therapy in Mental Health, 6,* 27–45.

Barris, R., Dickie, V., & Baron, K. B. (1988). A comparison of psychiatric patients and normal subjects based on the model of human occupation. *Occupational Therapy Journal of Research, 8*(1), 3–23.

Barris, R., & G. Kielhofner, (1985). Adolescence. In G. Kielhofner, (Ed.). *A model of human occupation. Theory and application* (pp. 63–75). Baltimore: Williams & Wilkins.

Barris, R., Kielhofner, G., & Watts, J. (1983). *Psychosocial occupational therapy: Practice in a pluralistic arena.* Laurel, MD: Ramsco.

Barris, R., Kielhofner, G., Neville, A., Oakley, F., Salz, C., & Watts, J. (1985). Psychosocial dysfunction. In G. Kielhofner (Ed.). *A model of human occupation: Theory and application.* Baltimore: Williams & Wilkins.

Barris, R., Kielhofner, G., Martin, R. M. B., Gelinas, I., Klement, M., & Schultz, B. (1986). Occupational function and dysfunction in three groups of adolescents. *Occupational Therapy Journal of Research, 6*(5), 301–317.

Beck, A. T. (1997). The past and future of cognitive therapy. *Journal of Psychotherapy Practice and Research, 6*(4), 276–284.

Berry, D. S., & Pennebaker, J. W. (1993). Nonverbal and verbal emotional expression and health. *Psychotherapy and Psychosomatics, 59*(1),11–19.

Bjodstrup, B. (1986). Treating the chemically dependent adolescent. *Occupational Therapy Forum, 1*(5), 1–6.

Black, M. M. (1976). Adolescent role assessment. *American Journal of Occupational Therapy, 30*(2), 73–79.

Blakeney, A. B. (1985). Adolescent development: An application to the model of human occupation. *Occupational Therapy in Health Care, 2*(3), 19–41.

Blumenthal, S. J., & Kupfer, D. J. (1988). An overview of early detection and treatment strategies for suicidal behavior in young people. *Journal of Youth and Adolescence, 17*, 1–23.

Bonder, B. R. (1991). *Psychopathology and function.* Thorofare, NJ: Slack.

Brayman, S., & Kirby, T. (1982). The comprehensive occupational therapy evaluation. *In B. J. Hemphill (Ed.), The evaluative process in occupational therapy* (pp. 211–266). Thorofare, NJ: Slack.

Breden, A. K. (1992). Occupational therapy and the treatment of eating disorders. *Occupational Therapy in Health Care, 8* (2/3), 49–68.

Brent, D. A., Holder, D., Kolko, D., Birmaher, B., Baugher, M., Roth, C., Iyengar, S., & Johnson, B. A. (1997). A clinical psychotherapy trial for adolescent depression comparing cognitive, family, and supportive therapy. *Archives of General Psychiatry, 54*(9), 877–885.

Brent, D. A., & Kolko, D. J. (1998). Psychotherapy: Definitions, mechanisms of action, and relationship to etiological models. *Journal of Abnormal Child Psychology, 26*(1), 17–25.

Bridgett, B. (1993). Occupational therapy evaluation with patients with eating disorders. *Occupational Therapy in Mental Health, 12*(2), 79–89.

Brown, G. T., & Carmichael, K. (1992). Assertiveness training for clients with a psychiatric illness: A pilot study. *British Journal of Occupational Therapy, 55*(4), 137–140.

Bruce, M. A., & Borg, B. (1993). *Psychosocial occupational therapy. Frames of reference for intervention.* Thorofare, NJ: Slack.

Calabrese, R. L., & Adams, J. (1990). Alienation: A cause of juvenile delinquency. *Adolescence, 23*(98), 435–439.

Carlson, G. A. (1990). Bipolar disorders in children and adolescents. In Garfinkel, B., Carlson, G., & Weller, E. (Eds.), *Psychiatric disorders in children and adolescents.* Philadelphia: W.B. Saunders.

Carrey, N. J., Wiggins, D. M., & Milin, R. P. (1996). Pharmacological treatment of psychiatric disorders in children and adolescents. *Drugs, 51*(5), 750–759.

Connolly, J. (1989). Social self-efficacy in adolescence: Relations with self-concept, social adjustment, and mental health. *Canadian Journal of Behavioral Science, 21,* 258–269.

Courtney, C., & Escobedo, B. A., (1990). Stress management program: Inpatient-to-outpatient continuity. *American Journal of Occupational Therapy, 44*(4), 306–310.

Crespi, T. D., & Sabatelli, R. M. (1993). Adolescent runaways and family strife: A conflict-induced differentiation framework. *Adolescence, 28*(112), 867–877.

Dacey, J., & Kenny, M. (1997). *Adolescent development* (2nd ed.) Dubuque, IA: Brown & Benchmark.

Davis, G., & Hendren, R. L. (1993). What pediatricians should know about adolescent psychiatry. *Adolescent Medicine: State of the Art Reviews, 3* 381–145.

DeForest, D., Watts, J. H., & Madigan, M. J. (1991). Resonation in the model of human occupation: A pilot study. *Occupational Therapy in Mental Health, 11*(2/3), 57–71.

Donnelly, C. L., Maletic, V., & March, J. S. (1996). Anxiety disorders in children and adolescents. In D. X. Parmelee (Ed.), *Child and adolescent psychiatry* (pp. 97–119). St. Louis: Mosby.

Dryfoos, J. (1993). Schools as places for health, mental health, and social services. In Takanishi, R. (Ed.). *Adolescence in the 1990s: Risk and opportunity.* New York: Teachers College Press.

Ebb, E. W., Coster, W., & Duncomb, L. (1989). Comparison of normal and psychologically dysfunctional male adolescents. *Occupational Therapy in Mental Health, 9* (2), 54–74.

Ehrenberg, M. F., Cox, D. N., & Koopman, R. F. (1991). The relationship between self-efficacy and depression in adolescents. *Adolescence, 26,* 361–374.

Emery, L. J., & Huebner, R. A., (1996). Content revision in adolescent psychosocial occupational therapy. *Occupational Therapy in Health Care, 10*(2), 37–47.

Emslie, G. (1996). The AACAP News. *Journal of the American Academy of Child and Adolescent Psychiatry,* Jan.–Feb., 15.

Emslie, G. J., Rush, A. J., Weinberg, W. A., Gullion, C. M., Rintelman, J., & Hughes, C. W. (1997). Reoccurrence of major depressive disorder in hospitalized children and adolescents. *Journal of the American Academy of Child and Adolescent Psychiatry, 36*(6), 785–792.

Erickson, E. H. (1963). *Childhood and society* (2nd ed.). New York: Norton.

Erikson, E. H. (1968). *Identity, Youth, and Crisis.* New York: Norton.

Fanchiang, S., Snyder, C., Zobel-Lachiusa, J., Loeffler, C. B., & Thompson, M. E. (1990). Sensory integrative processing in delinquent-prone and non-delinquent-prone adolescents. *American Journal of Occupational Therapy, 47,* 630–639.

Gangl, M. L. (1987). The effectiveness of an occupational therapy program for chemically dependent adolescents. *Occupational Therapy in Mental Health, 7*(2), 67–89.

Garner, D. M., Rockert, W., Davis, R., Garner, M. V., Olmstead, M. P., & Eagle, M. (1993). Comparison of cognitive-behavioral and supportive-expressive therapy for bulimia-nervosa. *American Journal of Psychiatry, 150*(1), 37–46.

Giles, G. M. (1985). Anorexia nervosa and bulimia: an activity-oriented approach. *American Journal of Occupational Therapy, 39*(8), 510–517.

Gorman, C. (1997, May 5). Anatomy of melancholy. *Time,* 78.

Gorski, G., & Miyake, S. (1985). The adolescent life/work planning group: A prevention model. *Occupational Therapy in Health Care, 2*(3), 139–150.

Greydanus, D. E. (1986). Depression in adolescence. A perspective. *Journal of Adolescent Health Care, 7*(65), 109–120.

Harrison, M., & Newcorn, J. (1996). Psychiatric examination and diagnosis in children and adolescents. In D. X. Parmelee (Ed.), *Child and adolescent psychiatry* (pp. 237–244). St. Louis: Mosby.

Havighurst, R. J. (1951). *Developmental tasks and education.* New York: Logmans, Green.

Havighurst, R. J. (1972). *Developmental tasks and education.* (3d ed.). New York: David McCay.

Hayes, R. L., & Halford, W. K. (1993). Generalization of occupational therapy effects in psychiatric rehabilitation. *American Journal of Occupational Therapy, 47*(2), 161–167.

Henry, A. D., & Coster, W. J. (1997). Competency beliefs and occupational role behavior among adolescents: Explication of the personal causation construct. *American Journal of Occupational Therapy, 51,* 267–276.

Hoag, M. J., & Burlingame, G. M. (1997). Evaluating the effectiveness of child and adolescent group treatment: A meta-analytic review. *Journal of Clinical Child Psychology, 26*(3), 234–246.

Hodgman, C. H. (1996). Adolescent psychiatric conditions. *Comprehensive Therapy, 22*(12), 796–801.

Houston, J. (1996). What works: The search for excellence in gang intervention programs. *Journal of Gang Research, 3*(3), 1–16.

Howe, M., & Schwartzberg, S. (1994). *A functional approach to group work in occupational therapy.* Philadelphia: Lippincott.

Howe, M. C., & Schwartzberg, S. (1995). *A functional approach to group work in occupational therapy* (2d ed.). Philadelphia: Lippincott.

Hunington, D. D., & Bender, W. N. (1993). Adolescents with learning disabilities at risk? Emotional well being, depression, suicide. *Journal of Learning Disabilities, 26,* 159–166.

Institute of Medicine (1989). *Research on children and adolescents with mental, behavioral and developmental disorders.* Washington, D.C.: National Academy Press.

Jaffe, S. (1996). The substance-abusing youth. In Parmelee, D. X. (Ed.), *Child and adolescent psychiatry* (pp. 237–244). St. Louis: Mosby.

Johnson, M. T. (1987). Occupational therapists and teaching of cognitive behavioral skills. *Occupational Therapy in Mental Health, 7*(3), 69–81.

Josman, N., & Katz, N. (1991). A problem solving version of the Allen cognitive level test. *American Journal of Occupational Therapy, 45,* 331–338.

Kaplan, S. L., Hong, G. K., & Weinhold, C. (1984). Epidemiology of depressive symptomatology in adolescents. *Journal of the American Academy of Child and Adolescent Psychiatry, 23,* 91–98.

Kaslow, N., Deering, C. & Racusin, G. (1994). Depressed children and their families. *Clinical Psychology Review, 14*(1), 39–44.

Katz, N., Josman, N., & Steinmetz, N. (1988). Relationship between cognitive disability theory and the model of human occupation in the assessment of psychiatric and nonpsychiatric adolescents. *Occupational Therapy in Mental Health, 8*(1), 31–44.

Kielhofner, G. (Ed.) (1985). *A model of human occupation. Theory and application.* Baltimore: Williams & Wilkins.

Kielhofner, G. (Ed.) (1995). *A model of human occupation. Theory and application* (2d ed.). Baltimore: Williams & Wilkins.

Kielhofner, G. (1997). *Conceptual foundations of occupational therapy* (2d ed.). Philadelphia: F. A. Davis.

Kielhofner, G., Henry, A., & Walens, D. (1989). *A user's guide to the occupational performance history interview.* Rockville, MD: The American Occupational Therapy Association.

Kielhofner, G., Mallinson, T., & de las Heras, C. G. (1995). Methods of data gathering. In G. Kielhofner (Ed.), *A model of human occupation. Theory and application.* (2d ed., pp. 205–231). Baltimore: Williams & Wilkins.

Kimball, R. O. (1986). Experiential therapy for youths: The adventure model. *Children Today, 15*(2), 26–31.

Kimmel, D. C., & Weiner, I. B. (1995). *Adolescence: A developmental transition.* New York: Wiley.

Kinsella, K. B., Anderson, R. A., & Anderson, W. T. (1996). Coping skills, strengths, and needs as perceived by adult offspring and siblings of people with mental illness: A retrospective study. *Psychiatric Rehabilitation Journal, 20*,(2), 24–32.

Klein, H. (1990). Adolescence, youth, and young adulthood. *Youth & Society, 21*(4), 446–471.

Knis, L. L. (1995,). Coping skills: The play's the thing. *OT Week, 9*(35), 18–19.

Kovacs, M., & Goldston, D. (1991). Cognitive and social cognitive development of depressed children and adolescents. *Journal of the American Academy of Child Psychiatry, 30,* 388–392.

Kowatch, R. A., Emslie, G. J., & Kennard, B. D. (1996). In D. X. Parmelee (Ed.), *Child and adolescent psychiatry* (pp. 121–140). St. Louis: Mosby.

Lancaster, J., & Mitchell, M. (1991). Occupational therapy treatment goals, objectives, and activities for improving low self-esteem in adolescents with behavioral disorders. *Occupational Therapy in Mental Health, 11*(2/3), 3–22.

Lasko, D. S., Field, T. M., Gonzalez, K. P., Harding J., Yando, R., & Bendell, D. (1996). Adolescent depressed mood and parental unhappiness. *Adolescence, 31*(121), 49–57.

Leary, S. (1994). *Activities for personal growth: A comprehensive handbook of activities for therapists.* Sydney: MacLennan & Petty Pty. Limited.

Lederer, J. M., Kielhofner, G., & Watts, J. H. (1985). Values, personal causation and skills of delinquents and nondelinquents. *Occupational Therapy in Mental Health, 5*(2), 59–75.

Leigh, B. C., Shafer, J., & Temple, M. T. Alcohol use and contraception in first sexual experiences. *Journal of Behavioral Medicine, 18*(1), 81–95.

Lewinsohn, P. (1993). Psychosocial characteristics of adolescents with a history of suicide attempt. *Journal of the American Academy of Child and Adolescent Psychiatry, 32,* 60–68.

Lewis, S. A., Johnson, J., Cohen, P., Garcia, M., & Velez, C. N. (1988). Attempted suicide in youth: Its relationship to school achievement, educational goals, and socioeconomic status. *Journal of Abnormal Child Psychology, 16,* 459–471.

Lim, P. Y., & Agnew, P. (1994). Occupational therapy with eating disorders: a study on treatment approaches. *British Journal of Occupational Therapy, 57*(8), 309–314.

Lloyd, C. (1986). The process of goal setting using goal attainment scaling in a therapeutic community. *Occupational Therapy in Mental Health, 6*(3), 19–30.

Loeber, R. (1991). Oppositional defiant disorder and conduct disorder. *Hospital and Community Psychiatry, 42,* 1099–1102.

Lowe, M. R., Gleaves, D. H., DiSimone-Weiss, R. T., Furgueson, C., Gayda, C. A., Kolsky, P. A., Neal-Walden, T., Nelsen, L. A., & McKinney, S. (1996). Restraint, dieting, and the continuum model of bulimia nervosa. *Journal of Abnormal Psychology, 105*(4), 508–517.

Mann, D. (1998). New guidelines address substance abuse in children and adolescents. *Medical Tribune: Family Physician Edition, 39*(3).

Marcus, R. F. (1996). The friendships of delinquents. *Adolescence, 31*(121), 145–158.

Martin, J. E., (1991). Occupational therapy in bulimia. *British Journal of Occupational Therapy, 55*(2), 48–52.

Masse, L. C., & Tremblay, R. E., (1997). Behavior of boys in kindergarten and the onset of substance use during adolescence. *Archives of General Psychiatry, 54,* 62–68.

Matsutsuyu, J. (1969). The interest checklist. *American Journal of Occupational Therapy, 23,* 323–338.

McCauley, E., et al. (1993). Depression in young people: Initial presentation and clinical course. *Journal of the American Academy of Child and Adolescent Psychiatry, 32,* 714.

McColl, M. A., Friedland, J., & Kerr, A. (1986). When doing is not enough: The relationship between activity and effectiveness in anorexia nervosa. *Occupational Therapy in Mental Health, 6*(1), 137–150.

McGee, K., & McGee, J. (1986). Behavioral treatment of eating disorders. *Occupational Therapy in Mental Health, 6*(1), 15–25.

Mead, M. (1927/1949). *Coming of age in Samoa.* New York: Mentor Books.

Melia, M. A., & Weikert, K. (1989). Evaluation and treatment of adolescents on a short term unit. *Occupational Therapy in Mental Health, 7*(2), 51–66.

Morano, C. D., Cisler, R. A., & Lemerond, J. (1993). Risk factors for adolescent suicidal behavior: Loss, insufficient familial support, and hopelessness. *Adolescence, 28*(112).

Mosey, A. C. (1970). The concept and use of developmental groups. *American Journal of Occupational Therapy, 24,* 272–275.

Mosey, A. C. (1996). *Psychosocial components of occupational therapy.* Philadelphia: Lippincott-Raven.

Mufson, L., & Fairbanks, J. (1996). Interpersonal psychotherapy for depressed adolescents: A one-year naturalistic follow-up study. *Journal of the American Academy of Child and Adolescent Psychiatry, 35*(9), 1145–1155.

Mullen, D. J., & Hendren, R. L. (1996). The suicidal child or adolescent. In Parmelee, D. X. (Ed.), *Child and adolescent psychiatry* (pp. 225–235). St. Louis: Mosby.

Muuss, R. E. (1986). Adolescent eating disorder: Bulimia. *Adolescence, 21*(82), 257–267.

Nightingale, E. O., & Wolverton, L. (1993). Adolescent roleness in modern society. In Takanishi, R. (Ed.), *Adolescence in the 1990s: Risk and opportunity* (pp. 14–28). New York: Teachers College Press.

Oakley, F., Kielhofner, G., Barris, R., & Reichler, R. (1986). The role checklist: Development and empirical assessment of reliability. *Occupational Therapy Journal of Research, 6*(3), 157–170.

Offer, D., & Schonert-Reichl, K. A. (1992).

Debunking the myths of adolescence: Findings from recent research. *Journal of the American Academy of Child and Adolescent Psychiatry, 31*(6), 1003–1011.

Parmelee, D. X. (Ed.) (1996). *Child and adolescent psychiatry.* St. Louis: Mosby.

Paulson, C. P. (1980). Juvenile deliquency and occupational choice. *American Journal of Occupational Therapy, 34*(9), 565–571.

Payne, R. A. (1995). *Relaxation techniques: A practical handbook for the health care professional.* Edinburgh: Churchill Livingstone.

Pennington, V., & Sharott, G. W. (1985). The developmental tasks of adolescence and the role of occupational therapy. *Occupational Therapy in Health Care, 2*(3), 7–18.

Pezzulli, T. V. (1988). *Test-retest reliability of the role checklist with depressed adolescents in a short-term psychiatric hospital.* Unpublished master's thesis. Department of Occupational Therapy, Virginia Commonwealth University, Richmond, VA.

Pezzuti, L. (1979). An exploration of adolescent feminine and occupational behavior development. *American Journal of Occupational Therapy, 33*(2), 84–92.

Pezzuti, L. (1985). Self-concept/self-esteem development: Its relevance to occupational therapy. *Occupational Therapy in Health Care, 2*(3), 41–48.

Piaget, J. (1972). Intellectual evolution from adolescence to adulthood. *Human Development, 15,* 1–12.

Puskar, K. R., Lamb, J., & Tusaie-Mumford, K. (1997). Teaching kids to cope: A preventive mental health nursing strategy for adolescents. *Journal of Child & Adolescent Psychiatric Nursing, 10*(3), 18–28.

Rockwell, L. E., (1990). Frames of reference and modalities used by occupational therapists in the treatment of patients with eating disorders. *Occupational Therapy in Mental Health, 10*(2), 47–63.

Scarth, P. P. (1990). Services for chemically dependent adolescents. *Mental Health Special Interest Section Newsletter, 12,* 7–8.

Scheffel, D. L. (1996). Learning disorders. In Parmelee, D. X. (Ed.), *Child and adolescent psychiatry* (pp. 97–119). St. Louis: Mosby.

Schinke, S. P., Schilling, R. F., & Snow, W. H. (1987). Stress management with adolescents at the junior high transition: An outcome evaluation of coping skills intervention. *Journal of Human Stress, 13*(1), 16–22.

Schulenberg, J., & Ebata, A. T. (1994). United States. In Hurrelmann, K. (Ed.),

*International handbook of adolescence.* Westport, CT: Greenwood Press.

Schultz, S. (1997, April). *Treating students with behavioral disorders: Occupational adaptation model.* Institute presented at the annual meeting of the American Occupational Therapy Association, Orlando, FL.

Scott, A. H. (1984). Structuring goals via goal attainment scaling in occupational therapy groups in a partial hospitalization setting. *Occupational Therapy in Mental Health, 4*(2), 39–58.

Seiffge-Krenke, I. (1993). Coping behavior in normal and clinical samples: More similarities than differences? *Journal of Adolescence, 16*(3), 285–303.

Sholle-Martin, S. (1987). Application of the model of human occupation: Assessment in child and adolescent psychiatry. *Occupational Therapy in Mental Health, 7*(2), 7–22.

Smith, R. E. (1989). Effects of coping skills training on generalized self-efficacy and locus of control. *Journal of Personality and Social Psychology, 56,* 228–233.

Smyntek, L., Barris, R., & Kielhofner, G. (1985). The model of human occupation applied to pyschologically functional and dysfunctional adolescents. *Occupational Therapy in Mental Health, 5*(1), 21–39.

Sourander, A., Helenius, H., & Piha, J. (1969). Child psychiatric short-term inpatient treatment: CGAS as follow-up measure. *Child Psychiatry and Human Development, 27*(2), 93–104.

Steinberg, L. (1996). *Adolescence* (4th ed.) New York: McGraw-Hill.

Strober, M., et al. (1993). The course of major depressive disorder in adolescents I: Recovery and risk of manic switching in a follow-up of psychotic and non-psychotic subtypes. *Journal of the American Academy of Child and Adolescent Psychiatry, 32,* 34–42.

Takanishi, R. (1993). Changing views of adolescence in contemporary society. In R. Takanishi (Ed.), *Adolescence in the 1990s: Risk and opportunity.* New York: Teachers College Press.

Talbot, J. F. (1983). An inpatient adolescent living skills program. *Occupational Therapy in Mental Health, 3*(4), 35–45.

Temple, S., & Robson, P. (1991). The effect of assertiveness training on self-esteem. *British Journal of Occupational Therapy, 54*(9), 329–332.

Thompson, K. L., Bundy, K. A., & Wolfe, W. R. (1996). Social skills training for young adolescents: Cognitive and performance components. *Adolescence, 31*(123), 505–521.

Thompson, K. L., Bundy, K. A., & Broncheau, C. (1995). Social skills training for young adolescents: Symbolic and behavioral components. *Adolescence, 30*(119), 724–734.

Tubesing, D. A., & Tubesing, N. L. (1991). *Seeking your healthy balance: A do-it-yourself guide to whole person well-being.* Duluth: Whole Person Associates.

Waller, D. (1996). Eating disorders. In D. X. Parmelee (Ed.), *Child and adolescent psychiatry* (pp. 141–151). St. Louis: Mosby.

Weinberg, W. A. (1973). Depression in children referred to an educational diagnostic center: Diagnosis and treatment. *Journal of Pediatrics, 83,* 1065–1072.

Weissenberg, R. (1989). Home economics day: A program for disturbed adolescents to promote acquisition of habits and skills. *Occupational Therapy in Mental Health, 9*(2), 89–103.

Williamson, G. G., Szczepanski, M., & Zeitlin, S. (1993). Coping frame of reference. In P. Kramer & J. Hinojosa (Eds.), *Frames of reference for pediatric occupational therapy.* Baltimore: Williams & Wilkins.

Windle, M., Hooker, K., Lenerz, K., East, P. L., Lerner, J. V., & Lerner, R. M. (1986). Temperament, perceived competence, and depression in early and late adolescents. *Developmental Psychology, 22,* 384–392.

Wise, K. L., Bundy, K. A., Bundy, E. A., & Wise, L. A. (1991). Social skills training for young adolescents. *Adolescence, 26*(101), 223–241.

Wood, I. K. (1996). Conduct disorder and oppositional defiant disorder. In D. X. Parmelee (Ed.), *Child and adolescent psychiatry* (pp. 83–95). St. Louis: Mosby.

Yalom, I. D. (1970). *The theory and practice of groups.* New York: Basic Books.

Yalom, I. D. (1983). *Inpatient group psychotherapy.* New York: Basic Books.

Zito, J. M., & Safer, D. J. (1997). Sources of data for pharmacoepidemiological studies of child and adolescent psychiatric disorders. *Journal of Child and Adolescent Psychopharmacology, 7*(4), 237–53.

Zonnaveldt, A. (1969). Music therapy with adolescents. *Acta-Paedopsychiatrica, 36*(5), 127–130.

# 13

# *Children as Burn Patients*

Susan Miller Porr, MEd, MS, OTR

*To maintain one's aspirations in the face of grave adversity, to work hard, to contend successfully with the daily assault of an impaired body on a robust spirit, to be victorious over the long course of losses and threats that constitute disability—these are lessons for all of us, examples of what is best in our shared humanity. Each of us, even the most advantaged, has need of all the good examples we can find.*

—A. Kleinman (1988), p. 138

**KEY POINTS**

- Pediatric burn care is a specialized field drawing on the skills of multiple disciplines in both acute and rehabilitation situations.

- OTs are actively involved in the acute, rehabilitation, and outpatient phases of pediatric burn care.

- Burns are a leading cause of injury and death in young children, and prevention practices continue to need community attention.

## BEGINNINGS

"Don't play with matches!" "Watch, the cocoa will burn!" and "The stove is HOT!" are childhood admonitions most people can recall. For 60,000 children a year, the scolding comes too late or not at all and burns are the result (Attorri, Randolph, & Orrawin, 1993).

The area of pediatric burn care has become a clinical specialty all of its own in the past 20 years. Medical caregivers have realized that children's smaller sizes and rapid developmental changes have mandated healthcare delivery that is different from that needed by adults (Attorri et al., 1993). The multiple issues surrounding the care of children with burns call for the skills and expertise of the burn team as well as the support of family and community members. OTs have developed a unique niche in this care spectrum that includes both physical disabilities skills and the psychosocial understanding of children's development.

## THE CLINICAL PICTURE

In the United States over 2 million burn accidents are counted on an annual basis (Carvajal & Parks, 1988). Of this large number, 40 percent involve children. Most pediatric burns occur in the home, and the cause of the burn tends to be different for specific age groups. The more common causes of burns in different age groups are listed in the accompanying table.

| Age of the Child | Type of Burn |
| --- | --- |
| Infants and the very young | Sunburn |
| Toddlers | Scalds from hot liquids, i.e., pulling cord on coffeepot |
| Preschoolers | Flame burns from stoves or matches |
| Schoolage children | Match burns in elementary-age children |
| Adolescents | Burns from flammable liquids (experimenting and risk-taking behaviors) |

*Source:* Data from Archambeault-Jones & Feller, 1983; McLoughlin et al., 1980.

Recent literature on burns has noted, unfortunately, a rise in the number of burns resulting from abuse (Leveridge, 1991; Schanberger, 1983). The majority of these occur in children under the age of 5. The major concern in these instances is to protect the child when danger can be anticipated.

## BURN PHYSIOLOGY 101

A burn can be caused by excessive heat, chemicals, X ray, ultraviolet light, or electricity. The burn agent generally comes in contact with the child's skin first. Skin acts as both a barrier for disease and a climate control "blanket" for the rest of the body. When the body is exposed to excess heat the skin reacts in the following way: Blood vessels in the skin expand (attempting to cool the area) and redness is seen. If this doesn't cool the area, the body tries to get rid of more heat and in the process plasma leaks out of damaged blood vessels (this creates edema). If there is too much heat the cells die and the degree of destruction becomes more severe (Leveridge, 1991).

The extent of the destruction caused by a burn is often discussed in the language by "degrees" or by the thickness of the tissue destroyed (Fig. 13–1). The accompanying chart may be helpful in understanding this terminology. It is important to note that actual pain from a burn may be *inversely* related to the depth of the burn (Hamill, Rest, & Nielson, 1983). For example, a child with a third-degree burn has less pain because of the damage of the nerve endings in the skin and the subsequent loss of sensation.

|  | **Thickness** | **Appearance and Damage** | **Concerns** |
|---|---|---|---|
| First-degree burn | Superficial | Redness, on top skin layer (epidermis) | Painful, some swelling, usually heals on own |
| Second-degree burn | Partial thickness | Blistered "weepy" skin, major epidermal loss | Very painful, major risks of infection; contracture and scarring risks high |
| Third-degree burn | Full thickness | Entire skin gone | No sensation, grafts needed for new skin |

*Source:* Data from Attorri et al., 1993; Hamill et al., 1983.

The wound-healing process is a critical one to consider for all burn patients. Connective tissue, which is a major component of the dermal layer of the skin, goes through changes that can cause scarring, loss of range of motion (ROM), and loss of functional skill in a young patient with burns. Burn teams direct their therapy efforts toward preventing and/or minimizing these negative outcomes.

The connective tissue portion of the dermis is made up of *fibers* and

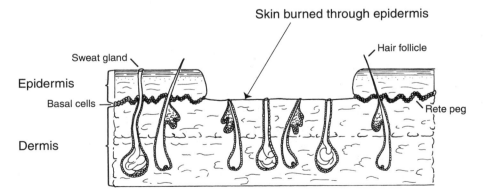

Figure 13–1 Burn through partial skin thickness. [*Source:* From Greenhalgh, D. G., & Staley, M. J. (1994). Burn wound healing. In R. L. Richard & M. J. Staley (Eds.). *Burn care and rehabilitation: Principles and practice* (p. 84). Philadelphia: F. A. Davis.]

*ground* (the gel-like "stuff" between the fibers that makes skin dense). There are three types of these connective fibers: (1) *collagen,* which makes skin strong and gives it stiffness, (2) *elastin,* which, like its name, gives skin elasticity and also forms a structure for other fibers to grow on; and (3) *reticulin,* which are fine fibers similar to collagen; reticulin fibers are the least numerous of the three in normal skin (Price, 1990).

In the early phases of the burn-healing process the skin makes an oversupply of collagen. This is then followed by a period in the healing where the collagen is broken down faster than it is made. This should end up in a even balance of collagen production. Unfortunately for many burn patients there is an "oversupply" of collagen, which produces *hypertrophic scarring.*

As experts have noted (Price, 1990; Staley & Richard, 1994), there are no predictors of whether excessive scarring will occur. Certain variables, among them race and location of the scar, may predispose patients toward excessive scarring. Interventions such as stretching and constant pressure can make changes in tissue when applied early in the rehabilitation program.

# OVERVIEW OF
# CLINICAL INTERVENTIONS:
# A TEAM APPROACH

As noted earlier in the chapter, the care of a child with burns is a team endeavor. Physicians, therapists, nurses, dietitians, and psychologists work along with other health-related personnel to provide a comprehensive approach to meeting the child and family's needs. The process for treating a child with burns begins in the often life-threatening acute stage and progresses through rehabilitation to outpatient care. This situation may span numerous years of a child's life.

In the acute phases a pediatric burn patient may need medical management to maintain a good airway (because of inhalation injury) and guard against "burn shock," which if unchecked, may be fatal (Morgan, 1991). Other early injury concerns include managing the child's fluid balance and temperature. The skin, which usually does these two jobs so well, has been compromised or is no longer there to work in the case of the burned child. Infection control is a major concern for burn patients in the acute phase. It is, in fact, the leading cause of death from burns in children (Attorri et al., 1993). In earlier years patients with burns were isolated to decrease infection risk; today better methods of controlling bacteria (i.e., with topical chemicals) and early surgical closing of wounds have decreased this medical practice (Constable, 1994; Johnson, 1994).

The rehabilitation process for children with burns involves working with scars; the ones that impede physical function and the emotional ones left on the psyche as a consequence of the trauma. There are many factors that come to play in the rehab process. These include: (1) the child's health status prior to the burn; (2) the severity of the injury and subsequent complications; and (3) the way the burn was treated immediately after the incident occurred (Reeves, Warden, & Staley, 1994). Families also play a major part in the rehabilitation process in regard to follow-up for appointments and as care managers after discharge.

Discharge planning is done in the final phases of the rehabilitation stay. The burn team will address with parents and caregivers any special instructions regarding protocols for special equipment or material (i.e., splints). Future surgery is often discussed at this time as children grow and require procedures to allow proper body growth. The community "re-entry" situation is also a concern for many parents and children. "Back-to-school" programs are often provided by therapists, psychologists, and other social support personnel. This allows for questions to be answered and for other children to prepare for their schoolmate's return.

A burn unit is more than a specialized facility for treatment. For many children it becomes their temporary home during a traumatic period in their lives. The people, not the place, make that unit a compassionate, caring refuge for successful recovery.

# INTERVENTION FROM THE OCCUPATIONAL THERAPY PERSPECTIVE

OTs are involved with pediatric burn patients from the intense acute stages to the outpatient follow-ups for splinting and other equipment and supply needs. As members of the burn team, OTs are concerned with ROM and positioning in the early stages of treatment. Occupational therapy rehab tasks include: (1) working on the child's everyday functional skills, such as feeding and dressing; (2) promoting strengthening and active ROM through play; and (3) often fitting and assisting with elastic pressure garments used for scar control. All of these tasks take place within the parameters of compassionate concern for the psychological state of young burn patients (Leveridge, 1991; Reeves et al., 1994).

# THE ASSESSMENT PROCESS

The assessment process is an ongoing one for the therapist working with the pediatric burn patient. Initial information available to the therapist includes the medical record and social and developmental information gathered from parent interview or other sources. This information provides background regarding the acute burn situation and the child's general status prior to the incident (Fader, 1988).

The physical components of the assessment may include an evaluation of the components listed in the accompanying table. Answering these questions will give the therapist a springboard for planning appropriate interventions for the child. Therapy goals are frequently focused on the areas of: (1) positioning, (2) improving functioning in daily life activities, and (3) reducing scarring and deformity. Although additional information is provided in these three areas, the therapist concentrating on pediatric burn care needs continuous updating in this field where technology and techniques are often changing.

| Component | Concerns |
| --- | --- |
| Actual wound site | How severe is the burn wound? (see following Therapeds Pointer) |
| Area surrounding the wound | What joints are involved? What is ROM? Is there swelling in the area? **Caution:** ROM may be limited by pain and swelling; proceed with care. |
| Child's present abilities | What activities of daily living (ADLs) are intact? Which need adaption or rehab? What is child's physical strength level? What is child's tolerance or endurance level at the present time for activity? |

*Source:* Data from Fader, 1988.

■ *THERAPEDS POINTER*

As noted earlier in the chapter, burn wounds are often defined by "degree" or thickness of tissue involved. The extent of the body surface that is involved is also another way of looking at the severity of a burn. This figure, total body surface area (TBSA), if often given in percentages in medical records, along with a chart indicating the areas of the body that are affected. For adults this TBSA figure is often in multiples of 9—hence "the rule of nines" (Fig. 13–2). For children (especially those under 5 years of age), the head and neck areas make up a much larger percentage of the TBSA than in adults. Burn estimate charts (Table 13–1) give a more accurate picture for children than the rule-of-nines diagram (McManus & Pruitt, 1991).

# INTERVENTION

## POSITIONING

Positioning of the child is an early concern for the OT treating a burned child. Many children prefer the fetal position, which is also known as the "position of comfort." This position, with the child's neck in flexion, elbows in flexion, arms pronated, and knees flexed, usually promotes contractures (Apfel, Ir-

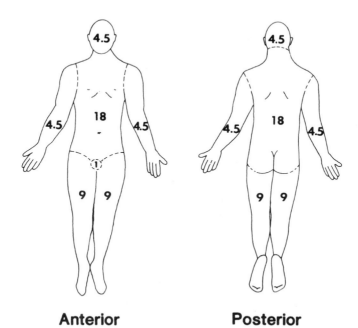

**Anterior**          **Posterior**

Figure 13–2 Rule of nines. [*Source:* From Miller, S. F., Richard, R. L., & Staley, M. J. (1994). Triage and resuscitation of the burn patient. In R. L. Richard & M. J. Staley (Eds.). *Burn care and rehabilitation: Principles and practice* (p. 109). Philadelphia: F. A. Davis.]

Table 13–1  **Child Burn Size Estimation Table (Percent Total Body Surface Area)**

| Burn Area | Age (years) | | | | |
| --- | --- | --- | --- | --- | --- |
| | **1** | **1–4** | **5–9** | **10–14** | **15** |
| Head | 19 | 17 | 13 | 11 | 9 |
| Neck | 2 | 2 | 2 | 2 | 2 |
| Anterior trunk | 13 | 13 | 13 | 13 | 13 |
| Posterior trunk | 18 | 18 | 18 | 18 | 18 |
| Genitalia | 1 | 1 | 1 | 1 | 1 |
| Upper extremity (each) | 9 | 9 | 9 | 9 | 9 |
| Lower extremity (each) | 14.5 | 15.5 | 17.5 | 18.5 | 19.5 |

*Source*: Reproduced from Miller, Richard, & Staley (1994), with permission.

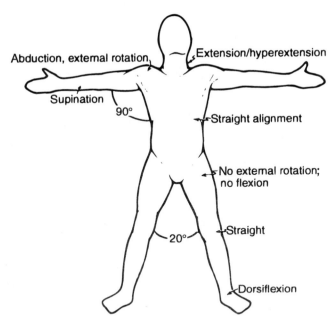

Figure 13–3 Positioning to prevent contracture. [*Source:* From Apfel, L. M., Irwin, C. P., Staley, M. J., & Richard, R. L. (1994). Approaches to positioning the burn patient. In R. L. Richard & M. J. Staley (Eds.). *Burn care and rehabilitation: Principles and practice* (p. 223). Philadelphia: F. A. Davis.]

win, Staley & Richard, 1994). Children do not readily lie in contracture-reducing positions (Fig. 13–3). Contracture, a shortening or tightening of a skin area, is a normal process in wound healing (Robson & Kucan, 1983). Other medical issues that need to be considered in positioning a child include good positioning for respiration and positions that decrease pressure and stretching of grafted and "donor sites" (places skin was taken from). At times the neck, ear, and axilla areas may need to be evaluated for special positioning depending on the location of the burns (Fader, 1988).

## SPLINTING

Splinting involves the use of customized forms to maintain a body part in a certain position. Splints can be used in all phases of the burn recovery process from the acute phase to later reconstructive surgery. Each phase will raise specific concerns for the therapist regarding the type of splint to be used and the reason for its application (Daugherty & Carr-Collins, 1994). For example, for patients with burns, splints may be used to provide pressure to an area of the body for scar-control purposes as well as for positioning. Although splints may provide both positioning and scar control for a child with burns, a delicate balance must be struck. The child's needs for functional mobility, that is for ADL, and the long-term costs of immobility must be considered when splinting a child (Lemaster, 1983).

## ▮▮▮ FROM THE BOOKSHELF

Reginald Richard and Marlys Staley have collaborated to produce an excellent text on rehabilitation issues in treating patients with burns. *Burn Care and Rehabilitation* (1994; F. A. Davis) has numerous contributors who are OTs working on burn units. The chapter on splinting by Daugherty and Carr-Collins is comprehensive and up-to-date as a resource. For those considering work in this field, this book is a superb professional reference for the library.

Splinting today has been positively influenced by the use of thermo-plastics (plastic splint materials that become moldable when heated). Although materials for splints have changed, the basic designs have stood the test of time (Daugherty & Carr-Collins, 1994). Splints commonly used with pediatric patients include neck conformer splints, hand splints, and knee and elbow splints (Doane, 1989).

### ▮ *THERAPEDS POINTER*

Splints for children with burns may be made out of a variety of materials. The accompanying chart highlights some of the more common materials used in pediatric splinting for burns.

| Splinting Materials for Burns | |
|---|---|
| Low-thermal plastics (low-heat plastics) | Most popular for splints for pediatric burns as they are easy to mold and to clean. |
| High-heat plastics | Often are used for face masks (clear color) to provide pressure to decrease scarring; children seem to prefer these clear plastics. |
| Silicone | Like the plastics above but more flexible; used to make pressure molds under elastic pressure masks for face; parents seem to like these as they are more difficult for a child to remove. |
| Foams | Two types of foam: open-cell and closed-cell foams are often used in conjunction with other materials to make splints; closed-cell foams can be cleaned; open-cell foams are not easily cleaned. |

*Source:* Data from Fader, 1988.

Splinting children comes with its own challenges; those with anxiety about being hurt or resistant to sitting still for the process make this task a true challenge for the therapist. This is where both the psychological and the physical realms of occupational therapy training truly come into play!

Once the decision to splint a pediatric patient has been made, parameters beyond actual splint fabrication need to be considered. Concerns regarding children's thinner skin and the possible hypermobility of joints (extra flexible) need to be addressed by the therapist. Young children may also have problems tolerating dynamic splints (those with movable parts) that may readily be used by an older child or an adult (Reeves et al., 1994).

It is *very important* to leave complete written instructions for all caregivers and parents regarding the use of the splints. Pictures and illustrations are also helpful in the education process as a visual reference for others (Leman & Ricks, 1994). When feasible, wearing instructions may be written directly on the splint in permanent marker (Reeves et al., 1994). This may include directional labels for application (i.e., "top," "thumb side . . .") (Daugherty & Collins-Carr, 1994). Instructions should include the wearing schedule, why the splint is being used, correct splint application, and any additional precautions necessary for safe, effective splint usage.

## SCAR CONTROL

The formation of excessive scar tissue (hypertrophic scars) is an ongoing concern with pediatric burn patients. The formation of this excessive scar tissue is related to the damaged skin's responses in the wound-healing phase (Price, 1990). As noted earlier, there is an increase in the amount of collagen (a "building material" of new skin). This collagen seems to be sticky and tends to "clump" in bundles rather than form smooth skin surfaces (Malick & Carr, 1980). The hypertropic scarring, which has a lumpy, thickened appearance, has serious cosmetic and functional movement consequences for many individuals with burns.

OTs are often involved from the beginning with burn scar management via positioning and splinting discussed above. Elastic pressure garments (i.e., those manufactured by Jobst) have been used successfully for many burn situations to provide consistent pressure to scarred areas over long periods of time. These garments, when used according to a strict wearing protocol, have been very successful in decreasing nodular scar formation (Malick & Carr, 1980; Staley & Richard, 1994).

The garments themselves are custom-tailored for each patient, and fitting them requires training and accurate measurement. The clothing is similar to "body suit" pieces made from high-pressure elasticized fabric. They fit like a second skin but should allow children to move freely about in their daily activities. Because of healing changes and children's rapid growth, these garments must be monitored *at least* monthly for fit. Written instructions for their care should be provided to the family, and often two sets of the garments are provided to the child (one to wash and one to wear).

Additional pressure to scars in specific areas such as the hands and face is sometimes provided by specialized splints, molds, and masks. The discussion of these specific splints is beyond the scope of this text, but therapists working in burn care are encouraged to pursue additional information in this area when working with pediatric burn cases.

## FUNCTIONAL LIVING SKILLS

OTs working with children who have been burned are responsible for assessing and encouraging increased independence in their young patients. Basic self-care activities, with a physician's approval, should be started early in the child's recovery process (Doane, 1989). Working with children on feeding and dressing skills may require temporary adaptations. In the independent-feeding area the use of spoons with built-up or longer handles will encourage self-feeding. It is important to wean the child away from these adaptions as soon as possible to encourage continued functional achievements.

Allowing the child to help with dressing changes encourages independence and a sense of control in a situation where this is not always possible. In considering dressing skills, clothing may need adaptions to fit over dressings and splints. Methods for donning and doffing garments may also be altered because of decreased hand function or ROM limitations.

Play activities are frequently motivators for young children and allow them to work on skills in an enjoyable way. Initial therapy may focus on increasing a child's active ROM through play activities and games that encourage these movements. Basketball activities with lightweight balls and varied hoop heights encourage range while making "2 pointers." When medically safe, blowing bubbles and using wands ("pop the big bubbles," "move the wand to make more bubbles") provide play with a purpose. These toys are enticing tools for encouraging work on hand movements and oral and facial flexibility. Bicycles and tricycles may promote increased ROM as well as strengthening and coordination in the patient's lower extremities (Reeves et al., 1994). Creative ideas are often only limited by a therapist's imagination and the medical concerns for the child. In choosing therapy tasks for children with burns there are some special issues to consider:

1. Arts and crafts and play materials must be evaluated for their possible contamination risks to the burn site.
2. Trauma to graft sites via overly energetic movements must be avoided. In the "fever" of the game this may be a very real concern!
3. As in all therapy activities, the appropriateness of the play materials must be viewed in regard to the child's age and cognitive skills; for example, small game parts and items such as balloons present a choking hazard for younger children (Reeves et al., 1994).

With older children, puzzles and game boards may be modified to promote fine motor movements in a social, cooperative context. Hobbies and age-appropriate interests (i.e., computer games) also offer opportunities to combine therapy and recreation when they can be graded for physical demands and cognitive complexity.

# PSYCHOSOCIAL CONCERNS: THE SCARS THAT DON'T SHOW

The psychosocial adjustment of the child with severe burns should be considered a long-term goal. A patient with burns is required to deal with stressors such as pain, disfigurement, and functional limitation, which may impact on that adjustment process (Bryant, 1996). Unlike adults, the age factor plays into the child's ability to handle this difficult situation. Although toddlers may exhibit separation anxiety, their grade school counterparts appear agitated and angry. Adolescents dealing developmentally with "control" issues may rebel and be noncompliant at therapy or simply withdraw from all of the demands. Adolescents also tend to have more difficulty with depression in the long-term adjustment period (Moss, Everett & Patterson, 1994).

In a study of 60 pediatric patients with burns (Robert et al., 1997), several general themes regarding psychological adjustment were revealed. These survivors, as a group, shared some universal concerns regarding their recovery and life to come. The five thematic areas that emerged through sentence completion tasks for this group included: (1) a preoccupation with health (illness vs. wellness), (2) the internal struggle of acceptance (i.e., anger vs. determination, (3) successful reconstruction of a "new life map," and the related topics of (4) changing relationships, and (5) redefining the world.

Each child, in this adjustment period, copes differently with issues such as those just noted. Roberts et al. (1997) found that all burn-care professionals can be called on to help in this adjustment. Educating the child as to what is "normal" in a traumatic situation and acknowledging that others have shared this dilemma provides reassurance to these young people. Statements such as "other children worry about . . ." and "people usually have many new concerns after a burn accident" (Roberts et al., 1997, p. 53) may open dialogue of discussing internal conflict.

Specific occupational therapy tasks may also help these young burn survivors with the psychological healing process. Games and activities where children can demonstrate competence help to build self-esteem. Relaxation techniques may be used to reduce anxiety in these children when they are used properly (Doane, 1989). Outings into the community may also be planned as children prepare to re-enter the world. Providing a "safe group" with which to travel when going to the mall or the local hamburger stand gives support. A chance to reflect with others on the unit afterward on "how it went" may also provide insights for future ventures into the "life after the burn." All of these tasks help children to build the comfort zone needed before one is discharged to home, family, and awaiting friends.

---

■ *THERAPEDS POINTER*

Children who have undergone traumatic situations frequently demand from professionals special skills when handling the emotional and psychological issues. The following points to consider may make the positive difference to a young patient on the burn unit.

---

**A Little Child Psychology Helps**

- Develop trust with the child and be truthful, in advance, about the nature of a treatment or procedure.

- Have a place on the unit where children can play with *no* treatment allowed—a "safe haven."

- Give children choices in therapy and treatment, but *only* when they can have a choice!

- Crying is allowed, but beware of behaviors (i.e., kicking, thrashing) that may compromise the safety of an intervention.

- Use "peer buddies" to help patients, especially adolescents, through the traumatic times. (The "been there—done that" rapport of teenage burn patients may be notably supportive.)

- Consider the use of "cooperation contracts" with challenging young patients.

---

*Source:* Data from Fader, 1988; Reeves et al., 1994.

The ultimate goals of the rehabilitation program for the child with burns are to promote independent functioning and to return him or her to the home and community setting with the social and psychological support for a successfully re-entry.

# DISCHARGE PLANNING

"Going home" for the pediatric burn patient is a memorable day. Children often spend weeks and months on a burn unit, and discharge planning involves all members of the team. Proper written instructions regarding all special splints, materials, and equipment should be reviewed and provided to parents. Frequent outpatient follow-up is needed to monitor such concerns as pressure garment fit and scar healing. Preparing families ahead of time for needed reconstructive or cosmetic surgeries in the future is also done before discharge.

Therapists, along with social workers or psychologists, are often involved in school reentry programs mentioned earlier in the chapter. The child can also be involved with the planning process as a partner in the re-entry process. Programs may include video materials, lectures, and "share and tell" examples such as splints and/or pressure garments. Explanations regarding how the burn happened, the hospitalization process, and special equipment and procedures (i.e., face masks, skin care) can be shared with staff and students (as appropriate) at this time (Leman & Ricks, 1994). It is important to remind all involved that a child is still a child and getting back to normal is a prime goal for these children.

Follow-up for pediatric burn patients should continue until they are developmentally full grown (Leman & Ricks, 1994). A primary school child may appear to have recovered fully and then several years later may run into difficulties. Growth spurts, scar changes, and psychological issues may all occur at a later date; children with burns are long-term follow-up candidates (Doane, 1989).

## A WORD ABOUT PREVENTION

The *Project Burn Prevention: Final Report* (McLoughlin et al., 1980) noted that one study found that 90 percent of burns resulted from the "way people behave." For children the behaviors may be spurred by curiosity, exploratory needs, or impulsivity. Although "round the clock" vigilance may be the only perfect, but not feasible, solution to preventing burns, some actions can be helpful. National regulations regarding the flammability of children's sleepwear are already in place. Home measures such as installing smoke detectors and reducing temperatures on hot-water heaters may further reduce burns from fire and scalding. Burn prevention advocates also look toward a future with mandated "kidproofing" on cigarette lighters and requirements on building sprinkler systems. As healthcare providers to families and children, therapists have an excellent opportunity to alert parents to the home hazards that cause burns.

## WRAPPING IT UP

OTs working with pediatric burn patients must call on a broad repertoire of therapeutic skills. The clinical expertise areas of splinting, positioning, and scar management should be combined with the compassion and caring needed for handling traumatized children.

From the "high-pressure" stages of acute care medicine to the final discharge planning, OTs providing services to burn units need specialized expertise. They must be knowledgeable about the nature of the burn trauma, the developmental status of the child, and the clinical protocol that will allow for maximizing a child's return to functional independence.

### CASE STORY

Brad is a 5-year-old boy who has been admitted to your burn unit from a small local emergency room (ER) about 3 hours away. Preliminary medical information indicates he was burned on his body by flames from a match fire started in his kitchen. Figure 13–4 and the burn surface area chart indicate the extent of the burns as noted by the ER staff. As the therapist you are concerned about positioning and splinting. Using the accompanying graphics and the reference chart in the chapter assess the following:

1. What is the approximate total body surface area (TBSA) involved in the burn? _____%
2. What medical concerns and conditions should you consider when planning positioning for Brad? (There could be several!)
3. What joints and/or appendages may be of particular concern regarding splinting, contractures, and functional mobility?

Burn diagram: Age 5 Sex-M Wt.: 40 lb.

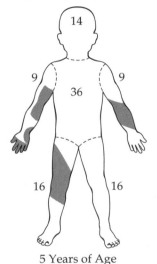

5 Years of Age

▰ Burns

Chart information*: Brad X. 5 yrs. 3 mos.

S: "I told him to never play with matches" by distraught parent; incident occurred 15 minutes prior to 911 call

O: Child conscious, no difficulty in breathing; may be in shock, TBSA chart completed; patient is in notable pain

A: TBSA charted; majority 2nd-degree burns; left hand more severe (2–3?); airway intact

P: 1. treat for shock

   2. evac to burn unit

   3. pain management

Also see burn estimates, age 5–9 yrs (Table 13–1).

Figure 13–4 Brad's burns. [*Source:* Adapted from Malik, M. (1983). Functional restoration burns. In H. L. Hopkins & H. D. Smith (Eds.), *Willard and Spackman's occupational therapy* (6th ed.). Philadelphia: J. B. Lippincott.]

*This chart is in SOAP note form where S = subjective information, O = objective information, A = assessment, and P = plan.

# Real-Life Lab

**1.** An 18-month-old female infant has been admitted to the burn unit with second-degree burns to her back and arms. Grafting donor sites* have included her buttocks. The burn team has asked for an OT to design a "bed frame" to maintain the child in prone position with hips flexed slightly to allow for good positioning and decreased pressure on the graft donor sites (buttocks). Sketch below what you might consider making and list possible materials (i.e., foam, sheepskin, splinting materials) needed for the fabrication.

| Bed "Working Plan" | Materials and Supplies |
| --- | --- |
| | |

**2.** You have been working with a 4-year-old girl who has marked facial scarring secondary to a facial burn from a kerosene heater fire (Fig. 13–5). Your therapy plan includes activities to increase flexibility in the mouth and cheek areas. Brainstorm with colleagues several play-type activities that would include movement in this facial area. (Food for thought: imitation, straws, "dress-ups"). Remember to address development concerns regarding age and safety.

| Activity Description | What Will This Do? Why Is It Helpful? |
| --- | --- |
| | |

*Donor sites are places skin was taken from for grafts.

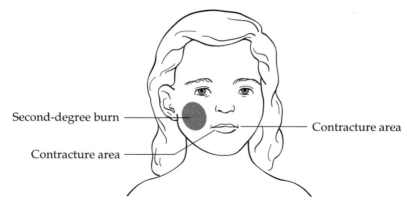

Second-degree burn

Contracture area

Contracture area

Figure 13–5  Facial area burns.

# References

Apfel, L. M., Irwin, C. P., Staley, M. J., & Richard, R. L. (1994). Approaches to positioning the burn patient. In R. L. Richard & M. J. Staley (Eds.). *Burn care and rehabilitation: Principles and practices* (pp. 221–242). Philadelphia: F. A. Davis.

Archambeault-Jones, C., & Feller, I. (1983). Burn nursing is nursing. In Wachtel, T. L., Kahn, V., & Hugh, H. A. (Eds.), *Current topics in burn care* (pp. 187–202). Rockville, MD: Aspen Systems Corporation.

Attorri, R. J., Randolph, J. G., & Orrawin, T. (1993). Burns in children. In P. R. Holbrook (Ed.). *Textbook of pediatric critical care* (pp. 1092–1101). Philadelphia: W. B. Saunders.

Bryant, R. A. (1996). Predictors of post-traumatic stress disorder following burns injury. *Burns: Journal of the International Society for Burn Injuries, 22* (2), 89–92.

Carvajal, H. F., & Parks, D. H. (Eds.). (1988). *Burns in children: Pediatric burn management.* Chicago: Year Book.

Constable, J. D. (1994). The state of burn care: Past, present, and future. *Burns, 20* (4), 316–324.

Daugherty, M. B., & Carr-Collins, J. A. (1994). Splinting techniques for the burn patient. In R. L. Richard & M. J. Staley. (Eds.). *Burn care and rehabilitation: Principles and practices* (pp. 242–323). Philadelphia: F. A. Davis.

Doane, C. B. (1989). Children with severe burns. In P. N. Pratt & A. S. Allen (Eds.). *Occupational therapy for children* (pp. 524–534). St. Louis: C. V. Mosby.

Fader, P. (1988). Preserving function and minimizing deformity: The role of the occupational therapist. In H. F. Carvajal & D. H. Parks (Eds.). *Burns in children: Pediatric burn management* (pp. 324–344). Chicago: Year Book.

Greenhalgh, D. G., & Staley, M. J. (1994). Burn wound healing. In R. L. Richard & M. J. Staley (Eds). *Burn care and rehabilitation: Principles and practices* (pp. 70–102). Philadelphia: F. A. Davis.

Hamill, W. T., Rest, S., & Nielson, J. (1983). Stress management in burn cases. In T. L. Wachtel, V. Kahn, & H. A. Frank (Eds.). *Current topics in burn care* (pp. 203–206). Rockville, MD: Aspen Systems Corporation.

Johnson, C. (1994). Pathologic manifestations of burn injury. In R. L. Richard & M. J. Staley. *Burn care and rehabilitation: Principles and practices* (pp. 29–48). Philadelphia: F. A. Davis.

Kleinman, A. (1988). *The illness narratives: Suffering, healing, and the human condition.* New York: Basic Books.

Leman, C. J., & Ricks, N. (1994). Discharge planning and follow-up burn care. In R. L. Richard & M. J. Staley (Eds.). *Burn care and rehabilitation: Principles and practices* (pp. 447–472). Philadelphia: F. A. Davis.

Lemaster, J. E. (1983). Rehabilitation of the burn-injured patient. In T. L. Wachtel, V. Kahn, & H. A. Frank (Eds.). *Current topics in burn care* (pp 217–230). Rockville, MD: Aspen Systems Corporation.

Leveridge, A. (Ed.). (1991). *Therapy for the burn patient.* London: Chapman & Hall.

McLoughlin, E., Vincem, C. H., Lee, A.,

MacKay, A., Halpern, J., & Crawford, J. D. (1980). *Project Burn Prevention: Final Report*. (Contract #C-75-0107) Washington, D.C.: U.S. Consumer Product Safety Commission.

Malick, M. (1983). Functional restoration-burns. In H. L. Hopkins & H. D. Smith (Eds.). *Willard and Spackman's occupational therapy* (6th ed.) (pp. 479–493). Philadelphia: J. B. Lippincott.

Malick, M. H., & Carr, J. A. (1980). Flexible elastomer molds in burn scar control. *The American Journal of Occupational Therapy (34)*, 603–608.

McManus, W. F., & Pruitt, B. A. (1991). Thermal injuries. In E. E. Moore, K. L. Mattox & D. V. Feliciano (Eds.). *Trauma* (2d ed.). Norwalk, CT: Appleton & Lange.

Miller, S. F., Richard, R. L., & Staley, M. J. (1994). Triage and resuscitation of the burn patient. In R. L. Richard & M. J. Staley, (Eds.). *Burn care and rehabilitation: Principles and practices* (pp. 105–118) Philadelphia: F. A. Davis.

Morgan, B. (1991). Pathology of burns. In A. Leveridge (Ed.). *Therapy for the burn patient* (pp. 10–15). London: Chapman & Hall.

Moss, B. F., Everett, J. J., & Patterson, D. R. (1994). Psychologic support and pain management of the burn patient. In R. L. Richard & M. J. Staley (Eds.). *Burn care and rehabilitation: Principles and practices* (pp. 475–498). Philadelphia: F. A. Davis.

Price, H. (1990). Connective tissue in wound healing. In L. C. Kloth, J. M. McCulloch, & J. A. Feedar (Eds.). *Wound healing: Alternatives in management* (pp. 31–42). Philadelphia: F. A. Davis.

Reeves, S. U., Warden, G., & Staley, M. J. (1994). Management of the pediatric burn patient. In R. L. Richard & M. J. Staley (Eds.). *Burn care and Rehabilitation: Principles and practice* (pp. 499–530). Philadelphia: F. A. Davis.

Robert, R., Berton, M., Moore, P., Murphy, L., Meyer, W., Blakeney, P., & Herdon, D. (1997). Applying what burn survivors have to say to future therapeutic interventions. *Burns: Journal of the International Society for Burn Injuries, 23* (1), 50–54.

Robson, M. C., & Kucan, J. O. (1983). The burn wound. In T. L. Wachtel, V. Kahn, & H. A. Hugh (Eds.). *Current topics in burn care* (pp. 55–63). Rockville, MD: Aspen Systems Corporation.

Schanberger, J. E. (1983). Inflicted burns in children. In T. L. Wachtel, V. Kahn, & H. A. Frank (Eds.). *Current topics in burn care* (pp. 179–186). Rockville, MD: Aspen Systems Corporation.

Staley, M. J., & Richard, R. L. (1994). Scar management. In R. L. Richard & M. J. Staley (Eds.). *Burn care and rehabilitation: Principles and practices* (pp. 380–418). Philadelphia: F. A. Davis.

# 14

# *Children with Traumatic Brain Injury*

Susan Miller Porr, MEd, MS, OTR

*. . . my son died in that automobile accident and the individual that survived was a completely new individual that I had to learn to love all over again.*

—Mother of a son with TBI (Deutsch, 1991, p. 2–8)

## KEY POINTS

- Children with traumatic brain injury (TBI) come in all ages, shapes, and colors, and the recovery pattern is an individual one for each child.
- Recent research indicates that children, despite their "plastic" nervous systems, do not seem to fare better in the recovery period than their adult counterparts.
- Recovery from TBI goes in stages from acute to rehabilitation to community re-entry.
- OTs have intervention roles with children in all stages of the TBI recovery process.

## BEGINNINGS

Child restraint seats, bicycle helmets, and seat belt laws all have one thing in common (Bruce, 1990; Giles, 1994)—they have helped to reduce the incidence of traumatic brain injury (TBI) in children over the past several years. Despite these efforts this childhood trauma still remains a major public health concern (Bruce, 1990).

TBI is one of the leading causes of death and disability in children (Bruce, 1990; Molnar & Perrin, 1992). The improvements in trauma medicine have kept children alive who have received near-fatal injuries from auto accidents, falls, and gunshot wounds (Struck, 1994). This medical progress has presented occupational therapy with new therapy challenges. For many of these children the complex and far-reaching effects of pediatric TBI have a critical impact on the rest of their lives (Molnar & Perrin, 1992). OTs have skills to offer these children in all stages across the life span.

# THE CLINICAL PICTURE

TBI may be defined as an insult to the brain. ("Head injury" is another term often used to describe a TBI.) TBI is caused by an external force or motion that damages the living brain tissue. In most cases of TBI there is a change in the level of the person's consciousness. This change could be a period of amnesia or a degree of coma (RehabNET—NH Resource, 1997).

There are two categories of TBI. In a *closed-brain injury* rapid acceleration and deceleration of the head "throws" the brain against the skull in a forceful manner. This movement of the brain inside the skull may cause compression of the brain. Stretching, twisting, and/or rotation of the brain tissue may also occur. Closed-brain injuries are the more common type of TBI. They tend to cause more diffuse types of damage to the brain, and results are highly variable from person to person (Molnar & Pyrone, 1992; RehabNET—NH Resource, 1997).

Actual physical damage to the brain tissue from an outside source (i.e., from a gunshot wound) may also occur (Aicardi, 1992; Bell, 1994). This type of brain injury, where an object actually enters the brain, is known as an *open-brain injury*. These injuries tend to be more localized, and results from the injury are more predictable (RehabNET—NH Resource, 1997). Of concern in an open-brain injury are the risks of infection, possible tissue death (necrosis), brain swelling, and the body's reaction to the damaging object (e.g., bullet) (Molnar & Perrin, 1992).

These damaging forces of TBI may be caused by an auto accident, a fall from a height, or a sports-related injury (e.g., a fall from a bicycle). The actual mechanics of the trauma may also lead to secondary problems, both in the brain and in other body systems. When the central "command-and-control system" for the body is damaged, the outlying systems, which depend on that control, are also in jeopardy. Table 14–1 helps to sort out those signs and symptoms that are primary to the brain itself and those that are secondary to the actual injury.

The clinical picture for a TBI is highly variable. In children, the cause of the trauma varies with age. Males are consistently found to sustain a head injury two times more often than their female peers, but there is presently no

Table 14–1 **Signs and Symptoms of Primary and Secondary Brain Injury**

| Primary Damage to the Brain | Secondary Injury and/or Concerns |
|---|---|
| Bruising of brain tissue | Brain swelling and intracranial pressure changes |
| Damage to brain tissue or atrophy of brain tissue | Aberrant development in the child who is still in an uncompleted stage of development |
| Bleeding in the brain | General malfunctions in other organ systems (e.g., respiratory system) |
| Actual damage to areas of the brain, e.g., the cranial nerves | Problems of disturbed blood flow and oxygen to the brain |
| Damage to the vascular system in the brain | Seizures |

*Source:* Data from Aicardi, 1992; Hutchison, 1992; Johnson, Uttley, & Wyke, 1989; and Molnar & Perrin, 1992.

researched explanation as to *why* this pattern occurs (Bruce, 1990). Males between the ages of 15 to 24 are at the greatest risk for TBI because of motor vehicle accidents (Conti, 1993). Younger children experience TBI from accidental falls in most cases. Unfortunately, *nonaccidental* head injury (i.e., shaken baby trauma, see Therapeds Pointer following) is the most common type of TBI in children under the age of 2. This often results in one of the most severe types of TBI (Aicardi, 1992).

■ *THERAPEDS POINTER*

"Shaken babies" often have repeated acceleration and deceleration of the brain in the skull when handled by parents or caregivers in an abusive manner. These children often have poor outcomes from TBI because of: (1) the repetitive nature of their injury, (2) the long time period before medical help is sought (because the custodian "hopes" the child will get better), and (3) the reluctance of medical personnel to accept child abuse as the cause of the injury (i.e., a comatose child in the ER) (Bruce, 1990; James, 1993).

# TBI: THE ACUTE PHASE

The child who sustains a TBI will go through several phases of recovery depending on the extent of the injury and the individual recovery pattern. These injuries are often classified as mild, moderate, or severe, depending on the length of loss of consciousness and subsequent amnesia surrounding the event. In a mild head injury loss of consciousness is brief. In a moderate situation the period of unconsciousness may be longer and responsiveness is decreased. In a severe TBI the child may be in a coma for days, weeks, or indefinitely.

The use of a rating scale for determining the level of the brain injury is commonly seen in trauma centers. The *Glasgow Coma Scale* (*GCS*) (Jennett & Bond, 1975) has been used to determine the extent of an individual's head injury. This scale is based on responses from the patient that include verbal responses and motor indications of awareness (Giles, 1989).

---

### ■ *THERAPEDS POINTER*

The *Glasgow Coma Scale* has been widely used to quantify the extent of a patient's injury following TBI. It looks at three different responses: (1) eye movements, (2) verbal responses, and (3) limb movements. After the scale was presented, practitioners working with children noted those changes that needed to be made to the scale if it was to be appropriate for children. The result was the *Pediatric Coma Scale* (*PCS*) (Simpson & Reilly, 1982). Table 14–2 compares the scoring for the adult scale (*GCS*) with the scoring for the pediatric scale (*PCS*). Although the scoring for eye responses and motor responses is the same, verbal responses are scored differently.

In both the *PCS* and the *GCS* the scores in each of the three sections are added to get a total score. The higher the number of the total score the better the predicted prognosis is for the patient.

---

Table 14–2 **Comparison of *Glasgow Coma Scale* (*GCS*) and *Pediatric Coma Scale* (*PCS*) in Scoring Areas**

| *Eyes Open Response* | | | *Best Verbal Response* | | | *Best Motor Response* | | |
|---|---|---|---|---|---|---|---|---|
| **GCS** | **Score** | **PCS** | **GCS** | **Score** | **PCS** | **GCS** | **Score** | **PCS** |
| Open spontaneously | 4 | Same as adult | Oriented | 5 | Oriented | Obeys commands | 5 | Same as adult |
| Open to speech | 3 | " | Confused | 4 | Words | Localizes to pain | 4 | " |
| Open to pain | 2 | " | Inappropriate words | 3 | Vocal sound | Flex to pain | 3 | " |
| No response | 1 | " | Incomprehensible sounds | 2 | Cries | Extends to pain | 2 | " |
| | | | None | 1 | None | None | 1 | |

*Source:* Data from Cockrell, 1996; Simpson & Reilly, 1982.

The *Glasgow Coma Scale* is not used with infants because infants are developmentally unable to make the required responses (Coster, Haley, & Baryza, 1994). Hutchison (1992), instead, indicated that coma is present in babies who do not open their eyes or cry.

Children who are in a coma usually need to have an airway established, are medically managed with IV lines, and are frequently seen in the intensive care unit (ICU). The length and extent of the coma are highly unpredictable for each child (Hutchison, 1992). At this point in the recovery period medical teams are focused on preservation of life and prevention of secondary problems (see Table 14–1). OTs may be involved with positioning, range of motion (ROM) exercises, and sensory stimulation programs (in some cases) for these pediatric patients.

Each child with TBI emerging from the acute phase (coma) to the post acute phase will provide a personal profile of information. It is also important to note that recovery may slow or stop at any point in the process (Conti, 1993). As children to move into the rehabilitation stages of TBI recovery, the medical team moves from acute care management to assessment of the child's functional status. This may take place in the hospital or in a rehabilitation center.

# TBI AND REHABILITATION: CHILDREN IN THE HEALING PROCESS

Once a child with TBI is medically stable, medical team members can move to further assessment of the child's status. A head injury often impacts a child in numerous physical, social, behavioral, and cognitive ways. In assessing children following TBI, the name of the game is flexibility. Ylvisaker et al. (1990) emphasize the need of all professionals to "integrate their assessments, to focus on issues of functional significance, and to consistently relate assessment findings to normal development" (p. 558).

Physical changes may included increased muscle tone (spasticity) in one or more limbs and/or ataxia (irregularity in muscle coordination). Motor skills may also be impacted by sensory loss due to nerve damage. Furthermore, functional motor performance may be hampered by neglect (the brain's inattention to a particular body part). These forementioned changes may, for example, impact on a child's mobility or on the swallowing skills needed for feeding and eating (Jaffe, Brink, Hays, & Chorazy, 1990).

Social and behavioral problems for children with TBI are often intertwined. In the early recovery phase negative behaviors such as agitation or aggressiveness (i.e., kicking or biting) may be seen. Other antisocial behaviors may be exhibited by some children. Sleep patterns may also be interrupted in some of these pediatric patients (Aicardi, 1992). Later issues may surround a child's depression over loss of skills or low self-esteem (Jaffe et al., 1990). It has been noted that it is these behavioral changes rather than the physical changes that are more difficult for families to cope with in the recovery period (Coster, Haley, & Baryza, 1994).

Cognitive changes in children with TBI are most commonly lasting markers of the injury (Bell, 1994). Although actual intellectual scores (IQs) may improve, other areas of cognition may present long-term problems (Jaffe et al., 1990). Difficulty with memory seems to be a consistent problem for most patients with head injuries. The information-processing speed for many children may be slowed as they work through both new and old information. Attention to task and shifting attention from task to task may also be problematic for some children. The executive functions the brain performs may also be impaired. These include judgment, impulse control, insight, and the ability to do long-term planning (Sohlberg & Mateer, 1989).

Language issues are also present for many children with TBI. These needs are related to expressive language in the areas of word finding (coming up with the right word), labeling (giving the item a name), and organizing spoken language (Hutchison, 1992; Jaffe et al., 1990). However, the prognosis for recovery of these language skills seems to be good (Jaffe et al., 1990).

It is important to remember that the "rehab/recovery" phase for a TBI may last as long as several years after the initial brain insult. Although children do make recovery over these times periods, they do not appear to make greater gains than their adult counterparts as was earlier thought (Sohlberg & Mateer, 1989). In very young children this may be attributed to the more "diffuse" nature of their head injuries (Hutchison, 1992). Others feel children may not do as well as adults because they lose the strategies to acquire certain skills (i.e., abstract reasoning) that may already be in an adult's skill repertoire (Molnar & Perrin, 1992).

Overall the outcome predicted for children with TBI should be one of "cautious optimism" (Gans, Mann, & Ylvisaker, 1990, p. 614). OTs with team roles throughout the recovery process offer children interventions for moving toward optimal performance.

## INTERVENTION FROM THE OCCUPATIONAL THERAPY PERSPECTIVE

OTs as team members participate in the recovery program of children with TBI in several different ways. They may intervene in the acute phase with positioning and splinting needs, in the rehabilitation span with social skills and motor skills remediation, and in school and community re-entry with programming transitions. Communication among therapists in these varied settings may also help to promote more efficient transitions for the child with TBI.

## ASSESSMENT

The assessment plan a therapist uses will depend on the setting in which the therapist works. Regardless of the setting, it is important to remember to keep the plan flexible, because the path of recovery for each child with TBI is highly variable. In assessing children following a head injury, determine first the goal of the assessment. Ylvisaker et al. (1990) recommend measuring baseline performance (what the child does today) and charting strengths and needs of the child and then looking to see how these impact on the child's functional performance.

---

### ■ *THERAPEDS POINTER*

### ASSESSMENT: WHERE TO START AND WHAT TO USE

Children with TBI present unique challenges to the assessing therapist. Because a brain injury presents itself as a continuum of disability both within an individual over time and between different children at the same time, choosing tools for evaluation is often unique for each case. As the OT one wants to get a "total" picture of how the child functions in his or her roles as well as a feel for the underlying performance components that may impact that child's overall daily performance (Case-Smith, 1997). Below are listed some of the tools one may choose from to assist with evaluation. Observations, interviews with parents and others (i.e., teachers, caregivers), and record and chart reviews also add valuable pieces to the evaluation puzzle.

Tests that assess the performance and functioning of a child in a specific setting, or environment, or role:

- *The Wee-FIM* (Center for Functional Assessment Research, 1993)
- *The Functional Independence Measure* (*FIM*) (Center for Functional Assessment Research, 1986)
- *The Pediatric Evaluation of Disabilities Inventory* (*PEDI*) (Haley, Coster, Ludlow, Haltiwanger, & Andrellos, 1992)
- *The Vineland Adaptive Behavior Scales* (Sparrow, Ball, & Cicchetti, 1984)
- *The Hawaii Early Learning Profile* (*HELP*) (Furuno, O'Reilly, Hosaka, Inatsuka, Allman, & Zeisloft, 1985)

---

Data from Case-Smith, 1997; Cockrell, 1996

---

The therapist also needs to assess the components that are the foundations of functional performance to determine other areas for remediation or adaption (Table 14–3). The child with a TBI may have deficits in one or more performance components.

The following example below uses clinical observations and parent interview to obtain information for evaluating a child's feeding status. These are nonstandardized tools one may use for evaluation.

Table 14–3 **Tests of Functional Performance Used in Assessment of TBI**

| Sensory Processing | Visual perception/ Visual Motor Skills | Psychosocial Skills | Motor Skills |
|---|---|---|---|
| *Sensory Integration and Praxis Tests (SIPT)* (Ayres, 1989) | *The Test of Visual Motor Skills (TVMS)* (Gardner, 1986) | *Adolescent Role Assessment* (Black, 1981) | *Peabody Developmental Motor Scales (PDMS)* |
| *DeGangi-Berk Test of Sensory Integration* (Berk & DeGangi, 1983) | *The Developmental Test of Visual Motor Integration (VMI)* (2d ed.) (Hammill, Pearson, & Voress, 1993) | *NPI Interest Inventory* (Matsutsuyu, 1981) | *Bruininks-Oseretsky Test of Motor Proficiency (BOTMP)* (Bruininks, 1978) |
| | *Motor Free Visual Perception Test (MVPT)* (Colarusso & Hammill, 1972) | | |

*Source:* Data from Briggs & Agrin, 1981; Case-Smith, 1997.

Assessment goal: To determine status of feeding skills using spoon for a 4-year-old child with moderate TBI
Tools: observation, parent interview
Findings:

| Baseline Performance | Strengths | Needs | Foundation Components |
|---|---|---|---|
| Child sits without support in a small chair at the table to eat | Independent sitting in chair | | Balance and trunk strength appropriate for task |
| Child gets food into mouth with fair accuracy because of "shakiness" | Motor sequence for hand-to-mouth pattern intact | Better control owing to ataxia | Neuromotor control compromised |
| Eating a small bowl of applesauce takes 15 minutes with numerous verbal cues | No gagging; oral motor patterns appropriate | Attention to task impaired; consider less distractible environment | Selective and sustained attention impacted |

In reviewing the findings, the therapist noted needs in the areas of attention and neuromotor control. The ataxic quality in the child's movements may decrease further on in the recovery, and the use of wrist weights or a weighted spoon may provide a temporary compensation. Oral-motor skills appeared to be intact. Feeding in a low-stimulus environment (i.e., a desk with preschool buddy) rather than a more distracting one (preschool group table) may decrease eating time.

The changeable nature of head injury offers therapists numerous opportunities to assess their young charges. As several authors have noted (Conti, 1993; Sohlberg & Mateer, 1989) there is no one "recipe for success," and what looks like a deficit today may be a child's strength or asset next week. For most assessment information regarding a young patient with TBI, the only certainty may be change!

# INTERVENTIONS

## THE ACUTE PHASE OF INJURY

The therapist involved in the acute management phase with a young child with TBI may be focused on maintaining ROM. The child may be in a coma and spasticity may require sustained stretching of limbs. A ROM program will help to prevent contractures, and frequent repositioning helps to prevent decubitus ulcers (bedsores) (Molnar & Perrin, 1992). In some cases inhibitive casting may be done as a form of positioning for children in a coma. The ankle, wrist, and hand joints are frequently considered for this specialized casting technique (Gans et al., 1990; Molnar & Perrin, 1992).

## REHABILITATION

When a child with TBI enters the rehabilitative phase of recovery, assessment of present skills is again necessary. The therapy goals for each child will be different depending on the individual and the level of recovery. One also needs to consider the child "before" the accident. Some issues (e.g., poorer attention, behavior) may have been part of the child's personal repertoire prior to the head injury (Hutchison, 1992).

OTs are the team members involved with fostering a child's functional independence in his or her life roles. This may include activities of daily living (ADL) for dressing and feeding, play and leisure skills for engaging with peers, and the organizational and management skills needed to function in school each day. What skills a child practices are dependent on the age of the child and the amount of motor involvement noted (Molnar & Perrin, 1992). The cognitive components of skills also have to be considered when teaching or reteaching activities such as dressing, safely crossing the street, or preparing a backpack for school. The completion of these functional tasks goes beyond the motor skills needed to carry out the activity. For example, consider the following scenario:

---

**CASE STORY**

The child is a 9-year-old boy with TBI in a rehabilitation setting. His task is to pack clothes for swimming class in a backpack. The task demands the motor skills to open the backpack, stuff the appropriate clothes into the pack (9-year-olds do it that way), and close the pack.

---

When observing the boy completing the task, consider these questions that go beyond just doing the activity and impact both on the quality and completeness of the task.

| Question | Cognitive Component |
| --- | --- |
| Does the child stay on task to finish? | Attention |
| Can he remember the sequence for opening the backpack? | Memory |
| Does he know what to do if there's a knot in the backpack drawstring? Does he recognize and select appropriate items? | Problem solving |
| Are all the items in the pack so it will close? | Organization |
| Is the task completed in a reasonable amount of time? | Efficiency |

*Source:* Data from Ylvisaker et al., 1990.

When interventions and time do not yield the results a child needs to function well in a setting, then compensations and/or adaptations may be used. For example, a pocket-size electronic datebook may help a high school student keep track of schedules and assignments. A first-grader may switch to Velcro closure shoes to make herself an independent dresser, since preinjury shoe-tying skills are not in place. A preschooler who walked may need a wheelchair for mobility in the community with family. (Do consider equipment that "grows" with the child in this situation!) All of these scenarios represent OT interventions that go beyond the treatment session to make life for children and their families workable.

## RE-ENTRY INTO LIFE

TBI impacts on numerous important aspects of a child's life. It influences the way that youth lives, works, and plays in his or her community. It often challenges the way one socializes as a family member. Lastly, TBI and its aftermath may determine the way one functions in the community at large for months or years to come (Fralish, 1991).

**Discharge planning.** Children with TBI go home to families, friends, and neighborhoods. It is important for this transitional phase to be planned out ahead of the actual homecoming to make the process a smooth one for all concerned. The use of a "home pass" may help to troubleshoot areas for families and youth prior to the actual discharge to home (Bontke, Brockman, Cilio, Robert, & Worthington, 1991). This short-term visit home allows for additional questions and concerns to be considered and perhaps resolved before the homecoming date.

Discharge planning is a major first step and depends on the cognitive and physical recovery of the child at the point of departure from the hospital or rehabilitation center (Molnar & Perrin, 1992). Healthcare personnel need to provide both information and education to the family and community regarding the nature of TBI and the way it is impacting the child. Upon discharge, families should be aware that their child's ability to handle the daily routine of life is impaired. Whether that impaired functioning is temporary or permanent is an unknown. Changes in the child's status either for the positive or the negative may occur for months or years after the TBI. Staff, friends, and family working with a child with TBI need to recognize that deficits not present at discharge may occur later, because the child's developmental sequence of acquiring skills has been altered by the injury (Lehr, 1989).

**The family.** As demonstrated in the opening quote of this chapter, the child with TBI who comes home to family may be a "stranger" to both parents and siblings. Families may be as devastated by the injury as the patients themselves. To assist with the transitions, both counseling and education for the family are recommended. Counseling helps families to handle the "emotional side of the house," whereas education provides information and instruction regarding the practical day-to-day issues of dealing with the child with TBI (Deutsch, 1991). It is important to include the *whole* family in these counseling and educational sessions; the family balance is disrupted when one member has a brain injury. Siblings need to deal with their "new" brother or sister and their feelings regarding the trauma's impact on their own lives.

Research (Shaw, 1991) has shown that families need different kinds of information at different stages of their child's recovery. In the acute phase family services are focused on information regarding TBI, patient care issues, and the prognosis for the child. As rehabilitation progresses, family concerns are focused on managing their child's behavior problems, learning ways to interact with their child, and planning discharge needs *with* the professional team. Unmet needs of families in regard to services for TBI are still present (Shaw, 1991) years after the acute phase has past. Concerns regarding public awareness, employment and recreational opportunities, and financial issues surface as community re-entry becomes more complete.

Discharge planning will vary with each individual child. The age of the child, the level of recovery at the time of discharge, and the supports available to the family in the local community all need to be considered in the process.

**Young children.** Young children and infants often follow a daily routine at home. Parents and siblings may best know the preinjury child. For this age, family-centered interventions may be the most beneficial (Coster, Haley, & Baryza, 1994). Determining how the child's TBI impacts on the family and home routines will be important as the child is reintroduced to life at home. The focus may need to be on supporting the parents who will end up with the main responsibilities of caretaking for a child of this age. Parents of children with TBI are dealing not only with the emotional stress of the trauma but also with the anxiety of what the future holds for their child. This may also be compounded by the need for moms and dads to "reorganize" their parenting skills to deal with the physical and psychological changes that they encounter in their child (Molnar & Perrin, 1992).

**School re-entry.** Educational planning for children with TBI is paramount for school-aged children. OTs in the school and rehabilitation settings need to communicate with each other well prior to a child's return to school. Therapists, along with nurses, often become the medical liaisons for teaching staff, whose background is not health-care–oriented.

Integrating a child back into the school setting is, again, a team effort, with OTs helping to explain to others the functional impact of TBI, assisting schools and students with adaptations in the program and the environment, and integrating therapy goals well to optimize educational progress and avoid fragmentation in programming (Savage & Wolcott, 1988). When it is appropriate (with parental consent), a student's peers may also be educated regarding their classmate's injury. Basic information regarding the brain and changes a TBI can cause may help children to become more comfortable with an old friend who may seem "new."

The actual educational program for a child with TBI is highly individualized. Both progress in the child's recovery and the developmental level of the child will determine skills to be acquired in the educational environment. It has been noted that younger students who have not mastered the basics of reading, writing, and math may be more significantly impacted by the effects of the brain injury (Lehr, 1989).

More research needs to be done in the area of educating the child with TBI (Lehr, 1989). Questions are still unanswered regarding a "best approach" for teaching these students. Is it better to work on deficit areas or strength areas? Should a general learning strategy be used or does a task specific approach bring better results? As more information in the educational arena becomes available, these and other related questions will be answered and programs for students with TBI will benefit from this knowledge.

## ▓▓▓ FROM THE BOOKSHELF

These two books are *very* different but both enlightening!

*An Educator's Manual: What Educators Need to Know About Students with Traumatic Brain Injury* (Savage & Wolcott, 1988). This is an excellent resource for both rehabilitation therapists and school therapists. It gives an overview of TBI in lay language and provides case studies and strategies for developing a workable education program.

*Accident* (Steele, 1994) is a novel but accurately highlights the medical, familial, and social issues surrounding a teenager's head injury following an auto accident. A great break from anatomy notes!

---

**The adolescent with TBI: Special concerns.** Adolescents with TBI present their families, schools, and communities with special issues. Within the pediatric population teenagers are the highest-risk group for TBI (Fryer, 1989). This fact, coupled with the reality that normal adolescence is a time of turbulence, may complicate and multiply the re-entry issues for a teenager with a TBI.

Adolescents are working on independence issues. The family and the educational systems provide the background for sorting out social, vocational, and self-evaluation dilemmas. When the skills to meet these challenges are altered by disability, teens face the "double whammy" of proceeding through a difficult life stage with altered social, behavioral, cognitive, and physical competencies (Fryer, 1989).

In the school setting, a student with TBI may surprise staff and peers because he or she "looks good" physically but is not performing well in the academic and social arenas (Furlonger & Johnson, 1989). Academically these teens need assessments that show what they do and don't know and *how* they process information to learn. This information needs to be integrated with an evaluation of other psychosocial and behavioral abilities. This idea of "fitting in" and having friends has been cited as a long-term problem for teenagers with TBI (Fryer, 1989). In some cases this issue is magnified as adolescents turn to socially unsanctioned behaviors (Fryer, p. 266). Sexual acting out, substance abuse, and violent acts may lead to criminal behaviors. The root of these problems is often impulsive behavior or decreased self-control—both common residual effects of TBI. Esposito and Esposito (1990) account from a family perspective the challenges of helping to remake the future of an adolescent athlete son following a TBI. It becomes for all involved a search for a new and meaningful life.

# CONSIDER K.C.: A CASE STORY

The story of K.C. follows a child with TBI through acute phases into her re-entry into school. The various phases of her recovery include evaluation strategies, results, and the interventions an OT may use. It is important to remember that OT interventions are not done in isolation. As Howard (1991) notes, many of the important goals for a child with TBI are not discipline-specific. Needs in areas such as *organization* impact on everyday activities from dressing for school to completing home chores to keeping school assignments organized for homework. Programs where communication across the "team" exists and activities are meaningful to the child will best meet goals.

---

**CASE STORY**

K.C. is an 11-year-old child with a TBI. She sustained the injury in the past summer while riding on a haywagon pulled behind a tractor at her uncle's farm. A fall from the wagon resulted in a head injury that caused loss of consciousness and required emergency transport to the local general hospital. K.C. was medically stabilized there and moved to a major university hospital in a nearby town that had a pediatric unit. She was in a coma for 2 weeks, participated in rehabilitation for 4 weeks, and had a "homecoming" 2 weeks after the beginning of the new school year. She has been placed in a sixth-grade class with her peers. (Prior to her accident K.C. was an "A and B" student, enjoyed journal writing and young author activities, and had daily chores to perform around her home. She participated in bike hikes and swimming outings with her friends in the summer months.) Table14–4 lists the evaluations, results and OT interventions with K.C.

As one can see the assessment and intervention process for a child with TBI is on a continuum and involves many settings and many people. K.C. will most likely need this process to continue as new challenges of school, vocational choice, and the social interactions of adolescence remain on the horizon.

---

# WRAPPING IT UP

The trauma of a brain injury impacts a child in many complex ways. The changes within the child that are physical, intellectual, and/or social interplay with the family and community issues resulting from the trauma.

OTs are challenged to understand the recovery process from head injury. Although specific literature regarding OTs' roles with TBI is limited, available information is used for planning interventions. Therapists must then integrate that information with the child's strengths and needs to determine what is best for their young patients and their families in their unique setting.

Table 14–4 **Occupational Therapy: From Acute to Re-entry with K.C.**

| The Acute Phase (coma) | Rehabilitation Unit | Return to Home and School |
|---|---|---|
| | *EVALUATION AREAS* | |
| ROM and muscle tone assessments<br>Clinical observations of position in bed<br>Awareness level (*PCS* rating) | Independence in daily living tasks (*Vineland Adaptive Scales*)/ observation of tasks in therapy settings and at bedside<br>Interest inventory and personal interview with K.C. regarding upcoming re-entry | Level of independence in home setting (home visit observations and family follow-up interview)<br>Level of independence in school setting (classroom observations, staff interview, fine motor and visual motor testing (*BOTMP, VMI,* and handwriting samples)<br>Level of involvement in age-appropriate leisure skills (interview with K.C.) |
| | *RESULTS OF EVALUATION* | |
| Passive ROM on the left side limited; increased muscle tone in hand, wrist, and arm areas (left side)<br>*PCS* rating at second week: eyes 3, motor 4, verbal 4 | Feeding and toileting skills essentially independent<br>Difficulty with fasteners on clothing and with ordering in dressing sequence<br>Attention to tasks limited (5–10 minutes) without prompts<br>Memory for personal information, i.e., address, birthday, impaired<br>Limited repertoire of interests in relation to pre-TBI status<br>Observed K.C.'s difficulties reading "body language" in small peer groups | Home visit went well; minor needs with fastening closures on back pack and jeans; efficiency reported "ok" if clothing is prepped night before; parents noted K.C. seemed not to be listening to directions<br>School independence for mobility is within normal limits; transitioning between activities is problematic according to teachers; K.C. is about 1 year behind in math skills and reading comprehension activities; written work seems to be laborious; *BOTMP* scores and *VMI* scores below age expectations (scores in 8 yrs 2 mos–10 yrs 6 mos. range in *BOTMP* composite). Handwriting sample (cursive) is legible; speed of written output appears to be slowed because of processing and visual motor needs |

*continued on next page*

Table 14–4 *continued*

| The Acute Phase (coma) | Rehabilitation Unit | Return to Home and School |
|---|---|---|
| | *OT INTERVENTIONS* | |
| Discuss use of multi-sensory stimulation with team | Work with fine motor tasks to increase left hand manipulative skills | Talk with parents and K.C. about acceptable clothing changes (i.e., sweats instead of jeans) to aid in dressing; plan a daily home program with buttoning practice on old jeans |
| Talk with unit staff about positioning of K.C. to prevent contractures | Adapt clothing fasteners to increase present level of dressing ADL | Talk with family about structuring directions and slowing speed down to allow for K.C.'s slowed process time |
| Consult with physical therapist about splinting for left hand | Introduce K.C. to new activities via small group to increase leisure repertoire | In school share results of OT evaluation with child study team; collaborate with teaching staff to structure transitions for K.C. (i.e., have buddy help with materials, give cues ahead of change, organize folders for subjects in order of daily use) |
| | Work on personal information tasks in context of therapy activities, i.e., filling out mail-away requests for desired items; develop with K.C. a personal info card to keep in her purse or backpack as cue | Include K.C. in "writers' workshop" group that works on handwriting and writing skills; consider use of a word prediction program for school computer to speed up writing process for K.C. |
| | Consult with recreation therapist about small group leisure skills session to work on social skills in meaningful context | Have lunch with K.C. once a month in lunch buddy program to check progress outside of school leisure activities; encourage parents and family to investigate community swim program and local bike club to foster old interests in group setting with limits set for safety |

## CASE STORY

Jane is a 4-year-old preschooler who has been on the ICU for 2 weeks with a TBI secondary to a fall from a kitchen counter. She is in a coma, is being fed intravenously, and receives daily ROM exercises to prevent limitations of movement and contractures. Her eyes will open to pain, she cries at times, and motorically she will flex her right leg when a painful stimulus is introduced.

Jane's mother has been living at the hospital since the accident and has asked what she can do to be more useful. She also reports that two older siblings are distressed at home and want to see their sister. Jane's father, a second-shift factory worker, has been managing the home situation with the assistance of friends and extended family.

1. According to the information above what would be Jane's scores on the Pediatric Coma Scales?
   Eyes Open Response _____
   Best Verbal Response _____
   Best Motor Response _____
2. What strengths does Jane's family appear to have according to the brief scenario above?
3. At the end of the third week Jane comes out of her coma. She has mild spasticity on her left side and exhibits some confusion in following oral directions and attending to short tasks (1–3 minutes). What would be the primary areas you, as the OT, would want to assess in this situation? What is one activity you might bring for a bedside therapy session given this information? (Remember Jane's age and noted difficulties with direction and attention.)
4. Two techniques of intervention sometimes used with patients with TBI are: (1) *multisensory stimulation* and (2) *inhibitive casting.* Choose one of these interventions, research what it is, and cite any pros and cons found in the literature regarding the technique. Share the information with your colleagues.

*Note:* The references *Pediatric Rehabilitation* (2d ed.) (Molnar, 1992) and *Rehabilitation of the Adult and Child with Traumatic Head Injury* (2d ed.) (Rosenthal, Griffin, Bond, & Miller, 1990) are good starting points for this search.

---

# Real-Life Lab

**1.** You are an OT in the school setting. The multidisciplinary team (MDT) at your high school has received a referral on a 10th-grade student who is transferring into the district next month. The boy is 9 months' post–head injury and has been receiving special education to assist with classroom work. The student moves from class to class independently and ADLs are essentially independent. He has had the greatest difficult with tracking his schedule and completing academic work. A student with a TBI is a "first" for this team. There are lots of questions. The team asks you, as the therapist with some medical background, to explain "exactly what is a traumatic brain injury?" The team leader hands you a piece of construction paper and a marker and you proceed to explain TBI to the group complete with pictures!

**2.** Role play this situation with several of your colleagues. How will you draw a diagram others can understand?

**3.** What kinds of analogies could you use to help others understand how the brain works? (e.g., the brain is like a . . . computer . . . a file cabinet . . . a telephone switchboard).

**4.** Research pocket electronic data books. How could one of these assist a student with TBI to be more independent in the school setting? How might you determine if this is usable for this particular student? (Think assessment here!)

---

# References

Aicardi, J. (1992). *Diseases of the nervous system in childhood*. London: Mac Keith Press.

Ayres, A. J. (1989). *Sensory integration and praxis tests (SIPT)*. Los Angeles, CA: Western Psychological Services.

Bell, T. A. (1994, June). Understanding students with traumatic brain injury: A guide for teachers and therapists. *School system special interest section newsletter: American Occupational Therapy Association*.

Berk, R. A., & DeGangi, G. A. (1983). *DeGangi-Berk test of sensory integration*. Los Angeles, CA: Western Psychological Services.

Black, M. M. (1981). Adolescent role assessment. In A. K. Briggs & A. R. Agrin (Eds.). *Crossroads: A reader for psychosocial occupational therapy* (pp. 126–132). Rockville, MD: American Occupational Therapy Association.

Bontke, C. F., Brockman, N., Cilio, M. P., Robert, V., & Worthington, L. (1991).

Acute care and rehabilitation. In P. M. Deutsch & K. B. Fralish (Eds.). *Innovations in head injury rehabilitation* (pp. 4-1–4-23). New York: Matthew Bender.

Briggs, A. K. & Agrin, A. R. (Eds.). (1981). *Crossroads: A reader for psychosocial occupational therapy*. Rockville, MD: American Occupational Therapy Association.

Bruce, D. A. (1990). Scope of the problem— early assessment and management. In M. Rosenthal, E. R. Griffith, M. R. Bond, & J. D. Douglass (Eds.). *Rehabilitation of the adult and child with traumatic brain injury* (2d ed.) (pp. 521–538). Philadelphia: F. A. Davis.

Bruininks, R. (1978). *Bruininks-Oseretsky test of motor proficiency*. Circle Pines, MN: American Guidance Service.

Case-Smith, J. (1997). Pediatric assessment. *OT Practice, 2* (4), 24–39.

Center for Functional Assessment Research, SUNY—Buffalo (1986). *Functional independence measure (FIM)*, Buffalo: UB Foundation Activities.

Center for Functional Assessment Research, SUNY—Buffalo (1993). *Wee-FIM*. Buffalo: UB Foundation Activities.

Cockrell, J. (1996). Pediatric brain injury rehabilitation. In L. J. Horn & N. D. Zasler (Eds.). *Medical rehabilitation of traumatic brain injury* (pp 171–196). Philadelphia: Hanley & Belfus.

Colarusso, R. P., & Hammill, D. D. (1972). *Motor-free visual perception test*. Novato, CA: Academic Therapy.

Conti, G. E. (1993). Traumatic brain injury. In R. A. Hansen & B. Atchison (Eds.). *Conditions in occupational therapy: Effect on occupational performance* (pp. 155–168). Baltimore: Williams & Wilkins.

Coster, W. J., Haley, S., & Baryza, M. J. (1994). Functional performance of young children after traumatic brain injury: A 6-month follow-up study. *The American Journal of Occupational Therapy, 48,* 211–218.

Deutsch, P. M. (1991). Family centered rehabilitation. In P. M. Deutsch & K. B. Fralish (Eds.). *Innovations in head injury rehabilitation* (pp. 2-1–2-10). New York: Matthew Bender.

Esposito, E. F., & Esposito, F. W. (1990). A family perspective. In P. Wehman (Ed.). *Vocational rehabilitation for persons with traumatic brain injury* (pp. 323–333). Rockville, MD: Aspen.

Folio, R. & Fewell, R. (1983). *Peabody developmental motor scales and activity cards*. Allen, TX: DLM Teaching Resources.

Fralish, K. B. (1991). Characteristics of persons with head injury. In P. M. Deutsch & K. B. Fralish (Eds.). *Innovations in head injury rehabilitation*. New York: Matthew Bender.

Fryer, J. (1989). Adolescent community integration. In P. Bach-y-Rita (Ed.), *Traumatic brain injury* (pp. 255–286). New York: Demos Publications.

Furlonger, D., & Johnson, D. A. (1989). Return to school. In D. A. Johnson, D. Uttley, & M. A. Wyke (Eds.). *Children's head injury: Who cares?* (pp. 147–162). Philadelphia: Taylor and Francis.

Furuno, S., O'Reilly, K. A., Hosaka, C. M., Inatsuka, T. T., Allman, T. L., & Zeisloft, B. (1985). *Hawaii early learning profile (HELP)*. Palo Alto, CA: VORT Corp.

Gans, B. M., Mann, N. R., & Ylvisaker, M. (1990). Rehabilitation management approaches. In M. Rosenthal, E. R. Griffith, M. R. Bond, & J. D. Miller (Eds.). *Rehabilitation of the adult and child with*

*traumatic head injury* (2d ed.) (pp. 593–615). Philadelphia: F. A. Davis.

Gardner, M. (1986). *Test of visual motor skills*. San Francisco: Health Publishing.

Giles, G. M. (1989). Demonstrating the effectiveness of occupational therapy after severe brain trauma. *The American Journal of Occupational Therapy, 43,* 613–614.

Giles, G. M. (1994). The status of brain injury rehabilitation. *The American Journal of Occupational Therapy, 48,* 199–205.

Haley, S., Coster, W., Ludlow, L. H., Haltiwanger, J. T., & Andrellos, P. J. (1992). *Pediatric evaluation of disability inventory (PEDI)*. Boston: Department of Rehabilitation Medicine, New England Medical Center Hospital.

Hammill, D. D., Pearson, N. A., & Voress, J. K. (1993). *Developmental Test of Visual Perception* (2d ed.). Austin, TX: PRO-ED.

Howard, M. E. (1991). Interdisciplinary team treatment in acute care. In P. M. Deutsch & K. B. Fralish (Eds.). *Innovations in head injury rehabilitation* (pp. 3-1–3-26). New York: Matthew Bender.

Hutchison, H. T. (1992). Traumatic encephalopathies. In R. B. Davis (Ed.). *Pediatric neurology for the clinician* (pp. 169–184). Norwalk, CT: Appleton & Lange.

Jaffe, K. M., Brink, J. D., Hays, R. M., & Chorazy, A. (1990). Specific problems associated with pediatric head injury. In M. Rosenthal, E. R. Griffith, M. R. Bond, & J. D. Miller (Eds.). *Rehabilitation of the adult and child with traumatic brain injury* (pp. 539–557). Philadelphia: F. A. Davis.

James, H. E. (1993). Head trauma. In P. R. Holbrook (Ed.). *Textbook of pediatric critical care* (pp. 201–208). Philadelphia: W. B. Saunders.

Jennett, B., & Bond, M. (1975). Assessment of outcome after severe brain damage. *Lancet* (March), 480–484.

Johnson, D. A., Uttley, D., & Wyke, M. A. (Eds.) (1989). *Children's head injury: Who cares?* Philadelphia: Taylor & Francis.

Lehr, E. (1989). Community reintegration after traumatic brain injury: Infants and children. In P. Bach-y-Rita (Ed.), *Traumatic brain injury* (pp. 223–254). New York: Demos Publications.

Matsutsuyu, J. S. (1981). The interest check list. In A. K. Briggs & A. R. Agrin (Eds.). *Crossroads: A reader for psychosocial occupational therapy* (pp. 181–186). Rockville, MD: American Occupational Therapy Association.

Molnar, G. E. (Ed.) (1992). *Pediatric*

*Rehabilitation* (2d ed.). Baltimore: Williams & Wilkins.

Molnar, G. E. & Perrin, J. (1992). Head injury. In G. E. Molnar (Ed.). *Pediatric rehabilitation* (2d ed.). (pp. 254–292). Baltimore: Williams & Wilkins.

RehabNET-NH Resource Manual (1997). *Overview of TBI.* Salem, NH: Northeast Rehabilitation Hospital. [http://www.rehabnet.com/resource/tbiover. htm]

Rosenthal, M., Griffith, E. R., Bond, M. R., & Miller, J. D. (Eds). (1990). *Rehabilitation of the adult and child with traumatic brain injury.* Philadelphia: F. A. Davis.

Savage, R. C., & Wolcott G. F. (Eds.). (1988). *A educator's manual: What educators need to know about students with traumatic brain injury.* Southborough, MA: National Head Injury Foundation.

Shaw, L. R. (1991). Sequencing family services in response to changing needs. In B. T. McMahon & L. R. Shaw (Eds.). *Work worth doing: Advances in brain injury rehabilitation* (pp. 375–395). Orlando: Paul M. Deutsch.

Simpson, D., & Reilly, P. (1982). Paediatric coma scale. *Lancet* 2 (pt. 1) (July–September), 450.

Sohlberg, M. M. & Mateer, C. A. (1989). *Introduction the cognitive rehabilitation: Theory and practice.* New York: Guilford Press.

Sparrow, S. S., Ball, D. A., & Cicchetti, D. V. (1984). *Vineland adaptive behavior scales.* Circle Pines, MN: American Guidance Service.

Steele, D. (1994). *Accident.* New York: Dell Publishing.

Struck, M. (1994, June). From the editor. *School system special interest section newsletter: American Occupational Therapy Association,* p. 1.

Ylvisaker, M., Chorazy, A., Cohen, S. B., Mastrilli, J.P., Molitor, C. B., Nelson J., Szekeres, S. F., Valko, A. S., & Jaffe, K. M. (1990). Rehabilitative assessment following head injury in children. In M. Rosenthal, E. R. Griffith, M. R. Bond, & J. D. Miller (Ed.). *Rehabilitation of the adult and child with traumatic brain injury* (2d ed.) (pp. 558–583). Philadelphia: F. A. Davis.

# 15

# *Children with Cancer*

Susan Miller Porr, MEd, MS, OTR

This chapter is in memory of
LINDA MILLER COCHRAN
March 12, 1954–November 23, 1996

*No matter what happens, whether the cancer never flares up again or whether you die, the important thing is that the days you have had, you will have lived.*

—Gilda Radner

*At the age of nine, Jana Haislip was diagnosed with leukemia.*
*"My heart was ripped away," her father, Jackie, said.*
*"You see, she was our only child."*
*When told, Jana looked directly at her doctors and asked,*
*"Am I going to die?"*
*No, said a young doctor getting down on his knees to meet her gaze.*
*"You're going to live and have 18 grandchildren."*
*School opened the other day in her hometown of Robersonville, North Carolina. Jana, now 13, attended cheerleading tryouts.*
*"I didn't make it," she confided to me.*
*A tough break, I agreed, but, as her mother said to me, "Isn't it nice to have normal problems?"*
*Jana has no remaining trace of the disease.*
            —C. Newman, *National Geographic* (March, 1995, p. 131)

## KEY POINTS

- Survivors of cancer in the pediatric population are the norm rather than the exception because of major strides in cancer interventions in the past two decades

- Children tend to get different kinds of cancer than do adults.
- A diagnosis of cancer impacts on the child and the entire family system in which the child lives.
- Side effects from cancer treatments have their own set of medical management issues with which cancer survivors must contend.
- Research suggests that pediatric oncology is a new intervention area for occupational therapists who are using functional approaches in their programs.

# BEGINNINGS

Childhood cancer, which once rang a death knell of despair for parents and children, has become a more hopeful situation. Childhood cancer has evolved from an inevitably fatal diagnosis to a life-threatening chronic disease over the past several decades (Varni, Katz, Colegrove, & Dolgin, 1993). Although medical management, treatment protocols, and rehabilitation for children with cancer continue to emerge, today new "quality-of-life" issues have been added to the programs as children who survive cancer live to be adults.

Cancer as a disease has been recognized for a long time. The word *carcinoma* comes from the Greek *karkinoma,* meaning crab. Hippocrates (400 B.C.) used this word to describe the spreading actions of cancer which were, to him, like the outreaching claws of that crustacean (McAllister, Horowitz, & Gliden, 1993).

The role of the OT in treating children with cancer is a developing one. As survivors of cancer grow to be teens and adults, new needs in the psychosocial as well as the physical arenas offer unique challenges for therapists involved with children.

# THE CLINICAL PICTURE

Diagnosis of cancer in a child is rare (Fernbach, 1990). Annually, about 6000 pediatric cancer diagnoses are made (compared to 900,000 diagnoses each year in adults). The causes of cancer are also different in adults versus children. In many cases, adult cancers are attributed to long exposure to toxins (e.g., cigarettes, the sun). Although tentative links to genetics, radiation, and chemicals have been made, the etiology of most childhood cancers is largely unknown (Bair, 1990; Morgan, 1994). Children tend to get cancers of the blood and lymphatic tissues (leukemias and lymphomas), the central nervous system (CNS) (brain tumors), and connective tissues (sarcomas). The forementioned progress in treatment is gratifying, but cancer is still the leading cause of death from disease in children from the ages of 1 to 18 (Fernbach, 1990).

The development of a cancer is a multistep process involving cells whose growth and development has gone helter-skelter. These cells, which grow with chromosomal rearrangements, multiply quickly and invade normal cells through their cell membranes. If these cancerous cells move through membranes into a circulating system (i.e., blood or lymph) they may land at a new organ or tissue site. This movement to the new site is known as *metastasis.*

Signs and symptoms, treatment modalities, and interventions and remissions vary for each type of cancer associated with children. Cancer treatments often combine surgery, radiation, and chemotherapy. The type of treatment protocol used is often dependent on the patient's medical status and the type and stage of the tumor. The measure of success in treating children with cancer is twofold. The medical remission of the cancer, the period where the child is tumor- or disease-free, is the common marker for determining a "cure." This period of total remission is different for each cancer. A child who is tumor-free for 2 years with one type of cancer may be considered cured; a longer period of remission may be needed before a patient with a different type of cancer is considered disease-free. A second measure of success in treating young patients with cancer is their ability to resume a normal lifestyle without after effects of the disease or the treatment protocols (Simone, 1987). The effects of cancer treatments themselves require medical management and may have long-term implications for children who survive their cancers (Morgan, 1994). What follows is a quick overview of the cancers more commonly encountered in pediatric occupational therapy practice.

## LEUKEMIAS

Leukemias are the most common cancers seen in children. They originate in bone marrow where incomplete immature cells proliferate. These dysfunctional cells crowd out normal blood-producing cells and cause organs to enlarge.

Acute lymphoblastic leukemia (ALL), the most common cancer in children (Mahoney, 1990), is one of the "good news" stories in the cancer world. There has been a major jump in the cure rate for this cancer, with 60 percent of newly diagnosed children being disease-free for 5 years. Before 1970, the survival rate for patients with ALL was about 10 percent. Of those children with ALL who are not cured, infection remains a major concern, as their immune systems are suppressed because of chemotherapy treatments (Mauer, 1986). ALL is seen more often in boys than in girls, with the peak age for diagnosis being between 3 and 4 years of age (Morgan, 1994). Symptoms of the disease unfortunately present much like those of many nonspecific childhood illnesses: a possible virus that does not resolve, irritable behavior, fever, and a lack of appetite (Mahoney, 1990; Mauer, 1986). Bleeding may be seen also. A definitive diagnosis is made by examining bone marrow samples.

The distant second runner to ALL in diagnosis is acute myelocytic leukemia (AML). This leukemia tends to be seen more often in teenagers than in children. It presents with symptoms very similar to ALL: fatigue, a history of recurrent infections, and fever (Mauer, 1986). One red flag that may alert doctors to this condition is spongy, bleeding gums, which is the result of the leukemia cells invading this area of the body. The prognosis for children with AML is poorer than for those with ALL. First remissions may last less than a year, and death from infections following chemotherapy regimens is a major concern (Mauer, 1986).

Treatment for leukemias is generally a 2- to 3-year process using combination chemotherapy. In the *induction* therapy phase, drugs are used to get rid of the malignant cells. This is done to encourage remission where there are no abnormal cells found upon bone marrow aspiration. In the *consolidation* phase of the regimen, radiation and chemotherapy may be used in combination to get rid of the abnormal cells that may be found in the meninges (the connective tissue membranes enclosing the brain and spinal cord). After this phase there is usually a *maintenance* therapy phase during which chemotherapy may be done on a daily or weekly basis to "catch" cancer cells and prevent a relapse (return of the cancer) (Albano, Greffe, Odom, & Stork, 1995; Bair, 1990; Morgan, 1994). Although the duration of this maintenance therapy is still being debated, most children with ALL will get 3 years of postremission therapy (Berenson & Gale, 1990). Essentially, all of the drugs used in chemotherapy have the potential for creating significant side effects in young patients. These issues are discussed later in this chapter with the iatrogenic effects of other forms of cancer therapy. (Iatrogenic refers to the negative outcomes caused by the treatment or medical management situation, not the disease itself. For example, the anemia induced by chemotherapy is an iatrogenic outcome of the treatment.)

## BRAIN TUMORS

Brain tumors are the second most common type of cancer reported in children and teenagers. Like most other pediatric cancers, the cause of the brain tumors is usually unknown. Because brain tumors are rare, a diagnosis may be made late. Most pediatricians may see two children with brain tumors in their entire medical career (Albano et al., 1995). The signs and symptoms of brain tumors are also variable depending on the site of the tumor and the age of the child. These complaints—headaches, irritability, visual disturbances, and vomiting—mimic those seen in many childhood illnesses. In children with brain tumors the intensity of these symptoms often increases over a 2-month period. Mahoney (1990) reported that 85 percent of the children with a primary brain tumor will have abnormal ocular or neurological examination results 2 to 4 months following the onset of headache symptoms.

---

■ *THERAPEDS POINTER*

Computed tomography (CT) and magnetic resonance imaging (MRI) have provided the technology for medicine to "look inside" the body for diagnostic purposes with greater accuracy than ever before!

CT is a method for looking at soft tissues of the body. X-ray beams scan through a body part (e.g., the brain) and a computer calculates the amount of the x ray that is absorbed at each point. From this computerized picture a radiologist can study both normal and abnormal soft tissue structures.

In MRI (also known as nuclear magnetic resonance [NMR]) an electromagnetic field—like a giant magnet—stimulates the atomic nuclei within a person's body. When stimulated, these nuclei give off energy that is picked up by receivers and charted. This chart, again, provides a picture for diagnostic purposes, which is more accurate than an x ray for showing particular abnormalities in the body (information from Rothenberg & Chapman, 1994).

---

Diagnosis of brain tumors may be done with computed tomography (CT) or with magnetic resonance imaging (MRI) (Albano et al., 1995; Mahoney, 1990). After the diagnosis is made and the location and size of the tumor have been determined, surgical removal is often the initial treatment of choice (Cooper, 1992). This may be combined with radiation depending on the age of the child. There are major long-term effects of radiation on developing brains. (Albano et al., 1995). If used the radiation treatment may lead to later cognitive deficits and learning problems (Albano et al., 1995; Morgan, 1994). Studies have found that children who were younger than the ages 4 to 6 when given radiation have the most notable changes in IQ and memory (Kun & Moulder, 1989). Some forms of chemotherapy have also been used with brain tumors. These also raise concerns regarding future neuropsychological problems for young patients with cancer. The ultimate goal of treatment is to eliminate the tumor with the fewest short-term and long-term negative effects.

With surgery of brain tumors comes postoperative concerns and problems. Following brain surgery one may see decreased range of motion in the neck area of the young patient. Insult to the brain may also result in hemiparesis or ataxia (lack of coordinated muscle action seen as staggering gait). A residual tumor or surgery may block the flow of cerebral spinal fluid (CSF). In these cases a shunt may be used to decrease intracranial pressure (Morgan, 1994). These medical interventions all take a notable toll on the body of a young patient who is dealing both with the direct and indirect effects of a cancerous brain tumor.

The strides in neuro-oncology have not been as great as those in other areas of pediatric cancer. However, new methods of providing radiation therapy have been studied. There are also new chemotherapy agents being tried that may better penetrate the CNS (Albano et al., 1995). Despite these steps forward "the outlook for cure or preservation of a normal lifestyle remains poor for children with high-grade brain tumors" (Albano et al., p. 1159). (*High-grade brain tumor* refers to a tumor that is aggressive and has already metastasized.)

## LYMPHOMAS

Lymphomas are cancers of the spleen or the lymph nodes. This group of cancers is the third largest group of childhood cancers reported. The two kinds of lymphomas seen are Hodgkin's disease (HD) and non–Hodgkin's lymphoma (NHL). The etiology of both is unknown (Murphy & Thompson, 1986).

HD presents clinically as a painless progressively enlarging lymph node, usually first found in the neck area. Like many of the other cancers, symptoms may also include those associated with so many other childhood illnesses; fever, weight loss, and nausea (Murphy & Thompson, 1986). It is unlikely to see HD in a child before the age of 7. It then increases in prevalence in youths until their mid-20s.

NHL presents differently depending on the site of the tissues involved. For example, a child with NHL in the abdomen may have stomach complaints. The teenager with node involvement in the chest area may have wheezing and a cough. For unknown reasons NHL is seen three times more often in males than in females. It is seen most frequently in young patients between the ages of 7 and 10. Unlike its cousin HD, NHL metastasizes more rapidly and in a more disorganized manner.

Diagnosis of lymphomas requires both medical history and laboratory testing. In some cases laparoscopic surgery is done to see if the spleen is involved in the cancer. Following diagnosis, treatment is begun using a combination of radiation and chemotherapy. When the appropriate stage of cancer is determined and chemotherapy and radiation are used in combination, the majority of children with HD are cured (Murphy & Thompson, 1986). The prognosis for children with NHL has improved dramatically in the past two decades because of intense combination chemotherapy. Today 80 to 90 percent of the children with NHL who are treated with multiple drug chemotherapy get a complete remission (Murphy & Thompson, 1986).

Later concerns for children who have been treated include infections (from a weakened immune system because of chemotherapy), weight loss, and sterility (in males). Other side effects of treatment for the lymphomas may be injury to normal tissue and decreased bone growth (Murphy & Thompson, 1986).

## SARCOMAS

Other cancers that are seen less frequently in children are *bone tumors,* also known as sarcomas. *Osteosarcomas* are found in the long bones of the body such as leg bones (femur or tibia) or the arm (humerus). These cancers tend to be seen more often in teenagers than in younger children. Of concern is their tendency to rapidly metastasize to the lungs (Morgan, 1994).

*Ewing's sarcoma* is seen in the long bones but may also present itself in the pelvis or the ribs. This sarcoma is also more often seen in adolescents than in younger patients. The treatments for the two sarcomas may initially be different. Ewing's tumors respond well to radiation therapy. The osteosarcomas may require amputation of the limb with a wide margin of "good tissue" removed to be certain of total cancer removal. This treatment has notable implications for therapy following the surgery.

# CANCER SURVIVORS: THE AFTERMATH OF TREATMENT

The long-term side effects of a cancer treatment are both psychological and physical. Despite improving cure rates, young patients and their families continually deal with the worry "Will it come back?" It has been reported that 3 to 20 percent of the children originally diagnosed with some type of cancer will have a second malignancy within 20 years of their original diagnosis (Albano et al., 1995). This is 10 times the norm when peers are age-matched.

As was previously noted, the effects of surgery, radiation, and chemotherapy may also have long-term implications for these children as they resume their functional roles as playmates, school peers, and family members. Table 15–1 highlights some of the short-term issues and long-term concerns regarding these treatments.

Table 15–1. **Interventions and Side Effects**

| **Treatment** | **Radiation** | **Chemotherapy** | **Surgery** |
|---|---|---|---|
| Short-term concerns | Hair loss<br>Nausea<br>Suppressed immune system | Hair loss<br>Nausea<br>Suppressed immune system<br>Weight loss | Decreased ROM<br>Pain<br>Muscle atrophy<br>Sensory change |
| Long-term issues | Cognitive deficits<br>Slowed growth<br>Endocrine complications<br>Gastric problems (ulcer) | Toxic effects on many major body systems (heart, liver, lungs, kidneys) | Neuropsychological problems<br>Behavioral changes<br>Balance and motor skill changes |
| Implications for function | Self-esteem regarding body changes<br>Decreased motivation because of nausea and fatigue<br>Medical monitor for size<br>Sterile conditions for immunosuppressed<br>Learning problems | Increased risk for heart failure, liver problems<br>Grade exercise<br>Monitor fatigue and vital signs<br>Hand function changes from peripheral neuropathy<br>(All implications from radiation column also apply) | Learning and social skills problems<br>Changes in functional skills as a result of limb amputation |

Data from Albano et al., 1995; Bair, 1990; Morgan, 1994.

Considering the long-term side effects of cancer treatment may be as important as considerations for the cancer itself. Medical researchers have identified late effects of cancer treatment in as many as 40 percent of the children who survive their initial cancers (Albano et al., 1995). This information emphasizes the importance of the team approach when working with children who have cancer. The cancer and its aftermath impact on all the domains of a child's life. The multidisciplinary team is the recommended choice for optimal care. As Sahler (1990) put it so well:

*"Unquestionably, there is a distinct and distinctive role for each person included in the constellation of those working with the child who has cancer. It is only by working together that eventually we shall find and apply all the treatments necessary to truly cure us of cancer." (p. 8)*

---

**■ *THERAPEDS POINTER***

A bone marrow transplant (BMT) is a medical process involving the transfusion of bone marrow to provide healthy bone marrow cells for a patient with cancer. The cells may be taken from the patient (autologous BMT) or from a matched (compatible) donor. The entire BMT process can take 4 to 6 weeks and involves several steps: (1) initially the patient gets massive chemotherapy and radiation doses to clear out any remaining cancer cells; (2) the healthy bone marrow is "harvested" from the compatible donor in a surgical process in the operating room; and (3) finally the patient receives the treated bone marrow. (*Note:* If the patient is "donating" his or her own bone marrow, this harvesting process is done *prior* to the massive chemotherapy and the harvested bone marrow is treated so that cancer cells are eliminated.)

Following the procedure *strict* isolation is maintained while the grafting of the cells takes place and new bone marrow cells are made. Complications regarding rejection of cells, infection, and drug side effects are common. It takes several months for a full immune system recovery following BMT.

BMT plays a role in treatment when patients have relapsed during another treatment or within 6 months after treatment. For these patients it may be a "last-chance cure." (Information from Albano et al., 1995; Cooper, 1992; Morgan, 1994)

---

# INTERVENTION FROM AN OCCUPATIONAL THERAPY PERSPECTIVE

OTs who work with children with cancer may see them in one of several phases of their disease. In the acute stages these children may be seen in the hospital following surgery or later as outpatients after chemotherapy treatments. Therapists working in the schools may intervene with these young patients as they return to their former environment. Each setting provides challenges for assessment and opportunities for intervention. In all settings sharing information and opening communications foster cohesive team efforts for that particular child. Specific points regarding assessment and intervention in the hospital, the outpatient setting, and transition are discussed in the following sections.

## THE HOSPITAL SETTING

Therapists working with children with cancer in this setting address issues related to acute care. The medical management issues following surgery (e.g., for brain tumor or amputation) or chemotherapy impact on assessment and intervention. In the *assessment* phase therapists need to do a thorough chart review to determine the disease status, types of surgery that have been done, chemotherapy drugs that may have been used, and sites of radiation. Side effects of any chemotherapy are also important to consider in assessment. Information regarding shunts (to decrease intracranial pressure) should also be reviewed. Lab information regarding blood cell counts may also impact on the type of intervention that is allowed or feasible for a child (Morgan, 1994). All of this information will provide valuable pieces to the assessment puzzle.

Each particular child's case will determine the type of evaluation and intervention to be provided. *Interventions* may be based on results of ROM (range of motion) and muscle strength testing, sensory testing, upper extremity skills assessment, and play and leisure skills. The psychosocial status of the child also needs to be a key consideration in intervention. Self-esteem and coping strategies may also be intervention targets in therapy.

In many cases the effects of cancer treatments may cause fatigue or nausea, which may decrease a child's motivation to participate in either assessment or therapy. In these cases adopting a "go with the flow" attitude makes the process more workable for all.

---

■ *THERAPEDS POINTER*

A note of caution! Children with cancer in these acute phases may be immunosuppressed as a result of chemotherapy or radiation, which affect white blood cell counts. In these cases if sterile protocols are in place they need to be followed. Hospital team practices will determine to what extent the young patient may be protected. These policies may include handwashing techniques, visitor screenings, and infection control practices for both staff and guests of the patient (Campbell & Foody, 1995; Morgan, 1994). Of particular concern to these children is exposure to chicken pox and the virus that causes it (varicella zoster). It is important to take precautions with any communicable disease that might put the young immunosuppressed patient at risk (Randolph, Leum, & Buschel, 1995).

Precautions regarding resistive movements (e.g., "Push hard against my hands—show me how strong you are") should also be heeded because children with low platelet levels may bleed or bruise easily.

## THE OUTPATIENT SETTING

Children may be seen in an outpatient setting for follow-up therapy or interventions required from long-term effects of the cancer or treatment (see Table 15–1). In this setting *assessment* may include some of the more common tools such as *The Peabody Developmental Motor Scales* (Folio & Fewell, 1983), visual perceptual testing, and observations of play and fine motor skills. A more global picture of the child's functional status in the home and school may be obtained by using a functional inventory tool such as the *Pediatric Evaluation of Disability Inventory (PEDI)* (Haley, Coster, Ludlow, Haltiwanger, & Andrellos, 1992). The PEDI provides functional skills information as well as evidence of modification and adaptation that may have been done. Interventions may be designed to foster those strengths the child is exhibiting, remediate for "need" areas, and provide compensations (i.e., adaptive equipment) when warranted.

---

### ■ *THERAPEDS POINTER*

Hand function in children may be temporarily affected by a peripheral neuropathy. This is a common side effect from the heavy doses of chemotherapy given to patients with cancer. A child with this condition may have a weaker grasp, a wrist drop, and changed sensory feedback in wrists and hands. Interventions may include adaptations in fine motor tasks, precautions regarding poorer sensations (e.g., watching out for extreme heat or cold), and wrist splinting (for wrist drop). On the bright side, this condition is usually seen only for the duration of the chemotherapy. Patients usually see a return of normal function once the chemotherapy has been discontinued (Cook & Burkhardt, 1994; Morgan, 1994).

---

Some of the psychosocial issues surrounding a cancer diagnosis may also be addressed in the outpatient setting. Occupational therapy programs may provide children and adolescents with coping skills for their medical treatments and social transitions. Working with groups on self-esteem "maintenance" for a changing body (e.g., hair loss, disfigurement) and peer support also assists these children with return to their normal occupations in life

(Curtin, 1993). Social skills training (Varni et al., 1993) has also been effective in helping young patients with cancer to re-enter into their life roles. Skills such as social problem solving and assertiveness training may provide the tools for a smooth re-entry.

## THE TRANSITION: BACK TO SCHOOL

The child with cancer returns to school in many ways as a changed person. As cancer becomes a more curable disease, *quality-of-life* rather than *life-limiting* issues becomes important to these young people. Returning to school is often encouraged as soon as it is realistic for many cancer survivors (Varnie et al., 1993). School therapists can play both educator and liaison roles in this vital transition back to school. School transition programs include the child, the school, and the family. Children may be helped by sessions that emphasize coping, assertiveness, and social skills. Integration back to the classroom has also been improved when school peers and staff have had cancer demystified (Varni et al., 1993; Sahler, 1990). Information regarding the child's treatment, side effects (hair loss, nausea), and notable changes (cognitive issues, amputation) all prepare the school and the student for the first day back.

School therapists may act as liaisons to the hospital once a child is in a classroom program. They may also be alert to problems the child may be having academically (new learning problems) or physically (fatigue, hand function decrements), that may be related to the student's cancer or treatment. This information may be shared with (given family permission) and discussed by the multidisciplinary team in the school setting.

## DON'T FORGET THE FAMILY

A diagnosis of cancer impacts not only the pediatric patient but also the entire family. Parents, siblings, and extended families all feel the effects of the serious illness (Sargent et al., 1995). Parents must deal not only with the diagnosis, but the routine changes, financial burdens, and the stresses of caring for a very sick child (Sahler, 1990). Couples (Gaes, Gaes, & Bashe, 1992) have noted that the cancer crisis puts stress on the best of marriages and may threaten to undo the "I do's" of less-than-sturdy relationships. Continued nurturing of this relationship is paramount during this time of crisis. Drawing on the support of extended family (e.g., grandparents, cousins) and friends often provides a lifeline for parents regardless of their marital status.

Siblings often feel the impact of a life-threatening disease with more force than is realized. Each child's reaction in the family is as unique as that individual child's personality (Gaes et al., 1992). Emotions among siblings run the gamut from fear to jealousy; from overprotection of the ill child to withdrawal from the family scene (Gaes et al., 1992; Schechter, 1997). The

Table 15–2. **Common Sibling Reactions During Cancer Crisis**

| Physical Signs in Siblings | Psychological and Behavior Signs in Siblings |
|---|---|
| Psychosomatic illness (headache, stomachache) | Immature, "babyish" behavior |
| Changes in sleep patterns (oversleeping, nightmares) | Defiant or aggressive behavior |
| Bed wetting | Changes in school performance from becoming the model student to refusal to go to school |
| Changes in eating patterns (either overeating or undereating) | |

*Source*: Data from Gaes et al., 1992; Simone, 1987.

silent calls for "help" from siblings may be reflected overtly as numerous different behaviors, both physical and psychosocial in nature. (Table 15–2).

Brothers and sisters also feel the changes in the household routine. There is decreased time spent as a family unit, and possibly greater parental expectations to pitch in on the home front (e.g., more chores, increased babysitting duties) without the "perks" of parental attention. Siblings may also experience anxieties about getting the cancer themselves and the fear of death (Sargent et al., 1995). The emotional roller coaster of pediatric cancer takes the whole family for a precarious ride.

## ▟▐▌ FROM THE BOOKSHELF

*I Want to Grow Hair, I Want to Grow Up, I Want to Go to Boise* by Erma Bombeck (1989) is a must read for anyone who works with children who have cancer. It handles the physical, emotional, and familial aspects of dealing with the disease in that style that is only Erma Bombeck's.

*Gentle Willow* (Mills, 1993) is a book geared toward children to help them deal with the concept of death; this may be an outcome for some pediatric patients with cancer.

*You Don't Have to Die: One Family's Guide to Surviving Childhood Cancer* (Gaes et al., 1992) is an excellent resource covering family issues, written by a family that knows from experience. It covers an array of topics from the informational to the emotional.

## WHEN A CHILD IS DYING OF CANCER

For many of us children represent irrepressible excitement, hope, and new beginnings. We don't expect them to die . . . but sometimes they do. Although the majority of youth diagnosed with cancer will be in the survivor category, there will be children who will die.

Therapists, as health-care providers, can provide supportive services to terminally ill children with cancer (Morgan, 1994). This may occur within the framework of a hospice setting. The philosophy of hospice places emphasis on the *quality* of life when the *quantity* of life is limited. Hospice is an idea rather than a place. Models for hospice care are flexible and run the gamut from units in acute care facilities, to freestanding hospices, to home-centered support (Picard & Magno, 1982).

Hospice services are provided nationwide for pediatric patients (*Hospice*, 1995). Families of homebound children may need help with positioning and transfers. Adaptations may be required for activities of daily living (e.g., feeding). OTs also have the skills to offer psychosocial support to families in this most difficult of times. Hospice personnel need to handle each child's needs on an individual basis. One child may benefit from the planning of a special celebration in his or her last days (Schechter, 1997). Another youth may need to be engaged in the routine and familiar activities of daily life as much as medical conditions permit (Picard & Magno, 1982). Asking questions and active listening will help therapists to decide with their young patients what is most life enhancing for that particular child and family.

In the event of a child's death, hospice services are extended to a grieving family for up to 13 months after the death (Whitacre, 1992). Follow-up support to the family via telephone or home visits may be offered by the hospice or medical facility (Simone, 1987). In summary, there is no timetable for grief and no one way to process the emotions surrounding the loss of a child.

# WRAPPING IT UP

OTs working with children will be likely to come in contact with a child who has had cancer. As the cure rate for pediatric cancers improves, children will be seen in many settings for therapy interventions. Knowledge of the disease, its medical management, and long-term implications are important for occupational therapy treatment planning. With a holistic approach to intervention, OTs have much to contribute to the health and quality of life for children with cancer.

My personal thanks to Alison Longbottom, PT, and Cindy Kaapana, OTR/L, Mary Bridge Children's Hospital and Health Center, Tacoma, WA, for sharing their professional experience and expertise regarding pediatric oncology.—SMP

## CASE STORY

As an OT you have been following Stephen for 3 years through the pediatric rehabilitation clinic. He is now 8 years old and in the second grade at a local elementary school. Stephen is a cancer survivor; he had a malignant brain tumor removed as an infant and still demonstrates some of the effects of the cancer and surgery. He walks with a walker, has mild hemiparesis in his left arm, and some notable speech and language deficits. His parents have reported that he is independent for most age-appropriate ADLs (toileting, dressing, personal hygiene, feeding) with the exception of fasteners (buttons, zippers). The parents have noted Stephen is going to participate in an outdoor camping overnight with Cub Scouts this spring. They have raised some concerns regarding his needs for assistance in this new experience.

1. How would you go about helping them anticipate problems in this setting?
2. What would you as a therapist guess would be concern areas for Stephen on this overnight?
3. What concrete steps could be taken before the outing to "troubleshoot" for Stephen and reduce the parents' level of concern? (Think barriers, environment, and communication here.)

## Real-Life Lab

You are working with a 6-year-old child who is terminally ill with cancer. A last resort cure via a bone marrow transplant was unsuccessful and she is rapidly declining. The home health nurse reports difficulties with feeding and maintaining nutritional intake. The presence of seizure activity has also been documented. The parents have indicated decreased awareness in their daughter at different times during the day. The family is interested in hospice care so that her final days can be spent at home.

**1.** In your local area research the availability of a hospice program. How does one access the program? How does one qualify for services? What are the costs? What services are provided to patients and families?

**2.** Visit a local bookstore or library to check resources for siblings of dying children. Read one book or article and critique it for your colleagues.

   **a.** To what age level is the book geared?

   **b.** What features help to explain dying to the reader?

   **c.** Does it offer coping strategies? Which ones?

# References

Albano, E. A., Greffe, B. S., Odom, L. F., & Stork, L. C. (1995). Neoplastic disease. In W. W. Hay, J. R. Groothuis, A. R. Hayward, & M. J. Levin (Eds.). *Current pediatric diagnosis and treatment* (pp. 1152–1177). Norwalk, CT: Appleton & Lange.

Bair, F. E. (Ed.) (1990). *The cancer sourcebook* (Vol. 1). Detroit, MI: Omnigraphic.

Berenson, J. R., & Gale, R. P. (1990). Acute

lymphoblastic leukemia. In C. M. Haskell (Ed.). *Cancer treatment* (3rd ed.) (pp. 606–620). Philadelphia: W. B. Saunders.

Bombeck, E. (1989). *I want to grow hair, I want to grow up, I want to go to Boise*. New York: Harper & Row.

Campbell, L. R., & Foody, M. C. (1995). Administrative issues for the inpatient BMT unit. In P. C. Buschel & M. B. Whedon (Eds.). *Bone marrow transplantation: Administrative and clinical strategies* (pp. 39–68). Boston: Jones and Bartlett.

Cook, A., & Burkhardt, A. (1994). The effect of cancer diagnosis and treatment on hand function. *American Journal of Occupational Therapy, 48*, 836–839.

Cooper, G. M. (1992). *Elements of human cancer*. Boston: Jones and Bartlett.

Curtin, C. (June, 1993). The story of Danny: Pediatric oncology program. Program presented at the American Occupational Therapy conference, Seattle, WA.

Fernbach, D. J. (1990). General considerations. In F. A. Oski, C. D. DeAngelis, R. D. Feigin, & J. B. Warshaw (Eds.). *Principles and Practices of Pediatrics* (pp. 1564–1565). Philadelphia: J. B. Lippincott.

Folio, M. R. & Fewell, R. R. (1983). *Peabody developmental motor scales and activity card (manual)*. Allen, TX: DLM Teaching Resources.

Gaes, G., Gaes, C., & Bashe, P. (1992). *You don't have to die: One family's guide to surviving childhood cancer*. New York: Villard Books.

Haley, S. M., Coster, W. J., Ludlow, L. H., Haltiwanger, J. T., & Andrellos, P. J. (1992). *The pediatric evaluation of disability inventory*. Boston: New England Medical Center and PEDI Research Group.

*Hospice* (1995). A special kind of caring [pediatric special issue]. *6* (5).

Kun, L. E., & Moulder, J. E. (1989). General principles of radiation therapy. In P. A. Pizzo & D. G. Poplack (Eds.). *Principles and practice of pediatric oncology* (pp. 233–262). Philadelphia: J. B. Lippincott.

Mahoney, D. H. (1990). Malignant brain tumors in children. In F. A. Oski, C. D. DeAngelis, R. D. Feigin, & J. B. Warshaw (Eds.). *Principles and practices of pediatrics* (pp. 1583–1587). Philadelphia: J. B. Lippincott.

Mauer, A. M. (1986). The leukemias of childhood. In V. C. Kelley (Ed.). *Practice of pediatrics* (Vol. 5) (pp. 1–30). Philadelphia: Harper & Row.

McAllister, R. M., Horowitz, S. T., & Gliden, R. V. (1993). *Cancer*. New York: Basic Books.

Mills, J. C. (1993). *Gentle willow: A story for children about dying*. New York: Magination Press.

Morgan, C. R. (1994). Pediatric oncology. In J. S. Tecklin (Ed.). *Pediatric physical therapy* (2d ed.) (pp. 187–207). Philadelphia: J. B. Lippincott.

Murphy, S. B., & Thompson, E. I. (1986). The lymphomas. In V. C. Kelley (Ed.), *Practice of pediatrics* (Vol. 5) (pp. 1–15). Philadelphia: Harper & Row.

Newman, C. (March, 1995). North Carolina's Piedmont. *National Geographic, 87(3)*, 114–138.

Picard, H. B., & Magno, J. B. (1982). The role of the occupational therapist in hospice care. *The American Journal of Occupational Therapy, 36*, 597–589.

Randolph, S., Leum, E., & Buschel, P. (1995). Long term complications of BMT. In P. C. Buschel & M. B. Whedon (Eds.). *Bone marrow transplantation: Administrative and clinical strategies* (pp. 323–349). Boston: Jones and Bartlett.

Rothenberg, M. A., & Chapman, C. F. (1994). *Dictionary of medical terms for the nonmedical person* (3d ed.). Hauppauge, NY: Barron's Educational Series.

Sahler, O. J. (1990). Caring for the child with cancer and the family: Lessons learned from children with acute leukemia. *Pediatrics in Review, 12* (1), 6–8.

Sargent, J. R., Sahler, O. J., Roghmann, K. J., Mulhern, R. K., Barbarian, O. A., Carpenter, P. J., Copeland, D. R., Dolgin, M. J., & Zeltzer, L. K. (1995). Sibling adaptation to childhood cancer collaborative study: Siblings' perceptions of the cancer experience. *Journal of Pediatric Psychology, 20*, 151–164.

Schechter, D. (March 4, 1997). Going up to God: What Jonathan taught us. *Family Circle*, 48–50.

Simone, J. V. (1987). Pediatric oncology. In A. M. Rudolph (Ed.). *Pediatrics* (18th ed.) (pp. 1094–1132). Norwalk, CT: Appleton & Lange.

Varni, J. W., Katz, E. R., Colegrove, R., & Dolgin, M. (1993). The impact of social skills training on the adjustment of children with newly diagnosed cancer. *Journal of Pediatric Psychology, 18*, 751–767.

Whitacre, J. D. (1992). *Confronting life-threatening illness: Maintaining control and establishing positive objectives*. Ann Arbor, MI: Pierian Press.

# Chronic Illness, Terminal Illness, and Closure

Susan Miller Porr, MEd, MS, OTR

*"Am I going to die?"*
*Yes, we are all going to die because that is simply what happens to us.*
*Sooner or later everything that lives will die. The real question is*
*"When?"*

—Menten (1995, p. 35)

**KEY POINTS**

- The issue of dying children is one almost all therapists working in pediatrics will encounter at some point in their professional experience.
- Bereavement and grief issues need to be addressed by OTs as they work with youth and families and personally resolve their own issues in this arena.
- Children with AIDS present with a clinical prognosis that requires OTs to work with and accept terminal stages of illness.
- The AIDS epidemic includes children and has presented a complex medicosocial issue for world health care.

# BEGINNINGS

This is the beginning on endings—a strange way to start a chapter, but then this chapter is different than most of the others in this book. Although it includes important clinical information on what is currently considered a terminal disease (AIDS), it also deals with the issue of dying patients, a piece of the occupational therapy training that seems to be neglected for many pediatric therapists.

Pediatric OTs often work with children who are at risk for dying. Premature infants in the neonatal unit, students with multiple disabilities in classrooms, and children with chronic conditions die, and therapists must contend with both their professional and personal feelings in this area. It is often easy to relegate this issue to the professional back burner until a child you consider "one of your own" dies.

This chapter reviews pertinent material regarding death and dying as these topics pertain to OTs who work with dying children, their families, and their circles of friends. Because increasing numbers of children with AIDS require therapy services, this chapter focuses on AIDS as an example of terminal illness in children. On the following pages the assessment and intervention roles that are emerging for OTs will be summarized. The opening material on death is pertinent for OTs working with children who die in many different settings. The OT who works with the teenager who dies suddenly following a head injury sees death in one setting. The home health-care provider who helps a family after their infant dies from cystic fibrosis complications deals with a different environment but the same topic—the death of a child. Both therapists need supports, strategies, and information regarding children and death.

# DEALING WITH DEATH: GRIEF AND BEREAVEMENT

Each person brings a different set of information and experiences into the situation of a dying child. Children, their parents and siblings, and the professional with whom they work all have their own repertoire of coping skills. Age, personal memories, and professional knowledge impact on how death is defined for each individual.

## CHILDREN AND DEATH

Children understand and perceive death differently, depending on their age. For children under the age of 3 the word "death" has no meaning. Children ages 3 to 6 see death as temporary. They want to know when the loved one will "come back." Six-year-olds begin to understand that death is final. They know that a person or animal is no longer "working" in the biological sense. Children under 7 also may feel that they are ill or dying because of something they may have done (Lansdown, 1994).

Children in the older elementary school years (ages 9–10) are able to be more philosophical about death and realize it is inevitable for all (Boyd-Franklin, Drelich, & Schwolsky-Fitch, 1995). They begin to view death in a similar way to adults (Buckingham, 1989). The realization that death is a "one-way experience that is inevitable" begins to take hold (Buckingham, 1989, p. 48).

Answering questions about death and dying is often difficult for adults working with dying children. Effective communication with children about death includes four key aspects (Lansdown, 1994): (1) Professionals need to be aware of the child's developmental level. (2) One should ascertain and appreciate the level of communication in the family regarding a child's illness and death. (3) Adults should acknowledge that effective communication can decrease a child's anxiety. (4) Communication may be verbal or it may be nonverbal (e.g., a hug). Other outlets for communication regarding feelings include play and art. Children may act out feelings such as anger, or "play act" medical procedures with dolls or toys. It is important that interpretation of play or art tasks be done by those trained to translate these nonverbal responses correctly (Lansdown, 1994).

As they understand death and illness, children begin to merge their ideas about death and illness in regard to themselves (Lansdown, 1994). They want to know the answers to questions like, "Am I ever going to get better?" "Can this disease kill me?" and eventually, "Am I going to die?" Children need to have honest answers to these difficult questions. As Menten (1995) notes, "Answers, like truth, are the night light that keeps the boogeyman away" (p. 40).

## ▞▊▌ FROM THE BOOKSHELF

*Where Is Heaven?* (Menten, 1995) is one of those little books one stumbles upon in the process of looking for something else. The author, who notes he has none of those fancy letters after this name, has worked in a hospital setting with children who are terminally ill. His sketches of these children dealing with dying are insightful, thought provoking, and full of the questions on death from candid kids. Put it on the shelf!

*The Fall of Freddie the Leaf* (Buscaglia, 1982) is a metaphorical story about death using a nature theme. It may provide a good springboard for dialogues on death with older elementary-school-aged children.

*On Children and Death* (1983) is Kübler-Ross's classic on the topic of children and dying.

*Be A Friend: Children with HIV Speak* (1994) compiled by Wiener, Best, and Pizzo, is a collection of art and writings done by children who are HIV-infected. It is reflective of children who are working through issues much bigger than themselves.

## FAMILIES AND THE DYING PROCESS

The process of dying is well explored in Kübler-Ross's (1969) classic work. The steps leading to the acceptance of death may include anger, rage, envy, resentment, and denial (Spiegal & Mayers, 1991), but there is no seven-step plan for grieving with a tranquility guarantee at the end of the process.

As parents see their child's health deteriorating, they may become isolated. It requires a delicate balancing act from professionals who work with these families to provide both hope and a truthful assessment when a child begins a downward spiral toward death. Often helping the parents to see themselves as competent care providers helps them to work though this difficult time (Spiegel & Mayers, 1991). Activities such as teaching a mother how to position a child for comfort allows her to regain a sense of control and know she is doing the best she can for her child.

After a child dies the grief reactions of family and friends are highly individualized. Some family members will be overcome with the emotions surrounding the death. Others will appear to be stoic throughout the early bereavement period, only to have a delayed grief reaction. Others in the child's circle of support may withdraw as they don't feel as if they "belong in the picture" anymore (Boyd-Franklin et al., 1995).

There is also no timetable for grieving. People will move through this process at their own pace. Coping skills and support systems also vary widely from person to person. With deaths (i.e., from AIDS) where secrecy and stigma may be attached to the death, a family may lose its main support pillars; the professionals who worked with their child and family as the health-care providers are no longer regular visitors (Boyd-Franklin et al., 1995).

The time following the death of a child is one of turmoil within the family system. How long this period of disturbance remains varies from family to family. Anniversaries of events (i.e., child's birthday, a special holiday) will trigger grief feelings for years after the child has died. It may be difficult for others outside the circle of support to understand the length and intensity of the entire bereavement process. As one health-care provider noted when a family member died of AIDS, she had only a few close friends and a bereavement group who gave her the needed support. They honored her need to grieve in her own personal way, "without a timetable" (Boyd-Franklin et al., p. 190).

Families do survive the deaths of their loved ones with varying degrees of success. By collecting the memories, the dreams, and the forgotten laughter, parents and friends continue their lives. The process may be slow, but the dreams live on.

## IN REGARD TO SIBLINGS

Brothers and sisters of children who are dying have many feelings. In the stages when their sibling is very ill, it is often they who deal with schedule changes, preoccupied parents, and guilt over "bad thoughts" regarding that sick brother or sister (Overbeck & Overbeck, 1997). Like the ill child, siblings need information regarding their family member's illness and its seriousness. This information, when given in an age-appropriate manner, helps to reduce anxiety and provides coping support (Trapp, 1994).

---

■ *THERAPEDS POINTER*

*School Alert!* When a family has to deal with a serious illness or a family death, contacting appropriate school personnel (e.g., teach-

ers, counselors) can provide valuable support for siblings in this setting. Parents and the school can collaborate regarding the following:

1. How questions at school about the sick child should be answered.
2. Ways to help siblings maintain or "return" to normal in their
   school and other peer-related activities during illness or following the death of a brother or sister.
3. Adults who can provide additional support for siblings who are
   stressed by their home situation and/or the grieving process.

Information from Overbeck & Overbeck (1997) and Trapp (1994).

---

Siblings need to be considered when a child dies. The loss of one's sibling, often one's confidante, playmate, and lifelong companion, is a traumatic situation for any child. Surviving children need time to grieve, supports to cope,
and happy memories to save for another time.

## THERAPISTS WORKING
## WITH CHILDREN WHO DIE

OTs working in pediatrics need to deal with the concept that children die, and
sometimes they die when we "expect it" and sometimes when we're caught
totally off guard. Whether in schools, hospitals, or clinic settings, therapists
*can* and *do* develop long-term relationships with "their kids" and the families
with whom they work. The need to balance the personal and professional relationship is important to prevent burnout in stressful situations such as a patient death.

Reactions to a child's death within the professional team may be as varied as those within the family itself. Speaking from both personal experience
and research information (Boyd-Franklin & Boland, 1995), it helps to think
about ways to cope with the death of a pediatric patient and reflect prior to
the event regarding one's own feelings on death. However, even with this
preplanning, the actual event is a difficult one, at best, for many health professionals. Realize that feeling professionally inadequate when a child dies is
not uncommon. Administrators can often assist in this area by providing support groups and/or in-services on this often-neglected topic.

Anger at the situation surrounding the death may also be seen (Boyd-
Franklin & Boland, 1995). The OT working with the teen who contracted AIDS
via unprotected sex might feel anger as the youth continues that practice after
"safe sex" counseling. Anger at the parent whose baby died after a recommendation to seek medical follow-up was not pursued may seem personally justi-
fied but is not professionally condoned. Knowing that the anger may surface
as a reaction to a child's death is one step in the professional coping process.

Putting closure on the emotional aspects of a child's death may also help
health-care providers deal with this aspect of being in a "helping profession."
Some programs dealing with terminally ill children have memorial services or

special rituals to remember a beloved friend who has died (Menten, 1995). Administrative leave to attend funerals or outside memorial services should seriously be considered for staffs who continually deal with crisis control and very sick children (Boyd-Franklin & Boland, 1995). Acknowledging the potential for burnout and providing staff development in the area of death and dying should be as critical as the new techniques for patient care. In conjunction with this education should be the availability of outside help for the professional on overload who needs to share experiences and feelings regarding a death or the processing of that issue (Boyd-Franklin & Boland, 1995).

In summary, dealing with death is a highly personalized and emotional issue for many people. Each individual, be it the parent, professional, or playmate, will be called upon to cope in his or her own best way while grieving a child's death.

## THE THERAPIST'S ROLE WITH DYING CHILDREN AND THEIR FAMILIES

OTs' roles with families may vary according to their personal and professional connections with that specific family. For example, the therapist who comes to provide palliative care (i.e., feeding and positioning strategies) through a hospice program may have a short-term but intense relationship with the child and family. The OT working with the school-aged child may have a long-term, year-to-year relationship with the student, family, and the circle of support.

The OT dealing with the family and child will most likely be one of many therapeutic disciplines involved in the child's complex care (Meyers & Weitzman, 1991). Clear communication and family-focused collaboration with other team members are important tenets of the OT's role. Encouraging quality of life for all family members to provide balance under the stresses of dealing with death may be a role for the OT on the team. This may help to counter the emotional and physical exhaustion brought on by the circumstances of dying children (Shannon, 1995). Finally, the therapist must be ever sensitive to the cultural, ethical, and familial issues surrounding death and dying (Meyers & Weitzman, 1991).

The following pages will address the topic of AIDS and children. This disease and its present terminal outcome provide a framework for therapists' thinking as they encounter the concepts of quality of life and "gentle closing" (Menten, 1995) of death for the children with whom they may work.

## AIDS: THE CLINICAL PICTURE

The cause of AIDS is the human immunodeficiency virus (HIV). This virus is a member of the Retroviridae family (Chadwick & Yogev, 1995). It infects the helper T lymphocytes, which are key players in the immune system. Active replication of HIV leads to the destruction of the immune system (Wade,

1991). Infection by the virus causes abnormalities in lymphocyte function and eventually leads to the demise of the patient (Shannon, 1995). AIDS is the most advanced stage of infection by HIV and the spectrum of health from asymptomatic to critically ill is seen in persons with HIV infections.

AIDS was originally described in 1981 and was observed in homosexual men (Moffet, 1989). As the AIDS epidemic moves into its second decade, there are increasingly wider impacts of the disease (Nicholas & Abrams, 1992). Worldwide, women account for 40 percent of the new AIDS cases (Joe, 1996). The rise in pediatric cases of AIDS parallels this noted increase in women infected with HIV (Carmichael, Carmichael, & Fischl, 1995).

AIDS has now become one of the top 10 causes of death in children between the ages of 1 and 5, as infected mothers transmit the virus to their children (Edelson & Noel, 1992). Sources indicate that the majority (81 to 89 percent) of pediatric AIDS cases are from this *vertical transmission* from mother to child. Although the exact biological mechanics of vertical transmission are not medically well understood, there may be three possible routes of transmission from infected mother to child: (1) *in utero* across the placenta from mother to child, (2) perinatal exposure to the infected mother's blood during the birthing process, and (3) postnatal via breast milk (Shannon, 1995).

---

■ *THERAPEDS POINTER*

Modes of Transmission for the AIDS Virus (So & Johnson, 1997)

| Horizontal Transmission (from Person to Person) | Vertical Transmission (from Mother to Child during Pregnancy or Perinatal Period) |
|---|---|
| 1. Sexual transmission (major mode worldwide) | 1. Transmission during pregnancy |
| 2. Blood and blood products<br>  A. Sharing of contaminated needles for injected drugs<br>  B. Transfusion of blood or blood products | 2. Transmission during the birthing process |
| 3. Transmission via organ transplantation | 3. Transmission via breast milk in postpartum period |
| 4. Occupational transmission in healthcare workers<br>  A. Skin puncture from needle or contact with contaminated blood to skin or mucous membrane<br>  B. Risk from this mode is documented 0.3% | |

Although transmission from mother to child is the most common route of infection in children, other modes of transmission are known. Exposure to contaminated blood products (i.e., transfusions*) and via sexual routes (Carmichael et al., 1995) are considered horizontal transmission modes for HIV. For young children, this latter horizontal mode is most often in the form of sexual abuse. Although fewer than 1 percent of the children with AIDS are exposed through sexual intimacy, this may become a more common avenue of exposure as adolescent AIDS increases (Edelson & Noel, 1992; Joe, 1996).

Heterosexual intercourse is *the* most common method of transmission of HIV in the adolescent population. It has also been noted that transmission is more likely to occur from male to female than from female to male (Wells et al., 1995).

The advent of AIDS prompted the development of formal guidelines for decreasing the risk of transmission to health-care workers while protecting the confidentiality of patients (Chanock, 1992). These guidelines, developed and supported by both the Centers for Disease Control and Prevention (CDC) and the Food and Drug Administration (FDA) are known as Universal Precautions. Universal Precautions constitute the guidelines, procedures, and plans regarding infection control. This concept supports the idea that all persons, blood, and most body fluids are considered to be potential carriers of infectious disease. Implementing Universal Precautions erases the uncertainty of working in situations where infection may be possible, by requiring all body fluids and blood to be treated as potentially infectious. It is important to remember that persons who are infectious cannot all be identified, and it may only take one exposure to become infected.

Workplaces, whether they are schools, hospitals, or clinics, regularly provide infection control training to staff. These in-service programs cover policies regarding things such as handwashing procedures and the use of personal protective equipment (i.e., gloves and gowns). In short, knowing the procedures and taking reasonable precautions provide a safer environment for all (*Bloodborne Pathogens*, 1992).

---

■ *THERAPEDS POINTER*

The basics regarding Universal Precautions apply to handling blood and body secretions containing visible blood. The idea is to protect individuals by barriers (gloves, gowns) when handling the noted body fluids or materials.

→Gloves are worn for handling blood, body secretions (vaginal, semen) and tissues obtained by puncture (i.e., cerebrospinal

---

*In the United States blood products have been screened for HIV antibodies since 1985. At the present time the risk to a recipient is very small. If a donor has been exposed to HIV before the antibodies appear in the blood and the donated blood screen is negative for HIV, there is a risk to the recipient. This risk is reported to be 1 in 40,000 units of blood transfused (Simonds & Rogers, 1992).

fluid); gowns may be needed where spattering of blood may occur (i.e., emergency room).

→Use of gloves does not apply to feces, nasal discharge, sweat, tears, urine, vomitus, or sputum *unless* blood is visible.

→Receptacles for disposing of contaminated materials should be tightly closed and childproof.

→Cleanup of contaminated surfaces should be done with household bleach solutions (HIV does not live well outside the body on environmental surfaces).

→Persons with open skin conditions should wear gloves; should skin become contaminated, wash with soap and water, check for open lesion contamination, and follow local infection control procedures

Information from Chanock, 1992.

---

Diagnosis of HIV in children comes via laboratory screening (see the following Therapeds Pointer). Those infants born to mothers who are known to be HIV-positive are often screened with the *enzyme-linked immunosorbent assay (ELISA)* method to determine their status. This screening determines if a person's blood serum has antibodies to HIV antigens (Stine, 1993). However, ELISA may not be reliable until after a baby is 15 to 18 months old, since immunoglobulin (IgG) from the mother passes easily across the placenta to the infant. If this IgG contains maternal HIV antibodies, positive lab results are a result of maternal antibodies in the child's system (Joe, 1996; Shannon, 1995). If the antibodies are passed from mother to child, and the child is not infected, the antibodies will disappear in the child between the ages of 9 and 15 months (CDC, 1994; Moffet, 1989). This happens in the majority of children born to mothers who are HIV-positive. Resources indicate that between 25 and 40 percent of children with mothers who are HIV-positive will actually be infected (Carmichael et al., 1995; Shannon, 1995).

---

■ *THERAPEDS POINTER*

The two more common tab tests used to screen for the presence of HIV in a person are the ELISA and the Western blot assay.

The ELISA is low-cost, standardized, and uses a blood sample. It provides quick results and looks for the presence of HIV antibodies. This makes it an indirect lab method for screening. That is, the HIV antibody presence *highly* suggests HIV infection.

The Western blot assay is considered the "gold standard" when determining the presence of HIV infection. It uses a lab process (gel electrophoresis) that gives more qualitative information regarding HIV than the ELISA. Because it is more costly and time consuming than the ELISA, the Western blot assay is used to confirm the ELISA results (Stine, 1993).

---

Although the clinical picture for each child is variable, children also tend to be affected by the virus differently than adults. This is thought to be because of the child with HIV is a "more immunologically naive organism" (Walker, 1995, p. 159). In children the incubation period from HIV infections to AIDS is much shorter than in adults. The infant infected perinatally will usually become symptomatic by the age of 3. In blood transfusion–related cases the situation is a little more prolonged, with the time from positive laboratory results to AIDS being slightly more than $3^1/_2$ years (Simonds & Rogers, 1992).

As noted earlier, the pattern of disease in children with HIV / AIDS is variable. At this time there seem to be two groups of children within the diagnosis. Flynn (1994) notes that those children who get opportunistic infections very young tend to have a poorer prognosis. Opportunistic infections are those diseases that would not normally occur in a person with a healthy immune system but become pathogenic in those with impaired immune systems (Stine, 1993). CNS encephalopathy and the noted infections cause the demise of more than half (52 percent) of this pediatric group before 3 years of age.

A second group of children who are HIV-positive tend to be older when exhibiting the disease and develop a more chronic, progressive type of disease pattern. In this second group prognosis is better and the large majority of these children (97 percent) remain alive at 3 years of age. Infants who develop HIV infection before a year appear to have the poorest prognosis of all. For these young patients the time between testing positive for HIV and the death of the infant averages 9 months, with 70 to 85 percent of this group dying before the age of 2 (Shannon, 1995).

At the present time there is no vaccine or cure for AIDS (Wells et al., 1995). As Wilfert and Pizzo (1994) noted, a child with HIV can "reasonably expect to survive a median of 7 to 8 years with supportive care and antiretroviral therapy" (p. 922).

The prognosis for adolescents with HIV-positive status differs from that of children. Adolescence, as a transition phase, shares both risk factors from children and adults. Younger adolescents, like children, tend to be infected via exposure to blood products or blood. In older teens a dramatic increase in HIV cases has been seen because of IV drug use and increased sexual activity (more like adults who are HIV-positive). Adolescents who are infected via sexual contact or the use of IV drugs may live 12 or more years after diagnosis (Joe, 1996). Sexual activity becomes linked with the potential for teenage pregnancy and the possibility of subsequent infected children (Simonds & Rogers, 1992). With the increased longevity of this group, psychosocial considerations include rehabilitation, life choices, and vocational transition (Joe, 1996). The situation is both medically complex and socially disconcerting for those working with adolescents today.

The child who is HIV-positive today presents differently from those youth who were seen in the first years of the AIDS epidemic. In earlier years children entered the medical "arena" with fully symptomatic AIDS. The clinical signs and symptoms of AIDS for this advanced stage include growth failure, chronic diarrhea, malignancies, and the presence of opportunistic infections that are persistent and recurrent (Arpadi & Caspe, 1991; Wade, 1991).

Today, as a result of increased awareness of HIV and AIDS, children are less sick when initially seen because they come to the attention of the medical clinician much earlier in the disease state than previously. The presence of an opportunistic infection, which suggests that the child's immune system is compromised, is one of the "red flags" alerting a clinician that HIV may be the cause (Pizzi & Hinds-Harris, 1990). The emerging clinical picture includes a wide variety of health problems in many body systems. Commonly seen problems include the aforementioned recurrent infections, involvement of the lymphatic system, presence of the "marker" pneumonia, *Pneumocystis carinii* pneumonia (PCP), and CNS dysfunction.

The CNS is a key target for HIV infection (Hanna & Mintz, 1995). Impaired neuropsychological and neurodevelopmental functioning is commonly associated with pediatric AIDS. Children with HIV and AIDS often present with developmental delays, motor dysfunction, and the loss of developmental milestones (Pizzi & Hinds-Harris, 1990). The way that the CNS is impacted may depend on the age of the child. Younger children tend toward the aforementioned milestone delays. In older youths an actual deterioration of already acquired skills (i.e., in cognitive or emotional areas) is seen (Hanna & Mintz, 1995).

One of the more common medical conditions seen in children compromised with HIV is PCP. This opportunistic infection is known as an AIDS-defining illness in children who are HIV-positive (Carmichael et al., 1995). (An AIDS-defining illness marks the onset of full-blown AIDS.) The onset of PCP is usually acute and accompanied by a fever and nonproductive cough. Another pulmonary disease seen in children with HIV infection includes the more chronic progressive lymphoid interstitial pneumonitis (LIP) (Shannan, 1995).

Abnormalities in all organ systems may be seen in children with HIV infection. Changes in cardiac structure and function may occur. Blood and bone marrow abnormalities may lead to anemia and lowered numbers of blood platelets. Painful and difficult swallowing, combined with gastrointestinal problems, may lead to wasting syndrome, which is often seen in patients with HIV infection. In this deterioration process, weight loss is accompanied by decreases in strength, appetite, and activity level (Rothenberg & Chapman, 1994). Chronic diarrhea, along with intermittent or constant fevers, is also associated with wasting syndrome in persons infected with HIV (CDC, 1994).

Children with AIDS are also seen with other noninfectious complications. These include cancers such as non-Hodgkin's lymphoma. Neuromuscular problems such as spasticity and low muscle tone may also be present. It should also be noted that intrauterine exposure to HIV may cause neurodevelopmental delays even though the child is *not* infected (Hanna & Mintz, 1995).

The Centers for Disease Control (CDC) developed a classification system for AIDS in children in the late 1980s. This was revised in 1994 by the CDC to place children with HIV infection into one of numerous categories based on the status of the child's health in three different areas (Shannon, 1995). The new classification system looks at (1) the state of the child's immune system (i.e., suppressed vs. not suppressed), (2) the level of clinical symptoms that are exhibited by the child, and (3) the child's infection status (HIV-positive or -negative) (CDC, 1994). The infection parameter of this "three-way" classification system is determined by laboratory testing (ELISA and Western blot) and the CDC's definition of HIV infection. Although further explanation is beyond the scope of this chapter, therapists working with children with HIV diagnoses will become familiar with this information as they review charts and interface with the medical community regarding their young charges.

---

■ *THERAPEDS POINTER*

The *New Illustrated Webster's* (1994) defines *ethics* as the "basic principles of right action." The answers in this study of how humans conduct themselves in "what's right or wrong" situations are *much* grayer than the black-and-white print of the definition on the page. As OTs dealing with people, emotions, and medical crises, ethical dilemmas will arise with certainty! To get into practice, discuss the following scenario with your colleagues:

> You are an OT in a developmental clinic working with a child who has fine motor delays. The chart indicates the child is HIV-positive and the parent has contacted you to talk. The mother indicates she knows her son's condition but does not want you to indicate this to the child in any manner. In the context of a therapy session this 7-year-old asks you if he is "sick enough to die."

How are you going to handle this situation?

---

As Mendez (1991) noted, the thrust of care for the child with HIV or AIDS needs to be family-centered and nonjudgmental. Team members may vary according to the child and family needs at any particular time. Roles may overlap and change as the disease dictates the life of the child.

## TEAM INTERVENTION: AN OVERVIEW

Medical personnel on the team are involved with initial diagnosis as noted. After the diagnosis of HIV or AIDS, a "three-pronged attack" is adopted for the child's care. This includes: (1) healthy child care, (2) care for medical crises (e.g., a PCP episode), and (3) continuous care needed for the chronic conditions associated with the disease state (Mendez, 1991).

### *Healthy Child Care*

Children who are as asymptomatic need typical "kid care" such as physicals and immunizations. Health precautions need to be taken regarding those immunizations that may be risky for immunocompromised persons. Physicians are most often the providers in this medical maintenance role (Carmichael et al., 1995). The nutritionist as a team member may also be called on to assist patients with nutrition counseling and the development of a healthy eating plan.

---

■ *THERAPEDS POINTER*

CDC has made formal recommendations for the immunization process of children with HIV infection. This is based on the child's disease status at the time of scheduled immunization. Children, whether they are symptomatic or asymptomatic, may receive vaccines for diphtheria, tetanus, and pertussis (DPT), the pneumococcal vaccine, and *Haemophilus influenzae* b (conjugate) vaccine (a type of flu vaccine). Live virus vaccines such as the oral polio vaccine should not be given to children with HIV infection regardless of their status. Instead, substitutions such as the inactivated (the virus is dead) polio vaccine are recommended.

All medical care recommendations should be determined by the child's individual medical care provider on a one-to-one basis.

---

*Source:* American Academy of Pediatrics (1997).

### *Medical Crisis and Management*

In the time of medical crisis many team members from nursing staff to social work may be involved with the child and the family. Because each case is different, there is no one "right" combination on the intervention team. From the medical standpoint, treatment of the specific condition's symptoms is done. For example, a child with an episode of severe diarrhea may require nutritional supplements administered by methods other than oral. Beyond acute care, the introduction of life-prolonging antiretroviral drugs is often seen.

Antiretroviral drug use treatment with children has been continuously evolving. The most common agent used in children with AIDS is zidovudine (Retrovir). Didanosine (Videx) is also approved for use in children over the age of 6 months (Carmichael et al., 1995). The use of azidothymidine (AZT) was approved for pediatric use in 1989 (Joe, 1996). In children, it is used to help extend and maintain periods of health, similar to the way it is used with adults.

---

■ *THERAPEDS POINTER*

AZT works by slowing or stopping the replication of HIV in cells. Researchers believe this process is targeted at the DNA synthesis of the virus. (This drug has actually been around awhile; it was used as an anticancer agent in the 1960s.)

The use of AZT in children has brought about positive changes, because it delays the suppression of the immune system by HIV. Decreases in opportunistic infections have been noted as well as improvements in motor, verbal, and mental skills (Stine, 1993). Unfortunately, AZT also may have serious side effects such as nausea, headaches, insomnia, and rashes. About 40% of those taking AZT also have anemia. Toxicity of bone marrow has also been seen in pediatric patients receiving AZT (Shannon, 1995).

---

## Chronic Care Issues

As children with HIV and AIDS live longer and more productively, the "quality-of-life" issues that surround any chronic illness become important. Meyers and Weitzman (1991) noted that pediatric HIV disease is the "newest chronic illness of childhood." Currently, children with the HIV virus have it for life, and the disease progression is one marked by deterioration. This pattern of deterioration may also be seen in childhood chronic diseases like muscular dystrophy.

The unpredictable nature of the disease's peaks and valleys makes it similar to other pediatric chronic illnesses such as asthma or some of the childhood cancers (Meyers & Weitzman, 1991). This uncertainty with the progression of the AIDS virus can be problematic for both staff and family. The terminal phase of this disease is not clear-cut; with each exacerbation, a new balance must be found. The juggling of active intervention strategies with the possibility that death is near is a major feat for both professionals and family members (Duggan, 1994).

There are specific concerns surrounding pediatric AIDS that make it unique in the chronic illness world. For the majority of children with AIDS, parents are ill or absent. AIDS is often associated with drug use, poverty, and minority populations (Flynn, 1994; Nicholas & Abrams, 1992). The characteristics of HIV disease call for the skills of other members of the intervention team. Social workers and psychologists become involved with emotional support and community service access for families and children. Therapists, both occupational and physical, are needed to intervene in the areas of rehabilitation and activities of daily living as life spans become longer for this population. OTs with background in both psychosocial and physical disabilities have skills to offer in both the mental and physical areas for these children. OT services are clearly appropriate . . . for children with HIV and AIDS (Joe, 1996, p. 15).

## INTERVENTION FROM THE OCCUPATIONAL THERAPY PERSPECTIVE

Working with children with HIV or AIDS may be a fact of life for pediatric therapists in many different settings. An OT in a developmental clinic may get a referral from a pediatric neurologist regarding a child's developmental delay. The therapist in the neonatal intensive care unit (NICU) may be seeing an infant who was exposed to HIV in utero. The OT in the school may be programming for the preschooler who is HIV-positive and entering the district for the first time. As Pizzi and Hinds-Harris (1990) note, there is a need for "holistic assessment of the child's functioning" (p. 107). Intervention strategies are then based on those assessment findings and the status of the child's health.

## ASSESSMENT

The assessment of the child with HIV or AIDS is similar to that done with other children presenting with conditions that cause developmental delays. The use of standardized tools will depend on the age and health status of the child. Assessment should include: (1) a chart review, (2) a developmental history, (3) clinical observations, and (4) information gathering (via interview, observations, and standardized tools) in the areas of childhood occupations such as school, activities of daily living (ADL), and play (Pizzi & Hinds-Harris, 1990). Other information that is specific to a particular case may also be needed for holistic assessment (i.e., the health status of caregiver).

As the role of occupational therapy continues to evolve, assessment tools expand. At the present time therapists have successfully used the *Bruininks-Oseretsky Test of Motor Proficiency (BOTMP)* (Bruininks, 1978) and the *First-STEP Screening Test for Evaluating Preschoolers* (Miller, 1993) for determining baseline skills and tracking progress in children with HIV or AIDS (Joe, 1996; Herzberg, 1996). The *Denver Developmental Screening Test* has also been used with younger children (Frankenburg, Fandal, Sciarillo, & Burgess, 1981). Herzberg (1996) noted that tests with a visual method for presenting results (i.e. a graph) were easier to use in explaining results to parents. The *Test of Visual Motor Integration (VMI)* (Beery & Buktenica, 1967) has also been used successfully for tracking progress in fine motor skills during antiretroviral therapy (Hanna & Mintz, 1995).

The chart that follows shows several different scenarios one might encounter as a therapist assessing a child who has HIV infection. The tools and tactics provide one option for evaluation; others may be dictated by environmental, professional, and child-related needs.

| Scenario | Assessment Tools/Tactics |
|---|---|
| A 4-year-old in city program for preschoolers with HIV-positive status; is generally a "well child at this point in time"; staff concerns are related to decreased attention span and poorer use of craft materials involving hand use | Observe the child during a morning craft "messy session" with paintbrush, paints (Note: Is attention to task age-level appropriate?)<br><br>Administer *FirstSTEP* (Miller, 1993) and score Talk with parent about present opportunities to manipulate materials at home<br><br>Address pattern of strengths and needs that emerges |
| High school student (female) recently contracted HIV infection through unprotected sexual contact; she is attending school and is able to maintain school day routine at this point in time; she is also receiving AZT for health maintenance; guidance counselor asks for OT assistance in "future planning" with this student | Discuss with counselor student's present academic level and performance<br><br>Interview student as to her vocational preferences, interests, experiences (i.e., unpaid or paid work, volunteer experiences)<br><br>Consider the use of a vocational preference test to assist with goals setting (The *PIVOT* manual by AOTA [Kirkland & Robertson, 1985] provides a wealth of basic information in this area)<br><br>Administer vocational and work evaluation, e.g., from the *McCarron Dial Evaluation System* (Dial, McCarron, & Amann, 1988) |
| Two-year-old with HIV-positive status (perinatal transmission) is living with an aunt in the home. Child has had notable failure to thrive since birth and nutritional and feeding needs have been a topic of concern. The OT following the child on a home health caseload has been asked for her input by nurse on the case. | Collaborate with the nurse concerning: past feeding history, present feeding patterns, weight-maintenance pattern (see Chapter 11)<br><br>Talk with aunt about feeding patterns during the day—what works and what doesn't<br><br>Observe aunt feeding child or watch child during a meal (if self-feeding skills are present)<br><br>Use a structured checklist (see Cook, 1991, pp. 66–67 for an example) to help organize feeding assessment<br><br>Consider outside consultation with nutritionist for additional nutritional information or do joint assessment with nutritionist |

Using the example of the high school student in the chart, one can plan some OT goals related to her strengths and needs as determined by the assessment. Goals should address needs, support and use strengths, and reflect the student's interest areas.

---

G   + Student has worked for pay in local rest home as aide (good job performance)

O   − Student has little idea about work options beyond above experience but likes "helping people"

A   − AZT also leaves her feeling "less than great" some days

L   *Goal:* Student will explore in Career Opportunities class three "helping professions" that allow for job flexibility (in light of possible changes in health status) and have community interviews visits with three persons in the respective fields. From this interview a "best choice" will be made by the student for additional exploration.

---

Assessment involves a series of processes from observation, to interview, to actual testing of the child or youth using specific tools of the trade. The information gathered in assessment provides the OT with direction for planning interventions. It is ongoing and continually tailored to meet the needs of the specific child at a specific time. The strategies for intervening with a child may also be influenced by cultural issues, the health status of the child, and the possibility that the caregiver for the child is also infected with HIV (Pizzi & Hinds-Harris, 1990).

---

■*THERAPEDS POINTER*

Moms and their children with AIDS are a major medical concern with far-reaching social implications. As noted before, the majority of HIV infection in children is through vertical transmission—from mother to child. Many children who are HIV-positive have caregivers whose own health is compromised. As Schable et al. (1995) noted from their research: "Mothers with HIV, often alone, are the primary caretakers of their children" (Abstract, p. 511). Demographic information also finds these mother are disproportionately from minority families for whom poverty and lack of access to the system are continual problems (Wilfert & Pizzo, 1994).

Issues for concern in these families include: (1) guardianship plans of children who survive parents, (2) parenting skills for parents who didn't have models, and (3) ongoing emotional support for sick parents dealing with sick children.

---

Addressing the issues unique to the HIV-AIDS condition will help to provide a more realistic, workable plan for both the child and the family.

## INTERVENTIONS:
## THE CUSTOMIZED APPROACH

The interventions used with children with HIV or AIDS are as varied as the youths and the settings from which they come. Areas of remediation and habilitation that are often the focus of OT concern include fine motor skills, play and social skills, and ADLs such as feeding. It is important for therapists working with children with HIV or AIDS to realize that these children may never attain some developmental milestones or other skills.

Interventions planned may also be influenced by the medical management of the child in reference to antiretroviral drug therapy. Research regarding the impact of antiretroviral drug intervention has been mixed. Hanna and Mintz (1995) noted positive qualitative changes in a child's fine motor skills following treatment with zidovudine (Fig. 16–1). Others have not

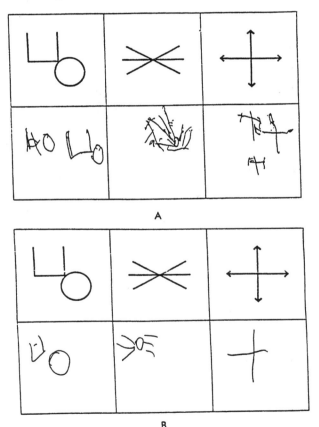

Figure 16–1 Comparison of graphomotor samples (Beery VMI) taken from child with PE (A) before treatment with zidovudine and (B) 6 months after treatment was initiated. (From Hanna & Mintz: Neurological and neurodevelopmental functioning in pediatric HIV infection. In Boyd-Franklin et al. [Eds]: Children, Families, and HIV/AIDS: Psychosocial and Therapeutic Issues. Guilford Press, New York, p. 42, 1995.)

seen the same positive changes in motor skills with other drugs. Wolters and associates (1994) noted improvements in all areas of children's adaptive behaviors except motor skills when treated with AZT. Motor skills involve both the CNS and peripheral nervous system. (AZT seems to not impact as notably on the peripheral nervous system as it does on the CNS.)

In the intervention process the therapist should foster functional competence for the child as he or she meets the obstacles and challenges of the surrounding environment. By matching the child's assessed needs with family-focused, therapist-generated strategies, positive changes are seen.

---

■*THERAPEDS POINTER*

Confidentiality, the guaranteed trust that information will remain private, is an important professional tenet to maintain in working with children who are diagnosed with HIV or AIDS. This includes information shared and not shared in written reports and the confidentiality of professional consultation.

The HIV or AIDS diagnosis is one that has been highly stigmatized by the media and children and families are protected by the idea that only those who "need to know" are informed. Parents often are in the dilemma of withholding information to protect their child and being concerned that disclosure is the way to get better care for their son or daughter. The controversy over who belongs in the need-to-know arena continues as children move between health departments, social services, and school districts for their programming. The bottom line is that confidentiality should be build into one's model for professional integrity! (Information from Joe, 1996; Santelli, Birn, & Linde, 1992).

---

The following scenarios provide examples of some possible OT challenges that may need intervention and problem-solving strategies. Every setting and each new child will present more "chances for OTs to excel" as they help children with HIV and AIDS tackle the everyday issues of life.

| The Scenario | OT Problem Solving and Intervention |
|---|---|
| A toddler is HIV-positive (exposed perinatally) and demonstrates mild spastic diplegia (right side) at developmental clinic assessment; concerns regarding feeding and nutrition arise | Determine through observation the child's present feeding skills, including finger feeding and spoon and cup use; determine oral motor status for safe feeding; discuss feeding goals with parent (see "The Holistic Feeding Observation" in Chapter 11) |
| Goal: Toddler will self-feed snack of cereal and juice using adapted utensils or cup for each morning snack 5×/week with minimal assistance. | Consult with nutritionist and parent about feeding and positioning strategies for the child at mealtime; for mother, request from nutritionist meals that are easy to prepare and cost-effective |
| | Order adaptive handle spoon and cup with "sippy" lid for fostering self-feeding |

| | |
|---|---|
| A kindergartner in new school program with inclusion model is having difficulty with dressing routine for outdoor play; referral to school OT is made by classroom teacher. | Observe the child in the dress-for-play routine; note skills and "gaps"<br><br>Discuss results with teacher—Is immediate independence for child a goal in the inclusion setting or should basic skills be built from present level? |
| Goal: Kindergartner will don and doff outdoor play coat independently and zip garment (with minimal adult assistance to engage separating zipper) during outdoor play activities each school day. | Provide short-term direct intervention with child concerning fine motor skills for zipping and buttoning. Leave written directions for staff about the steps you use in teaching the zipping and button routines to child.<br><br>Follow up to see if child is independent in routine or if material adaptions (e.g., Velcro coat fasteners) need to be made to expedite the process. |
| Inner-city community center requests OT services for "play-group" model, which provides services to children of HIV-positive mothers | Determine with center staff the model for the program; decide on "parent and child together" model<br><br>Contact center to provide transportation to encourage participation |
| Goals: In this model collaboration goals for the setting may be done. The OT may "own" such goals as: (1) provide staff workshop on scissors and scissors-readiness skills or (2) produce library reference list of craft books from *local* library appropriate to setting | Provide activity centers for the various ages of children with focus on inexpensive or free materials and modeling for parents<br><br>Close with healthy snack for all and play activity to take home; make suggestion for activity to do (e.g., newspaper hats, "paper balls," and paper telescopes) |
| A group of school-aged children enter program for new antiretroviral drug study; OT is asked to track progress for children in fine motor skills area related to school | *Each child has *Test of Visual Motor Integration* (*VMI*) (Beery & Buktenica, 1967) administered prior to treatment and 6 months after treatment has begun |
| Goals in the setting will probably already be dictated by drug study parameters. Score change in positive direction regarding the VMI and ETCH would most likely be the OT related goals; clinical observation re: handwriting changes in samples may also be valuable. | *Handwriting samples for school work are analyzed with the ETCH (Amundsen, 1995)<br><br>*A comparative evaluation of samples is done for research team (see Fig. 16–1) |

[Source for ideas: Herzberg (1996, April); Hanna & Mintz (1996).]

At the present time therapists working with children focus on the here and now (Joe, 1996). Interventions are directed toward the everyday accomplishments of childhood and adolescence: the preschooler who dresses himself; the second grader who begins cursive writing; and the youth who learns to roller blade for the first time. It must be acknowledged though, that for children with HIV and AIDS there is no cure. The clinical progression for AIDS is often unpredictable, with plateaus and periods where things seem OK (Hanna & Mintz, 1995; Joe, 1996). At this point in time, the course of the disease is eventually downhill.

Children and families living with HIV and AIDS deal with paradox on a daily basis. Although they attempt to live as "normal a life as possible," they must also prepare emotionally for the inevitable death (Boyd-Franklin et al., 1995). This continuous shift in focus has been compared to a roller coaster by family members and friends of persons with AIDS (Brown & Powell-Cope, 1991). The crisis times are punctuated by periods of relative calm and stability both with the disease and the family environment. Living with the uncertainty of where "the ride" will take one next is one of the major issues for persons dealing with death in this arena. It is a precarious thing to balance the issue that children live with AIDS and children die from AIDS.

## WRAPPING IT UP

OTs working in pediatrics will encounter in their career children who are dying or will die before adulthood. With the increase of HIV and AIDS in the pediatric population this encounter may arise more frequently than in the past. "Best practices" for assessment and intervention combined with the psychosocial support skills will continue to evolve as this practice with "high risk" children continues to expand.

### CASE STORY

Sherry is a 4-year-old preschooler who has AIDS. She was infected at birth and her mother has died. Sherry and her older sister Meg (8 years old) are presently living with her grandmother in a government housing area. Sherry has been on your home health caseload for the past year and you have been working both with the therapist in her preschool and with the grandparent at home, providing ADL and fine motor activities.

Sherry's physical health has recently taken a turn for the worse and she is not eating well, has had numerous tantrums, and seems to be "walking funny," according to her grandmother. These problems have all arisen in the past several weeks since your last consultation.

1. What information in this scenario would be red flags regarding Sherry's neurological status at this time?
2. What other members of the intervention team should be contacted for assisting Sherry and her family with this change in her health status?

3. How might you help Meg deal with this change in her sister Sherry's status? In light of her age, what might Meg be thinking about death?
4. What do you need to check into regarding confidentiality before acting on this case? (Think grandmother's preferences, "need to know," and what agencies are presently involved.)
5. Research the term "wasting syndrome" and find out the characteristics of this medical problem associated with AIDS.

## Real Life Lab

**1.** You are part of a preschool team that works with a multiaged (4–6 yrs.) program. You serve children with a variety of developmental diagnoses both of static and degenerative natures. One night after work you get a call from the lead teacher in the program. She tells you that Stephen, one of "your" children at the program with an unusual degenerative neurological condition (Batten disease), has died that day. In your telephone conversation you discuss how to tell the rest of the group about Stephen's death.

**a.** Who in the program can provide you with resources for this task?

**b.** What books, besides those listed in the Bookshelf Section, might be appropriate for opening this issue with your class of preschoolers? (Check with your local library, a bookstore, or your hospital pediatrics program for direction.)

**2.** Universal Precautions concepts provide the framework for agency guidelines on work practices regarding potentially infectious body fluids and personal protective equipment. Have a member of a local agency (i.e., hospital, school, day care) discuss with you how the worksite routines are enacted and monitored at his or her agency. Contacts may include infection control personnel, school nurses, or day care directors.

## References

American Academy of Pediatrics. (1997). Summaries of infectious diseases. In G. Peter (Ed.). *Red book: Report of the Committee on Infectious Diseases* (24th ed.) (pp. 293–295). Elk Grove Village, IL: Author.

Amundsen, S. (1995). *Evaluation tool of children's handwriting (ETCH)*. Homer, AL: OT Kids.

Arpadi, S., & Caspe, W. B. (1991). HIV testing. *Journal of Pediatrics, 119* (1-Pt. 2), S 8–13.

Beery, K., & Buktenica, N.A. (1967). *The*

*Beery-Buktenica test of visual motor integration (VMI)*. Cleveland: Modern Curriculum Press.

*Blood borne pathogens*. (1992). Virginia Beach: Coastal Video Communications Corp.

Boyd-Franklin, N., & Boland, M. G. (1995). Caring for the professional caregiver. In N. Boyd-Franklin, G. L. Steiner, & M. G. Boland (Eds.). *Children, families, and HIV/AIDS: Psychosocial and therapeutic issues* (pp. 216–231). New York: Guilford Press.

Boyd-Franklin, N., Drelich, E. W., & Schwolsky-Fitch, E. (1995). Death and dying/Bereavement and mourning. In N. Boyd-Franklin, G. L. Steiner, & M. G. Boland (Eds.). *Children, families, and HIV/AIDS: Psychosocial and therapeutic issues* (pp. 179–195). New York: Guilford Press.

Brown, M. A., & Powell-Cope, G. M. (1991). AIDS family caregiving: Transitions through uncertainty. *Nursing Research, 40,* 338–345.

Bruininks, R. (1978). *The Bruininks-Oseretsky test of motor proficiency.* Circle Pines, MN: American Guidance Service.

Buckingham, R. W. (1989). *Care of the dying child: A practical guide to those who help others.* New York: Continuum.

Buscaglia, L. F. (1982). *The fall of Freddie the leaf: A story of life for all ages.* Thorofare, NJ: Charles B. Slack.

Carmichael, C. G., Carmichael, J. K., & Fischl, M. A. (1995). *HIV/AIDS: Primary care handbook.* Norwalk, CT: Appleton & Lange.

Centers for Disease Control (CDC) (1994). Revised classification system for human immunodeficiency virus infection in children less than 13 years of age. *Morbidity and Mortality Weekly Report, 43* (RR-12), 1–10.

Chadwick, E. G., & Yogev, R. (1995). Pediatric AIDS. *Pediatric Clinics of North America, 42,* 969–992.

Chanock, S. (1992). Transmission of HIV infection: Implication for Policy. In A. C. Crocker, H. J. Cohen, & T. A. Kastner (Eds.). *HIV infection and developmental disabilities: A resource for service providers* (pp. 215–222). Baltimore: Paul Brookes.

Cook, D. G. (1991). The assessment process. In W. Dunn (Ed.). *Pediatric occupational therapy: Facilitating effective service provision* (pp. 35–72). Thorofare, NJ: Slack, Inc.

Duggan, C. (1994). HIV and AIDS. In A. Goldman (Ed.). *Care of the dying child* (pp. 42–51). New York: Oxford University Press.

Dial, J. G., McCarron, L., & Amann, G. (1988). *Perceptual motor assessment for children (Test Manual).* Dallas, TX: McCarron-Dial Systems.

Edelson, P. J. & Noel, G. J. (1992). *Handbook of pediatric infectious disease.* Boston: Little, Brown.

Flynn, P. M. (1994). Pediatric HIV infection and the primary care physician. Meeting unique needs. *Postgraduate Medicine, 95* (1), 59–60, 65–68, 72–74.

Frankenburg, W. K., Fandal, A. W. Sciarillo, W., & Burgess, D. (1981). The newly abbreviated and revised Denver Developmental Screening Test. *Pediatrics, 99,* 995–999.

Hanna, J., & Mintz, M. (1995). Neurological and neurodevelopmental functioning in pediatric HIV infection. In N. Boyd-Franklin, G. L. Steiner, & M. G. Boland (Eds.), *Children, families and HIV/AIDS: Psychosocial and therapeutic issues* (pp. 30–50). New York: Guilford Press.

Herzberg, G. (1996, April). Kids, AIDS, and occupational therapy. Presentation at the American Occupational Therapy Association Conference, Chicago, IL.

Joe, B. (1996, January 25). How AIDS affects our children. *OT Week,* pp. 14–16.

Kirkland, M., & Robertson, S. C. (1986). *PIVOT: Planning and implementing vocational readiness in occupational therapy.* Rockville, MD: American Occupational Therapy Association.

Kübler-Ross, E. (1983). *On children and death.* New York: Macmillan Publishing.

Kübler-Ross, E. (1969). *On death and dying.* New York: Macmillan.

Lansdown, R. (1994). Communicating with children. In A. Goldman (Ed.), *Care of the dying child* (pp 93–106). New York: Oxford University Press.

Mendez, H. (1991). Ambulatory care of HIV-seropositive infants and children. *Journal of Pediatrics, 119* (1-Pt. 2), S14–S20.

Menten, T. (1995). *Where is heaven? Children's wisdom on facing death.* Philadelphia: Running Press.

Meyers, A., & Weitzman, M. (1991). Pediatric HIV disease: The newest chronic illness of childhood. *Pediatric Clinics of North America, 38* (1), 169–194.

Miller, L. (1993). *FirstSTEP.* San Antonio: Psychological Corp.

Moffet, H. L. (1989). *Pediatric infectious diseases: A problem oriented approach* (3rd. ed.). Philadelphia: J. B. Lippincott.

*New illustrated Webster's dictionary of the English Language* (1994). New York: PMC Publishing.

Nicholas, S. W., & Abrams, E. J. (1992). The silent legacy of AIDS. Children who survive their parents and siblings [editorial; comment]. *Journal of the American Medical Association, 265,* 3478–9 and 3456–61.

Overbeck, B., & Overbeck, J. (1995). *Concerning siblings* [WWW document]. URL http://www.metronet.com/~tlc/siblings.htm. Dallas: TLC Group.

Pizzi, M., & Hinds-Harris, M. (1990). Infants and children with HIV infection: Perspectives in occupational and physical therapy. In J. J. Johnson & M. Pizzi (Eds.). *Productive living strategies for people with AIDS* (pp. 103–123). New York: Haworth Press.

Rothenberg, M., & Chapman, C. F. (1994). *Dictionary of medical terms for the nonmedical person* (3rd ed.). Hauppauge, NY: Barron's Educational Series.

Santelli, J. S., Birn, A. E., & Linde, J. (1992). School placement for human immunodeficiency virus-infected children: the Baltimore City experience. *Pediatrics, 89* (5-Pt 1), 843–848.

Schable, B., Diaz, T., Chu, S. Y., Caldwell, M. B., Conti, L. Alston, O. M., Sorvillo, F., Checko, P. J., Hermann, P., Davidson, A. J., et al. (1995). Who are the primary caretakers of children born to HIV-infected mothers? Results from a multistate surveillance project. *Pediatrics, 95,* 511–515.

Simonds, R. J., & Rogers, M. F. (1992). Epidemiology of HIV in children and other populations. In A. C. Crocker, H. J. Cohen, & T. A. Kastner (Eds.). *HIV infection and developmental disabilities: A resource for service providers* (pp. 3–13). Baltimore: Paul Brookes.

Shannon, L. (1995). Clinical perspectives and current trends of HIV infection in the newborn and child. *Neonatal Network, 14* (3), 21–34.

So, P., & Johnson, L. (1996). Acquired immune deficiency syndrome (AIDS). In R. E. Rakel (Ed.). *Conn's current therapy—1997* (pp. 46–61). Philadelphia: W. B. Saunders.

Spiegel, L., & Mayers, A. (1991).

Psychosocial aspects of AIDS in children and adolescents. *Pediatric Clinics of North America, 38,* 153–167.

Stine, G. (1993). *Acquired immune deficiency syndrome: Biological, medical, social, and legal issues.* Englewood Cliffs, NJ: Prentice-Hall.

Trapp, A. (1994). Support for the family. In A. Goldman (Ed.). *Care of the dying child* (pp. 76–92). New York: Oxford University Press.

Wade, N. (1991). Immunologic considerations in pediatric HIV infection. *Journal of Pediatrics, 119* (Part 2), S5–S7.

Walker, A. R. (1995). HIV infection in children. *Emergency Medicine Clinics of North America, 13,* 147–162.

Wells, E. A., Hoppe, M. J., Simpson, E. E., Gillmore, M. R., Morrison, D. M., & Wilsdon, A. (1995). Misconceptions about AIDS among children who can identify the major routes of HIV transmission. *Journal of Pediatric Psychology, 20,* 671–686.

Weiner, L. S., Best, A., & Pizzo, P. (Compilers). (1994). *Be a friend: Children who live with HIV speak.* Morton Grove, IL: Albert Whitman.

Wilfert, C. M., & Pizzo, P. A. (1994). A blueprint for care, treatment, and prevention of HIV/AIDS in children. *Pediatric Infectious Disease Journal, 13,* 920–923.

Wolters, P. L., Brouwers, P., Moss, H. A., & Pizzo, P. A. (1994). Adaptive behavior of children with symptomatic HIV infection before and after zidovudine therapy. *Journal of Pediatric Psychology, 19,* 47–61.

# *Index*

*Numbers followed by an "f" indicate figures; numbers followed by a "t" indicate tabular material.*